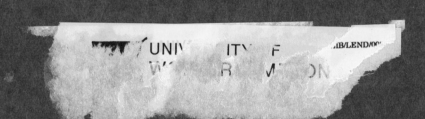

Disorders of

THROMBOSIS

&

HEMOSTASIS

Clinical and Laboratory Practice

Disorders of

THROMBOSIS

&

HEMOSTASIS
Clinical and Laboratory Practice

Rodger L. Bick, MD, FACP

Clinical Professor of Medicine, Division of Hematology Oncology, Department of Medicine
UCLA Center for the Health Sciences
Associate Member, Jonsson Comprehensive Cancer Center at UCLA
Medical Director, Regional Cancer and Blood Disease Center of Kern, Bakersfield, California
Chairman, Department of Medicine, Bakersfield Memorial Hospital
Medical Director, UCLA-Kern Cancer Program
Medical Director, California Coagulation Laboratories, Bakersfield, California
Fellow, American Society of Clinical Pathologists (FASCP)

ASCP Press
American Society of Clinical Pathologists
Chicago

Acquisitions & Development: Joshua Weikersheimer
Editor: Karen D. Johnson
Production Manager: Lisa Pollak

Notice: Medicine is an ever-changing science. As new research and clinical experience broaden our knowledge, changes in treatment and drug therapy are required. The author and the publisher of this work have checked with sources believed to be reliable in their efforts to provide information that is complete and generally in accord with the standards accepted at the time of publication. However, in view of the possibility of human error or changes in medical sciences, neither the author nor the publisher nor any other party who has been involved in the preparation or publication of this work warrant that the information contained herein is in every respect accurate or complete. For example and in particular, readers are advised to check the product information sheet included in the package of each drug they plan to administer to be certain that the information contained in this book is accurate and that changes have not been made in the recommended dose or in the contraindications for administration. This recommendation is of particular importance in connection with new or infrequently used drugs.

Library of Congress Cataloging in Publication Data
Bick, Rodger L.
Disorders of thrombosis and hemostasis: clinical and laboratory practice / Rodger L. Bick.
p. 352
Includes bibliographical references and index.
ISBN 0-89189-340-7
1. Blood—Coagulation, Disorders of. 2. Hemostasis. 3. Thrombosis. I. Title.
[DNLM: 1. Blood Coagulation Disorders. 2. Hemostasis. 3. Thrombosis. WH 322 B583db]
RC647.C55B54 1992
616.1'57—dc20
DNLM/DLC   91-33248
for Library of Congress   CIP

Printed on recycled paper.

Printed in the United States of America.

96 95 94 93   5 4 3 2

Dedicated With Love To

Shauna Nicole Bick

My Daughter
&
Joy In Life

Contents

Preface

Disorders of thrombosis and hemostasis are common to almost all medical specialties, and all physicians, laboratory scientists, and allied health professionals are all too aware of the catastrophic consequences of these diseases. Because the end results of these disorders often lead to considerable morbidity or in many instances mortality, it is of extraordinary importance for all those dealing with these diseases to be able to quickly diagnose conditions and treat patients with these defects. Providing rapid clinical and laboratory diagnosis and subsequent effective treatment requires an authoritative familiarity with principles of the etiology, pathophysiology, clinical and laboratory diagnosis, and management of disorders of thrombosis and hemostasis.

In this book, each particular disease or disease group has been approached in logical and sequential order, covering the etiology, pathophysiology, clinical and laboratory diagnostic aspects, and principles of medical and laboratory management. Using this approach, it is hoped the clinician of any particular medical specialty or the laboratory specialist, be it physician or technologist, can readily utilize this book as a working resource to rapid diagnosis and management principles.

This book was written with a sincere attempt to cover disorders of thrombosis and hemostasis in a logical, sequential, and practical manner, and it is my sincere desire that all using it will find it of benefit in ultimately rendering outstanding medical care to patients with these potentially devastating disorders.

Rodger L. Bick, MD, FACP

Acknowledgments

The author wishes to thank his administrative assistant, Ms. Mary Sue Smothers, for her invaluable editing and re-editing, compiling of the references, preparation of tables and figures, and final preparation of the book. A special thank you is due my office nurses, Karen Collier and Judy Barnes, and my associate, Dr. James Donovan, for fielding innumerable telephone calls and patient problems while this book was being written. A heartfelt thank you is due my many patients for not only allowing me to evaluate and study their diseases, but for their patience and understanding during the writing of this book. Lastly, a personal thank you is due my many ASCP workshop participants and the Hematology Oncology Postdoctoral Fellows at UCLA, all of whom have inspired me to continue to learn and write.

Physiology of Hemostasis

Mastering basic physiology of hemostasis is important for many reasons. First, one can interpret new testing modalities with confidence. Second, one can appreciate the enormously complex nature of most disease processes and the intermediary mechanism of disease involved in many seemingly unrelated disorders. Third, and essential for the clinician, one can evaluate the novel and specific pharmacologic interventions that are now being explored for treating disorders of hemostasis and thrombosis.

Figure 1-1 depicts an early scheme of the coagulation sequence that was developed by Davie and Ratnoff.[1,2] While fundamentally correct, this scheme is limited in scope because it does not address the important role of inhibitors, the interactions between different blood protein systems, and the key interactions between the blood proteins, the platelets, and the endothelial and vascular compartment.[3,4]

The three equally important anatomic compartments of hemostasis[3,4] are the following: the platelets, which must be normal in both number and function; the blood proteins, which include procoagulants, anticoagulants, and fibrinolytic proteins; and the vasculature, which remains the "last frontier" and least understood with respect to disorders of hemostasis and thrombosis. These three compartments are intricately interrelated, and disturbances of these delicately balanced interrelationships may lead to serious clinical consequences.[4]

Vascular Function

Normal vascular morphology comprises three discrete layers: the intima, media, and adventitia.[5-7] The intima has a monolayer of nonthrombogenic endothelial cells and an internal elastic membrane. The media has smooth muscle cells, and its size varies depending on the type (arterial or venous) and size of the vasculature. The adventitia is composed of an external elastic lamina or membrane and supportive connective tissue.

Figure 1-2 depicts an important pathophysiologic event: endothelial sloughing.[8,9] Endothelial sloughing may be induced by a wide variety of insults (triggers) including aci-

dosis, hypoxia, endotoxin, circulating antigen-antibody complexes, and many others.[10-14] Figure 1-3 depicts the first event that occurs after endothelial sloughing, with the subsequent exposure of subendothelial collagen and basement membrane. Platelets are immediately recruited to fill this endothelial gap.[15,16] Both subendothelial collagen and subendothelial basement membrane recruit platelets to form a primary hemostatic plug, thereby stopping blood from leaving the vascular compartment. As the primary hemostatic plug is formed, subsequent reparative events ensue. Smooth muscle or other cells from the media will differentiate, migrate through the internal elastic membrane, and then redifferentiate into new nonthrombogenic endothelial cells.[4] If this is a one-time event, then a normal reparative process is completed. Forming the primary hemostatic plug, however, may constitute an overwhelming event, leading to a large platelet/fibrin thrombus, impedence of blood flow, and resultant end-organ damage via ischemia.[4]

Figure 1-4 depicts another event that may happen when endothelial sloughing and damage occur: atherosclerotic plaque formation.[17-20] If this process occurs repeatedly in the same area over a protracted period of time, then as smooth muscle or other cells dedifferentiate and migrate into the intima of the vessel, compounds are released that attract macrophages, which then ingest cholesterol and other materials, and an atherosclerotic plaque will eventually develop.[21] These potential events are summarized in Figure 1-5.

Permeability, fragility, and vasoconstriction are properties of the vasculature.[4] Vascular permeability, if increased, results in blood leaving the vessel and manifests as petechiae and purpura or sometimes large ecchymoses. If increased vascular fragility occurs, the vasculature may rupture with ensuing petechiae and purpura, especially in the integument and mucous membranes, large ecchymoses, and potential serious deep-tissue hemorrhage. If vasoconstriction is inappropriately intense, the vessel may occlude because of thrombus formation. Vasoconstriction is controlled by local, neural, and humoral factors, the most important of these being humoral control. Those compounds that mediate humoral control of vasoconstriction are primarily com-

Figure 1-1. Cascade Scheme of Coagulation

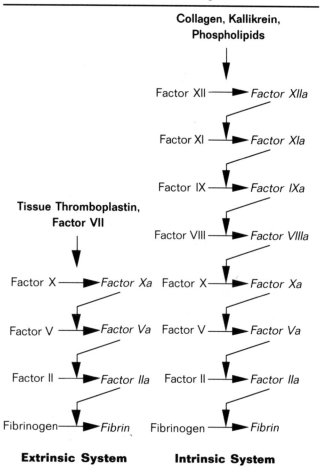

Extrinsic System   **Intrinsic System**

Figure 1-2. Endothelial Sloughing and Exposure of Blood to Subendothelial Collagen/Basement Membrane

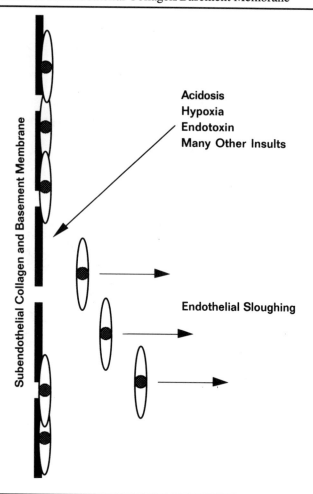

pounds released from platelets including epinephrine, nore-pinephrine, ADP, kinins, and thromboxanes.[22-24] Fibrin-(ogen) degradation products (FDPs), liberated when the fibrinolytic system acts on a fibrin clot, will also modulate vasoconstriction.[4]

Properties of the endothelium are summarized in Table 1-1. Endothelial cells contract when stimulated by histamine, serotonin, kinins, or thromboxanes. In addition, the endothe-

Table 1-1. Properties of the Endothelium and Subendothelium

Endothelium:
    Contraction by histamine, kinins, serotonin, and
      thromboxanes
    Synthesis of plasminogen activator activity
    Synthesis of VII:vWF factor
    Synthesis of protein C inhibitor

Subendothelium:
    Platelet activation and attraction
    Factor XII activation
    Factor XI activation

lial cell is the major site of high-molecular weight factor VIII biosynthesis (von Willebrand factor or ristocetin cofactor).[25,26] Low–molecular weight factor VIII or factor VIII coagulant activity (factor VIII:C) is synthesized by the hepatocyte and probably other cellular sites.[27] The endothelial cell provides one of the two key activation pathways of the fibrinolytic system through the synthesis and release of plasminogen activator.[28-31] Protein C activator and inhibitor appear to be synthesized and released by the endothelium.[32] The role of endothelial cell prostaglandin synthesis is discussed in later sections. Properties of the subendothelium are also shown in Table 1-1. Platelet attraction and subsequent activation occur when basement membrane or collagen is exposed. Subendothelial collagen can directly activate factor XII to factor XIIa and factor XI to factor XIa.[33,34] Clearly, any of these processes could give rise to a generalized activation of the hemostatic system.[14] Cellular interactions between the endothelium and other cells, including neutrophils and cells of the monocyte-macrophage system, are not only important in hemostasis but also in the mediation of inflammatory and immune responses.[35-37]

Figure 1-3. Platelets Filling Endothelial Gaps

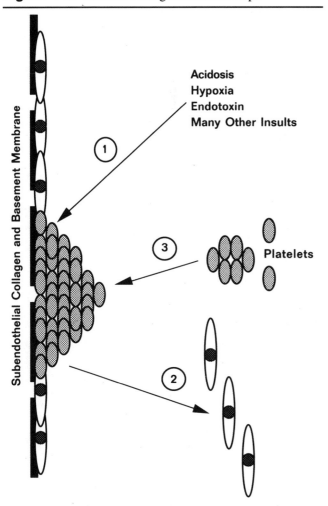

Figure 1-4. Endothelial Sloughing and Atheroma Formation

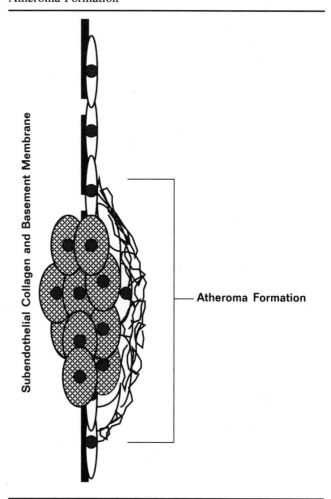

Platelet Function

Table 1-2 shows normal platelet morphology. This morphologic division, although somewhat artificial, facilitates the understanding of relevant biology. Generally, the platelet can be envisioned as being composed of three primary zones: a peripheral zone, a sol-gel zone, and an organelle zone.[38] The peripheral zone is composed of an extramembranous glycocalyx surrounding a plasma membrane, similar to any other trilamellar cellular plasma membrane. Under the plasma membrane is an open canalicular system. The sol-gel zone is composed of microtubules and microfilaments and a dense tubular system that contains primarily adenine nucleotides and calcium. In addition, the important contractile protein, thrombosthenin, is found in the sol-gel zone and is similar to actomyosin. The organelle zone is composed of dense bodies, alpha granules, mitochondria, and many other organelles found in other cellular systems, including lysosomes and endoplasmic reticulum. Alpha granules contain and release fibrinogen and lysosome enzymes, whereas dense bodies contain and release adenine nucleotides, sero-

tonin, catecholamines, and platelet factor 4.[39-42] Figure 1-6 is a transmission electron micrograph of a platelet showing many of these constituents and organelles. The open canalicular system, dense bodies, mitochondria, and lysosomes are apparent.

Table 1-2. Platelet Morphology

Peripheral Zone
    Glycocalyx
    Platelet membrane
    Open canalicular system

Sol-Gel Zone
    Microtubules and microfilaments
    Dense tubular system
    Thrombosthenin

Organelle Zone
    Dense granules
    Mitochondria
    Alpha granules

Figure 1-5. Vascular Damage and Consequences of Endothelial Cell Sloughing

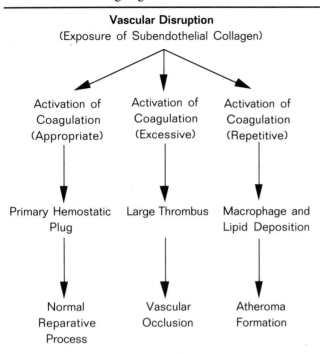

Vascular Disruption
(Exposure of Subendothelial Collagen)

Activation of Coagulation (Appropriate) → Primary Hemostatic Plug → Normal Reparative Process

Activation of Coagulation (Excessive) → Large Thrombus → Vascular Occlusion

Activation of Coagulation (Repetitive) → Macrophage and Lipid Deposition → Atheroma Formation

Figure 1-6. Platelet

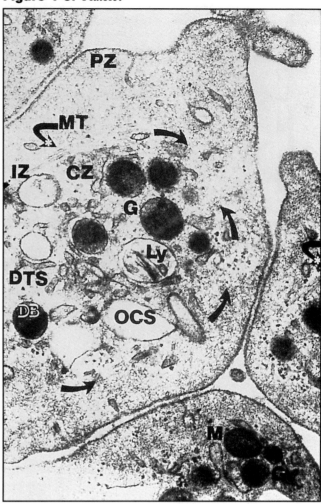

Table 1-3 summarizes the factors necessary for normal platelet function. An adequate number of platelets must be present for normal platelet function in vivo and in vitro, which is usually defined as approximately 100×10^9/L (100,000/mm³). In vitro and ex vivo tests of platelet function, with a platelet count of less than 100×10^9/L (100,000/mm³), will yield abnormal results; for example, prolonged template bleeding times and abnormal platelet aggregation profiles will usually be noted.[4] For normal function, platelets must have adequate energy metabolism and an adequate number of storage granules (with appropriate contents) capable of releasing their contents when appropriate stimuli are presented. Cationic proteins such as thrombasthenin must also be present. Membrane receptors must be responsive to appropriate stimuli. Platelets require divalent cations, the most important of which is calcium, and adequate physical conditions, such as pH and temperature.[4]

Table 1-3. Factors Necessary for Normal Platelet Function

Adequate number of platelets (> 100×10^9/L)
Adequate energy metabolism
Adequate number and contents of storage granules
Adequate storage granules and release
Adequate cationic proteins
Adequate membrane receptors and responsiveness
Adequate divalent cations (Mg++, Ca++)
Adequate physical conditions (pH, temperature)

Table 1-4 summarizes the common platelet proteins. Some are not platelet specific, including many plasma proteins found in or on platelets. Many of the coagulation proteins are found in or on platelets, including factors II, V, VII, VIII, IX, X, XI, XII, and XIII.[43,44] Sometimes these proteins

Table 1-4. Platelet Proteins

Nonspecific (Plasma) Proteins
Fibrinogen
Factors II, V, VII, VIII, IX, X, XII, and XIII
Albumin
Plasminogen
Complement components

Specific Platelet Proteins
Thrombosthenin
Platelet glycoproteins
Platelet factors 2 and 4
Platelet antiplasmin
Cathepsin A
Beta-thromboglobulin

Figure 1-7. Moderately Activated Platelet

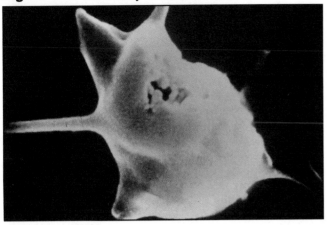

Table 1-6. Compounds Released From Platelets

Biogenic Amines
   Serotonin
   Epinephrine
   Norepinephrine
   Histamine

Adenine Nucleotides
   ADP
   ATP
   Cyclic AMP

Cations
   K+
   Ca++

Platelet Factors 3 and 4

Platelet Proteins
   Albumin
   Fibrinogen
   Platelet factor 4

Thromboxanes

are found in a slightly different molecular form in platelets when compared to plasma (eg, factor XIII). Platelet-specific proteins are also present and consist of thrombosthenin, platelet factor 4, beta-thromboglobulin, cathepsin A, and others.[4]

Table 1-5 depicts those platelet factors that have been identified and characterized. Thus far, platelet factors 1 through 7 are recognized. The most important of these are platelet factor 3 (or platelet membrane phospholipoprotein, so-called platelet thromboplastin) and platelet factor 4 (antiheparin factor), which has become an important molecular marker of hemostatic activity and platelet reactivity in particular.[45-48]

Table 1-6 summarizes the compounds released from platelets: the biogenic amines, including serotonin, catecholamines, and histamine; the all-important adenine nucleotides, including cyclic AMP, ADP, and ATP; various enzyme activities, including acid hydrolases; specific ions, including calcium, magnesium, and potassium; and platelet factors, including platelet factor 4, beta-thromboglobulin, platelet factor 3, and thromboxanes.[4] Platelet factor 3 is not actually released but most probably represents a conformational change in the platelet membrane, which makes an activity available that is referred to as platelet factor 3. In addition, other proteins including fibrinogen, other clotting factors, albumin, and other compounds are released from platelets during a release reaction.[4]

Many stimuli will induce a platelet release reaction,[49-52] including subendothelial collagen and basement membrane.

Table 1-5. Platelet Factors

Platelet factor 1:	Coagulation factor V
Platelet factor 2:	Thromboplastic material
Platelet factor 3:	Platelet thromboplastin
Platelet factor 4:	Antiheparin factor
Platelet factor 5:	Fibrinogen coagulant factor
Platelet factor 6:	Antifibrinolytic factor
Platelet factor 7:	Platelet cothromboplastin

Other potent inducers of a platelet release reaction are the following: thrombin, soluble fibrin monomer (fibrin monomer that has been solubilized by complexing with split products), FDPs (especially fragment X), endotoxin, circulating antigen-antibody complex, gamma globulin–coated surfaces, various viruses, ADP, catecholamines, and free fatty acids.[53-56] Many proteolytic enzymes, including trypsin, snake venoms, papain, and elastase, are used in vitro to study platelet release.[4] Other in vitro release reaction techniques include the use of centrifugation, cold fracture, latex particles, carbon particles, kaolin, and celite.[4]

Figure 1-7 is a scanning electron micrograph of a moderately activated platelet. As platelets become activated, they begin to contract and form pseudopods. During contraction the many intraplatelet compounds and granules are concentrated at the center of the platelet. As activation progresses, platelets become markedly contracted with pronounced pseudopod formation.[4] It is thought that during this event the platelet organelles, including alpha granules and dense bodies, are concentrated at the center of the platelet where organelle membranes disrupt, their contents are released and then transported outside the platelet via the open canalicular system. These compounds then interact with platelet membrane receptors of adjacent platelets, causing further platelet activation in a type of logarithmic amplification process by which numerous platelets become activated.[4] In addition, many of these compounds may interact with adjacent endothelium. Pseudopod formation enhances platelet-surface interaction (adhesion) and platelet-platelet interaction (cohesion).[4]

Figure 1-8 is a scanning electron micrograph of endothelium that has been made hypoxic. Endothelial cells are missing in several areas, having been sloughed because of

Figure 1-8. Hypoxic Endothelium

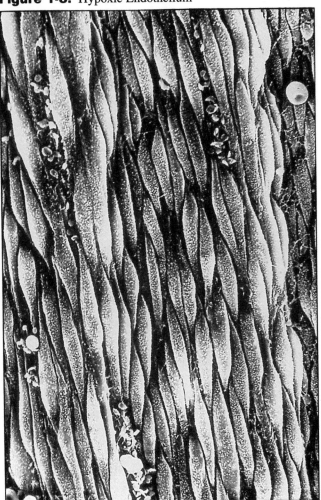

Figure 1-9. Abbreviated Platelet Function

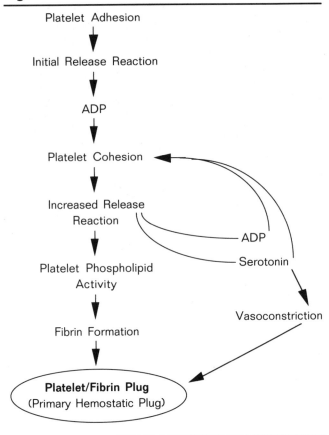

hypoxia. These endothelial cell gaps are filled by activated platelets, contracted and with marked pseudopod formation.

A summary of platelet function is presented in Figure 1-9. The first process that occurs during platelet activation is that of platelet adhesion.[4] Platelet adhesion refers to a platelet adhering to something other than another platelet (eg, a glass bead, other artificial surface, or collagen/basement membrane). Following platelet adhesion is an early release reaction with the release of intraplatelet ADP. This reaction is a reversible process, accounts for the primary wave on an aggregation pattern, and is called primary (reversible) aggregation. As the concentration of ADP increases, platelet cohesion (platelets adhering to other platelets) then occurs, causing more and more ADP and other compounds (including serotonin) to be released. These compounds not only activate adjacent platelets but also induce vascular constriction (to prepare for an effective primary hemostatic plug or primary platelet/fibrin plug). During this increased release reaction, when the ADP concentration reaches a critical point, an irreversible conformational change ensues in the platelet membrane, making available platelet factor 3 or platelet membrane phospholipid-type

activity. This material then serves as a primary surface mediating the formation of complexes in the coagulation protein sequence. The sequence of platelet cohesion, increased release reaction, and the conformational changes leading to the availability of platelet factor 3 is an irreversible process and accounts for the secondary wave seen on a platelet aggregation pattern.[4] In vivo, the result of this sequence is the formation of a platelet/fibrin plug, or primary hemostatic plug, the function of which is rendered most efficient by vasoconstriction induced by compounds released from platelets.

Simplified intraplatelet functional biochemical sequences are outlined in Figure 1-10. The key modulator of intraplatelet function is cyclic AMP.[57-59] The role of this compound is to combine with a cyclic AMP–dependent protein to generate a kinase activity. The role of this kinase is to phosphorylate a receptor protein, which then binds calcium. When intraplatelet calcium is bound, it is not available to thrombosthenin, rendering the platelet hypoaggregable and hypoadhesable. Epinephrine, thrombin, collagen, and serotonin inhibit the enzyme adenylate cyclase, which is responsible for the conversion of ATP to cyclic AMP. This inhibition results in a decrease in kinase concentration, a decrease in phosphorylated receptor protein, and an increase in ionized calcium concentration, which renders the platelet hyperaggregable.[4]

Figure 1-10. Simplified Intraplatelet Biochemistry

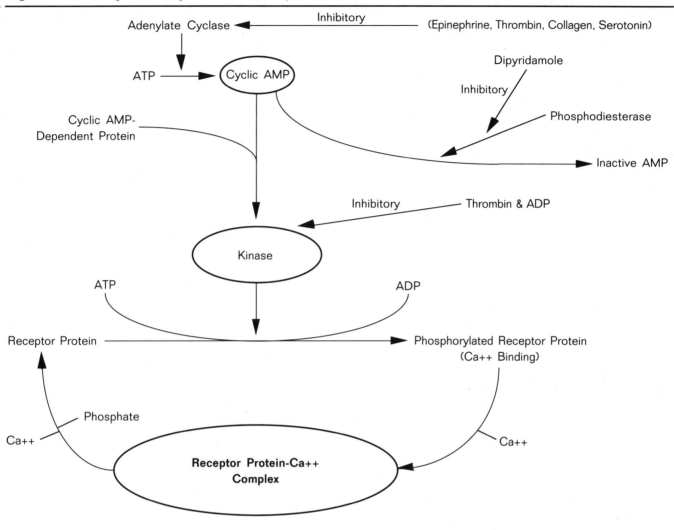

The enzyme responsible for converting cyclic AMP into an inactive form is phosphodiesterase.[60,61] One popular antiplatelet agent, dipyridamole, inhibits phosphodiesterase.[4] Caffeine and papaverine also inhibit it. In these instances, the concentration of cyclic AMP, kinase, and phosphorylated receptor protein will increase, intraplatelet calcium will become bound, and the platelet will be rendered nonfunctional.[4]

The role of prostaglandins and derivatives in platelet function are summarized in Figure 1-11. Platelet and endothelial cell membrane phospholipids are converted into arachidonic acid by the enzyme, phospholipase A_2,[62-64] which is activated by both thrombin and collagen. Arachidonic acid is converted into prostaglandin intermediates, prostaglandin G_2 (PGG_2), and prostaglandin H_2 (PGH_2) by the enzyme cyclo-oxygenase. In the platelet membrane, thromboxane synthetase converts PGH_2 into thromboxane A_2, one of the most potent aggregating agents described.[4] Thromboxane A_2 also has extremely potent vasoconstricting activity. In the endothelial cell, and in some subendothelial muscle cells, prostacyclin synthetase converts PGH_2 into prostacyclin, which is a potent aggregation inhibitor and a potent vasodilator.[65-67] Prostacyclin has been assessed in clinical trials for thromboembolic and vaso-occlusive disease.[68,69] Cyclo-oxygenase is inhibited by aspirin and sulfinpyrazone, two popular antiplatelet agents.[70] Current evidence suggests that the selectivity of these two antiplatelet agents is directed about 70% toward platelets and only 30% toward the endothelial cell with respect to prostacyclin synthesis. In addition, endothelium continues to synthesize prostaglandins, but platelets do not.[4]

Thromboxane A_2 is a potent inhibitor of adenylate cyclase, and prostacyclin is a potent stimulator of adenylate cyclase. Therefore, the presence of bleeding or thrombosis may depend on the relative concentrations of these two compounds. This represents an exquisite biologic system in which platelets are synthesizing and releasing into the adjacent milieu, a compound (thromboxane A_2) is inducing platelet aggregation, and alternatively the adjacent endothelium is synthesizing and releasing prostacyclin, which keeps platelets away from the endothelium and inhibits aggregation.[4]

Figure 1-11. Prostaglandins in Platelet/Endothelial Function

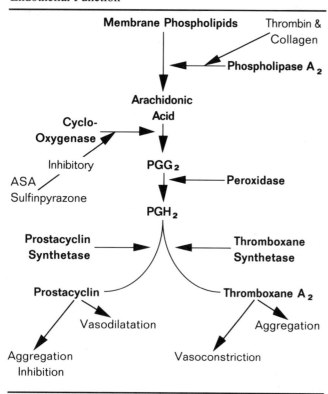

Platelet interactions with the vasculature (adhesion), other platelets (cohesion), and plasma protein reactions occur at the platelet membrane surface. These many interactions are mediated by various platelet membrane glycoproteins (PMGPs).[71] The major platelet membrane glycoproteins and their functions, where known, are summarized in Table 1-7. Platelet membrane glycoprotein Ia is complexed to PMGP IIa and functions to adhere platelets to subendothelial collagen independent of von Willebrand factor.[72] Platelet membrane glycoprotein Ib has a molecular weight of about 170,000 d and is composed of an alpha and beta subunit, one of which fixes it to the platelet membrane. PMGP Ib is complexed to PMGP IX and V.[73] PMGP Ib and IX are absent from platelets in Bernard-Soulier syndrome.[74] PMGP Ib serves as a receptor for von Willebrand factor; thus, subendothelial binding of von Willebrand factor to PMGP Ib is responsible for initial platelet adhesion to the subendothelial surface, the first step in platelet adhesion.[75] PMGP Ib is also the receptor for quinine and quinidine drug-dependent antibody present in quinine- and quinidine-induced thrombocytopenia.[76] PMGP Ib is also part of the thrombin receptor complex of platelets; PMGP V is of vital importance in thrombin activation of platelets.[77] In addition, the PMGP Ib/IX complex is an important thrombin receptor site.[78]

PMGP IIb/IIIa complex is found in platelet alpha granules as well as the membrane.[79] PMGP IIb has a molecular weight of about 125,000 d and PMGP IIIa about 93,000 d. PMGP IIb and IIIa appear to be subunits of a single glycoprotein; the subunits are heavily dependent on calcium binding of the complex, and PMGP IIb is a major calcium-binding protein for platelet function.[80] PMGP IIa/IIIb is absent or markedly reduced in Glanzmann's thrombasthenia, is the binding site for fibrinogen, and serves as the apparent binding site for PLA$_1$ antibody.[81,82] The binding of fibrinogen to PMGP IIb/IIIa is needed for optimal ADP-induced platelet aggregation. Glycoprotein G is also called thrombospondin; the molecular weight of this PMGP is about 180,000 d. Thrombospondin is partially responsible for thrombin- and collagen-induced aggregation.[83,84] Platelet membrane glyco-

Table 1-7. Platelet Membrane Glycoproteins

Glycoprotein	Function	Characteristic
Ia	von Willebrand-independent receptor for subendothelium	—
Ib	von Willebrand receptor	Missing in Bernard-Soulier syndrome; quinidine-antibody receptor
IIa		
IIb	von Willebrand and fibrinogen receptor	Missing in Glanzmann's thrombasthenia; PLA$_1$ antibody receptor
IIIa	von Willebrand and fibrinogen receptor	Missing in Glanzmann's thrombasthenia; PLA$_1$ antibody receptor
V	Thrombin receptor	Missing in Bernard-Soulier syndrome
IX		Missing in Bernard-Soulier syndrome

Table 1-8. Blood Protein Function: The Five Interactive Systems

Coagulation Protein System
Fibrinolytic Enzyme System
Complement System
Kinin System
Inhibitors of these Systems

proteins Ic and IIa have been identified but are as yet without known function in hemostasis.

Plasma Protein Function

Plasma protein function in hemostasis comprises numerous systems, the five most important of which are listed in Table 1-8. These systems consist of (1) the coagulation protein system, (2) the fibrino(geno)lytic system, (3) the kinin system, (4) the complement system, and (5) the inhibitors of these systems.[4] Kinin generation and complement generation (activation) are often not appreciated as important participants in thrombohemorrhagic disorders. Pathophysiologically, these systems assume extreme importance, especially in disorders such as disseminated intravascular coagulation (DIC).[85]

Coagulation Proteins

Coagulation proteins and their synonyms are summarized in Table 1-9. The Roman numeral system is most widely used and preferred, although in some instances no Roman numerals have been assigned to factors. Protein C has been referred to as factor XIV or autoprothrombin II-A; Fletcher factor is synonymous with prekallikrein; and Fitzgerald factor, also called William's factor, Flaujac factor, Reid factor, or Fujiwara factor, is known as high–molecular weight kininogen.[86-88] The chromosome locations containing genetic information for synthesis of almost all the coagulation factors are known[89,90] and summarized in Table 1-10.

The formation of a fibrin clot is best thought of as consisting of four key reactions; this concept is helpful to render the procoagulant system easily understandable. The first key reaction is contact activation, the second is the formation of factor Xa, the third is the formation of thrombin, and the fourth is the formation of fibrin (Table 1-11). Again, when recalling the blood coagulation system, appreciating these four key reactions is of help in remembering the entire system and the order and interplay of these reactions.

The contact activation phase of coagulation begins with the activation of Hageman factor or factor XII. Factor XII can be activated by many potential mechanisms, and several of these are depicted in Figure 1-12. Phospholipids, collagen, subendothelial collagen, and kallikrein (activated Fletcher factor) are capable of converting factor XII to factor

Figure 1-12. Mechanisms of Factor XII Activation

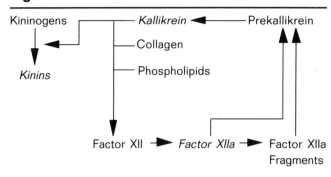

XIIa.[91-94] Active Hageman factor, also a serine protease, then converts factor XI into factor XIa. This reaction occurs very quickly in the presence of Fitzgerald factor (high–molecular weight kininogen) but very slowly without Fitzgerald factor, thus accounting for a significantly prolonged activated partial thromboplastin time in the absence of Fitzgerald factor.[95,96] The role of factor XIa, also a serine protease, is to convert factor IX (in the presence of calcium) into factor IXa. Factor IXa is the enzyme responsible for the second key reaction, the generation of factor Xa.[4] Factor XIIa itself can convert prekallikrein (Fletcher factor) into kallikrein, which can then convert more factor XII into factor XIIa.[4]

Figure 1-13 exemplifies how the second key reaction occurs. The formation of factor Xa is a five-component system and requires the following: (1) a substrate (factor X), (2)

Table 1-9. Coagulation Factors and Synonyms

Factor	Synonym
I	Fibrinogen
II	Prothrombin
V	Ac-globulin
VII	Prothrombin conversion accelerator
VIII:C	Antihemophilic factor
IX	Christmas factor (PTC)
X	Stuart-Prower factor
XI	Thromboplastin antecedent (PTA)
XII	Hageman (contact) factor
XIII	Profibrinoligase
Fletcher factor	Prekallikrein
Fitzgerald factor	High–molecular weight kininogen
Protein C	Xa inhibitor
Protein S	None

Table 1-10. Chromosomal Location Containing Coagulation Factor Information

Factor	Inheritance	Chromosome	Region
I	Autosomal dominant	4	q26-31
II	Autosomal dominant	11	p11-q12
V	Autosomal recessive	1	q21-25
VII	Autosomal recessive	13	q34
VIII:C	Sex-linked recessive	X	q28
vWF	Autosomal dominant	12	p12-13
IX	Sex-linked recessive	X	q27
X	Autosomal recessive	13	q34
XI	Autosomal recessive	4	q35
XII	Autosomal recessive	5	q33
XIII	Autosomal dominant	6	p24-25
Antithrombin III	Autosomal dominant	1	p23
Protein C	Autosomal dominant	2	q13-14
Protein S	Autosomal dominant	3	p21
Plasminogen	Autosomal dominant	6	q26-27
TPA	Autosomal dominant	8	p12
TPA-I-1	Autosomal dominant	7	q21-22
TPA-I-2	Autosomal dominant	18	q21-22
Antiplasmin	Autosomal recessive	18	?
Fletcher factor	Autosomal recessive	?	?
Fitzgerald factor	Autosomal recessive	?	?
Heparin cofactor II	Autosomal dominant	22	?

an enzyme (factor IXa), (3) a determiner or cofactor (factor VIII:C), (4) a surface (platelet factor 3), and (5) calcium ions.[44,97] The complex formed is bound together by calcium, depicted by the asterisks in Figure 1-13. The enzyme factor IXa cleaves a peptide from the substrate (factor X) with resultant exposure of an active serine site. Factor Xa is the product of this reaction. Factor VIII:C is then modified and rendered dysfunctional.

The third key reaction is the formation of thrombin. Figure 1-14 summarizes enzyme substrate complex formation for this reaction. This reaction is also a five-component sys-

Table 1-11. The Four Key Procoagulant Reactions

Contact Activation (Generation of IXa)
Generation of Factor Xa
Generation of Thrombin (IIa)
Generation of Fibrin

tem and requires the following: (1) a substrate (factor II), (2) an enzyme (factor Xa), (3) a determiner or cofactor (factor V), (4) a surface (platelet factor 3 or platelet membrane phospholipoprotein), and (5) calcium ions.[98-100] These components form an enzyme substrate complex on the phospholipid surface, and a product, thrombin, the new enzyme, is generated. Factor V, like factor VIII:C in the previous reaction, is modified and loses biologic activity. The role of the determiner/cofactor is to ensure that the correct enzyme and substrate enter into complex formation. For example, the presence of factor V enables the enzyme factor Xa to interact with the correct substrate, factor II, and not an inappropriate substrate. Likewise, in the second key reaction, the role of factor VIII:C as a determiner/cofactor is to ensure that the appropriate enzyme, factor IXa, reacts with the appropriate substrate, factor X.[4]

Figure 1-15 summarizes the second and third key reactions, emphasizing that both are similar five-component systems. Figure 1-16 exemplifies the necessity of stoichiometry

Figure 1-13. The Formation of Factor Xa

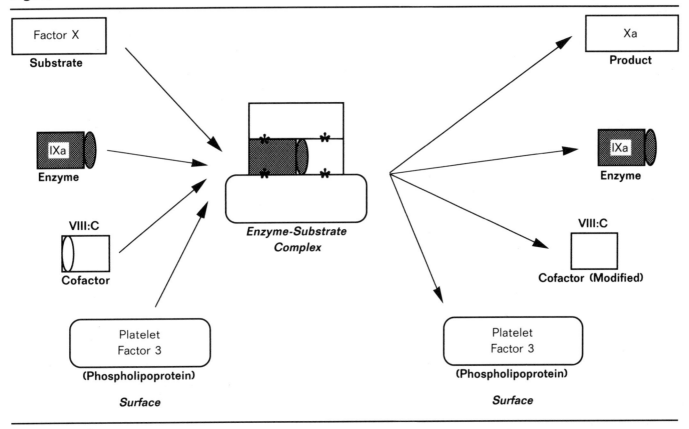

for these reactions. If the amount of prothrombin (substrate) is decreased, the amount of thrombin generated is decreased. If factor V concentration is decreased and other components stay the same, the amount of thrombin generated is decreased. If the concentration of the enzyme, factor Xa, is decreased, the amount of thrombin generated is decreased. If the amount of platelet factor 3 or platelet phospholipid available is decreased, the amount of thrombin generated is decreased. Thus, for these reactions to occur, all five components must be present in relatively normal concentrations and must be appropriately functional.[101] This stoichiometry also applies to the generation of factor Xa.

Platelet membrane phospholipid, or platelet factor 3, has many individual constituents. Four of these constituents are selectively active in the second and third key reactions (Table 1-12). Phosphatidylserine and phosphatidylinositol are active in the third key reaction, or thrombin generation, but have no activity in factor Xa formation.[4] Phosphatidylcholine and phosphatidylethanolamine have no activity in thrombin formation but are active in the formation of factor Xa.[4]

The two previous reactions, generation of factor Xa and factor IIa (thrombin), are dependent on many vitamin K–dependent factors: factors II, VII, IX, and X, protein C, and protein S. Prothrombin, the other prothrombin complex factors (VII, IX, and X), and proteins C and S can be synthesized in a normal form or a so-called plasma abnormal

form.[102-104] The role of vitamin K in synthesizing these vitamin K–dependent factors is to attach a calcium-binding prosthetic site postribosomally to each of these proteins.[4] In the absence of vitamin K (eg, a patient receiving warfarin therapy), calcium-binding sites are not attached. Although a complete protein is synthesized, calcium-binding sites are missing. This situation is depicted on the left-hand side of Figure 1-17. Normal vitamin K–dependent factor synthesis is depicted on the right-hand side of the figure, with the "x's" representing the calcium-binding prosthetic groups attached postribosomally by vitamin K. Thus, plasma abnormal prothrombin complex factors or normal plasma prothrombin complex factors can be synthesized, depending on the absence or presence of vitamin K. These abnormal vitamin

Table 1-12. Platelet Membrane Phospholipid (Platelet Factor 3) Selectivity in Procoagulant Activity

Phospholipid Component	Factor Xa Generation	Thrombin Generation
Phosphatidylethanolamine	Active	Not Active
Phosphatidylcholine	Active	Not Active
Phosphatidylinositol	Not Active	Active
Phosphatidylserine	Not Active	Active

Figure 1-14. The Formation of Thrombin (Factor IIa)

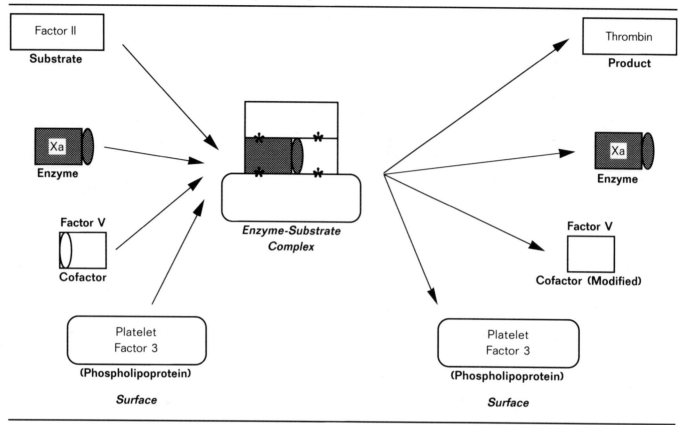

K–dependent factors are called "PIVKAs," or proteins induced by vitamin K absence or antagonists.[105] This important calcium-binding prosthetic group, attached to the pro-thrombin complex factors by vitamin K, is gamma-carboxyglutamic acid.

The fourth key reaction is the formation of fibrin. Figure 1-18 summarizes the conversion of fibrinogen to fibrin. The third key reaction generated thrombin; the primary role of thrombin is to remove two small peptides, fibrinopeptide A

Figure 1-15. Summary of the Second and Third Key Reactions: The Formation of Factor Xa and Thrombin

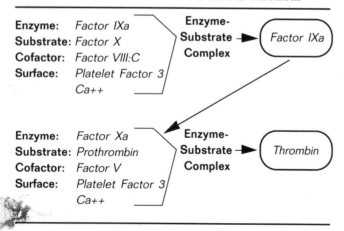

and fibrinopeptide B, from fibrinogen, leaving fibrin monomer.[106,107] Fibrin monomer begins to aggregate end to end and side to side; these aggregates are held together by hydrophobic bonds.[4] These fibrin monomer aggregates form soluble fibrin, which will dissolve in 5 mol/L urea or 1% monochloroacetic acid, both of which disrupt hydrophobic bonds.[4] The formation of soluble fibrin monomer aggregates, held together only by hydrophobic bonds, is called polymerization I. Another important role of thrombin is to activate factor XIII (profibrinoligase) to factor XIIIa (fibrinoligase). Factor XIIIa replaces hydrophobic bonds with peptide bonds, rendering insoluble fibrin.[108,109] This is called polymerization II. Figure 1-19 depicts fibrinogen. Fibrinogen is a dimer; each symmetric side is composed of three polypeptide chains: A-alpha, B-beta, and gamma.[110] The role of thrombin is to remove fibrinopeptides A and B proteolytically by cleaving at specific amino acid sites. Fibrinopeptide A is released rapidly, and fibrinopeptide B is released more slowly.[4] Fibrin monomer aggregation begins immediately after fibrinopeptide A is released, and the B peptide need not necessarily be released for fibrin monomer aggregation to occur.[4] Figure 1-20 illustrates polymerization I, the alpha and gamma chains held together by hydrophobic bonds before factor XIII (fibrinoligase) activation by thrombin. Figure 1-21 illustrates polymerization II with factor XIIIa having replaced hydrophobic bonds with peptide bonds. Fibrinopeptide A consists of 16 amino acids, and fibrinopeptide B consists of 14 amino

Figure 1-16. Stoichiometry in Coagulation Reactions

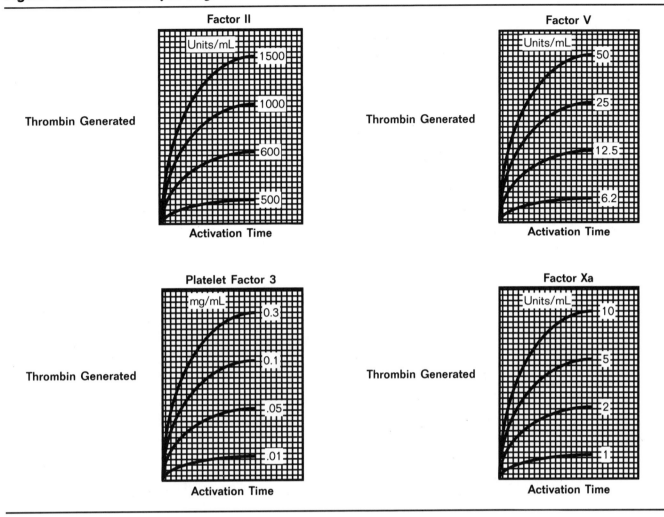

Fibrinolytic System

The fibrinolytic system, the second plasma protein system, is responsible for the destruction of a fibrin clot. It is generally thought that small amounts of fibrin are constantly and probably systemically being deposited, which is followed by lysis of these fibrin deposits.[111,112] Thus, the presence or absence of hemorrhage or thrombosis depends on a delicate balance between the procoagulant system and the fibrinolytic system.[113] Figure 1-22 summarizes the physiology of the fibrinolytic system. The fibrinolytic system consists of a proenzyme, plasminogen, which is converted via many mechanisms into the active enzyme, plasmin.[114] Plasmin, a serine protease, is not specific, like thrombin, and has equal affinity for both fibrinogen and fibrin, degrading both into fibrin(ogen) degradation products (FDPs).[115] Plasmin may biodegrade factors V, VIII, IX, and XI, corticotropin (ACTH), growth hormone, insulin, and probably many other plasma proteins.[113,116-119] There are two primary physiologic

(and pathologic) activation pathways for the fibrinolytic system: endothelial plasminogen activator[120] and Hageman factor activation.[121] Active Hageman factor converts a proactivator (plasminogen proactivator) into an activator, which then converts plasminogen into plasmin. This proactivator may be kallikrein.[4] Numerous poorly characterized tissue activators convert plasminogen to plasmin. Pharmacologic activators are currently used for therapeutic thrombolysis, including streptokinase, urokinase, tissue plasminogen activator (TPA), and acyl-plasminogen-streptokinase activator complex (APSAC).[122] Urokinase directly activates plasminogen into plasmin, and streptokinase forms a streptokinase-plasminogen complex, which then converts plasminogen into plasmin.[123]

Figure 1-23 summarizes the Hageman factor activation pathway for the fibrinolytic system. Numerous materials can convert Hageman factor into active Hageman factor, including collagen and phospholipids. Endotoxin, antibody-antigen complex, and other pathologic materials may also initiate this activation pathway, creating circulating plasmin.[91-93,124] Plasmin tends to be a self-perpetuating enzyme, a self-feed-

Figure 1-17. Vitamin K-Dependent Coagulation Factors and PIVKA Synthesis

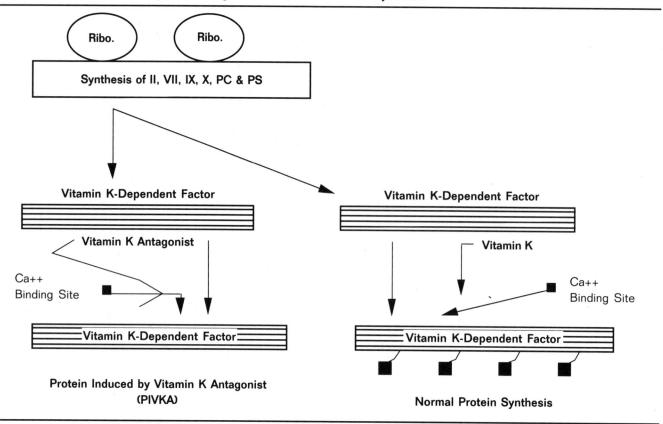

ing loop generating more plasmin once plasmin is generated via the Hageman activation pathway. The conversion of active Hageman factor into Hageman factor fragments by plasmin will then convert more proactivator to activator and convert more plasminogen to plasmin.[125,126]

The fibrinolytic system includes several primary inhibitors. Alpha-2-antiplasmin is a rapid inhibitor of plasmin activity, and alpha-2-macroglobulin is an effective, although slow, inhibitor of plasmin activity.[112,127] There are two known inhibitors of TPA: TPA-I-1 and TPA-I-2.[128,129] TPA-I-1 is found in endothelial cells, platelets, smooth muscle cells, and hepatocytes[130-133] and is a serine protease inhibitor similar to antithrombin III (AT III).[134] TPA-I-2 was first isolated from placental tissue and is also found in granulocytes

and monocyte-macrophage cells.[135,136] Like TPA-I-1, this inhibitor is similar to AT III.[137]

Although the primary activity of thrombin is to cleave fibrinopeptides A and B from fibrinogen, creating fibrin monomer, plasmin begins to biodegrade fibrinogen at the carboxy terminal end of the A-alpha chain to create degradation products. Figure 1-24 depicts the clinically significant FDPs. At the top of the figure, fibrinogen is depicted as being composed of the A-alpha, B-beta, and gamma chains, with the A peptide and the B peptide depicted as small circles. Fibrinogen and fibrin are first degraded into fragment X after plasmin-induced symmetric cleavage of the carboxy terminal end of the A-alpha chain. Subsequent digestion of fibrinogen and fibrin by plasmin is then asymmetric at the amino terminal end of one portion of the molecule, giving rise to a fragment Y and a fragment D. Following this plasmin digestion of the opposite amino terminal portion occurs, giving rise to another fragment D and a fragment E, or a so-called N-terminal disulfide knot.[138,139] Fragments X, Y, D, and E are the clinically significant FDPs measured by commercially available FDP assay kits.[113] Fragment E is the last fragment with antigenic determinants; thus, the utilizing antifibrinogen or anti-FDP latex particles (both commonly used in the kits) will not detect products digested beyond the fragment E stage.[115] This is important in disorders such as DIC. Thrombin clot tubes are supplied to clot out fibrinogen

Figure 1-18. Fibrin Formation

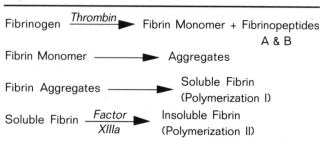

Figure 1-19. The Structure of Fibrinogen

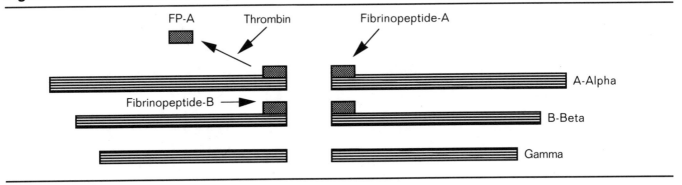

so that the antifibrinogen or anti-FDP latex particles will only react with the degradation products and not with fibrinogen itself. Fragments X and Y still contain fibrinopeptide A, and the thrombin will clot out fibrinogen and fragments X and Y. Therefore, FDP detection kits measure fragments D and E.

The FDPs are named in descending order of molecular weight with fibrinogen having a molecular weight of about 340,000 d, fragment X about 265,000 d, fragment Y about 155,000 d, fragment D about 95,000 d, and fragment E, the smallest and last of the fragments (with recognizable antigenicity), about 50,000 d.[113] The presence of FDPs may seriously compromise hemostasis by interference with fibrin monomer polymerization and platelet function.[113,140,141]

Complement Activation and Hemostasis

The next plasma protein system is complement and its interrelationships with coagulation. Complement activation is often not considered important in hemostasis; however, complement interactions with hemostatic components are of

major importance in many thrombohemorrhagic disorders. The complement system is capable of increasing vascular permeability, leading to hypotension and shock, which are common occurrences in DIC and other thrombohemorrhagic disorders.[142,143] Complement activation to the C8-C9 (attack) phase leads to osmotic lysis of red blood cells and platelets.[144,145] The lysis and disruption of red blood cells and/or platelets lead to release of procoagulant material, which usually accelerates a procoagulant process.[4] For example, if complement-induced red blood cell lysis occurs, red blood cell membrane phospholipoprotein and ADP are released, both of which serve as procoagulant- or coagulation-accelerating materials. Lysis of platelets leads to release of molecular materials, including ADP, which may also promote clotting activity and act as accelerators to the procoagulant system.

The complement system is a sequential activation pathway system similar to the procoagulation system and includes a primary activation pathway via activation of C1 and a so-called alternate or properdin activation pathway through the

Figure 1-20. Polymerization I (Soluble Fibrin)

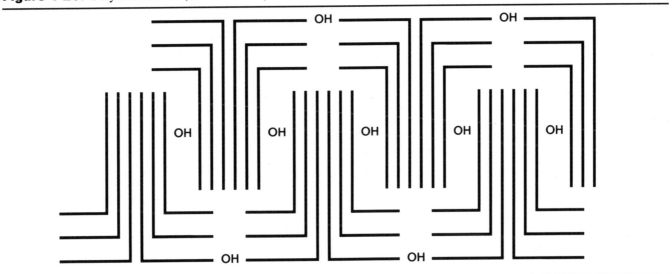

Figure 1-21. Polymerization II (Insoluble Fibrin)

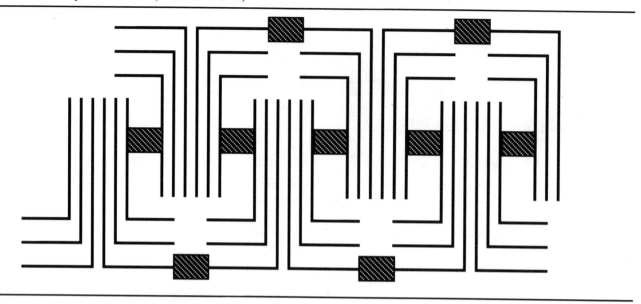

activation of C3 (Figure 1-25).[146,147] The activation of C1 through C5 is the activation phase, and the activation of C5 through C9 is the attack phase, leading to osmotic lysis. Figure 1-26 summarizes mechanisms of complement activation in the hemostasis system. Factor XII is converted into factor XIIa via numerous mechanisms including phospholipids, collagen, and kallikrein. Factor XIIa converts proactivator to activator, which converts plasminogen to plasmin. Plasmin is capable of directly activating C1 or C3, providing two independent pathways for plasmin activation of complement. In many instances of clinically significant thrombohemorrhagic

disease, plasmin-induced activation of the complement system leads to serious clinical consequences.[14,85,117]

Kinins and Coagulation

The next plasma protein system is the kinin system. Only recently has the importance of kinin generation during pathologic thrombohemorrhagic phenomena been appreciated.[4] Kinins are capable of vascular dilatation leading to hypotension, shock, and other potential end-organ damage.[148-150] Kinins increase vascular permeability with ensuing hypotension and shock. Figure 1-27 summarizes the interrelationships between Hageman factor, the fibrinolytic system, and the kinin system.[88] Like complement activation, activation of kinins centers around Hageman factor activation.

Figure 1-22. Physiology of Fibrinolysis

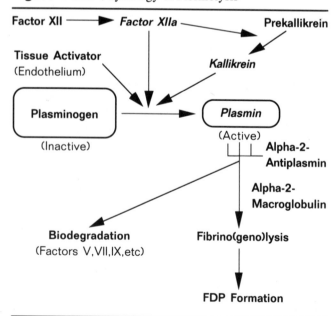

Figure 1-23. Factor XII-Dependent Activation of the Fibrinolytic System

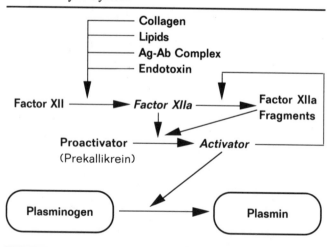

Figure 1-24. Formation of Fibrin(ogen) Degradation Products (FDPs)

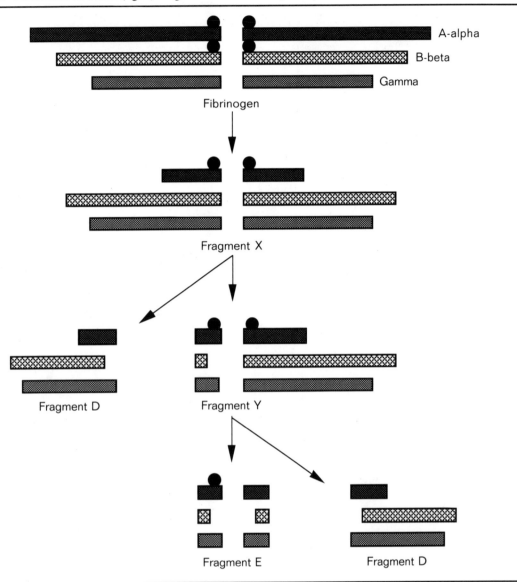

Factor XIIa converts prekallikrein (Fletcher factor) into kallikrein; kallikrein converts kininogens into kinins. Factor XIIa is converted into XIIa fragments by plasmin; these fragments also activate prekallikrein to kallikrein with ensuing generation of kinins.

Figure 1-28 illustrates the important interrelationships between the coagulation system, the fibrinolytic system, the complement system, and the kinin system. Hageman factor is converted to active Hageman factor by various compounds including collagen and phospholipids; active Hageman factor converts proactivator to activator; and activator converts plasminogen to plasmin. Plasmin activates C1 and C3, therefore activating the complement system. Active Hageman factor (or plasmin-induced Hageman factor fragments) converts prekallikrein to kallikrein, which converts kininogens to kinins. Kinin and complement activation

occur via these pathways in many thrombohemorrhagic disorders. These activation pathways often lead to serious clinical consequences.

Inhibitor Systems

The most important inhibitors of the procoagulant system are AT III, protein S, and protein C.[151,152] Table 1-13 summarizes the inhibitory mechanisms in hemostasis. Most of these inhibitory mechanisms are important physiologically, and some assume major importance in pathophysiology. First, factors V and VIII:C are inactivated by thrombin and by activated protein C (protein Ca) and protein S.[153,154] In addition, prothrombin activation and fibrin formation are inhibited by small fragments that are generated during the conversion of prothrombin to thrombin (profragments 1 and 2). Factor Xa is inhibited by modified protein C, and evi-

Figure 1-25. The Complement System

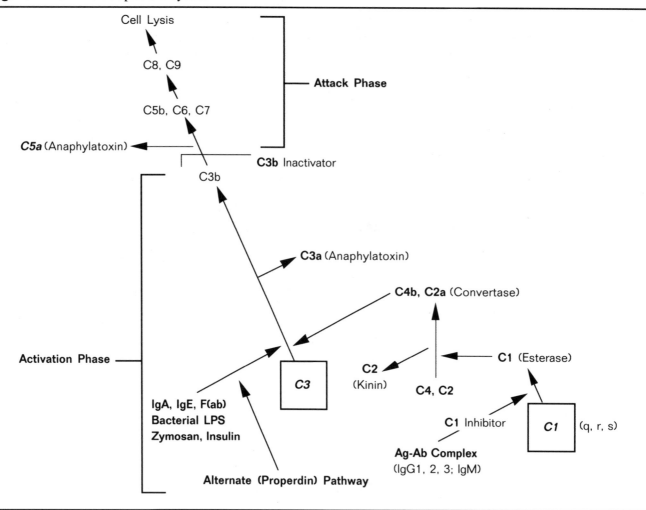

dence would suggest that alpha-1-antitrypsin may also be an inhibitor of factor Xa.[155] The serine proteases, including thrombin, factors Xa, IXa, XIa, and XIIa, and kallikrein, are

Table 1-13. Inhibitory Systems in Hemostasis

Inactivation of factors V and VIII by thrombin and activated protein C and protein S system

Inhibition of thrombin, factors Xa, IXa, XIa, XIIa, and kallikrein by antithrombin III

Inhibition of prothrombin activation and fibrin formation by prothrombin fragments

Inhibition of thrombin or factor Xa formation by suboptimal "complex" components

Inhibition of thrombin activity by absorbing to fibrin

Inhibition of fibrin monomer by polymerization and platelet function by fibrin(ogen) degradation products (FDPs)

inhibited by AT III.[156-159] The inhibitory activity of AT III is markedly enhanced by heparin.[160-162]

As fibrin is formed it absorbs thrombin, thus decreasing thrombin concentration. Inhibition of fibrin monomer polymerization and platelet function by FDPs may occur. If FDPs complex with fibrin monomer before polymerization, fibrin monomer becomes solubilized and unavailable for fibrin deposition. Later degradation products, especially fragments D and E, have a high affinity for platelet membranes and render platelets markedly dysfunctional. In some pathologic instances, this activity can lead to significant clinical hemorrhage via an FDP-induced platelet function defect.[113]

Figure 1-29 depicts a popular model of AT III and its inhibitory activity against serine proteases. Arginine-rich centers in AT III may react irreversibly with serine centers of serine proteases.[156,158] In this particular figure, thrombin is depicted; however, factor Xa, factor IXa, or other serine proteases could also have been illustrated. Serine proteases irreversibly react with arginine of AT III, and the complex is removed from the circulation. Heparin reacts with lysine

Table 1-14. Functions of Protein C

Inactivation of factors V and VIII:C (enhanced by protein S)
Enhancement of fibrino(geno)lysis by depressing inhibitors
Enhancement of epinephrine-induced platelet aggregation
Related to clot retraction by unclear mechanisms
Competitive inhibition of factor Xa (?)

Figure 1-26. Complement Activation in Hemostasis

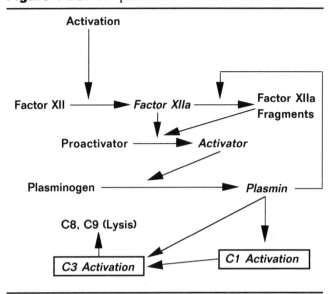

sites in antithrombin, making the arginine-rich center more available, thereby enhancing antithrombin inhibitory activity.

Table 1-14 summarizes the functions of protein C and protein S. Protein C is capable of the inactivation of factors V and VIII:C, which is accelerated by protein S.[153,154,163,164] Protein C enhances fibrinolysis by depressing fibrinolytic inhibitors or enhancing activators. Figure 1-30 depicts the protein C and S system.

Other Interactive Components

Many other interactive components of hemostasis, including the vascular proteoglycans, fibronectin, complement derivatives, neutrophils/monocytes, and other as yet unknown components, may have important roles in modulating hemostasis. With time, the interactive activities of these components will become clear; it is expected that many other components in the cellular and blood systems will be found to interact with the hemostasis system.

Fibronectin is a high–molecular weight glycoprotein that is found in its soluble form in plasma.[165] An insoluble form is found in connective tissue and basement mem-branes.[166] Fibronectin binds to collagen, fibrin, fibrinogen, and intact cells.[166-170] Fibronectin is synthesized by vascular endothelium and is also found in, and possibly synthesized by, the alpha granules of platelets.[171] Fibronectin is cleaved by thrombin and trypsin and coprecipitates with fibrin.[172,173] Fibronectin is cross-linked by factor XIIIa[172,173] and is covalently cross-linked to a fibrin clot by factor XIIIa. Fibronectin is necessary to support cell growth and the cellular migration into a fibrin clot and provides an extracellular matrix that eventually replaces a fibrin clot. Additional activities are the potentiation of plasminogen activators, thus mediating

Figure 1-27. Kinin Generation and Hemostasis

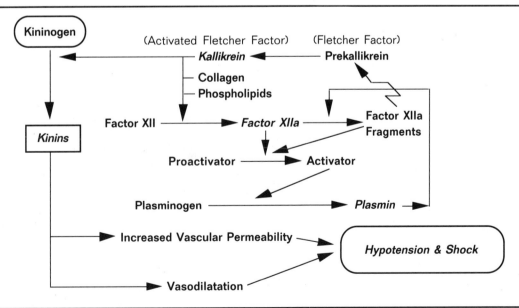

Figure 1-28. Interrelationships Between Coagulation, Fibrinolysis, Complement, and Kinins

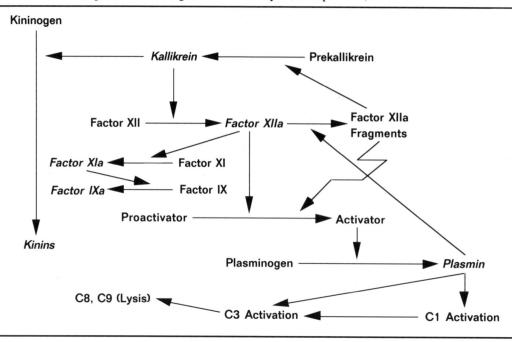

clot lysis and matrix turnover. Fibronectin mediates activation of platelets by damaged tissue, promotes opsonization of bacteria, and mediates attachment of bacteria to damaged tissues. The fibronectin associated with alpha granules of platelets is released by collagen- or thrombin-induced platelet aggregation; following release, fibronectin binds to the platelet surface. On the platelet surface, fibronectin mediates collagen-platelet adhesion and further stimulates collagen-induced platelet aggregation and release. Other activities of fibronectin include cellular binding, especially to fibroblasts, binding to bacteria where promotion of opsonization by neutrophils may occur (this requires factor XIIIa), and inhibition of the endothelial uptake of low-density lipoprotein. Fibronectin interacts intimately with fibrinogen and fibrin. As clot formation occurs, about 50% of plasma fibronectin is lost.[160] This is enhanced if clot formation occurs at less than 4°C. This loss is caused by cross-linking of fibronectin to the alpha chain of fibrin by factor XIIIa; fibronectin accounts for about 5% of the total protein of a fibrin clot. Fibronectin is necessary for cryoprecipitation of fibrinogen/fibrin complexes and accounts for the cryoprecipitation seen in DIC. The fibrin/fibronectin complex is necessary for the migration and adhesion of cells in an area of thrombus formation. Fibronectin is commonly decreased in DIC, in postoperative

Figure 1-29. Antithrombin III Inhibitory Activity

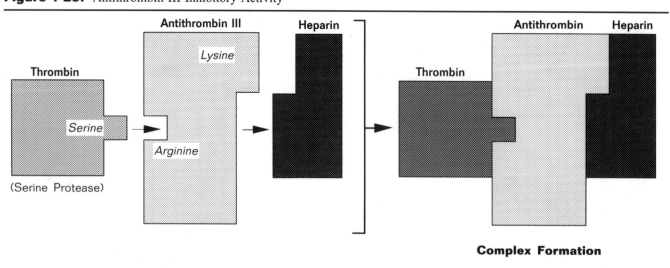

Figure 1-30. Protein C and S Activity

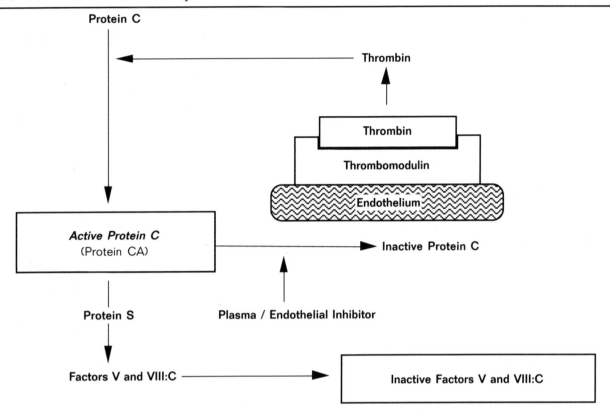

states, in patients sustaining major trauma and burns, and in patients with solid tumor metastases.[161] Fibronectin also interacts with collagen and other vascular proteoglycans. Fibronectin binds to collagen, which is mediated by cross-linking of fibronectin to collagen by factor XIIIa. In addition, fibronectin binds to heparin, endogenous heparan sulfate, hyaluronic acid, and chondroitin sulfate. Heparin may accelerate the binding of fibronectin to both fibrinogen and collagen; however, the binding of heparin to fibronectin does not change the anticoagulant nature of the bound heparin.[174]

Vascular proteoglycans are a heterogeneous group of high–molecular weight protein polysaccharides consisting of carbohydrate polymers (glycosaminoglycans) covalently linked to a protein core.[175] The common vascular proteoglycans are hyaluronic acid, chondroitin-4-sulfate, chondroitin-6-sulfate, dermatan sulfate, keratin sulfate, heparan sulfate, endogenous heparan sulfate, and heparin. Endogenous heparan sulfate differs from USP heparin in that it is a low-sulfated, D-glucuronic, acid-rich polysaccharide, whereas USP heparin is a highly sulfated, L-iduronic, acid-rich polysaccharide. The amount of each particular type of vascular proteoglycan depends on the type and portion of the vasculature evaluated. Most of the vascular proteoglycans are concentrated in the intimal layer of the vessel. The concentration of some vascular proteoglycans, especially dermatin and heparan sulfate, correlates closely with antithrombotic activity.

Selected vascular proteoglycans inhibit collagen- and thrombin-induced platelet aggregation and accelerate AT III inhibitory activity directed against thrombin and factor Xa. Vascular proteoglycans induce the release of platelet factor 4. The concentrations of vascular proteoglycans change with the development of atherosclerotic plaques. The physiologic role of vascular proteoglycans is thought to consist of supporting vascular integrity, maintaining the viscoelastic properties of vessels, regulating permeability of macromolecules from the plasma passing through the vessel wall, and regulating arterial lipid deposition. Vascular proteoglycans are potentially of importance in regulating hemostatic balance by modulating interactions of blood proteins and the vascular wall.

Several complement derivatives, especially C3a and C5a, may have importance in the hemostasis system.[4] These components not only regulate vascular tone but also may induce a neutrophil/monocyte release of elastases and collagenases, which is important in the degradation of fibrinogen, fibrin, and FDPs.[176] Complement derivatives modulate release of granulocyte/monocyte procoagulant activity, may modulate platelet reactivity, and influence the neutrophil/monocyte interaction with fibronectin.[177] Granulocytes and monocytes contain procoagulant activity, which may be released under pathologic conditions (such as acute leukemia) and interact with the hemostasis system.[178,179]

It can be reasonably foreseen that many other components of the cellular and blood protein system may be found to interact with, and perhaps be important to, the physiology and pathophysiology of hemostasis and thrombosis.

Summary

The importance of firmly mastering basic mechanisms of hemostasis is again stressed. Subsequent chapters will deal with specific disease states, more easily understood by appreciating basic physiology. A working knowledge of basic physiology of hemostasis enhances interpretation of testing modalities, affords the clinician a better understanding of thrombohemorrhagic diseases, provides a basis for therapeutic approaches, and serves as a tool for future development of improved diagnostic and therapeutic approaches.

References

1. Davie WE, OD Ratnoff: Waterfall sequence for intrinsic blood clotting. Science 145:1310, 1964.

2. Macfarland RG: An enzyme cascade in blood clotting mechanisms and its function as a biochemical amplifier. Nature 202:498, 1964.

3. Bick RL: Basic mechanisms of hemostasis pertaining to DIC, ch 1. In: RL Bick (Ed): Disseminated Intravascular Coagulation and Related Syndromes. CRC Press, Boca Raton, FL, 1983, p 1.

4. Bick RL: Basic physiology of hemostasis and thrombosis, ch 1. In: Disorders of Hemostasis and Thrombosis: Principles of Clinical Practice. Thieme, Inc., New York, 1985, p 1.

5. Crawford T: Blood and lymphatic vessels. In: WAD Anderson, JM Kissane (Eds): Pathology. CV Mosby, St. Louis, 1977, p 879.

6. Harker LA, R Ross: Pathogenesis of arterial vascular disease. Semin Thromb Hemost 5:274, 1979.

7. Lie JT: Normal structure of the vascular system and its reactive changes. In: JF Fairbairn, JL Ivergens, JA Spittel (Eds): Peripheral Vascular Diseases, ed 5. WB Saunders, Philadelphia, 1980, p 51.

8. Barnhart MI, ST Chen: Vessel wall models for studying interaction capabilities with blood platelets. Semin Thromb Hemost 5:112, 1978.

9. Wessler S, ET Yin: On the mechanism of thrombosis. Prog Hematol 5:112, 1978.

10. Bick RL: Vascular disorders associated with thrombohemorrhagic phenomena. Semin Thromb Hemost 5:167, 1979.

11. Mueller-Berghaus G: Pathophysiology of generalized intravascular coagulation. Semin Thromb Hemost 3:209, 1977.

12. Ryan TJ: The investigation of vasculitis. In: Microvascular Injury. WB Saunders, Philadelphia, 1976, p 333.

13. Bick RL: Vascular disorders associated with thrombohemorrhagic phenomena, ch 3. In: Disorders of Hemostasis and Thrombosis. Thieme, Inc., New York, 1985, p 44.

14. Mueller-Berghaus G: Pathophysiologic and biochemical events in disseminated intravascular coagulation: dysregulation of procoagulant and anticoagulant pathways. Semin Thromb Hemost 15:58, 1989.

15. O'Brian JR: The adhesiveness of native platelets and its prevention. J Clin Pathol 14:140, 1961.

16. Sheppard B, JE French: Platelet adhesion in the rabbit abdominal aorta following the removal of endothelium: a scanning and transmission electron microscopic study. Proc R Soc Lond 176:427, 1971.

17. Friedman RJ, ER Burns: Role of platelets in the proliferative response of the injured artery. Prog Hemost Thromb 4:2498, 1978.

18. Harker LA, SM Schwartz, R Ross: Endothelium and arteriosclerosis. Clin Haematol 10:283, 1981.

19. Roberts WC, VJ Ferrans: The role of thrombosis in the etiology of atherosclerosis (a positive one) and in precipitating fatal ischemic heart disease (a negative one). Semin Thromb Hemost 2:123, 1976.

20. Sinzinger H: Role of platelets in atherosclerosis. Semin Thromb Hemost 12:124, 1986.

21. McCoy L: Vascular function in hemostasis, ch 12. In: G Murano, RL Bick (Eds): Basic Concepts of Hemostasis and Thrombosis. CRC Press, Boca Raton, FL, 1980, p 5.

22. Fareed J, JM Walenga, RL Bick, EJ Bermes, HL Messmore: Impact of automation on the quantitation of low molecular weight markers of hemostatic defects. Semin Thromb Hemost 9:355, 1983.

23. Henry RL: Platelet function in hemostasis, ch 2. In: G Murano, RL Bick (Eds): Basic Concepts of Hemostasis and Thrombosis. CRC Press, Boca Raton, FL, 1980, p 17.

24. Triplett DA: The platelet: a review. In: DA Triplett (Ed): Platelet Function. ASCP Press, Chicago, 1978, p 1.

25. Ruggeri ZM, Zimmerman TS: von Willebrand factor and von Willebrand disease. Blood 70:895, 1987.

26. Zimmerman TS, Ruggeri ZM: von Willebrand disease. Hum Pathol 18:140, 1987.

27. White GC, Shoemaker CB: Factor VIII gene and hemophilia. Blood 73:1, 1989.

28. Astrup T: Fibrinolysis: an overview. In: JF Davidson, RM Rowan, MM Samama, PE Desnoyers (Eds): Progress in Chemical Fibrinolysis, vol 3. Raven Press, New York, 1978, p 1.

29. Kwaan HC: The role of fibrinolysis in disease states. Semin Thromb Hemost 10:71, 1984.

30. Pecket L: Fibrinolysis. N Engl J Med 273:966, 1965.

31. Todd AS: Histologic localization of fibrinolysis activator. J Pathol Bacteriol 78:281, 1959.

32. Mammen EF: Inhibitor abnormalities. Semin Thromb Hemost 9:42, 1983.

33. Walsh P: The effect of collagen and kaolin on the intrinsic coagulation activity of platelets. Evidence for an alternative pathway in intrinsic coagulation not requiring factor XII. Br J Haematol 22:393, 1972.

34. Wilner GD, HL Nossel, EL LeRoy: Activation of Hageman factor by collagen. J Clin Invest 47:2608, 1968.

35. Harlan JM: Consequences of leukocyte-vessel wall interactions in inflammatory and immune reactions. Semin Thromb Hemost 13:434, 1987.

36. Bevilacqua MP, MA Gimbrone: Inducible endothelial functions in inflammation and coagulation. Semin Thromb Hemost 13:425, 1987.

37. Nawroth PP, DM Stern: Endothelial cell procoagulant properties and the host response. Semin Thromb Hemost 13:391, 1987.

38. Henry RL: Platelet function. Semin Thromb Hemost 4:93, 1977.

39. Droller MJ: Ultrastructure of the platelet release reaction in response to various aggregating agents and their inhibitors. Lab Invest 29:595, 1973.

40. Stuart MJ: Inherited defects of platelet function. Semin Hematol 12:233, 1975.

41. White JG: Identification of platelet secretion in the electron microscope. Ser Haematol 6:429, 1973.

42. White JG: Interaction of membrane systems in blood platelets. Am J Pathol 66:295, 1972.

43. Nachman RL: Platelet proteins. Semin Hematol 5:18, 1968.

44. Seegers WH: Enzymes in blood clotting. J Med Enzymol (Jpn) 2:68, 1977.

45. Day NJ, H Stormorken, H Holmsen: Subcellular localization of platelet factor 3 and platelet factor 4. Proceedings of the 12th Congress International of the Society of Hematology, Mexico City, 1968, p 172.

46. Mammen EF: Physiology and biochemistry of blood coagulation. In: NU Bang, FK Beller, E Deutsch, EF Mammen (Eds): Thrombosis and Bleeding Disorders. Georg Thieme Verlag, Stuttgart, Germany, 1971, p 1.

47. Packham MA, JF Mustard: Platelet reactions. Semin Hematol 8:30, 1971.

48. Thomas DP, S Niewiarowski, VJ Ream: Release of adenosine nucleotides and platelet factor 4 from platelets of man and four other species. J Lab Clin Med 75:607, 1970.

49. Born GVR, MJ Cross: The aggregation of blood platelets. J Physiol 168:178, 1963.

50. Bull BS, MB Zucker: Changes in platelet volume produced by temperature, metabolic inhibitors, and aggregating agents. Proc Soc Exp Biol Med 120:296, 1965.

51. McLean JR, N Veloso: Changes of shape without aggregation caused by ADP in rabbit platelets at low pH. Life Sci 6:1983, 1967.

52. Zucker MB, J Peterson: Serotonin, platelet factor 3 activity and platelet aggregating agent released by adenosine diphosphate. Blood 30:556, 1967.

53. Davis RB, WR Mecker, WL Bailey: Serotonin release after injection of E. coli endotoxin in the rabbit. Fed Proc 20:261, 1961.

54. Des Prez RM, HI Horowitz, EW Hook: Effects of bacterial endotoxin on rabbit platelets. I. Platelet aggregation and release of platelet factors in vitro. J Exp Med 114:857, 1961.

55. Mueller-Eckhardt C, EF Luscher: Immune reactions of human blood platelets. I. A comparative study on the effects on platelets of heterologous antiplatelet antiserum, antigen-antibody complexes, aggregation gamma globulin, and thrombin. Thromb Diath Haemorrh 20:155, 1968.

56. Pfueller SL, EF Luscher: The effects of immune complexes on blood and their relationship to complement activation. Immunochemistry 9:1151, 1972.

57. Brodie GN, NL Bienziger, LR Chase: The effects of thrombin on adenylcyclase activity and a membrane protein from platelets. J Clin Invest 51:81, 1972.

58. Haslam RJ: Interactions of the pharmacological receptors of blood platelets with adenylate cyclase. Ser Haematol 6:333, 1973.

59. Salzman EW: Cyclic AMP and platelet function. N Engl J Med 286:358, 1972.

60. Cole B, GA Robison, RC Hartman: Effects of prostaglandin E and theophylline on aggregation and cyclic AMP levels of human blood platelets. Fed Proc 29:316, 1970.

61. Horlington M, PA Watson: Inhibition of 3' 5'-cyclic-AMP, phosphodiesterase by some platelet aggregation inhibitors. Biochem Pharmacol 19:955, 1970.

62. Gerrard JM, JG White: Prostaglandins and thromboxanes: "middlemen" modulating platelet function in hemostasis and thrombosis. Prog Hemost Thromb 4:87, 1978.

63. Hinman JW: Prostaglandins. Ann Rev Biochem 41:161, 1972.

64. Nalbandian RM, RL Henry: Platelet-endothelial cell interactions: metabolic maps of structure and actions of prostaglandins, prostacycline, thromboxane, and cyclic AMP. Semin Thromb Hemost 5:87, 1979.

65. Day CE: On the newly discovered role of prostaglandins in arteries and its implications for the control of atherosclerosis, platelets, and thrombosis. Artery 2:480, 1976.

66. Gryglewski RJ, S Bunting, S Moncada, RJ Flower, JR Vane: Arterial walls are protected against deposition of platelet thrombi by a substance (prostaglandin X) which they make from prostaglandin endoperoxides. Prostaglandins 12:685, 1976.

67. Moncada S, RJ Gryglewski, S Bunting, JR Vane: A lipid peroxide inhibits the enzyme in blood vessel microsomes that generate from prostaglandin endoperoxides the substance (prostaglandin x) which prevents platelet aggregation. Prostaglandins 12:715, 1976.

68. Gryglewski RJ, A Szczcklik, R Nizankowski: Antiplatelet action of intravenous infusion of prostacyclin in man. Thromb Res 13:153, 1978.

69. Hensby CN, PJ Lewis, P Hilgard, GP Mofti, J Hows, J Webster: Prostacyclin deficiency in thrombotic thrombocytopenic purpura. Lancet 2:748, 1979.

70. Turpie AGG: Antiplatelet therapy. Clin Haematol 10:497, 1981.

71. Berndt MC, Caen JP: Platelet glycoproteins. Prog Hemost Thromb 7:111, 1984.

72. Davies GE, Palek J: Platelet protein organization: analysis by treatment with membrane-permeable cross-linking reagents. Blood 59:502, 1982.

73. Berndt MC, C Gregory, BH Chong: Additional glycoprotein defects in Bernard Soulier syndrome: confirmation of genetic basis by parental analysis. Blood 62:800, 1983.

74. Clemetson KJ, JL McGregor, E James: Characterization of the platelet membrane glycoprotein abnormalities in Bernard-Soulier syndrome and comparison with normal by surface-labeled techniques and high-resolution two-dimensional gel electrophoresis. J Clin Invest 70:304, 1982.

75. Meyer D, HR Baumgartner: Role of von Willebrand factor in platelet adhesion to the subendothelium. Br J Haematol 54:1, 1983.

76. Kunicki TJ, N Russell, AT Nurden: Further studies of the human platelet receptor for quinine and quinidine-dependent antibodies. J Immunol 126:398, 1981.

77. Berendt MC, DR Phillips: Interaction of thrombin with platelets. Purification of the thrombin substrate. Ann N Y Acad Sci 370:87, 1981.

78. Ruggeri ZM: The platelet glycoprotein Ib-IX complex. Prog Hemost Thromb 10:35, 1991.

79. Gogstad GO, J Hagen, R Korsmo: Characterization of the proteins of isolated human platelet alpha granules, evidence for a

separate alpha granule pool of the glycoproteins IIb and IIIa. Biochim Biophys Acta 670:150, 1981.

80. Fujimura K, DR Phillips: Binding of Ca++ to glycoprotein IIb from human platelet plasma membranes. Thromb Haemost 50:251, 1983.

81. White JG: Inherited disorders of the platelet membrane and secretory granules. Hum Pathol 18:123, 1987.

82. McMillan R, D Mason, P Tani: Evaluation of platelet surface antigens: localization of the PLA$_1$ alloantigen. Br J Haematol 51:297, 1981.

83. Lawler J, RO Hynes: Structural organization of the thrombospondin molecule. Semin Thromb Hemost 13:245, 1987.

84. Santoro SA: Thrombospondin and the adhesive behavior of platelets. Semin Thromb Hemost 13:290, 1987.

85. Bick RL: Disseminated intravascular coagulation and related syndromes: a clinical review. Semin Thromb Hemost 14:299, 1988.

86. Coleman RW, A Bagdasarian, RC Talmo, CF Scott, W Seaven, JA Guimardes, JV Pierce, MP Kaplan: Williams trait: human kininogen deficiency with diminished levels of plasminogen proactivator and prekallikrein associated with abnormalities of the Hageman factor dependent pathway. J Clin Invest 56:1650, 1975.

87. Habel FM, HZ Movat: Kininogens of human plasma. Semin Thromb Hemost 3:27, 1976.

88. Murano G: The "Hageman connection" interrelationships of blood coagulation, fibrino(geno)lysis, kinin generation, and complement activation. Am J Hematol 4:303, 1978.

89. McKusick VA: Mendelian Inheritance In Man: Catalogs of Autosomal Dominant, Autosomal Recessive and X-Linked Phenotypes, ed 9. Johns Hopkins University Press, Baltimore, 1990.

90. Schriver CR, AL Beaudet, WS Sly: Blood and blood-forming tissue, pt 14. In: The Metabolic Basis of Inherited Disease. McGraw-Hill, New York, 1989, p 2107.

91. Kaplan AP, HL Meier, R Mandle: The Hageman factor–dependent pathways of coagulation, fibrinolysis, and kinin-generation. Semin Thromb Hemost 3:1, 1976.

92. Kaplan AP: Initiation of the intrinsic coagulation and fibrinolytic pathways of man: the role of surfaces, Hageman factor, prekallikrein, high molecular weight kininogen, and factor XI. Prog Hemost Thromb 4:127, 1978.

93. Meyer KL, JV Pierce, RW Coleman, AP Kaplan: Activation and function of human Hageman factor. J Clin Invest 60:18, 1977.

94. Ratnoff OD, H Saito: Coagulation factors and the role of surfaces in their activation. Ann N Y Acad Sci 283:88, 1977.

95. Griffin JH, CG Cochrane: Recent advances in the understanding of contact activation reactions. Semin Thromb Hemost 5:254, 1979.

96. Wiggins RC, BN Bouma, CG Cochrane, JH Griffin: Role of high–molecular weight kininogen in surface-binding and activation of coagulation factor XI and prekallikrein. Proc Natl Acad Sci USA 74:4636, 1977.

97. Irwin JF, WH Seegers, TJ Andary, LF Fekete, E Novoa: Blood coagulation as a cybernetic system: control of autoprothrombin C (Xa) formation. Thromb Res 6:431, 1975.

98. Seegers WH, G Murano: Blood coagulation: a cybernetic system. Pol Arch Med Wewn 55:1, 1976.

99. Seegers WH, HI Hassouna, D Hewett-Emmett, TJ Andary: Prothrombin and thrombin: selected aspects of thrombin formation, properties, inhibition, and immunology. Semin Thromb Hemost 1:211, 1975.

100. Seegers WH, N Sakuragawa, LE McCoy, JA Sedensky, FA Dombrose: Prothrombin activation: ac-globulin, lipid, platelet membrane, and autoprothrombin c (Xa) requirements. Thromb Res 1:293, 1972.

101. Seegers WH: Prothrombin complex. Semin Thromb Hemost 7:291, 1981.

102. Denson KWE: The levels of factors II, VII, IX, and X by antibody neutralization techniques in the plasma of patients receiving phenindione therapy. Br J Haematol 20:643, 1971.

103. Pereira M, D Couri: Studies on the site of action of dicoumarol on prothrombin synthesis. Biochim Biophys Acta 237:348, 1971.

104. Stenflo T: Vitamin K, prothrombin, and gamma-carboxy-glutamic acid. N Engl J Med 296:624, 1977.

105. Mackie MJ, AS Douglas: Drug-induced disorders of coagulation, ch 17. In: OD Ratnoff, CD Forbes (Eds): Disorders of Hemostasis. WB Saunders, Philadelphia, 1991, p 493.

106. Huseby RM: Conformational structure of the fibrinopeptides related during fibrinogen to fibrin conversion. Physiol Chem Phys 5:1, 1973.

107. Walz DA, WH Seegers, J Reuterby, LE McCoy: Proteolytic specificity of thrombin. Thromb Res 4:713, 1974.

108. Alami SY, JW Hampton, GH Race, RJ Speer: Fibrin stabilizing factor (factor XIII). Am J Med 44:1, 1968.

109. Ratnoff OD: The molecular basis of hereditary clotting disorders. Prog Hemost Thromb 1:39, 1972.

110. Seegers WH: Fibrinogen. Semin Thromb Hemost 7:281, 1981.

111. Winman B, A Hamsten: The fibrinolytic enzyme system and its role in the etiology of thromboembolic disease. Semin Thromb Hemost 16:207, 1990.

112. Aoki N, PC Harpel: Inhibitors of the fibrinolytic enzyme system. Semin Thromb Hemost 10:24, 1984.

113. Bick RL: The clinical significance of fibrinogen degradation products. Semin Thromb Hemost 8:302, 1982.

114. Castellino FJ: Biochemistry of human plasminogen. Semin Thromb Hemost 10:18, 1984.

115. Bang NU: Physiology and biochemistry of the fibrinolytic system. In: NU Bang, KF Beller, E Deutch, EF Mammen (Eds): Thrombosis and Bleeding Disorders. Academic Press, New York, 1971, p 292.

116. Bick RL: Disseminated intravascular coagulation, ch 2. In: RL Bick (Ed): Disseminated Intravascular Coagulation and Related Syndromes. CRC Press, Boca Raton, FL, 1983, p 31.

117. Bick RL: Disseminated intravascular coagulation and related syndromes, ch 6. In: Disorders of Hemostasis and Thrombosis: Principles of Clinical Practice. Thieme, Inc., New York, 1985, p 157.

118. Ratnoff OD, GB Naff: The conversion of C1s to C1 esterase by plasmin and trypsin. J Exp Med 125:337, 1967.

119. Robbins KM: Present status of the fibrinolytic system. In: J Fareed, HL Messmore, J Fenton, KM Brinkhous (Eds): Perspectives in Hemostasis. Pergamon Press, New York, 1980, p 53.

120. Bachmann F, KO Kruithof: Tissue plasminogen activator: chemical and physiological aspects. Semin Thromb Hemost 10:6, 1984.

121. Kaplan AP, F Austin: The fibrinolytic pathway of human plasma. Isolation and characterization of the plasminogen proactivator. J Exp Med 135:1378, 1972.

122. Robbins KC, GH Barlow, G Hguyen: Comparison of plasminogen activators. Semin Thromb Hemost 13:131, 1987.

123. Bick RL: Thrombolytic therapy, ch 14. In: Disorders of Hemostasis and Thrombosis: Principles of Clinical Practice. Thieme, Inc., New York, 1985, p 365.

124. Stump DC, FB Taylor, ME Neshein: Pathologic fibrinolysis as a cause of clinical bleeding. Semin Thromb Hemost 16:260, 1990.

125. Goldsmith GN, H Saito, OD Ratnoff: The activation of plasminogen by Hageman factor (factor XII) and Hageman factor fragments. J Clin Invest 21:54, 1978.

126. Kaplan AP, KF Austen: A prealbumin activator of prekallikrein. II. Derivation of activators of prekallikrein from active Hageman factor by digestion with plasmin. J Exp Med 133:696, 1971.

127. Schreiber AD: Plasma inhibitors of the Hageman factor dependent pathways. Semin Thromb Hemost 3:43, 1976.

128. Loskutoff DJ, M Sawdey, J Mimuro: Type 1 plasminogen activator inhibitor. Prog Hemost Thromb 9:87, 1989.

129. Astedt B, I Lecander, T Ny: The placental type plasminogen activator inhibitor: PAI-2. Fibrinolysis 1:203, 1987.

130. Sprengers ED, JH Verheijen, VMW van Hinsbergh, et al: Evidence for the presence of two different fibrinolytic inhibitors in human endothelial cell culture medium. Biochim Biophys Acta 801:163, 1984.

131. Sprengers ED, HMG Princen, T Kooistra, et al: Inhibition of plasminogen activators by conditioned medium of human hepatocytes and hepatoma cell line. J Lab Clin Med 105:751, 1985.

132. Booth NA, JA Anderson, B Bennett: Platelet release protein which inhibits plasminogen activators. J Clin Pathol 38:825, 1985.

133. Laug EW: Vascular smooth muscle cells inhibit the plasminogen activators secreted by endothelial cells. Thromb Res 53:165, 1985.

134. Philips M, AG Juul, S Thorsen, et al: Purification and characterization of reactive and non-reactive plasminogen activator inhibitor-1 from human placenta. Thromb Haemost 58:2, 1987.

135. Kopitar M, B Rozman, J Babnik, et al: Human leukocyte urokinase inhibitor: purification, characterization and comparative studies against different plasminogen activators. Thromb Haemost 54:750, 1985.

136. Vasalli JD, JM Dayer, A Wohlwend, et al: Concomitant secretion of prourokinase and of plasminogen activator–specific inhibitor by cultured human monocytes-macrophages. J Exp Med 159:1653, 1984.

137. Bachmann F: Fibrinolysis. In: M Verstraete, J Vermylen, R Linjnen, J Arnout (Eds): Thrombosis and Haemostasis. Leuven University Press, Leuven, Belgium, 1987, p 277.

138. Kudryk B, D Collen, KR Woods, B Blomback: Evidence for localization of polymerization sites in fibrinogen. J Biol Chem 249:3322, 1974.

139. Murano G: The molecular structure of fibrinogen. Semin Thromb Hemost 1:1, 1974.

140. Kowalski E: Fibrinogen derivatives and their biological activity. Semin Hematol 5:45, 1968.

141. Marder VJ, NR Shulman: High molecular weight derivatives of human fibrinogen produced by plasmin: mechanism of their anticoagulant activity. J Biol Chem 244:2120, 1969.

142. Rosse WF: Complement. In: WJ Williams, E Beutler, AJ Erslev, RW Rundles (Eds): Hematology. McGraw-Hill, New York, 1977, p 87.

143. Ruddy S, I Gigli, KF Austen: The complement system in man, I: activation, control, and products of the reaction sequences. N Engl J Med 278:489, 1972.

144. Mayer MM: The component system. Sci Am 229:54, 1973.

145. Mueller-Eberhard HJ: Complement. Ann Rev Biochem 44:667, 1975.

146. Gotze O: Proteases of the properdin system. In: E Reich, DB Rifkin, E Shaw (Eds): Proteases and Biological Control. Cold Spring Harbor Symposium, Cold Spring Harbor, NY, 1975, p 255.

147. Pillimer L, L Blum, IH Lepow: The properdin system and immunity. I. Demonstration and isolation of a new serum protein, properdin, and its role in immune phenomena. Science 120:279, 1954.

148. Bennett B, D Ogston: Role of complement, coagulation, fibrinolysis, and kinins in normal haemostasis and disease. In: AL Bloom, DP Thomas (Eds): Haemostasis and Thrombosis. Churchill-Livingstone, London, 1981, p 236.

149. Ryan JW, US Ryan: Biochemical and morphological aspects of the actions and metabolism of kinins. In: JJ Pisano, KF Austin (Eds): Chemistry and Biology of the Kallikrein-Kinin System in Health and Disease. DHEW Pub #76-791, US Department of Health, Education, and Welfare, Bethesda, MD, 1974, p 315.

150. Van Arman CG, HR Bohidar: Role of the kallikrein-kinin system in inflammation. In: JJ Pisano, KF Austin (Eds): Chemistry and Biology of the Kallikrein-Kinin System in Health and Disease. DHEW Pub #76-791, US Department of Health, Education, and Welfare, Bethesda, MD, 1974, p 471.

151. Comp PC: Hereditary disorders predisposing to thrombosis. Prog Hemost Thromb 8:71, 1986.

152. Joist JH: Hypercoagulability: introduction and perspective. Semin Thromb Hemost 16:151, 1990.

153. Esmon CT: Protein-C: biochemistry, physiology, and clinical implications. Blood 62:1155, 1983.

154. Seegers WH: Protein C and autoprothrombin II-A. Semin Thromb Hemost 7:257, 1981.

155. Scully MF, V Ellis, VV Kakkar: Studies of anti-Xa activity. Thromb Res 29:387, 1983.

156. Bick RL: Clinical relevance of antithrombin III. Semin Thromb Hemost 8:276, 1982.

157. Rosenberg RD: The effect of heparin on factor XIa and plasmin. Thromb Diath Haemorrh 33:51, 1975.

158. Rosenberg RD, P Damus: The purification and mechanism of action of human antithrombin-heparin cofactor. J Biol Chem 248:6490, 1973.

159. Seegers WH: Antithrombin III. Semin Thromb Hemost 7:263, 1981.

160. Jaques LB, NM McDuffie: The chemical and anticoagulant nature of heparin. Semin Thromb Hemost 4:277, 1978.

161. Rosenberg RD: Biologic actions of heparin. Semin Hematol 14:427, 1977.

162. Seegers WH: Antithrombin III theory and clinical applications. Am J Clin Pathol 69:367, 1978.

163. Fyrand O, ND Solum: Heparin precipitable fraction (HPF) from dermatological patients: studies on the non-clottable components; identification of cold-insoluble globulin as the major nonclottable component. Thromb Res 8:659, 1976.

164. Matsuda M, T Saida, R Hasegawa: Cryofibrinogen in the plasma of patients with skin ulcerative lesions of the legs: a complex of fibrinogen and cold-insoluble globulin. Thromb Res 9:541, 1976.

165. Mosseson MW: Cold-insoluble globulin (CIg): a circulating cell surface protein. Thromb Haemost 38:742, 1977.

166. Pearlstein E, LI Gold, A Garcia-Pardo: Fibronectin: a review of its structure and biological activity. Mol Cell Biochem 29:103, 1980.

167. Couchman JR, MR Austria, A Woods: Fibronectin-cell interactions. J Invest Dermatol 94:7, 1990.

168. Ruoslahti E, A Vaheri: Interaction of soluble fibroblast surface antigen with fibrinogen and fibrin: identity with cold insoluble globulin of human plasma. J Exp Med 141:497, 1975.

169. Moser DF: Fibronectin. Prog Hemost Thromb 5:111, 1980.

170. Zucker MB, M Mosseson, M Broekman, KL Kaplan: Release of platelet fibronectin (cold-insoluble globulin) from alpha granules induced by thrombin or collagen: lack of requirement for plasma fibronectin in ADP-induced platelet aggregation. Blood 54:8, 1979.

171. Moser DF, PE Schad, HK Kleinman: Cross-linking of fibronectin to collagen by blood coagulation Factor XIIIa. J Clin Invest 64:781, 1979.

172. Mosseson MW, RA Umfleet: The cold-insoluble globulin of plasma. J Biol Chem 254:5728, 1970.

173. Wagner DD, RO Hynes: Domain structure of fibronectin and its relationship to function. J Biol Chem 254:6746, 1979.

174. Wight TN: Vessel proteoglycans and thrombogenesis. Prog Hemost Thromb 5:1, 1980.

175. Bick RL: Pathophysiology of hemostasis and thrombosis. In: WA Sodeman, TA Sodeman (Eds): Pathologic Physiology: Mechanisms of Disease, ed 7. WB Saunders, Philadelphia, 1985.

176. Goldstein IM, HD Perez: Biologically active peptides derived from the fifth component of complement. Prog Hemost Thromb 5:41, 1980.

177. Mueller-Berghous G: Pathophysiologic and biochemical events in disseminated intravascular coagulation: dysregulation of procoagulant and anticoagulant pathways. Semin Thromb Hemost 15:58, 1989.

178. Lisiewicz J: Disseminated intravascular coagulation in acute leukemia. Semin Thromb Hemost 14:339, 1988.

179. Galloway MJ, MJ Mackie, BA McVerry: Combinations of increased thrombin, plasmin, and nonspecific protease activity in patients with acute leukemia. Haemostasis 13:322, 1983.

C H A P T E R
2

Assessment of Patients With Hemorrhage

isorders of hemostasis are myriad and permeate all domains of pathophysiology and clinical medicine. Although many disorders of hemostasis are straight-forward and simple, many are multifaceted and remarkably complex with respect to pathophysiology, diagnosis, and management. Disorders of hemostasis can be appropriately compartmentalized into hereditary and acquired, with acquired defects being much more common than hereditary defects (Table 2-1). Moreover, all hereditary and acquired defects can be compartmentalized into defects of the vasculature, the platelets, or the coagulation proteins. Generally, the inherited defects of hemostasis tend to be simple, restricted to one hemostasis compartment, and commonly limited to one coagulation protein, particularly in most cases of coagulation protein disorders. In contrast, acquired disorders of hemostasis tend to be multifaceted in etiology and in pathophysiology, involve more than one coagulation factor, and frequently tend to involve other or all the hemostatic compartments. When assessing a patient with a bleeding disorder or a bleeding history, a methodical and perceptive approach to diagnosis is obligatory.

Obtaining the History

In extracting a current medical history from the patient, the chief complaint is traditionally solicited by first encouraging the patient to summarize the reasons he or she was referred. Precisely who uncovered this disorder and the date the condition was found is indispensable. If a physician first noted the disorder, then previous records can be obtained. It is important to learn if any therapy was administered for the condition. Often a patient will be referred for evaluation of a hemostatic problem, and it is found that the patient has recently been transfused with whole blood, fresh frozen plasma, or other blood components, potentially altering laboratory manifestations. The first meeting with the patient should involve briefly describing the problems in as precise a manner as possible. The patient should depict the primary symptomatology and describe how long the problem has been pre-

sent. Next, the patient should be asked about other medical conditions diagnosed and currently being treated. In this capacity, a specific drug history is of extreme importance, and all drugs and doses regularly or sporadically ingested by the patient should be elicited and recorded. Specific attention should be paid to eliciting a history of the ingestion of aspirin, aspirin-containing compounds, antihypertensives, cough medications, digitalis preparations, hormones, cortisone, insulin, diabetic medications, thyroid medications, narcoleptics, analgesics, weight-reducing medications, anticoagulants, dilantin, diuretics, antibiotics, barbiturates, tranquilizers, oral contraceptives, or any type of antidepressant. If the patient is not currently taking any of these medications, a history of former ingestion should be solicited.

A comprehensive medical history should be attained including childhood illnesses, such as mumps, measles, chicken pox, rheumatic fever, or scarlet fever, and other illnesses, such as coronary artery disease, heart disease of any type, hypertension, diabetes mellitus, emphysema, recurrent bronchitis, recurrent pneumonia, asthma, tuberculosis, herpes zoster, hepatitis, peptic ulcer disease, liver disease, jaundice, renal disease, hives, venereal disease, anemia, seizures, or mental disease. A rigorous history should be taken about the type of past bleeding the patient has experienced, especially if it has happened spontaneously. For example, attentive inquiries should be instituted about the development of petechiae or purpura to find out if bruises are spontaneous or accounted for and to detect if the patient had a childhood history of epistaxis, umbilical stump bleeding, gingival bleeding with toothbrushing, or easy and spontaneous bruising.

A thorough surgical history should be taken. In this context, the association of bleeding or the necessity of blood transfusions should be clarified with each particular surgical procedure. Details regarding past trauma, dental extraction and associated bleeding, and the necessity of transfusions should be illuminated. When obtaining this history the patient should be specifically asked regarding a transfusion reaction or any type of untoward experience happening with respect to transfusions. It may be expected that the patient, if truly demonstrating a bleeding problem, may need transfu-

Table 2-1. Classification of the Hemorrhagic Disorders

Vascular Compartment
    Hereditary
    Acquired
    Drug induced

Platelet Compartment
    Quantitative
        Hereditary
        Acquired
        Drug induced
    Qualitative
        Hereditary
        Acquired
        Drug induced

Blood (Coagulation) Protein Compartment
    Hereditary (quantitative or qualitative)
        Single factor defects (common)
        Multiple factor defects (rare)
    Acquired (quantitative or qualitative)
        Single factor defects (rare)
        Multiple factor defects (common)

Multiple Compartment Defects
    Disseminated Intravascular Coagulation
    Primary Fibrinolytic Syndromes

sions of one type or another eventually. The patient should be asked about serious injuries or accidents, especially those that have required hospitalization, and the presence and nature of any particular bleeding associated with injuries or accidents should be annotated. The patient should be subjected to a careful allergic history, especially allergies to any particular medications.

Next, a specific review of systems should be accrued including a meticulous history about the type, site, and severity of any type of bleeding problems, such as the presence of petechiae and purpura (including spontaneous manifestations), easy or spontaneous bruising, gingival bleeding with toothbrushing, epistaxis, especially during childhood, and the development of any mucosal membrane bleeding (gastrointestinal bleeding, genitourinary bleeding, hemoptysis, or blood-tinged sputum). A history of any type of deep tissue bleeding, including intracranial hemorrhage, intra-articular bleeding, deep muscle bleeding, or any other similar type of bleeding, should be noted when obtaining a comprehensive review of systems. Besides this, the patient should be asked about complaints of generalized weakness, chills, drenching night sweats, weight loss, loss of appetite, unexplained fevers, unexplained skin rashes, and an exact description of rashes, poorly healing sores, or enlarging moles. The patient should be asked about frequent, recurrent, or localized headaches, dizziness, or the loss of consciousness. A history of blurred vision, double vision, or persistent scotomata, tinnitus, hearing loss, or sore tongue is also important. The patient should be asked about oral mucosal

bleeding, the wearing of dentures, frequent upper respiratory tract infections, difficulty in swallowing, or any unexplained hoarseness. A history of cervical pain or the recognition of supraclavicular or cervical adenopathy, chronic cough, hemoptysis, blood-tinged sputum, coughing spells, shortness of breath, paroxysmal nocturnal dyspnea, orthopnea, angina-type chest pain, heart disease of any type, hypertension, the presence of intermittent or persistent tachycardia and palpitations, and the presence and persistence of ankle edema should be noted. A history of preprandial or postprandial epigastric distress, epigastric pain, nausea, emesis, hematemesis, melena, hematochezia, or any changes in bowel habits within the previous six months should be recorded. A history of hematuria, pyuria, frequency and urgency of urination, renal disease, renal stones, or port wine–colored urine is also obtained. The presence or absence of joint pain, back pain, or bone pain should be documented and the specific areas noted.

In the female patient, the age of beginning menstruation, the age of first pregnancy, and the presence or absence of continued menses and of menopause, including the year menopause stopped, should be recorded. A careful history about the degree and length of menstrual periods is of key importance. The prior ingestion of oral contraceptives, the presence or absence of excessive vaginal discharge, recurrent vaginal infections, intramenstrual bleeding, or the noting of nodules, discharge, or irritation of the breasts should be elicited. The number of children born needs to be defined, as well as any potential or real bleeding problems in any of her children that might have been manifest at birth, spontaneously, or in association with surgery. The patient should be asked if she bled unusually during delivery and whether blood transfusions were needed. In the male patient, a history of difficulty in urination, prostatic disease, and circumcision, including the presence or absence of unusual bleeding with circumcision, should be noted.

For a personal history, it is of obvious importance to ask the patient about the use of tobacco and the form used. An ethanol history is also often difficult to take but needs to be precisely defined in the patient with a potential or real disorder of hemostasis. This should include the type of alcohol and the daily amount ingested. Questions regarding special diets or food faddism should also be carefully elicited as the patient may potentially be nutritionally deficient, including vitamin K deficiency. A careful occupational history, especially about exposure to radiation, industrial toxins, pesticides, benzene, carbon tetrachloride lead, or any other potential marrow-damaging agent, should be recorded.

An attentive family history, including the birth date, birthplace, status of health of the parents, or, if dead, the age they died and the cause of death, should be recorded. The patient should be carefully asked about any bleeding tendencies in the mother, father, or any siblings. Since many inherited disorders are sex-linked and may skip several generations, a careful history regarding bleeding tendencies in maternal and paternal grandparents, aunts, uncles, and cousins should be obtained. If married, the general health of the spouse should be recorded. Of more importance, however, is to ask regarding the general health of the patient's children, and in this capacity, it is of obvious importance to take an attentive bleeding history, because bleeding disorders may be manifest in any of the children. The patient should be specifically asked if any children have any type of bleeding tendency, including easy or spontaneous bruising, the noting of petechiae or purpura, or any other type of bleeding. In addition, if the bleeding history in children is negative, the patient should be specifically asked if any of the children have been stressed by surgery or trauma. In this capacity, it is again important to ask if any relative, either maternal or paternal including the great grandparents, grandparents, aunts, uncles, and cousins, has had any type of bleeding disorder, real or imagined. A family history of the presence or absence of cerebral vascular disease, hypertension, tuberculosis, diabetes mellitus, thyroid disease, gout, arthritis, coronary artery disease, other heart disease, pulmonary disease, peptic ulcer disease, chronic inflammatory conditions, renal disease, or anemia should be elicited. In this capacity, it is again stressed that the clinician should carefully ask the patient about any type of bleeding tendency in any immediate or remote family members. After eliciting a complete history, the clinician should summarize by asking the patient if there are any additional points of information that the patient wishes to tell.

Physical Examination

Once the history is obtained, a careful and thorough physical examination is performed. Occasionally the physical examination will be preferentially directed by points mentioned in the history. First, the vital signs of the patient should be noted and recorded, including the right brachial blood pressure, pulse rate and regularity, respiratory rate, temperature, weight, height, and body surface area. During this time a careful general inspection of the patient is done to get a general idea of the health of the patient. A general examination of the patient will usually immediately demonstrate changes associated with chronic illness, including sallowish skin, tenting of the skin, loss of subcutaneous supportive tissue, or symmetric muscle wasting. Attentive examination of the entire integumentary system should occur, carefully searching for petechiae, purpura, ecchymoses, nonpulsatile, pinpoint, or nodular telangiectasia, and other signs of a systemic bleeding disorder. A careful examination of the fingernail beds, perioral areas, and the sublingual areas are important.

Examination of the eyes should include a careful inspection of the vasculature, looking for arteriovenous (A-V) fistulae, vascular conjunctival abnormalities, bulbar and palpebral conjunctival erythema, petechiae, purpura, telangiectasia, or the presence of bulbar conjunctival icterus. A careful ophthalmoscopic examination should also be performed, looking carefully at the vasculature for signs of hemorrhages, exudates, the formation of A-V fistulae, or other abnormal arterial or venous formations. The oral mucosa and nasal mucosa should be carefully inspected. The nasal mucosa is inspected for signs of localized vascular defects or the presence of petechiae, purpura, or telangiectasia. The oral mucosa is carefully examined, and patients should always be asked to remove dentures. Special attention is directed to searching for petechiae, purpura, telangiectasia, hemorrhagic bullae, or other signs of a platelet defect, vascular defect, or other coagulopathy. It is important to note the presence or absence of lateral papillae, always to look under the tongue for sublingual telangiectasia, and to inspect the gums for hyperplasia or the presence of petechiae, purpura, or hemorrhagic bullae. In addition, the circumoral area should be inspected for the presence or absence of perioral telangiectasia; for this, female patients are asked to remove lipstick. Weber and Rinne tests should be done to assess hearing, and the auditory canals should be inspected for any signs of blood, abnormal vascular malformations, or the presence of petechiae, purpura, or telangiectasia. The presence or absence of supraclavicular, cervical, submental, and axillary adenopathy and epitrochlear, inguinal, and deep iliac adenopathy should next be ascertained. Following this, the presence or absence of sternal, cervical, thoracic, or lumbosacral spine tenderness, costovertebral angle tenderness, or rib tenderness should be assessed. The chest is then examined to ascertain if it is clear to percussion and auscultation, to prove the presence or absence of rhonchi, localized wheezing, or rales, and to document the presence of adequate diaphragmatic excursion bilaterally. Palpation and auscultation of the heart need to be performed carefully, especially listening for murmurs that may be indicative of a chronic underlying anemia secondary to a hemorrhagic tendency. All women older than 25 years of age need to have a careful breast examination performed. Following this, the carotid and femoral arteries and the abdominal aorta should be palpated and auscultated for the presence or absence of bruits. An assessment of carotid pulses, brachial pulses, radial pulses, ulnar pulses, femoral pulses, dorsalis pedis pulses, and posterior tibial pulses should occur. The abdominal examination should include attentive percussion and palpation of the liver and spleen, including an attempt to elicit hepatic or splenic tenderness and to auscultate the left upper quadrant for splenic rubs. Bowel sounds should be recorded, the entire abdomen should be palpated for evidence of any masses or aortic aneurysm, and the presence or absence of direct or indirect inguinal hernias should be searched for at this time. Following this, an examination of the genitalia should occur. A rectal examination should be done in any adult patient with a real or imagined potential bleeding disorder, and the stool sample should be examined and tested for occult blood.

The extremities are next carefully evaluated, looking for changes in the integument including petechiae, purpura, or telangiectasia, which may sometimes be pinpoint and require the use of a magnifying glass. While inspecting the integument, the fingernail and toenail beds should be carefully inspected for underlying petechiae (splinter hemorrhages), purpura, and telangiectasia. Any vascular malformations of the skin should be noted and recorded. While inspecting the extremities and integument, the presence or absence of muscle wasting, chronic hemosiderin deposits, especially in the lower extremities, or any changes compatible with varicosities or chronic venous insufficiency, including the presence or absence of ankle edema, should be noted. The presence of chronic hemosiderin deposits should alert one to the potential presence of a chronic extravasation of blood from the vasculature, which suggests a potential for simple chronic venous insufficiency or, alternatively, a chronic quantitative or qualitative platelet defect, or a vascular defect affecting either the small or large vessels, or both. The presence or absence of an ashen complexion needs to be noted. The neurologic examination is usually done last and should consist of a general assessment of the cerebrum and cerebellum and evaluation of biceps, triceps, brachioradialis, patellar and Achilles tendon reflexes. Vibratory sensation and pinpoint sensation of the lower extremities should be tested. Information regarding function or dysfunction of cranial nerves II through XII would have been gathered in previous parts of the examination.

Often, the presence or absence of a disorder of hemostasis can be documented with about 90% accuracy with the completion of a careful history and physical examination. The history and physical examination, including attentive questioning of the patient with respect to site, severity, and type of hemorrhage (petechiae, purpura, and ecchymoses vs deep tissue bleeding vs telangiectasia) should allow for categorization of the type of defect present in greater than 90% of patients. This allows one to only subject the patient to selected laboratory testing procedures and shields one from chaotic ordering of innumerable unnecessary laboratory procedures. Once the history, physical, and type of bleeding are carefully delineated, the clinician will usually have a specific diagnosis or several diagnoses in mind and many others will have been ruled out. At this time, the clinician will have a good idea whether this is a hereditary or acquired hemostasis disorder.

Following the evaluation and the impressions of the clinician, directed laboratory screening and subsequent definitive laboratory tests are usually ordered. A tremendous amount of time and money can be wasted on laboratory hemostasis testing procedures; therefore, the testing procedures should be strongly directed by the initial clinical impression based on a sound history and physical examination. When a history and physical are done, the clinician will have developed a strong suspicion whether the condition represents a hereditary or an acquired disorder and whether the disorder involves the vasculature, the platelets, or the blood protein system, or alternatively, if it is a multiple hemostatic compartment defect (eg, DIC-type syndromes) and involves several or all of the hemostatic compartments. With this clinical impression, the clinician then orders appropriate laboratory testing modalities to confirm the presence or absence of a suspected defect or defects and to learn the severity of the defect thought to be present.

Laboratory Testing

Laboratory screening tests for compartmentalizing a specific type of defect into that of the vasculature, the platelets, or the blood proteins, or a combination thereof, can be done using five simple screening tests: platelet count, template bleeding time, evaluation of the peripheral blood smear, prothrombin time, and partial thromboplastin time (Table 2-2). Often, all the screening tests will not be needed as the clinician will, based on the clinical evaluation, have a strong working diagnosis, which might have eliminated defects of the vasculature, platelets, or coagulation factors. If only one compartment is suspected to be at fault, only tests appropriate to that particular hemostatic compartment are necessary. If the results of these are negative, other hemostatic compartments are then evaluated in instances where the first clinical impression was incorrect. In most circumstances, the eliciting of a careful history, the performance of a careful physical examination, the conceptualization of a working diagnosis, and the directed and specific ordering of laboratory tests to confirm or rule out the diagnosis will lead to a correct diagnosis and will define the severity of the defect suspected.

The approach to a patient with a potential or real bleeding disorder must be logical and sequential and must be preceded by a careful clinical examination of the patient instead of the indiscriminate ordering of many laboratory tests of hemostasis. If a strong working diagnosis is not suggested by the history or physical examination, the five laboratory screening tests may be needed to define the hemostatic compartment or compartments harboring the defect. If a vascular or platelet defect is present, the template bleeding time will usually be prolonged; exceptions are noted in hereditary hemorrhagic telangiectasia, the allergic vasculitides, and the vascular defects associated with paraprotein disorders, in which the template bleeding time may be normal despite a significant vascular defect (Table 2-3).

The finding of a prolonged template bleeding time or prolonged aspirin tolerance test with a normal platelet count suggests platelet or vascular dysfunction. The aspirin tolerance test will help distinguish between a questionable or borderline template bleeding time with a strongly suggestive

Table 2-2. Screening Tests of Hemostasis

Complete blood and platelet count
Peripheral blood smear evaluation
Template bleeding time
Prothrombin time
Partial thromboplastin time (activated)

Table 2-3. Screening Test Result Versus Compartment Containing the Hemostasis Defect

	Vascular disorder	Platelet function	Platelet number	Blood proteins
Platelet count	Normal	Normal	Abnormal	Normal
Template bleeding time	Abnormal	Abnormal	Abnormal	Normal*
Prothrombin time	Normal	Normal	Normal	Abnormal or normal**
Partial thromboplastin time	Normal	Normal	Normal	Abnormal or normal**

* Except von Willebrand syndrome
** Prothrombin time and/or partial thromboplastin time will be prolonged depending on factor involved; factor XIII deficiency and alpha-2-antiplasmin deficiency not detected by prothrombin time or partial thromboplastin time

history. An attentive examination of the blood smear, often neglected by clinicians, is paramount and may reveal findings suggestive of an associated blood dyscrasia, such as leukemia, leukocytosis, shistocytosis, reticulocytosis, or other underlying condition, to account for the hemostatic defect. In this regard, up to 50% of patients with acute leukemia may initially present with easy and spontaneous bruising and petechiae and purpura. During a careful evaluation of the blood smear, platelet morphology and number should be noted. If the template bleeding time is prolonged and the platelet count is normal, one must differentiate between a platelet function defect or vascular defect. At this point platelet aggregation or lumi-aggregation should be done to diagnose differentially between a platelet function defect and a vascular defect.

If a clinically significant coagulation protein abnormality is present either the prothrombin time, activated partial thromboplastin time, or both, will be prolonged, except in factor XIII deficiency or alpha-2-antiplasmin deficiency. In multiple compartment defects, such as DIC with secondary fibrinolysis, many tests of hemostasis may be abnormal, including the prothrombin time, the partial thromboplastin time, the template bleeding time, the platelet count, and platelet aggregation. Primary fibrinolytic syndromes will present with the same findings, except platelets may be normal in number. More sophisticated techniques for making a specific differential diagnosis from the laboratory standpoint are found in appropriate chapters in discussions following disease categories.

Bleeding resulting from a vascular disorder may call for a careful clinical and laboratory evaluation to undercover an underlying primary disease, such as Cushing's syndrome, scurvy, the allergic vasculitides, or a malignant paraprotein disorder. If no primary disease can be found, the template bleeding time and platelet function studies will help to define the vascular nature of a disorder. In this regard, the template bleeding time should usually not be performed in association with obvious bleeding or obvious thrombocytopenia, since unnecessary bleeding may occur. Since the template bleeding time and aspirin tolerance test may be abnormal in conditions other than vascular disorders, further studies are necessary to establish the diagnosis and to diagnose differentially a vascular disorder from a platelet function defect. When initial screening tests suggest a platelet disorder, a platelet count must be done. If the count is low, the bone marrow should next be examined if the cause of thrombocytopenia is not obvious. If the platelet count is normal, however, platelet aggregation studies need to be done to help define the qualitative abnormalities that are most probably present in the platelets.

Clinically significant coagulation factor abnormalities are almost always diagnosed from the initial prothrombin time and/or partial thromboplastin time. Factor XIII deficiency and alpha-2-antiplasmin deficiency, however, will not be detected by the prothrombin time or partial thromboplastin time. The ability to do these assays by totally automated instrumentation using premeasured small amounts of reagents has greatly enhanced their accuracy and convenience for use by physicians in private practice environments and outpatient facilities when ambulatory patients need examination. Reagents, however, should be carefully chosen. Comparative studies have shown that some commercial reagents do not perform as adequately as screening tests of hemostasis.

Summary

When examining a patient with a bleeding disorder or a bleeding history, a systematic and logical approach to the clinical and laboratory diagnosis is imperative. A simple and workable approach is to regard the hemostasis system as being composed of three hemostatic compartments: the vasculature, the platelets, and the coagulation proteins. Generally, for normal hemostasis to occur all three of these compartments must be intact. Platelets must be normal in both number and function, and coagulation proteins must be quantitatively and qualitatively normal. Often, a defect in only one hemostatic compartment can be corrected by overcompensation of the other two compartments, and clinically significant bleeding may or may not follow. For example, disruption of the vasculature, as in minor trauma or surgery, may not lead to pathologic bleeding if platelet number and function and coagulation proteins are intact and function properly to overcome this insult. Commonly, abnormalities in two of the three hemostatic systems must be present for significant pathologic bleeding to occur. Hemophiliacs often do not bleed (coagulation protein abnormality) unless another of the hemostatic compartments is disrupted (eg, interruption of the vasculature by surgery or trauma), thus inducing a defect in two of the three hemostatic compartments. Once one can discern which compartment or combination of compartments contains a defect, a thorough evaluation of this compartment can then be carried out from both the clinical and laboratory standpoints.

In the vast majority of instances, a clinical examination of the patient including a careful history will compartmentalize a defect of hemostasis with greater than 90% accuracy. If the patient has petechiae and purpura, one can assume the vasculature or platelets (either number or function) are at fault. Petechiae and purpura almost never arise from coagulation protein disorders alone. Platelet function defects, thrombocytopenia, and vascular defects are most commonly characterized by petechiae and purpura, easy and spontaneous bruising, gingival bleeding with toothbrushing, and mild to moderate mucosal membrane bleeding. Alternatively, single or multiple coagulation protein abnormalities are usually manifest by deep tissue bleeding, including intramuscular bleeding, intra-articular bleeding, and intracranial bleeding in association with moderate to severe mucosal membrane bleeding, and the development of large subcutaneous ecchymoses. A careful history should pinpoint a family history of bleeding, a personal history of bleeding, and the type, site, and severity of bleeding that has occurred. Obviously, patients should be thoroughly questioned about drugs for the detection of drug-induced platelet dysfunction, drug-induced thrombocytopenia, or drug-induced vascular defects.

Probably no area of laboratory medicine is more confusing to the clinician than hemostasis. Rapid growth in the understanding of hemostasis and blood proteins involved with hemostasis, the superfluity in terminology, the potpourri of techniques purported to measure the same factors, and the mysticism of reagents used, such as "thromboplastin" and "activators," serve to nurture this bewildering state of affairs. Even to the present time, no global agreement exists on even such a routine procedure as the prothrombin time, despite more than three decades of international committee meetings. Tables 2-1, 2-2, and 2-3 classify the bleeding disorders according to pathogenetic mechanisms and outline laboratory screening procedures that will simplify a systematic approach to the categorization of most bleeding disorders. Although a bleeding disorder can usually be defined without the aid of laboratory screening tests but merely with a meticulous history and physical examination, the diagnosis needs to be confirmed and the severity of the defect needs to be delineated using appropriate laboratory testing modalities. However, the choice and interpretation of these tests should always be predicated on the basis of major clinical data solicited by performing an attentive history and conducting a rigorous physical examination. Although a complete history should be taken, particular emphasis should be directed to the family history and drug ingestion (conspicuous or surreptitious). A history of obstetric and surgical events associated with unusual bleeding calls for a search for defects in hemostasis. Vascular defects are usually associated with easy and spontaneous bruising, petechiae and purpura, usually dependent, and mild to moderate bleeding from mucous membranes. Alternatively, platelet defects, although also associated with easy and spontaneous bruising and mild to moderate mucosal membrane bleeding, are usually associated with petechiae and purpura that are symmetric instead of dependent. In contrast, the blood protein defects rarely, if ever, present as petechiae and purpura, except von Willebrand's syndrome, but are usually associated with large subcutaneous ecchymoses, moderate to severe mucosal membrane hemorrhage, and deep tissue bleeding. Thrombocytopenias, hereditary or acquired, may be caused by the following: (1) bone marrow failure, (2) maturation/metabolic defects, or (3) peripheral platelet loss. More commonly bleeding may be caused by platelet dysfunction, either hereditary or acquired. Coagulation protein abnormalities, whether hereditary or acquired, may result from absent, decreased, or abnormal synthesis of a clotting factor or the development of antibodies against these factors.

In liver disease or suspected drug-induced bleeding (especially if caused by particular antibiotics), a therapeutic trial of vitamin K may prove useful in selected patients. In life-threatening situations, specific hemotherapeutic agents may be necessary to establish the diagnosis and to manage hemorrhage (eg, the use of prothrombin complex concentrates in selected clinical situations where a diagnosis is strongly suspected but not yet confirmed, and bleeding is so severe that the physician cannot wait for confirmatory evidence from the laboratory).

The recognition of inhibitors to specific clotting factors has increased greatly in recent years. Inhibitors may develop in up to 10% of hemophiliacs but also occur in postpartum females, in patients with autoimmune disorders, and in association with other well-defined disease entities. Occasionally they may occur spontaneously with no obvious associated condition. Patients with most acquired defects, including both DIC-type syndromes and primary fibrinolytic syndromes, and patients with chronic liver disease will harbor multiple coagulation factor abnormalities and multiple hemostatic compartment-type defects. After recognizing the underlying disease process, the laboratory evaluation of such patients should be guided by knowing the types of hemorrhagic syndromes that occur in particular clinical disorders. In our era of intemperate polypharmacy, drug-induced bleeding must be strongly considered, the classic example being aspirin ingestion. A host of other drugs, alone or in combination, may induce bleeding tendencies and not always by the same mechanisms. Drugs should be suspected when one or more defects can be demonstrated, without other obvious cause, and should especially be suspected when the discontinuation of medication causes hemostasis test results to return to normal. Careful initial clinical examination of the patient, including a painstakingly solicited history and a diligently performed physical examination, is the mainstay of diagnosis in the patient with a suspected or real hemorrhagic disorder. After this is performed an initial clinical impression or working diagnosis is formulated and is most often correct in the vast majority of instances (up to 90% of patients). Following the formulation of a working diagnosis or first impression, laboratory testing procedures, carefully chosen and based on the logical and sequential clinical examination of the patient, are selectively ordered to document the presence or absence of the defect and to delineate the severity. In this regard, a simple screening battery to assess all hemostasis compartments consists of a peripheral blood smear evaluation, platelet count, template bleeding time, prothrombin time, and activated partial thromboplastin time.

CHAPTER
3

Vascular Bleeding Disorders

isorders of the vasculature are common, although often unappreciated, causes of bruising and bleeding. Petechiae and purpura are hallmark findings of vascular disorders, and patients with vascular disorders often have mild to moderate mucosal membrane bleeding, often manifest as bilateral epistaxis, gastrointestinal bleeding, or genitourinary bleeding. Patients often present with a history of easy and spontaneous bruising or gingival bleeding with toothbrushing. Many individuals without vascular bleeding disorders experience occasional gingival bleeding with toothbrushing; however, if a patient relates that the gums bleed almost daily with toothbrushing, a vascular or platelet defect is probable. Another clinical clue to the presence of a vascular disorder is the finding of dependent petechiae and purpura primarily found on the extremities and usually absent from the torso. This is a characteristic of vascular bleeding, whereas platelet defects are typically associated with symmetric petechiae and purpura found on the extremities and torso. Common clinical findings of vascular disorders are summarized in Table 3-1.[1-3] The primary laboratory screening test for a vascular disorder or a platelet function defect is the standardized template bleeding time.[4]

Vascular disorders are best categorized as hereditary, acquired, and drug induced (Table 3-2). The hereditary vascular disorders generally are the hereditary collagen vascular diseases, and most are clinical oddities. The exception to rarity is Osler-Weber-Rendu disease (hereditary hemorrhagic telangiectasia), which is quite common. Alternatively, the acquired vascular disorders are very common, and all clinicians should be familiar with them. The importance of becoming familiar with acquired vascular disorders is severalfold: when a patient presents with dependent petechiae and purpura and easy or spontaneous bruising, the patient should be examined for acquired vascular disorders. If an individual has one of the acquired disorders known to be associated with vascular defects and will undergo surgery or sustains trauma, it should be assumed the patient has a systemic vascular defect that might lead to clinically significant thrombohemorrhagic problems.

Vascular disorders may present in bizarre and varied ways. Determinants of varied clinical presentations are summarized in Table 3-3. First, there are many potential host responses to a vascular disorder. For example, simply an antigenic response, only activation of the coagulation system, only activation of the fibrinolytic system, only activation of kinins, only activation of complement, or activation of any combination of these pathways may occur. Vascular insults, injuries, or diseases occur in varied severities. A mild vascular insult (disorder) will usually lead only to serum effusion, which clinically is interpreted as bullae and erythema. If the insult (disease) is more pronounced, however, both serum and blood may effuse from the vasculature, giving rise to bullae, erythema, and wheals in association with petechiae and purpura. If the insult is severe, not only will there be effusion of blood, but endothelial cell death, petechiae and purpura, gross hemorrhage, often large ecchymoses, and small or large vessel thrombosis will also occur. When the myriad host responses to a vascular disorder are integrated with severity of the vascular disorder or insult, it is apparent how many seemingly similar vascular disorders may present with varied clinical findings.

Hereditary Vascular Disorders

The hereditary vascular disorders include Ehlers-Danlos syndrome, Marfan's syndrome, osteogenesis imperfecta, pseudoxanthoma elasticum, homocystinuria, giant cavernous hemangiomas and the Kasabach-Merritt syndrome (the combination of giant cavernous hemangiomas and disseminated intravascular coagulation), and hereditary hemorrhagic telangiectasia.

Ehlers-Danlos Syndrome

The Ehlers-Danlos syndrome (ED syndrome) is a rare connective tissue disorder inherited by autosomal dominance.[5] Interestingly, one of the earliest descriptions of this syndrome may have concerned the violin virtuoso Paganini,

Table 3-1. Common Signs and Symptoms in Vascular Diseases

Petechiae and purpura (usually dependent)
Large ecchymoses
History of easy bruising
History of spontaneous bruising
Gingival bleeding
Mucosal membrane bleeding
    Pulmonary
    Gastrointestinal
    Genitourinary
    Epistaxis

Table 3-2. Classification of Vascular Disorders

Hereditary
  Ehlers-Danlos syndrome
  Marfan's syndrome
  Osteogenesis imperfecta
  Pseudoxanthoma elasticum
  Homocystinuria
  Giant cavernous hemangiomas
  Hereditary hemorrhagic telangiectasia

Acquired
  Collagen (autoimmune) vascular disorders
    Systemic lupus
    Scleroderma
    Rheumatoid arthritis
    Dermatomyositis
    Polyarteritis
    Mixed connective tissue disease
  Cushing's syndrome
  Diabetes mellitus
  Infectious purpuras
  Drug-induced purpuras
  Malignant paraprotein disorders
    Myeloma
    Waldenström's macroglobulinemia
  Benign paraprotein disorders
    Amyloidosis
    Cryoglobulinemia
    Essential monoclonal gammopathy
  Circulating immune complex disorders
  Autoerythrocytic sensitization
  Drug-induced vasculitis

Immune Mediated
  Cryoglobulinemia
  Sjögren's syndrome
  Proliferative glomerulonephritis
  Lymphoma and lymphoid leukemia
  Chronic infection or inflammation
  Malignant hypertension
  Viral infection
  Subacute bacterial endocarditis
  Allergic vasculitis
  Drug-induced vasculitis
  Collagen diseases
    Systemic lupus
    Mixed connective tissue disease
    Scleroderma
    Dermatomyositis
    Polyarteritis
    Rheumatoid arthritis

because this disorder was thought to contribute to his remarkable dexterity and talent. The ED syndrome is characterized by extreme vascular fragility, skin fragility, hypermobile joints, and molluscoid pseudotumors of the knees and elbows. Bleeding may be highly variable; however, easy and spontaneous bruising is a hallmark of this syndrome. Patients commonly have gingival bleeding with toothbrushing and severe bleeding after dental extraction. Petechiae, purpura, gastrointestinal bleeding, and hemoptysis are often present. In some instances, the bleeding diathesis may be severe enough to suggest hemophilia. Some patients may have associated platelet function defects and the characteristic vascular defects.[6] Other characteristics commonly noted in this syndrome are blue sclerae and angioid streaks. Aortic insufficiency and the "floppy" mitral valve syndrome may occur. The common laboratory findings are a prolonged template bleeding time and sometimes abnormal platelet aggregation if the patient has an associated platelet function defect. The basic pathology of the ED syndrome is poorly understood but is thought to represent a decrease in collagen and an increase in elastic tissue. The collagen from these patients is thought to contain an abnormal amino acid composition.[7] A prolonged template bleeding time is classically present. Characteristics of Ehlers-Danlos syndrome are summarized in Table 3-4.

Marfan's Syndrome

This syndrome is well described and the most well known of the hereditary collagen vascular disorders. It is inherited as an autosomal dominant trait and is characterized by skeletal defects (long extremities and arachnodactyly), cardiovascular abnormalities (ascending aortic aneurysm and/or dissection), and ocular defects, usually manifest as ectopia lentis.[8,9] Hyperextensible joints are uniformly present. Of all the hereditary collagen vascular disorders, Marfan's syndrome is least characterized clinically by a hemorrhagic diathesis. However, many patients have easy and spontaneous bruising, and some may have a poorly characterized platelet function defect as well. A prolonged template bleeding time may be present.[4] The characteristics are summarized in Table 3-5.

Osteogenesis Imperfecta

Osteogenesis imperfecta (brittle bones and blue sclerae syndrome) is also one of the more common hereditary collagen vascular disorders and is inherited as an autosomal dominant trait. This disorder is characterized by a patchy lack of bone matrix. However, the existing matrix undergoes normal

Table 3-3. Variable Determinants of Clinical
Manifestations in Vascular Disorders

Potential Host Response
    Allergic reaction
    Coagulation activation
    Fibrinolytic activation
    Kinin activation
    Complement activation
    Other enzyme activation
    Migration of leukocytes

Potential Severity of Defect
    Mild: serum effusion with bullae and erythema only
    Moderate: serum and blood effusion with bullae,
        erythema, wheals, petechiae, and purpura
    Severe: effusion of blood and endothelial cell death
        with petechiae, purpura, gross hemorrhage,
        and thrombosis

calcification. Osteogenesis imperfecta is clinically manifest as deformed and brittle bones that fracture easily. Skin and subcutaneous hemorrhages are characteristic.[10] Death often occurs at birth, resulting from intracranial hemorrhage caused by an abnormal calvarium coupled with a vascular hemorrhagic diathesis. Easy and spontaneous bruising, hemoptysis, epistaxis, and intracranial bleeding are common in osteogenesis imperfecta. An abnormal template bleeding time is characteristic.[11] Many patients have been described with abnormal platelet function as defined by aggregation studies. The basic pathophysiology of osteogenesis imperfecta is characterized by the inability of reticulin to mature into collagen; the collagen demonstrates an abnormal amino acid composition. Characteristics of this syndrome are summarized in Table 3-6.

Pseudoxanthoma Elasticum

Pseudoxanthoma elasticum (PE syndrome), unlike the other hereditary vascular diseases, often does not become

Table 3-4. Ehlers-Danlos Syndrome

Clinical Findings
    Autosomal dominant trait
    Vascular and skin fragility
    Easy and spontaneous bruising
    Gingival and dental bleeding
    Petechiae and purpura
    Gastrointestinal tract bleeding
    Hemoptysis
    Blue sclerae and angioid streaks
    Molluscoid pseudotumors
    Mitral valve prolapse

Laboratory Features
    Prolonged template bleeding time
    Platelet dysfunction (storage pool type)

Table 3-5. Marfan's Syndrome

Clinical Findings
    Autosomal dominant trait
    Easy and spontaneous bruising
    Systemic bleeding uncommon
    Ectopia lentis
    Arachnodactyly
    Hyperextensible joints
    Ascending aortic aneurysms
    Dissecting aortic aneurysms

Laboratory Findings
    Prolonged template bleeding time
    Platelet dysfunction in some

manifest until the second or third decade of life.[12] This rare disorder is inherited as an autosomal recessive trait. The PE syndrome is commonly characterized by significant hemorrhage since abnormal elastic fibers involve the entire arterial system. Hemorrhage may happen in any organ but most commonly involves the skin, eyes, kidneys, and gastrointestinal tract. Patients with PE syndrome have a marked tendency to easy and spontaneous bruising, commonly have petechiae and purpura, and have a marked predisposition to thrombosis, especially cerebral vascular thrombosis, acute myocardial infarction, and peripheral vascular occlusion with resultant gangrene and loss of extremities. Other clinical characteristics include relaxed, inelastic, and redundant skin in facial, neck, axillary, orbital, and inguinal areas. Hyperkeratotic plaques develop in these areas, and subcutaneous calcinosis is also common. Death is frequently caused by gastrointestinal hemorrhage.[4] Excessive uterine bleeding and intra-articular bleeding with formation of characteristic hemarthroses are common. The basic vascular pathology of this disorder is unclear but thought to be because of metabolic (enzyme) defects in elastic fibers.[4] This syndrome is summarized in Table 3-7.

Table 3-6. Osteogenesis Imperfecta Syndrome

Clinical Findings
    Autosomal dominant trait
    Easy and spontaneous bruising
    Subcutaneous bleeding
    Intracranial bleeding
    Epistaxis
    Hemoptysis
    Death at birth due to central nervous system bleeding
    Deformed and brittle bones
    Patchy lack of bone matrix

Laboratory Findings
    Prolonged template bleeding time
    Platelet dysfunction in some

Table 3-7. Pseudoxanthoma Elasticum Syndrome

Clinical Findings
  Autosomal recessive trait
  Easy and spontaneous bruising
  Petechiae and purpura
  Mucosal membrane bleeding
  Severe gastrointestinal bleeding (may be fatal)
  All bleeding may be severe
  Intraocular bleeding
  Intra-articular bleeding
  Relaxed, inelastic, and redundant skin in axillae, neck, and
      inguinal areas
  Hyperkeratotic plaques
  Subcutaneous calcium deposits
  Becomes manifest in second or third decades of life

Laboratory Findings
  Prolonged template bleeding time
  Platelet dysfunction in some

Figure 3-1. Thermogram of Patient With Giant Cavernous Hemangiomas

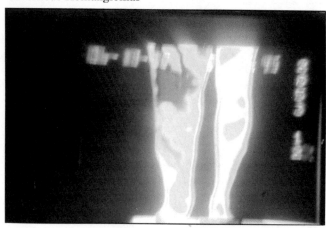

Homocystinurea

Homocystinurea is a rare inborn error of metabolism, inherited as an autosomal recessive trait and showing molecular heterogeneity.[13] Patients have decreased levels of cystathionine beta-synthetase leading to characteristic homocystinemia, methioninemia, and homocystinurea. Patients characteristically demonstrate ectopia lentis, varying degrees of mental retardation, and skeletal deformities, including osteoporosis with resultant biconcave vertebrae, scoliosis, and pes cavus.[14] Striking and unusual vascular changes are noted. Histologically, significant fibrosis of the intima and frayed muscle fibers in the media of arteries are found. Veins may also harbor these fibrous changes. Clinically, patients sustain arterial and venous thrombi; carotid artery thrombosis is a common event. On both the arterial side and the venous side, both large and small vessels may be involved with thrombosis and resultant occlusions. Widespread atheromatous changes occur in patients at an early age.[15] Homocystine-induced endothelial cell damage with resultant patchy endothelial cell sloughing and subsequent platelet-induced intimal proliferation of smooth muscle media cells occur, leading to widespread atheroma formation. The disease may be managed and complications somewhat aborted by treatment with large doses of pyridoxine. Thrombotic manifestations have been successfully controlled with combination platelet suppressive therapy consisting of dipyridamole and aspirin.[4]

Giant Cavernous Hemangiomas and the Kasabach-Merritt Syndrome

Hemangiomas are usually congenital, although they may not become clinically obvious until the patient is several years of age. They are more common in females and may be of three types: capillary, cavernous, or capillary-cavernous mixtures.[16] Cavernous forms are less common than capillary types but are more often associated with systemic thrombohemorrhagic problems. Cavernous hemangiomas are benign vascular tumors with dilated thin-walled vessels and sinuses lined by abnormal endothelium. The most common sites of involvement are the gastrointestinal tract, bones, liver, integument of the face and neck, and various mucosal membrane surfaces, including the oral mucosa.[17] Hemangiomas of the extremities may often involve the skin, subcutaneous tissue, and adjacent bone.[4] Many thrombi may form in these cavernous hemangiomas, and many patients may develop a local or disseminated intravascular coagulation syndrome.

The association of giant cavernous hemangiomas and DIC is called the Kasabach-Merritt syndrome, named after the two investigators who originally noted this association.[18] The DIC may be low grade but frequently progresses to a fulminant form. Some patients develop a life-threatening fulminant DIC with attempted surgical resection of these hemangiomatous masses.[19] Other patients develop DIC spontaneously. Disseminated intravascular coagulation can often be controlled with heparin, usually delivered subcutaneously. Occasionally, however, local radiation therapy or injections of sclerosing agents have been reported to be beneficial.[19,20] Patients may develop localized but extensive deep vein thrombosis in association with giant cavernous hemangiomas. The thermograms and venograms of such a patient are shown in Figures 3-1 and 3-2. When examining patients with giant cavernous hemangiomas, proper laboratory evaluation to determine the presence or absence of DIC should be instituted. The occurrence of DIC may significantly change morbidity or mortality, and the clinician may wish to consider appropriate prophylactic therapy for low-grade DIC, such as low-dose heparin or platelet-suppressive therapy, to abort a more fulminant form. Surely, any patients with giant cavernous hemangiomatous lesions considered candidates for corrective surgery should be examined for DIC, and the DIC syndrome should be corrected before surgery is performed. Treatment is symptomatic; however, steroids may also be of benefit in decreasing the size of hemangiomatous lesions.[4]

Figure 3-2. Venogram of Patient With Giant Cavernous Hemangiomas

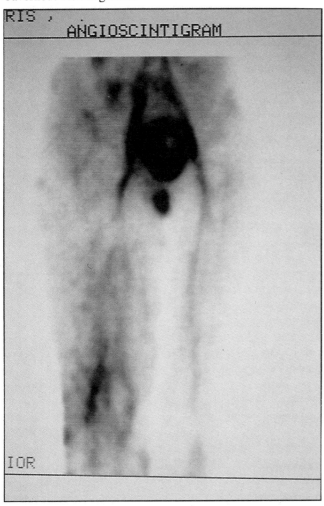

Hereditary Hemorrhagic Telangiectasia

Hereditary hemorrhagic telangiectasia (HHT) (Osler-Weber-Rendu disease) is a common disorder and is the most common hereditary vascular disorder leading to a hemorrhagic diathesis.[21-23] The disorder is inherited as an autosomal dominant trait, with 70% of affected individuals having a contributory family history.[4] The homozygous state is thought to be lethal. The gene responsible for HHT is somehow linked to blood group O.[4] The hallmark characteristic of this disease is epistaxis, which may be profuse and usually begins in early childhood. The classic telangiectatic lesions of HHT may not appear until later in life, commonly the second or third decade. The classic diagnostic triad of HHT includes a hereditary basis, telangiectasia, and bleeding from telangiectatic lesions.[4] Chronic blood loss, commonly from the gastrointestinal or genitourinary tract, is often severe enough for patients to present as having iron-deficient anemia of unknown etiology.

The telangiectatic lesions of HHT may be of three types: pinpoint, nodular, and spiderlike.[24] Unlike telangiectasia associated with chronic liver disease, those of HHT are nonpulsatile.[4] Telangiectasia and bleeding usually increase with advancing age, although epistaxis often decreases with age.[4] The origin of bleeding in HHT may be covert, but common causes are gastrointestinal or genitourinary tract hemorrhage, hemoptysis, or heavy menstrual flow. About 20% of patients develop A-V fistulae of the pulmonary vasculature.[25] An inordinately high incidence of Laennec's-type cirrhosis is noted in these patients.[4] Hamartomas of the liver and spleen may also be associated with HHT.[26] The basic pathophysiology of HHT is poorly understood. Most investigations have shown elastic fibers to be missing from the vascular walls.

Few characteristic laboratory findings are present in HHT. The template bleeding time may be normal or abnormal, depending on the integrity of the vasculature in the particular area where the test is performed.[4] The diagnosis is suggested by a history of recurrent bilateral epistaxis usually first noted in early years, occult gastrointestinal bleeding, and nonpulsatile pinpoint, nodular, or spiderlike telangiectasia, most commonly found in the skin, in sublingual and perioral areas, in the buccal mucosa, or under the fingernails.[4]

Hereditary hemorrhagic telangiectasia is often associated with other defects in hemostasis. Abnormal platelet function is present in many patients with HHT.[27,28] A poorly defined defect in the fibrinolytic system may occur.[29,30] Of major importance, and often unappreciated, is an associated DIC syndrome. Disseminated intravascular coagulation is often present in a low-grade form but periodically may become fulminant. If tested for, DIC is found in about 50% of patients with HHT; one study,[31] however, did not find DIC in a population of patients with HHT.[32] In some patients, bleeding may be severe enough that spontaneous intra-articular bleeding and resultant hemarthroses develop. HHT may be somewhat similar to the syndrome of giant cavernous hemangiomas and DIC, and hence, a "mini"-Kasabach-Merritt syndrome manifests in some patients, although it is often not recognized.[4] When DIC occurs, treatment should be targeted at stopping or blunting the process before a fulminant stage is attained.[19] Characteristics of HHT are depicted in Table 3-8.

Therapy for uncomplicated HHT depends on the particular clinical situation and the age of the patient. Localized epistaxis can often be controlled with local supportive measures and vasoconstrictive nasal sprays. However, electrocauterization may become necessary. Some instances of bleeding in HHT, such as gingival bleeding with toothbrushing, spontaneous bruising, and gastrointestinal/genitourinary tract bleeding, can sometimes be controlled with carbazochrome salicylate.[33] This agent is usually used in a dosage of 5 to 10 mg orally every three to four hours during waking hours and is without significant toxicity. High-dose estrogens may be used to scarify telangiectatic lesions and control bleeding. This modality, however, should be used as a last resort, especially in younger patients.[34]

Specific therapy for significant bleeding associated with congenital vascular defects, other than HHT, is generally not

Table 3-8. Hereditary Hemorrhagic Telangiectasia

Clinical Findings
    Autosomal dominant trait
    70% with contributory family history
    Epistaxis in early childhood
    Easy and spontaneous bruising
    Occult mucosal membrane bleeding
    Telangiectasia of skin and mucosal surfaces
    Pulmonary A-V fistulae
    Hamartomas of liver and spleen
    Laennec's cirrhosis in many
    Telangiectasia usually increases with age
    Bleeding may decrease with age in some

Laboratory Findings
    Template bleeding time often normal
    Platelet dysfunction in 50%
    Low-grade DIC in 50%

satisfactory and depends primarily on supportive measures and control of the underlying disease process.

Acquired Vascular Defects

It is important to be familiar with these acquired vascular defects because they are common. Patients presenting with easy and spontaneous bruising, petechiae and purpura, especially dependent, and other suggestive historical and physical findings should be suspected of having and be examined for the disorders associated with acquired vascular defects. Alternatively, if an individual has one of these disorders and is going to have surgery or experiences trauma, it can be assumed a vascular defect is probably present and significant hemorrhagic or thrombotic problems may follow. The common acquired diseases associated with systemic vascular problems leading to systemic hemorrhagic problems include the collagen vascular disorders, circulating immune complex disorders, multiple myeloma, Waldenström's macroglobulinemia, cryoglobulinemia, amyloidosis, Cushing's syndrome, diabetes mellitus, the allergic (Henoch-Schönlein) purpuras, numerous infectious agents, and drug-induced vascular defects.[4] Table 3-9 depicts several mechanisms by which these vascular defects occur.

In collagen vascular disorders, the vascular hemorrhagic defect is thought to be caused by poor vascular support from intrinsic collagen abnormalities. In Cushing's syndrome it is thought that the vascular disorder and typical hemorrhage occurring are caused by abnormal mucopolysaccharides in perivascular supporting tissue. All the paraproteins, including IgA, IgM, and IgG, have an affinity for attachment to the vascular endothelium and lead to a vascular hemorrhagic problem. This is most commonly noted with IgM and IgG$_3$ paraproteins. Paraproteins may occlude the vasa vasorum of affected vasculature, again giving rise to hemorrhage.[4]

Aspirin is commonly regarded as a platelet function inhibitor; however, aspirin is also an effective inhibitor of acetylcholine esterase, and this inhibition leads to a vascular bleeding problem.[35] If trauma (or microtrauma in the form of a template bleeding time) ensues in a patient taking a regimen of aspirin, prolonged vascular bleeding may occur. The usual vascular response to trauma is constriction. With vascular trauma, acetylcholine esterase degrades acetylcholine, which keeps the vessel dilated. Trauma-induced release of catecholamines will then constrict the vessel. If the patient is taking aspirin and the vasculature is severed, acetylcholine esterase is inhibited, acetylcholine cannot be degraded, and inadequate vascular constriction results.[4] Prolongation of the template bleeding time after aspirin ingestion may be the result of the vascular, instead of the platelet, inhibitory effect.[4]

Malignant Paraprotein Disorders and Amyloidosis

The many thrombotic and hemorrhagic tendencies in patients with malignant paraprotein disorders and amyloidosis, be they primary or secondary, are well recognized. These disorders can present with a wide clinical spectrum of hemorrhagic and thrombotic manifestations, depending on host response, size and site of the vasculature involved, and response of the particular end organ. Many mechanisms for the vascular complications of malignant paraprotein disorders have been proposed, and only the salient features of most of these mechanisms will be discussed here. Increased circulating levels of IgG and IgM, which are complement fixing and may lead to histamine release, chemotaxis of leukocytes, and platelet aggregation and release, can give rise to increased vascular permeability, serum and blood effusion, and sometimes small vessel thrombosis. Hyperviscosity in the malignant paraprotein disorders is a well-known cause of stasis and resultant ischemia and acidosis. This leads to increased vascular permeability, the consequences of which may be retinal hemorrhage and exudates, epistaxis, petechiae and purpura, and hemorrhage into other organs, including vital organs. Necrotizing vasculitis may occur via unclear mechanisms in malignant paraprotein disorders. Obviously, the clinical manifestations, whether they be thrombosis, hemorrhage, or a combination thereof, will depend on site and severity of the necrotizing vasculitis. When the malignant paraprotein disorders are associated with cryoglobulinemia (IgG and IgM paraprotein disorders), paraprotein is commonly found in the walls of the small vessels, which may lead to a frank vasculitis. Again, the clinical manifestations obviously range from effusions, bullae, petechiae and purpura, or frank end-organ damage (especially glomerulonephritis) to ischemia, cellular death, and end-organ failure. In all malignant paraprotein disorders a high incidence of thrombosis is noted, especially manifest as diffuse recurrent deep venous thrombosis, thromboembolism, pulmonary emboli, and renal vein thrombosis.[36,37] The mechanisms leading to this are unclear but need not be related to the development of hyperviscosity, except in cases of retinal vein thrombosis.[38]

Disseminated intravascular coagulation is also often seen in patients with malignant paraprotein disorders. Whether this association is because of endothelial damage by paraprotein or by other unexplained mechanisms is unclear. The fibrino(geno)lysis occurring in patients with malignant paraprotein disorders is also initiated through unclear mechanisms and might represent fibrinolysis secondary to DIC, fibrinolysis secondary to endothelial damage, or the result of deranged endothelial plasminogen activator activity.[39]

Amyloidosis further complicates the vascular changes of malignant paraprotein disorders and is associated with increased hemorrhage or thrombosis via disruptions of the vasculature. Classically, primary amyloidosis is of unknown etiology or associated with malignant paraprotein disorders. Primary amyloidosis characteristically involves the skin, tongue, heart, and gastrointestinal tract, whereas secondary amyloidosis is seen with chronic inflammatory/infectious diseases and typically involves the liver, spleen, kidney, and adrenal glands.[40] However, many cross-overs and mixtures of the two are commonly seen, and sometimes one cannot precisely define amyloidosis as being primary or secondary.[40] Despite the many proposed mechanisms for vasculitis in primary and secondary amyloidosis, the precise mechanisms remain unclear. Vascular hemorrhage is a classic hallmark of amyloidosis and is manifest as petechiae and purpura, ecchymoses, easy and spontaneous bruising, spontaneous hemorrhage into lymph nodes, recurrent hematuria, and spontaneous hemorrhage into vital organs.[4] Several proposed pathophysiologic events leading to generalized vasculitis have included antigen-antibody complex–induced endothelial damage or deposits of amyloid on the endothelium and in the perivascular areas.[41] Endothelial and perivascular amyloid deposits are more commonly appreciated in the secondary forms, especially in arterioles, which leads to both a hemorrhagic and thrombotic tendency. In secondary amyloidosis, amyloid deposits are noted along the endothelium. Intimal deposits start in the intima and progress to the media, with amyloid being deposited in parallel with reticulum fibers instead of around the collagen fibers, as is more frequent in primary amyloidosis. In primary amyloidosis, the deposits are usually seen along the collagen with progression from the adventitia to the media of arterioles and veins. The same process appears to occur in veins, possibly accounting for the thrombotic tendencies seen in individuals with amyloidosis.

In some patients with systemic amyloidosis, acquired factor X deficiency occurs.[42-47] In two patients similarly affected, an acquired combined deficiency of factors IX and X was noted.[47] Furie and associates[48] explored the mechanisms of factor X deficiency in amyloidosis using ^{131}I-labeled factor X. A triphasic plasma clearance pattern was noted; 85% of the labeled factor X cleared in less than 30 seconds, the next 10% cleared in less than 90 seconds, and the remaining 5% was absent after 10.5 hours. Subsequent surface scanning of the patients 24 hours after the labeled infusion revealed high concentrations in the liver and spleen. This observation, coupled with the rapid clearance of the

Table 3-9. Acquired Vascular Disorders: Proposed Mechanisms

Cushing's Syndrome: Loss of mucopolysaccharides in perivascular supporting tissues

Paraprotein Diseases: Coating of endothelium by paraprotein and occlusion of vasa vasorum

Allergic, Drug, and Infectious Vasculitis: Immune-complex–induced vascular and perivascular injury

Autoimmune Diseases: Collagen and connective tissue abnormalities in vascular supportive tissue

Diabetes Mellitus: Basement membrane thickening with porosity, decreased proteoglycans, and lipohyaline deposits

label on initial transit in the circulation, led these investigators to conclude that factor X is deposited at prior tissue sites of amyloid. These patients should respond to therapeutic infusions with factors II, VII, IX, and X concentrates; however, only a transient correction by concentrates in factor X–deficient cases of amyloidosis is noted.[4] The wide variability of hemorrhagic and thrombotic manifestations in patients with paraprotein disorders and amyloidosis will depend on the particular end organ involved and the degree of vascular permeability and/or occlusion.

Patients with malignant paraprotein disorders and amyloidosis may develop a diffuse vascular disease that may manifest as hemorrhage, thrombosis, or both. A high variability of end-organ damage may be seen. These patients may experience significant vascular bleeding and bleeding from obvious other causes when subjected to surgery or trauma. When examining patients with vascular disorders, malignant paraprotein defects or amyloidosis should be considered in the differential diagnosis. When a selective acquired factor X deficiency in an adult is found, underlying systemic amyloidosis should be strongly suspected.

Autoimmune Disorders and Vascular Defects

Immunologic diseases associated with circulating immune complexes, especially those associated with circulating cryoglobulins, are of paramount importance because these disorders are associated with a diffuse vasculitis and resultant thrombosis or hemorrhage. At least three potential mechanisms by which circulating immune complexes, circulating cryoglobulins, or circulating antibodies may lead to vasculitis have been described: (1) the production of an antibody that is directed specifically against the endothelium[49] (this is the least common operative mechanism); (2) the production of a nonspecific antibody or immune complex that nonspecifically attacks and damages endothelium and other cellular systems[50]; and (3) the generation of an antibody or immune complex that attaches to and damages perivascular tissues (including basement membrane) and secondarily causes endothelial damage and increased vascular perme-

Table 3-10. Common Infectious Agents Associated With Vasculitis

Bordetella pertussis
Chlamydia
Clostridium tetani
Coccidioidomycosis
Corynebacterium diptheriae
Cytomegalovirus
Epstein-Barr virus
Escherichia coli
Hepatitis virus
Influenza virus
Leprosy
Malaria
Mycobacteria
Pseudomonas aeruginosa
Salmonella typhi
Staphylococcus
Streptococcus
Subacute bacterial endocarditis
Syphilis
Tuberculosis

ability.[51] The vascular responses and clinical manifestations are variable and depend on severity, duration, and degree of repetition of endothelial or periendothelial insult and damage.[52] If the attack is mild, then increased vascular permeability, fibrin deposition, and a fibrinolytic response will occur, which lead to minimal hemorrhage and thrombosis.[4] If, however, the insult is persistent, excessive endothelial damage, depletion of fibrinolytic enzymes and endothelial fibrinolytic activators, increased fibrin and platelet deposition, more pronounced thrombosis or hemorrhage, and more enhanced and perpetuated endothelial damage will occur. In yet more severe insults to the endothelium or surrounding tissue by antibody, immune complex, or cryoglobulins, endothelial cell death, sloughing, and more severe thrombosis, hemorrhage, and end-organ failure may follow. Antibody directed specifically against the endothelium is a rare mechanism of autoimmune-induced vasculitis and is limited to the allergic purpuras (Henoch-Schönlein, etc) and polyarteritis nodosum.[49] Future immunologic investigations may define other disorders in this class. The other two mechanisms of immune complex–induced vasculitis are more common and are seen in a wide variety of autoimmune disorders. In many of these diseases, circulating immune complexes (IgG and IgM) attach to the endothelium, fix complement, and induce migration of leukocytes, which disintegrate and destroy the vessel.[53] For example, antistreptococcal antibody attaches to the glomerular endothelium or basement membrane, giving rise to subsequent renal vascular damage.[54] An extension of this is Goodpasture's syndrome, in which antibody or immune complexes are directed against both renal and pulmonary basement membrane with associated resultant endothelial damage and thrombohemorrhagic manifestations.

Many infectious agents are known to be associated on rare occasions with vasculitis and the attendant clinical manifestations; these include numerous bacterial, viral, and mycoplasma infections. The mechanisms, where known, include the induction of nonspecific anti-endothelial antibody by the invading organism, the inducement of specific anti-endothelial antibody by the invading micro-organism, and the development of circulating immune complexes.[55-58] Table 3-10 lists the most common infectious agents associated with vasculitis.

In most circulating immune complex diseases, the injury is nonspecific, and not only the endothelium but many other cellular systems are damaged. Diseases with circulating antibody–, immune complex–, or cryoglobulin-induced vasculitis are many and include collagen vascular disorders, drug reactions, serum sickness, and a large group of seemingly unrelated disorders. Table 3-11 summarizes pathophysiologic mechanisms.

Malignant Hypertension, Eclampsia, Cushing's Disease, Diabetes Mellitus, and Vascular Defects

In patients with malignant hypertension, advancing age, or diabetes mellitus, lipohyaline material is deposited in the subendothelium of arteries and arterioles.[4] In malignant hypertension, fibrinoid necrosis is another characteristic feature. As constant unrelenting damage occurs, the vessels eventually develop increased vascular permeability with plasma seepage and fibrin deposition. This leads to thrombosis and thromboembolism, a common clinical manifestation in these disorders.[59] The resultant downstream capillary stasis leads to the development of chronic purpura and local hyperpigmentation of the skin, resulting from chronic hemosiderin deposits. Authoritative reviews have detailed more completely the pathophysiologic events in these disorders.[60-62] The findings in eclampsia are similar to those previously described, with the development of hypertension and localized intravascular coagulation (fibrin deposition) in the placental and renal microcirculation.[63,64] Some women develop classic findings of either chronic or acute DIC with any or all the clinical manifestations of DIC.[19,65]

The vascular changes of Cushing's disease are poorly defined but include loss of subcutaneous elastic tissues leading to inadequate endothelial cell support, increased vascular permeability and fragility, and loss of elastic tissue in the vascular walls.[4] Advanced atherosclerotic changes occur in larger vessels.[66] Easy and spontaneous bruising and a marked increase of thrombosis and thromboembolic disease are seen in most patients with Cushing's syndrome.[4] Many patients with Cushing's syndrome experience profuse bleeding, because of a vascular defect, when undergoing surgery or trauma.[4]

Behçet's Syndrome

Behçet's syndrome is characterized by a typical triad of aphthous stomatitis, genital ulcerations, and iritis.[67,68] Many

Table 3-11. Immune-Associated Vascular Disease: Proposed Mechanisms

Anti-endothelial cell antibody and endothelial cell destruction

Immune complex (IgG and IgM) attachment to endothelium with complement fixation, migration of leukocytes, and destruction of the vessel

Immune complex (IgG and IgM) attachment to basement membrane or perivascular supportive tissue with increased vascular permeability or other damage

Table 3-12. Common Drugs Associated With Vascular Defects

Aspirin
Allopurinol
Arsenicals
Chloramphenicol
Chlorthiazide
Chlorpropamide
Digoxin
Estrogens
Furosemide
Gold
Heparin
Indomethacin
Iodine
Isoniazid
Meprobamata
Methyldopa
Piparazine
Quinidine
Quinine
Reserpine
Sulfonamides
Tolbutamide
Warfarins

patients develop recurrent deep venous thrombosis of unexplained pathophysiologic origin, usually involving large veins, the saphenous veins, or the superior and inferior vena cava.[69] Many develop a widespread, poorly defined arteritis.[70] Patients may demonstrate fibrinoid necrosis of the arterial tree.[71] Case reports have documented impaired fibrinolysis, and some patients have responded to thrombolytic therapy.[72] Except for the finding of impaired endothelial fibrinolytic activity, thus far the pathophysiologic mechanisms for recurrent deep venous thrombosis, arteritis, and hemorrhage, usually manifest as petechiae and purpura, are unclear.

Vascular Defects Associated With Cardiopulmonary Bypass

Poorly understood defects in the vasculature may happen during or after cardiopulmonary bypass surgery (CPB). A syndrome of mild to moderate nonthrombocytopenic purpura accompanied by splenomegaly and atypical lymphocytosis following CPB has been noted.[73] In this syndrome, purpura is usually benign, self-limiting, and frequently manifest only after the patient has been discharged from the hospital. One patient has been described who developed post-CPB classic glomerular nephritis of the type seen with the allergic vasculitides. Fatal purpura fulminans may also occur following CPB.[74] An inflammatory vasculitis may be associated with cardiopulmonary bypass, although the mechanisms remain unclear.

Drug-Induced Vasculitis

Drug-induced vasculitis is common in clinical medicine and often neglected as a cause of petechiae and purpura, skin necrosis, or frank gangrene. Drugs may induce vasculitis by many mechanisms, most of which do not significantly differ from the mechanisms operative in circulating immune complex disorders. Frequently, however, the precise mechanisms by which drugs induce vasculitis are poorly understood. Drugs may induce vascular defects by several mechanisms, including the development of a specific antivessel antibody,[75] the development of circulating immune complexes sometimes associated with cryoglobulinemia,[76] and more rarely, drug-induced independent changes in vascular permeability. A characteristic, catastrophic, and well-characterized vasculitis associated with warfarin anticoagulants has been well doc-

umented.[77-82] This vasculitis and not uncommonly hemorrhagic skin vasculitis as manifested by hemorrhagic skin infarction sometimes have been associated with intravascular coagulation.[78,80] Most warfarin derivatives have been incriminated: 90% of patients have been women, and gangrene of the breast has occurred in at least 25% of cases reported in the literature. Nalbandian and coworkers have described the histologic features of this syndrome, showing perivascular accumulations of inflammatory cells involving mainly the venules with extensive thrombosis of the draining veins with little or no invasion of arterioles.[78] Typically, the clinical picture develops three to 10 days after starting therapy and bears little relationship to the prothrombin time. Many patients are protein C, protein S, or antithrombin III deficient, and it is thought that a short period of hypercoagulability occurs, resulting from initial imbalance of the procoagulant and anticoagulant systems of these patients when starting warfarin therapy.[83,84] However, some patients with this disorder have normal protein C, protein S, and antithrombin III levels, and in these instances the mechanism may be that of a direct toxic effect on the endothelium by warfarin. Many patients respond to heparin therapy.[78,83,84] The most common drugs causing vascular problems are listed in Table 3-12.

Laboratory Findings

The primary laboratory screening test for a vascular disorder or a platelet function defect is the standardized tem-

Table 3-13. Laboratory Assessment of Vascular Disorders

Screening Tests
  Template bleeding time
  Aspirin tolerance
  Petechiometer test*
  Platelet aggregation
  Duke bleeding time**
  Tourniquet test**

Definitive Tests
  Autoimmune evaluation*
  Paraprotein evaluation*
  Vascular biopsy*
  Cryoglobulins*
  Cold agglutinins*
  Prostacycline assays***
  TPA assay***
  TPA-inhibitor assay***

* When indicated
** No longer used
*** Efficacy not yet known

plate bleeding time.[85,86] A standardized template bleeding time is usually not done in young individuals, especially infants and children younger than 15 years of age. A normal range has not been established for this age group and undue scar formation may be expected in this population. Prolonged bleeding times in children are common and therefore difficult, if not impossible, to interpret. In these instances the petechiometer test should be used. If an individual demonstrates a borderline template bleeding time, in the 10- to 12-minute range, with a positive or suggestive history, the aspirin tolerance test is useful.[87] The aspirin tolerance test consists of giving 600 mg of aspirin and repeating the template bleeding time in the opposite antecubital fossa two hours after taking the aspirin. The bleeding time in most individuals will be prolonged by about two to three minutes. The ingestion of 600 mg of aspirin, however, will unmask an underlying vascular or platelet function defect and render the repeat bleeding time about three times longer than the baseline template bleeding time, usually 20 to 30 minutes.[4]

Once an abnormal template bleeding time, abnormal petechiometer test, or abnormal aspirin tolerance test has been shown in the appropriate clinical setting with a normal platelet count, the differential diagnosis is then between a platelet function or a vascular defect.

To make this differential diagnosis, platelet function testing must be performed. The definitive test to differentiate between vascular and platelet defects is platelet aggregation. Platelet aggregation and lumi-aggregation will be discussed in chapter 4. An abnormal template bleeding time and normal platelet function as defined by platelet aggregation define a vascular disorder. Once a vascular defect has been documented, more definitive tests, including an evaluation

for autoimmune disease, paraprotein disorders, possibly a connective tissue or vascular biopsy, or other similar modalities, will often be needed to make a definitive diagnosis.[4]

The presence of a vascular disorder is usually documented in the hematology laboratory. Once the presence of a vascular disorder has been established, however, the specific diagnosis usually falls outside the realm of the hematology laboratory, and other types of laboratory procedures, including special biopsies and staining, are needed for a definitive diagnosis.[88,89] Table 3-13 summarizes the laboratory evaluation of vascular defects, including older methods and newer methods.[90] The Duke bleeding time is usually no longer done; the Ivy bleeding time (nonstandardized Ivy bleeding time) is also usually no longer done; and the Tourniquet test has been abandoned by most laboratories.[4] Newer methods available are the standardized template bleeding time (TBT),[91] the aspirin tolerance test[92] (which is only performed with a borderline or slightly prolonged template bleeding time, in the presence of a suggestive history), or alternatively the petechiometer test in younger individuals.[93] More definitive tests then needed, after documenting the probable presence of a vascular disorder, are platelet aggregation to rule out a platelet function defect as the cause of a prolonged template bleeding time, abnormal aspirin tolerance test results or abnormal petechiometer test results, and then more definitive tests for a specific diagnosis.[4]

The TBT is less painful and is associated with less scar formation than the nondisposable bleeding time devices. The cuts should always be made cephalocaudad (from elbow to wrist) and should never be made horizontally or across the arm for several reasons. Most clinical studies establishing normal and abnormal ranges for the standardized TBT have used cuts made in the cephalocaudad direction. The natural skin lines are cephalocaudad, and, consequently, if cuts are made horizontally (across the arm) prolonged template bleeding times often result and more scar formation occurs. Many laboratories have been reluctant to do template bleeding times because of the invasive nature of the test and potential scar formation. Significant scar formation can easily be avoided with attention to proper technique, such as correct bandaging for prevention of scars. Following completion of the template bleeding time a butterfly bandage should be placed over the cuts, barely opposing the two cut edges without pinching the skin. A butterfly dressing is placed over the wound, and the patient is instructed to remove the dressing 24 hours later. Patients should always be asked about a family or personal history of keloid formation, and, if present, a TBT should not be done or the potential scars accepted. With correct technique and correct bandaging of the TBT performed in adults, few patients will be left with significant scars. Template bleeding times should not be done in infants or patients in their early to mid-teenage years, because no normal ranges have been established and significant scar formation may result.

The petechiometer is an alternative to template bleeding times in children, older individuals, or patients with a personal or family history of keloid formation. The petechiometer applies a defined amount of suction to the skin, petechiae develop, and the number of petechiae formed are then recorded. This is done by laying a glass microscope slide over the suction area and carefully counting the number of petechiae. The levels considered to be normal are 0 to 10 petechiae per cm^2 after 50-cm vacuum for 60 seconds. When more than 10 petechiae per cm^2 develop, strong evidence for a vascular (or platelet) defect exists.[94] Recently, synthetic substrate assays for tissue (endothelial) plasminogen activator activity have become available.[95-97] Assays for vascular thromboxane derivatives are now available.[98] However, it is not yet clear if these assays are of clinical usefulness in evaluating vascular bleeding problems.

Summary

This chapter has summarized the more important disease entities that may be accompanied by or lead to a disorder of hemostasis or thrombosis via alterations of the vasculature. The vascular component of hemostasis is often overlooked by clinicians caring for patients with disorders of hemostasis and thrombosis. The vasculature is intricately related to the coagulation protein system and to platelets when involved in a thrombohemorrhagic diathesis.

References

1. Bick RL: Vascular disorders associated with thrombohemorrhagic phenomena. Semin Thromb Hemost 5:167, 1979.

2. Bick RL: A systemic approach to the diagnosis of bleeding disorders. In: G Murano, RL Bick (Eds): Basic Concepts of Hemostasis and Thrombosis. CRC Press, Boca Raton, FL, 1980, p 81.

3. Bick RL: Vascular disorders. In: G Murano, RL Bick (Eds): Basic Concepts of Hemostasis and Thrombosis. CRC Press, Boca Raton, FL, 1980, p 89.

4. Bick RL: Vascular disorders associated with thrombohemorrhagic phenomenon, ch 3. In: Disorders of Hemostasis and Thrombosis. Thieme, Inc., New York, 1985.

5. Johnson SA, EF Falls: Ehlers-Danlos syndrome: a clinical and genetic study. Arch Dermatol (suppl) 60:82, 1949.

6. Roberts HR, FG Kroncke: Tests of platelet activity: application to clinical diagnosis. In: KM Brinkhous, RW Shermer, FK Mostofi (Eds): The Platelet. Williams and Wilkins, Baltimore, 1971, p 365.

7. Pinnell SR, SM Krane, J Kenzora, MJ Glincher: A new heritable disorder of connective tissue with hydroxylysine-deficient collagen. N Engl J Med 286:1013, 1972.

8. Anderson M, RH Pratt-Thomas: Marfan's syndrome. Am Heart J 46:911, 1953.

9. Futcher PH, H Southworth: Arachnodactyly and its medical complications. Arch Intern Med 61:693, 1938.

10. Albright JA, EA Miller: Osteogenesis imperfecta. Clin Orthoped 159:2, 1981.

11. Seibel BM, IA Briedman, SO Schwartz: Hemorrhagic disease in osteogenesis imperfecta: studies of platelet function defect. Am J Med 22:315, 1957.

12. Polimer IJ: Pseudoxanthoma elasticum and gastrointestinal hemorrhage. J Maine Med Assoc 58:76, 1967.

13. Mudd SH, HL Levy, F Skovby: Disorders of transsulfuration, ch 23. In: CR Schriver, AL Beaudet, WS Sly, D Valle (Eds): The Metabolic Basis of Inherited Disease. McGraw-Hill, New York, 1989, p 693.

14. Valle D, GS Pai, GH Thomas, RE Pyeritz: Homocystinuria due to cystathionine beta-synthetase deficiency: clinical manifestations and therapy. Johns Hopkins Med J 146:110, 1980.

15. Carey MC, DE Donovan, O Fitzgerald, FD McAuley: Homocystinuria, I: a clinical and pathologic study of nine subjects in six families. Am J Med 45:17, 1968.

16. Burbank MK, JA Spittell: Tumor of blood and lymph vessels, ch 2. In: JL Juergens, JA Spittell, JF Fairbairn (Eds): Peripheral Vascular Diseases. WB Saunders, Philadelphia, 1980, p 679.

17. Allen PW, FM Enzinger: Hemangiomata of skeletal muscle: analysis of 89 cases. Cancer 28:8, 1972.

18. Kasabach HH, KK Merritt: Capillary hemangioma with extensive purpura. Am J Dis Child 59:1016, 1940.

19. Bick RL: Disseminated intravascular coagulation and related syndromes: a clinical review. Semin Thromb Hemost 14:299, 1988.

20. Edgerton MT: The treatment of hemangiomas: with special reference to the role of steroid therapy. Ann Surg 183:517, 1976.

21. Hans FM: Multiple hereditary telangiectasia causing hemorrhage (hereditary hemorrhagic telangiectasia). Bull Johns Hopkins Hosp 20:63, 1909.

22. Osler W: On multiple hereditary telangiectasia with recurrent hemorrhages. Q J Med (Oct):53, 1907.

23. Osler W: On telangiectasia circumscripta universalis. Bull Johns Hopkins Hosp 12:33, 1901.

24. Osler W: On a family form of recurrent epistaxis associated with telangiectasia of the skin and mucous membranes. Bull Johns Hopkins Hosp 12:33, 1901.

25. Hodgsum CH, RL Kaye: Pulmonary arteriovenous fistula and hereditary hemorrhagic telangiectasia. Dis Chest 43:449, 1963.

26. Fitz-Hugh T: Splenomegaly and hepatic enlargement in hereditary hemorrhagic telangiectasia. Am J Med Sci 181:261, 1931.

27. Bick RL, LF Fekete: Hereditary hemorrhagic telangiectasia and associated defects in hemostasis. Blood 52:179, 1978.

28. Quick AJ: Telangiectasia. In: AJ Quick (Ed): Hemorrhagic Diseases and Thrombosis. Lea and Febiger, Philadelphia, 1966, p 285.

29. McDervitt TJ, AS Toh: Epistaxis: management and prevention. Laryngoscope 47:1109, 1967.

30. Ryan AJ: Control of bleeding in familial telangiectasia. Meriden Hosp Bull 7:1, 1958.

31. Bick RL: Hereditary hemorrhagic telangiectasia and disseminated intravascular coagulation: a new clinical syndrome. Ann N Y Acad Sci 370:851, 1981.

32. Steel D, EG Bovill, E Golden: Hereditary hemorrhagic telangiectasia: a family study. Am J Clin Pathol 90:274, 1988.

33. Stitch MH: Carbazochrome salicylate therapy in hereditary hemorrhagic telangiectasia. N Y State J Med 59:2725, 1959.

34. Koch HJ, GL Escher, JS Lewis: Hormonal management of hereditary hemorrhagic telangiectasia. JAMA 149:1376, 1952.

35. Quick AJ: Hemostasis then and now, ch. 1. In: AJ Quick (Ed): The Hemorrhagic Diseases and the Pathology of Hemostasis. Charles C Thomas Publishers, Springfield, IL, 1974, p 3.

36. Lachner H: Hemostatic abnormalities associated with paraprotein abnormalities. Semin Hematol 10:125, 1973.

37. Bick RL: Acquired circulating anticoagulants and defective hemostasis in malignant paraprotein disorders, ch 10. In: G Murano, RL Bick (Eds): Basic Concepts of Hemostasis and Thrombosis. CRC Press, Boca Raton, FL, 1980, p 205.

38. Snapper I: Neurological complications. In: I Snapper, A Kahn (Eds): Myelomatosis. University Park Press, Baltimore, 1971, p 226.

39. Bick RL, CA Klein, LF Fekete, WL Wilson: Alterations of hemostasis associated with malignant paraprotein disorders. Transactions of the American Society of Hematology, 1976, p 63.

40. Gallo G, M Picken, J Buxbaum: The spectrum of monoclonal immunoglobulin deposition disease associated with immunocytic disorders. Semin Hematol 26:234, 1989.

41. Snapper I: Amyloidosis. In: I Snapper, A Kahn (Eds): Myelomatosis. University Park Press, Baltimore, 1971, p 238.

42. Triplett DA, NU Bang, CS Harms, MD Benson, JP Miletich: Mechanisms of acquired factor X deficiency in primary amyloidosis. Blood 50:285, 1977.

43. Galbraith PA, N Sharma, WL Parker, JM Kilgour: Acquired factor X deficiency. Altered plasma antithrombin activity and association with amyloidosis. JAMA 230:1658, 1974.

44. Glenner GG: Factor X deficiency and systemic amyloidosis. N Engl J Med 297:108, 1977.

45. Howell M: Acquired Factor X deficiency associated with systematized amyloidosis: report of a case. Blood 21:739, 1963.

46. Krause JR: Acquired Factor X deficiency and amyloidosis. Am J Clin Pathol 67:170, 1977.

47. McPherson RA, JW Onstad, RT Vgoretz, PL Wolf: Coagulopathy in amyloidosis: combined deficiency of Factor IX and X. Am J Hematol 3:225, 1977.

48. Furie B, E Green, BC Furie: Syndrome of acquired Factor X deficiency and systemic amyloidosis. N Engl J Med 297:81, 1977.

49. Stefanini M, IB Mednicoff: Demonstration of antivessel antibodies in serum of patients with anaphylactoid purpura and polyarteritis nodosa. J Clin Invest 33:967, 1954.

50. Dixon FJ, JJ Vazques, WD Weigle, CG Cochrane: Pathogenesis of serum sickness. Arch Pathol 65:18, 1958.

51. Pierson KK: Leukocytoclastic vasculitis viewed as a phase of immune-mediated vasculopathy. Semin Thromb Hemost 10:196, 1984.

52. Markowitz AS, CF Lang: Streptococcal related glomerulonephritis. J Immunol 92:565, 1964.

53. Cochrane CG: Mediators of the arthus and related syndromes. Prog Allergy 11:1, 1967.

54. Freedman P, NP Meister, HJ Lee, EA Smith, BS Co, BD Midas: The renal response to streptococcal infections. Medicine 49:433, 1970.

55. Parish WE: Studies on vasculitis, I: immunoglobulins, beta-1-C, C-reactive protein, and bacterial antigens in cutaneous vasculitis lesions. Clin Allergy 1:97, 1971.

56. Parish WE: Studies on vasculitis, II: some properties of complexes formed of antibacterial antibodies from persons with or without cutaneous vasculitis lesions. Clin Allergy 1:111, 1971.

57. Tanaseanu S, S Purice: The systemic vasculitides. Med Interne 27:167, 1989.

58. Bigby M, RS Stern, KA Arndt: Allergic cutaneous reactions to drugs. Primary Care Clin Office Prac 16:713, 1989.

59. Ashton N: The eye in malignant hypertension. Trans Am Acad Ophthalmol Otolaryngol 76:17, 1972.

60. Farber EM, EA Hines, H Montgomery, W Craig: Arterioles of skin in essential hypertension. J Invest Dermatol 9:215, 1947.

61. Kazmier FJ, P Didisheim, VF Fairbanks, J Ludwig, WS Payne, EJW Bowie: Intravascular coagulation and arterial disease. Thromb Diath Haemorrh (suppl) 36:295, 1969.

62. Ryan TJ: The investigation of vasculitis. In: TJ Ryan (Ed): Microvascular Injury. WB Saunders, Philadelphia, 1976, p 333.

63. Morris RN, P Vassalli, FK Beller, RT McCluskey: Immunofluorescent studies of renal biopsies in the diagnosis of toxemia of pregnancy. Obstet Gynecol 24:32, 1964.

64. Robboy SJ, MC Mihm, RW Coleman, JD Minna: The skin in disseminated intravascular coagulation: prospective analysis of 36 cases. Br J Dermatol 88:221, 1973.

65. Bick RL, SM Scates: Disseminated intravascular coagulation: a review. Lab Med, 1991, In press.

66. Forsham PH: The adrenal cortex. In: RL Williams (Ed): Textbook of Endocrinology. WB Saunders, Philadelphia, 1968, p 287.

67. Behcet H: Uber die rezidivierende apthose durch ein virus verursachte geschwure am mund, am auge und an den genitalien. Dermatol Wochenschr 105:1152, 1937.

68. Haim S, JD Sobel, R Freidman-Birnbaum: Thrombophlebitis and a cardinal symptom of Behçets syndrome. Acta Dermatol Venereol 54:299, 1974.

69. Nazzarro P: Cutaneous manifestations of Behçets disease: clinical and histological findings. Proceedings of the International Symposium of Behçets Disease, Karger, Basel, 1966, p 15.

70. Hills EA: Behçets syndrome with aortic aneurysms. Br Med J 4:152, 1967.

71. Sakuri M, T Miyaji: Behçets disease from the point of view of vascular pathology. Folia Ophthalmol Jpn 22:903, 1971.

72. Chajek T, M Fainard: Behçets disease with decreased fibrinolysis and superior vena caval occlusion. Br Med J 1:782, 1973.

73. Behrendt PM, SE Epstein, AG Marrow: Postperfusion nonthrombocytopenic purpura: an uncommon sequel of open heart surgery. Am J Cardiol 22:631, 1968.

74. Bick RL: Disseminated intravascular coagulation, ch. 2 In: G Murano, RL Bick (Eds): Basic Concepts of Hemostasis and Thrombosis. CRC Press, Boca Raton, FL, 1980, p 31.

75. Calabrese LH, BA Michel, DA Bloch: The American College of Rheumatology 1990 criteria for the classification of hypersensitivity vasculitis. Arthritis Rheum 33:1108, 1990.

76. Criep LH, CG Cohen: Purpura as a manifestation of penicillin sensitivity. Ann Intern Med 34:1219, 1951.

77. Nalbandian RM, IJ Mader, JL Barrett, JF Pierce, EC Rupp: Petechiae, ecchymoses, and necrosis of skin induced by coumarin cogeners. JAMA 192:603, 1965.

78. Nalbandian RM, FK Beller, AK Hamp, RL Henry, PL Wolf: Coumarin necrosis of the skin treated successfully with heparin. Obstet Gynecol 38:395, 1971.

79. Nudelman HL, RL Kempson: Necrosis of the breast: a rare complication of anticoagulant therapy. Am J Surg 111:728, 1966.

80. Comp PC, JP Elrod, S Karzenski: Warfarin-induced skin necrosis. Semin Thromb Hemost 16:293, 1990.

81. Cole MS, PK Minifee, FJ Wolma: Coumarin necrosis: a review of the literature. Surgery 103:271, 1988.

82. Becker CG: Oral anticoagulant therapy and skin necrosis. In: S Wessler, CG Becker, Y Nemerson (Eds): The New Dimensions of Warfarin Prophylaxis. Plenum Press, New York, 1987, p 217.

83. Francis RB: Acquired purpura fulminans. Semin Thromb Hemost 16:310, 1990.

84. Adcock DM, J Bronza, RA Marler: Proposed classification and pathologic mechanisms of purpura fulminans and skin necrosis. Semin Thromb Hemost 16:333, 1990.

85. Rodgers RP, J Levin: A critical reappraisal of the bleeding time. Semin Thromb Hemost 16:1, 1990.

86. Burns ER, C Lawrence: Bleeding time: a guide to its diagnostic and clinical utility. Arch Pathol Lab Med 113:1219, 1989.

87. Bick RL, T Adams, WR Schmalhorst: Bleeding times, platelet adhesion, and aspirin. Am J Clin Pathol 65:65, 1976.

88. Fairbairn JF: Clinical manifestations of peripheral vascular disease. In: JF Fairbairn, JL Juergens, SA Spittell (Eds): Peripheral Vascular Diseases. WB Saunders, Philadelphia, 1980, p 3.

89. Ryan TJ: The investigation of vasculitis. In: TJ Ryan (Ed): Microvascular Injury. WB Saunders, Philadelphia, 1976, p 333.

90. Bick RL: Clinical hemostasis practice: the major impact of laboratory automation. Semin Thromb Hemost 9:139, 1983.

91. Mielke CH, MM Kaneshiro, LA Maher, SI Rappaport: The standardized normal ivy bleeding time and its prolongation by aspirin. Blood 34:204, 1969.

92. Quick AJ: Salicylates and bleeding: the aspirin tolerance test. Am J Med Sci 252:265, 1966.

93. Sienco. The Petechiometer: package insert. Sienco, Inc., Morrison, CO, 1990.

94. Bick RL: Pathophysiology of Hemostasis and Thrombosis. In: WA Sodeman (Ed): Pathologic Physiology. WB Saunders, Philadelphia, 1985.

95. Bachmann F, I Egbert, KO Kruithof: Tissue plasminogen activator: chemical and physiological aspects. Semin Thromb Hemost 10:6, 1984.

96. Ranby M, B Norrman, P Wallen: A sensitive assay for tissue plasminogen activator. Thromb Res 27:743, 1982.

97. Wiman B, G Mellbring, M Ranby: Plasminogen activator release during venous stasis and exercise as determined by a new specific assay. Clin Chim Acta 127:279, 1983.

98. Messmore HL, JM Walenga, J Fareed: Molecular markers of platelet activation. Semin Thromb Hemost 10:264, 1984.

CHAPTER
4

Qualitative (Functional) Platelet Disorders

The common clinical findings of qualitative or quantitative platelet defects are petechiae and purpura, mild to moderate mucosal membrane bleeding, including bilateral epistaxis and gastrointestinal, pulmonary, and genitourinary tract bleeding, and a history of easy and spontaneous bruising.[1] Gingival bleeding with toothbrushing is a common clinical manifestation of platelet dysfunction or thrombocytopenia.[2] As discussed in chapters 2 and 3, gingival bleeding with toothbrushing can be a normal finding if it occurs occasionally; however, if a patient relates this occurring numerous times per week, then a platelet function defect, thrombocytopenia, or vascular defect is likely. Platelet function defects or thrombocytopenia are characteristically associated with petechiae and purpura, which are usually symmetric (ie, found throughout the integumentary system) and are usually found on the extremities as well as the torso. These findings are different than the noting of dependent petechiae and purpura, which are more characteristically associated with vascular disorders.[3,4] Clinical findings of platelet defects are summarized in Table 4-1. Typical petechiae and purpura are depicted in Figure 4-1.

Platelet defects are most easily divided into quantitative and qualitative types. The qualitative disorders, the platelet function defects, are further divided into hereditary and acquired types. Quantitative defects are best divided into the following: (1) thrombocytopenia due to decreased production and metabolic/maturation defects, including the hereditary, congenital, and infantile thrombocytopenias associated with decreased platelet production, the acquired platelet production defects, and drug-induced nonimmune thrombocytopenias; (2) acquired thrombocytopenia due to increased destruction, increased consumption, or peripheral loss; and (3) thrombocytosis and thrombocythemia. Hyperactive platelets associated with, leading to, or formed as a consequence of hypercoagulability and thrombosis constitute an additional category of abnormal platelet function.

Table 4-2 summarizes platelet defects, which are divided into qualitative (functional) vs quantitative types (ie, thrombocytopenia, thrombocytosis, and thrombocythemia).

An expensive and laborious platelet function work-up should not be instituted until normal platelet counts have been documented. Attempting to study platelet function in association with thrombocytopenia is usually fruitless.[5] Platelet function defects are best divided between those that are hereditary and those that are acquired. As with vascular defects, the hereditary forms of platelet function defects are clinical oddities and extremely rare.[5] However, the acquired forms are common, are associated with many common acquired diseases, and often lead to clinically significant bleeding problems frequently encountered in clinical practice.[5]

Table 4-3 depicts traditional tests of platelet number and function, especially the older tests. First, and extremely important in assessing platelets, a careful evaluation of the peripheral blood smear should be performed for a quantitative estimation of the number of platelets and an evaluation of platelet morphology. This is an often neglected simple modality performed in the hematology laboratory, and certainly the peripheral blood smear should be carefully evaluated in patients presenting with easy or spontaneous bruising and/or petechiae and purpura. Many clinical clues may be obtained from an evaluation of platelet morphology, such as noting abnormal granularity in the gray platelet syndrome, the large platelets and borderline thrombocytopenia of Bernard-Soulier syndrome, or the many "large bizarre" platelets or young platelets indicative of rapid platelet turnover and decreased platelet survival. An examination of the peripheral blood smear may actually lead to the specific diagnosis accounting for petechiae and purpura or easy bruising (eg, an acute or chronic leukemia). In addition, a quantitative platelet count should always be performed. Only with a normal platelet count can a platelet function defect be defined.[5] In the past, platelet adhesion in glass bead columns by a wide variety of techniques had been advocated to assess platelet function. Experience with this technique, however, has been far less than satisfactory and the procedure should not be used.[6,7] Although of clinical curiosity and historical interest, in vitro platelet adhesion testing by glass bead techniques is unreliable and has no clinical relevance.[6,7]

Table 4-1. Clinical Findings of Platelet Defects

Petechiae and purpura (usually symmetric)
Mild to moderate mucosal membrane bleeding
    Gastrointestinal
    Genitourinary
    Pulmonary
    Epistaxis
History of easy and spontaneous bruising
Frequent gingival bleeding with toothbrushing

Figure 4-2 depicts the standardized template bleeding time device, which is the primary screening test for platelet and vascular function.[8,9] Once a normal platelet count is documented with a suggestive or contributory history (petechiae, purpura, and easy and spontaneous bruising), the differential diagnosis is between a vascular defect and a platelet function defect, both of which will frequently, but not always, cause prolongation of the standardized TBT.[3,10-12]

Figure 4-3 depicts the standard petechiometer, which is used in children.[13] The template bleeding time has not been standardized in children and tends to leave scars. Thus, template bleeding times are used to screen for a platelet function or vascular defect in adults, and the petechiometer test is used in children. These two tests are only done in association with a normal platelet count and positive or suggestive history.[11,13] Although the TBT is useful as a simple screening test for platelet function, it is somewhat unreliable, and, thus, the noting of a normal template bleeding time certainly does not rule out the presence of a clinically significant platelet function defect. If the template bleeding time is normal and a suggestive history is obtained or platelet dysfunction is suspected on clinical grounds, platelet aggregation or lumi-aggregation should immediately be performed.

Hereditary Platelet Dysfunction

The hereditary platelet function defects are divided into the following: (1) platelet adhesion, typified by the Bernard-

Figure 4-1. Typical Petechiae and Purpura

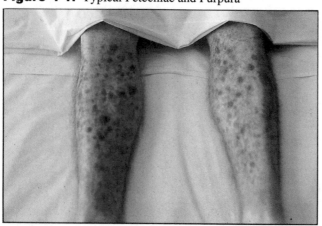

Table 4-2. Types of Platelet Disorders

Qualitative
  Hereditary
    Adhesion defects
      Bernard-Soulier syndrome
      Impared adhesion to collagen
    Aggregation defects
      Primary
        Glanzmann's thrombasthenia
        Essential athrombia
      Secondary
        Storage pool diseases
        Isolated defect (most common type)
          Tar baby syndrome
          Hermansky-Pudlak syndrome
          Chédiak-Higashi syndrome
          Wiskott-Aldrich syndrome
        Aspirinlike defect
          Cyclo-oxygenase deficiency
          Thromboxane synthetase deficiency
        Release reaction defects
          Hereditary collagen disorders
          Glycogen storage disease
          May-Hegglin anomaly
          Hurler's syndrome
          Hunter's syndrome
    Factor deficiencies
      Isolated platelet factor 3 deficiency
      Severe coagulation factor deficiencies
        Afibrinogenemia
        Factor VIII:C deficiency
        Factor IX:C deficiency
  Miscellaneous
  Acquired
    Associated with other diseases
    Presence of fibrin(ogen) degradation products
    Disseminated intravascular coagulation
    Primary fibrinolytic system activation
    Liver disease
      Acute
      Chronic
    Diabetes
    Uremia
    Waldenström's macroglobulinemia
    Multiple myeloma
    Amyloidosis
    Myeloproliferative and myelodysplastic syndromes
    Drug induced
Quantitative
  Hereditary
    Megakaryocytic
    Amegakaryocytic
  Acquired
    Megakaryocytic
    Amegakaryocytic
    Drug induced
  Thrombocytosis and thrombocythemia
    Benign
    Malignant
  Hyperactive and prethrombotic

Figure 4-2. Standard Template Bleeding Time Device

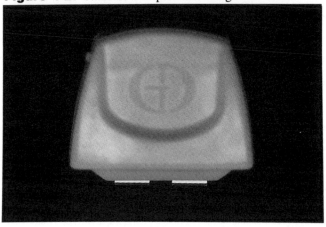

Table 4-3. Laboratory Assessment of Platelet Defects

Peripheral smear evaluation
Quantitative platelet count ✓
Template bleeding time ✓
Aspirin tolerance test ✓
Petechiometer test (children and elderly)
Platelet aggregation and lumi-aggregation
Platelet factor 3 availability
Platelet factor 4 release
Serotonin release
Platelet-associated antibodies

Soulier syndrome; (2) defects of primary aggregation, characterized by Glanzmann's thrombasthenia; and (3) defects of secondary aggregation, characterized by storage pool diseases as well as other more rare defects.[14] In addition, patients have been described with an isolated deficiency of

Figure 4-3. Standard Petechiometer

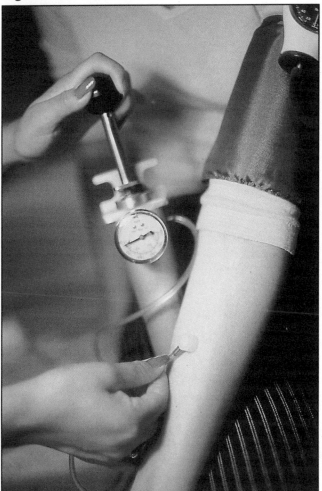

platelet factor 3, and patients with severe plasma coagulation protein deficiencies may have an associated platelet function defect. This is especially noted in severe afibrinogenemia, severe hemophilia A, and severe hemophilia B.[5] The accompanying platelet function defect seen in these patients exemplifies the importance of blood coagulation proteins for normal platelet function. The division of hereditary platelet function defects into those of adhesion, primary aggregation, or secondary aggregation is somewhat artificial, but it provides a convenient way to categorize the defects and to recall the laboratory manifestations.

Bernard-Soulier Syndrome

The Bernard-Soulier syndrome is inherited as an autosomal dominant trait and typifies a disorder of platelet adhesion. Heterozygotes are often asymptomatic. Superficially, the Bernard-Soulier syndrome can be mistaken for von Willebrand's disease. The clinical features are easy bruising, epistaxis, hypermenorrhagia, and petechiae and purpura[15-17]; these findings may also suggest von Willebrand's disease. During laboratory assessment, patients with Bernard-Soulier syndrome demonstrate abnormal adhesion as well as abnormal ristocetin-induced aggregation, and if only adhesion and ristocetin aggregation are performed one could mistake the patient as having von Willebrand's syndrome rather than the Bernard-Soulier syndrome. The distinction is made by more thoroughly evaluating the peripheral smear, which will usually demonstrate giant platelets and borderline thrombocytopenia in most, but not all, patients with Bernard-Soulier syndrome.[17,18] In addition, if von Willebrand's disease was suspected, factor VIII coagulation activity (factor VIII:C), factor VIII–related antigen (factor VIII:RAg), and ristocetin cofactor activity (factor VIII:RCo/factor VIII:vW) would also be performed and lead to the correct diagnosis.[19] Bernard-Soulier platelets are missing platelet membrane glycoproteins (PMGPs) Ib, V, and IX. Thus, it is important to recall the clinical and laboratory features of Bernard-Soulier syndrome, its superficial resemblance to von Willebrand's syndrome, and its manifestation as a hereditary adhesion defect of platelets. Table 4-4 summarizes the characteristics of the Bernard-Soulier syndrome.

Table 4-4. The Bernard-Soulier Syndrome

Clinical Manifestations
    Autosomal recessive
    Easy bruising
    Spontaneous bruising
    Epistaxis
    Hypermenorrhagia
    Petechiae and purpura (moderate)

Laboratory Manifestations
    Giant platelets
    Mild or moderate thrombocytopenia
    Abnormal template bleeding time
    Abnormal petechiometer test
    Abnormal ristocetin aggregation

Other aggregation normal
    Absence of PMGP Ib, V, and IX

Therapy
    Platelet concentrates for significant or life-threatening
      hemorrhage

Glanzmann's Thrombasthenia and Essential Athrombia

The primary aggregation disorders are Glanzmann's thrombasthenia, which is extremely rare, and essential athrombia, which is even more rare.[20-22] The clinical features are those usually expected with platelet dysfunction: easy and spontaneous bruising, subcutaneous hematomas, and petechiae.[20,23] Rarely, patients suffer intra-articular bleeding

Table 4-5. Glanzmann's Thrombasthenia and Essential Athrombia

Clinical Findings
    Autosomal recessive
    Petechiae and purpura
    Easy bruising
    Spontaneous bruising
    Mucosal membrane bleeding
    Large hematomas
    Intra-articular bleeding (rare)
    Decreasing severity with age

Laboratory Findings
    Prolonged template bleeding time
    Abnormal/absent primary aggregation with:
      ADP
      Epinephrine
      Thrombin
      Collagen
    Clot retraction
    Glanzmann's thrombasthenia: abnormal
    Essential athrombia: normal
    Absence of PMGP IIb/IIIa complex
    Therapy
    Platelet concentrates

Table 4-6. Hereditary Storage Pool Disease

Clinical Findings
    Variable inheritance
    Petechiae (uncommon)
    Purpura (uncommon)
    Mucosal membrane bleeding
    Epistaxis
    Easy bruising
    Spontaneous bruising
    Hematuria (common)

Laboratory Findings
    Abnormal template bleeding time
    Abnormal adhesion to collagen
    Absent aggregation to collagen
    Absent second aggregation curve to:
      Adenosine diphosphate
      Epinephrine
    Normal ristocetin aggregation
    Normal arachidonate aggregation (usually)

Therapy
    Platelet concentrates

with resultant hemarthroses. The bleeding tends to decrease in severity with age, as is the case with many of the hereditary hemostasis defects. The clinical and laboratory diagnostic features are depicted in Table 4-5 and consist of a prolonged standardized TBT, totally absent primary aggregation induced by ADP, thrombin, collagen, or epinephrine, abnormal platelet factor 3 availability, and abnormal clot retraction.[24,25] Glanzmann's platelets are missing the PMGP IIb/IIIa complex. All of these abnormalities are also noted for the even rarer related disorder, essential athrombia. In essential athrombia, however, clot retraction is normal.[22]

Therapy for these disorders is the infusion of platelet concentrates as needed for serious or life-threatening bleeding.[5] My general approach is to infuse platelet concentrates until bleeding stops rather than to rely on empiric monitoring of aggregation patterns or the template bleeding time. Bleeding in the vast majority of patients with a hereditary platelet function defect of any type will stop abruptly with the appropriate use of platelet concentrates.[26]

Hereditary Storage Pool Defects

Secondary aggregation disorders are more common than primary aggregation disorders and the most common types seen in this category are storage pool diseases.[27,28] In rare instances, storage pool defects are seen in patients with other rare clinical oddities, including the Wiskott-Aldrich syndrome,[29] the thrombocytopenia and absent radii syndrome (TAR baby syndrome),[30] the Hermansky-Pudlak syndrome,[31] and the Chédiak-Higashi syndrome.[32] Most patients with these rare clinical syndromes have an associated storage pool defect.[5] However, the majority of patients who present with a hereditary storage pool defect have no such asso-

Figure 4-4. Hereditary Storage Pool Defect: Platelet Aggregation Patterns

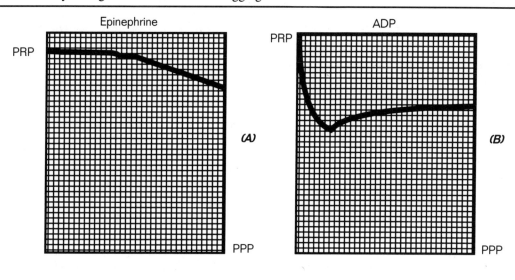

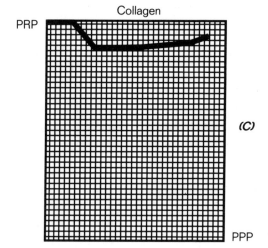

PRP = Platelet-Rich Plasma
PPP = Platelet-Poor Plasma

ciated disease and are otherwise perfectly normal.[33] The clinical features of secondary aggregation disorders are those expected with a platelet function defect and consist of mucocutaneous hemorrhages, hematuria, and epistaxis.[34] For unexplained reasons petechiae are less common than in other qualitative platelet disorders. Easy and spontaneous bruising are common complaints. During laboratory evaluation, patients with storage pool defects have absent epinephrine- and ADP-induced secondary aggregation waves, although the primary waves are present. Collagen-induced aggregation is absent or markedly blunted, and normal ristocetin-induced aggregation is typically noted.[35,36] A prolonged standardized template bleeding time is uniformly seen. The mainstay of therapy is the use of platelet concentrates if the patient bleeds. The clinical and laboratory features of hereditary storage pool disease are summarized in Table 4-6.

Figure 4-4 summarizes platelet aggregation findings in hereditary storage pool disease. This figure depicts a small primary wave induced by epinephrine (4A), primary aggregation induced by ADP, followed by disaggregation (4B), and a markedly blunted collagen-induced aggregation curve (4C). These findings are classic for hereditary storage pool defects. These patterns came from the mother of a patient who had initially presented to an emergency room with uncontrollable bilateral epistaxis. As soon as aggregation was performed, a diagnosis of storage pool disease was made. The patient was infused with platelets, and her profuse epistaxis ceased immediately. Following this, the mother and two siblings were examined and found to have the same defect.

Aspirinlike Defects

Another, more rare, secondary aggregation defect is that of the aspirinlike defect, which is inherited as an auto-

Table 4-7. Hereditary Aspirinlike Defect

Clinical Findings
    Easy bruising
    Spontaneous bruising
    Mucosal membrane bleeding
    Epistaxis

Laboratory Findings
    Abnormal template bleeding time
    Abnormal adhesion to collagen
    Absent secondary aggregation curves to:
        Adenosine diphosphate
        Epinephrine
    Absent aggregation to collagen
    Absent aggregation to arachidonate
    Absence of cyclo-oxygenase or thromboxane synthetase

Therapy
    Platelet concentrates
    Possibly steroids

somal dominant trait.[37] This disorder is extremely rare, with few patients described.[38-41] The clinical features are similar to other platelet function defects and consist of easy and spontaneous bruising, occasional spontaneous bleeding from mucosal membranes, epistaxis, hypermenorrhagia, and petechiae and purpura. From the laboratory standpoint these patients demonstrate a prolonged template bleeding time, an absent secondary wave to epinephrine, and absent collagen-induced aggregation. Therefore, they present with platelet aggregation patterns similar to the patterns seen in a patient who has ingested aspirin or another cyclo-oxygenase inhibitor.[42] This defect may be due to either a hereditary deficiency of the enzyme cyclo-oxygenase or a hereditary deficiency of the enzyme thromboxane synthetase.[43-45] Therapy, when clinically significant bleeding occurs, is the infusion of platelet concentrates. Some patients have improved with the use of steroids.[46] The features of this heterogeneous syndrome are summarized in Table 4-7. Platelet aggregation findings in the aspirinlike defect are seen in Figure 4-5.

More recently, a congenital platelet function defect has been described in a bleeding individual who had an inherited impairment of platelet membrane phosphatidylinositol metabolism. In this patient, the defect was characterized by clinical hemorrhage, delayed platelet aggregation to collagen, an absent epinephrine-induced second wave of platelet aggregation, and normal arachidonic acid–induced platelet aggregation.[47] The mode of inheritance and other clinical and laboratory features were not described.

Hereditary storage pool diseases are the most common of the otherwise rare hereditary platelet function defects and are usually not associated with one of the other rare clinical syndromes, such as Chédiak-Higashi or Wiskott-Aldrich syndromes. The other hereditary platelet function defects mentioned are extremely rare and are best classified as true clinical oddities.

Acquired Platelet Dysfunction

Many of the common acquired platelet defects are of significant clinical concern. Acquired platelet function defects are important because they are common causes of bleeding. Thus, many patients who have these underlying disorders are surgical candidates and may bleed profusely with surgery or trauma if an accompanying platelet function defect is present. Alternatively, if a patient develops unexplained hemorrhage attributable to a platelet function defect, the subsequent evaluation should include a search for these disorders often associated with acquired platelet dysfunction.

Uremia

Platelet function defects are almost universally found in patients who are uremic.[48-50] In uremic patients it is thought that circulating quanidinosuccinic[51,52] and/or hydroxyphenolic acids[53] interfere with platelet function by eradicating platelet factor 3 activity. Both of these compounds are dialyzable, and dialysis will often correct or improve platelet function. Other mechanisms of altered platelet function in uremia, including altered prostaglandin metabolism or intraplatelet nucleotides, have also been proposed.[54-60] Studies have demonstrated an abnormality in the interaction between von Willebrand factor and the platelet membrane glycoprotein IIb/IIIa complex in uremic patients; however, platelet membrane glycoproteins Ib, IIb, and IIIa are quantitatively normal in uremia.[61,62] These findings suggest a functional defect in the von Willebrand factor IIb/IIIa adhesive interaction. Figure 4-6 demonstrates lumi-aggregation patterns in a uremic patient. Like the other acquired platelet function defects, however, the aggregation pattern abnormalities are not uniform or characteristic, and essentially any combination of defects may be seen. Platelet concentrates are indicated for most instances of life-threatening bleeding in uremia; however, other modes of therapy that have been noted to correct the prolonged bleeding time in a variety of disorders will not only correct the bleeding time but also often control significant hemorrhage in uremic patients. These modalities are cryoprecipitate, DDAVP (intravenous, intramuscular, or intranasal), and estrogen compounds.[63-69] Dialysis also tends to correct the platelet function defect,[70-73] and the degree of correction toward normal appears to correlate with frequency of this procedure.[74] Platelet abnormalities noted in diabetes and other renal disorders, including hemodialysis and renal transplantation rejection, will be discussed in chapters 7 and 9.

Paraprotein Disorders

Many patients with malignant paraprotein disorders, including multiple myeloma, Waldenström's macroglobulinemia, or other monoclonal gammopathies, will demonstrate a platelet function defect.[75-79] This defect is due to the coating of platelet membrane by paraprotein, does not depend on the type of paraprotein, and occurs with IgA, IgM, or IgG monoclonal proteins. In addition, platelet

Figure 4-5. Aspirinlike Defect

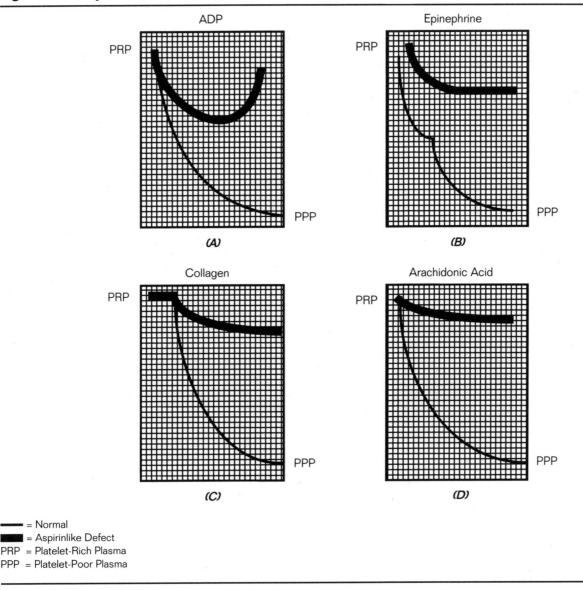

——— = Normal
■■■■ = Aspirinlike Defect
PRP = Platelet-Rich Plasma
PPP = Platelet-Poor Plasma

dysfunction by identical mechanisms can occur with benign monoclonal proteins. Almost all patients with malignant paraprotein disorders will demonstrate significant platelet dysfunction manifest by clinically significant bleeding as well as by abnormal results of platelet function with aggregation on lumi-aggregation testing. The template bleeding time is notoriously unreliable as a predictor of bleeding secondary to platelet dysfunction in paraprotein disorders. Lumi-aggregation patterns before and after plasmapheresis in a patient with IgA myeloma are depicted in Figure 4-7.

Myeloproliferative and Myelodysplastic Syndromes

Acquired platelet function defects are commonly seen in all of the myeloproliferative syndromes, especially essential thrombocythemia, agnogenic myeloid metaplasia, paroxysmal nocturnal hemoglobinuria, polycythemia rubra vera, chronic myelogenous leukemia, patients with refractory anemia and excessive blasts (RAEB syndrome), and other of the myelodysplastic syndromes and the sideroblastic or sideroachrestic anemias.[80-83] The platelet aggregation patterns noted in association with these syndromes are usually not characteristic, and essentially any combination of platelet aggregation defects may be seen.[5] The most common defects are abnormal aggregation and release to epinephrine, followed by abnormalities in collagen and ADP aggregation and release.[84-86] The template bleeding time is often abnormal but may not be a reliable guide to bleeding propensity in patients with myeloproliferative or myelodysplastic syndromes and associated platelet dysfunction.[84,85]

Figure 4-6. Platelet Function in Uremia (Lumi-Aggregation)

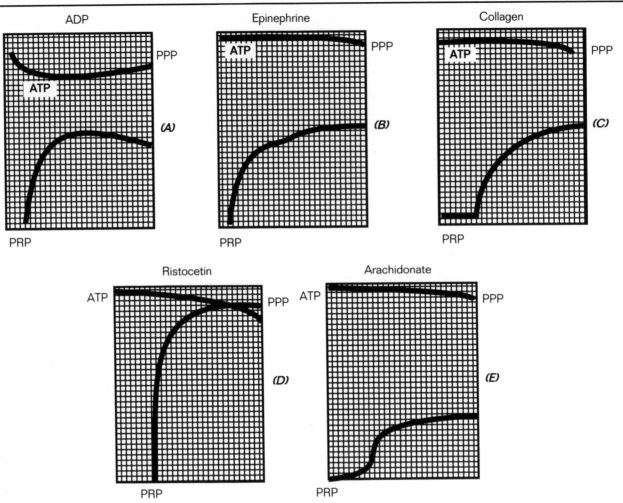

PRP = Platelet-Rich Plasma
PPP = Platelet-Poor Plasma
ATP = ATP Release

Cardiac Surgery

Patients undergoing cardiopulmonary bypass demonstrate the most severe platelet function defects.[87-91] Typical midbypass and postbypass lumi-aggregation patterns are seen in Figures 4-8 and 4-9. These defects will be discussed in detail in chapter 9.

Liver Disease

Platelet dysfunction in liver disease is multifaceted, very complex, and will be discussed in chapter 8.

Miscellaneous Disorders

Acquired platelet function defects are also seen in autoimmune disorders, including systemic lupus erythematosus, rheumatoid arthritis, scleroderma, and others.[92,93] Patients with immune-mediated thrombocytopenia commonly have associated severe platelet dysfunction due to coating of the platelet membrane by immunoglobulin. Thus, assessment of bleeding in patients with immune-mediated thrombocytopenias, such as immune/idiopathic thrombocytopenia purpura (ITP), must be made by evaluation of not only the absolute platelet count but also associated platelet function.[94] Figure 4-10 demonstrates platelet dysfunction in a patient with ITP.

The presence of fibrin(ogen) degradation products often induces a clinically significant platelet function defect.[95-97] The FDPs can be of any origin, including disseminated intravascular coagulation or primary hyperfibrino(geno)lytic syndromes.[98-101] The later degradation products, especially fragments D and E, appear to have a high affinity for the platelet membrane, attach to the membrane, and render a severe and clinically significant acquired platelet function defect. Patients with severe iron deficiency or severe folate or vitamin B_{12} deficiency may also demonstrate a platelet function defect, which may or may not lead to clinically sig-

Figure 4-7. Platelet Dysfunction in Multiple Myeloma (Lumi-Aggregation)

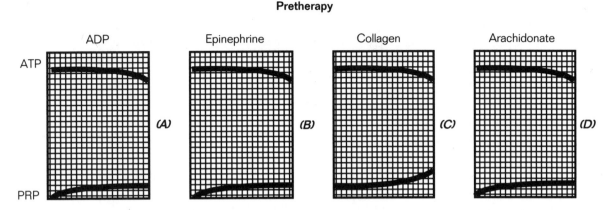

Pretherapy

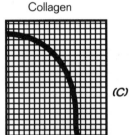

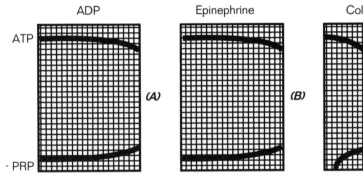

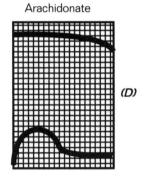

Posttherapy
(Plasmapheresis)

PRP = Platelet-Rich Plasma
ATP = ATP Release

nificant hemorrhage.[102,103] Drug-induced platelet function defects are commonly noted and are a common cause of easy and spontaneous bruising, petechiae and purpura, and bleeding associated with surgery or trauma.[104] Unlike the rare hereditary platelet function defects, the acquired platelet function defects do not demonstrate typical platelet aggregation abnormalities when patterns are studied. For example, one can study many patients with chronic myelogenous leukemia, and all patients will likely have abnormal aggregation patterns. However, many different varieties of abnormalities will usually be noted.

Drug Induced

The common clinical drugs that may cause a clinically significant platelet function defect and hemorrhage are numerous. The number of drugs interfering with platelet function as defined by laboratory tests (aggregation or lumi-aggregation) is much more extensive. Therefore, this review will be restricted to commonly used drugs reported to cause clinically significant hemorrhage in patients. The three most common mechanisms by which drugs interfere with platelet function, in descending order of prevalence, are the follow-

ing: drug interference with the platelet membrane or membrane receptor sites, drug interference with prostaglandin biosynthetic pathways, and drug interference with phosphodiesterase activity.[105,106]

Drugs Interfering With Platelet Membrane Receptors

The most common drugs interfering with platelet membrane function or receptors are Elavil,[107] Tofranil,[108] Sinequan,[109] thorazine,[110] cocaine,[111] xylocaine,[112] Isuprel,[113] propanolol,[114] Keflin,[115] ampicillin,[116] carbenicillin,[117] penicillin,[118] Benadryl,[119] Phenergan,[120] and alcohol.[121] Other drugs inducing platelet dysfunction by this mechanism are Regitine,[122] Dibenzyline,[122] Reserpine,[123] dihydroergotamine,[124] morpramine,[108] Aventyl,[108] stelazine,[125] procaine,[126] Nupercaine,[126] Furadantin,[127] Nafcillin,[128] moxalactam,[129] ticarcillin,[130] dextran,[131] and hydroxyethyl starch.[132]

Drugs Inhibiting the Prostaglandin Pathways

The most common drugs interfering with platelet prostaglandin synthetic pathways are aspirin,[133] indomethacin,[134] phenylbutazone,[135] Motrin,[136] Naprosyn,[92] sulfinpyrazone,[137] furosemide,[138] and varapamil.[139] Less commonly used

Figure 4-8. Cardiopulmonary Bypass Surgery Lumi-Aggregation Patterns

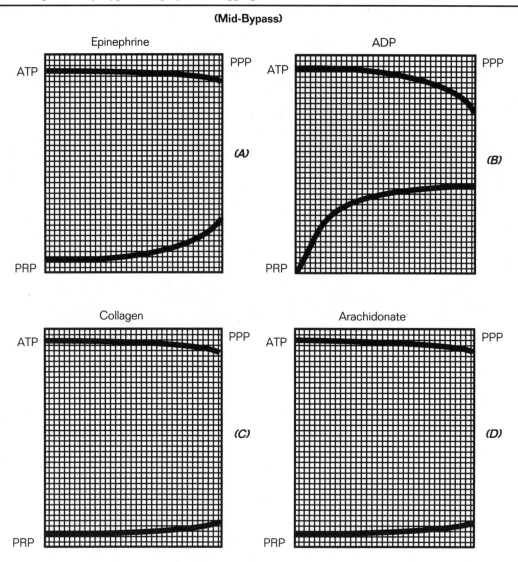

(Mid-Bypass)

PRP = Platelet-Rich Plasma
PPP = Platelet-Poor Plasma
ATP = ATP Release

drugs that share this mechanism of inducing platelet dysfunction are hydralazine,[140] quinacrine,[141] Nalfon,[105] Ponstel,[142] tocoferol,[143] hydrocortisone,[144] methylprednisolone,[145] and cyclosporin A.[146]

Drugs Inhibiting Platelet Phosphodiesterase Activity

The most common drugs interfering with platelet phosphodiesterase activity and inducing platelet dysfunction are caffeine,[147] dipyridamole,[148] aminophylline, theophylline, and papaverine.[149-151] Vinblastine, vincristine,[152] and colchicine[153] interfere with the platelet contractile protein, thrombosthenin.

Drugs With Unknown Mechanisms of Action on Platelet Function

Acetazolamine,[154] ethacrynic acid,[154] Areomycin,[155] Plaquenil,[156] dicoumarol,[157] nitroprusside,[158] Periactin,[159] glycerol guaiacolate,[160] and heparin[161-164] interfere with platelet function by unclear mechanisms. Nitroglycerine induces platelet dysfunction by interference with platelet cyclic-AMP.[165]

Classification of Drugs Interfering With Platelet Function

Anti-inflammatory drugs are extremely common offenders of platelet dysfunction. Aspirin, colchicine, Motrin,

Figure 4-9. Cardiopulmonary Bypass Surgery Lumi-Aggregation Patterns

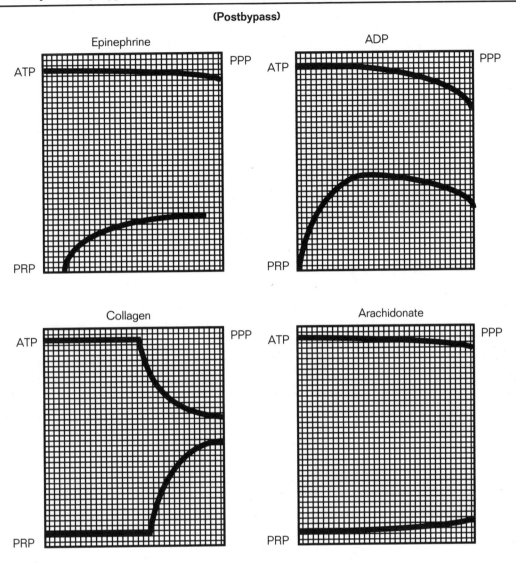

(Postbypass)

PRP = Platelet-Rich Plasma
PPP = Platelet-Poor Plasma
ATP = ATP Release

Indocin, and sulfinpyrazone are the most common. Any non-steroidal anti-inflammatory drug (NSAID) is capable of inducing significant platelet dysfunction, and all appear to inhibit the prostaglandin pathway.[94] Sulfinpyrazone and aspirin are used pharmacologically to suppress platelet function and have the same mode of action, and both drugs inhibit cyclo-oxygenase, therefore inhibiting the eventual platelet synthesis of thromboxane A_2. These drugs, therefore, inhibit endothelial cell synthesis of prostacyclin. It is thought, however, that the inhibitory selectivity of these drugs is approximately 70% against platelet cyclo-oxygenase and 30% against endothelial cyclo-oxygenase, thus accounting for the antithrombotic rather than prothrombotic action of these agents.[166-170]

Psychiatric drugs may also inhibit platelet function. The phenothiazine-related drugs, including Thorazine and Stelazine, may inhibit platelet function and lead to a clinically significant platelet function defect. In addition, the tricyclic amines interfere with platelet function. Numerous cardiovascular drugs are known to interfere with platelet function, including clofibrate, dipyridamole (Persantine), nicotinic acid, papaverine, propranolol, and the newer calcium-blocking drugs, including Varapamil. Newer agents, such as the new generation beta-blocking drugs and diltiazem, inhibit platelet function.[171] Sodium nitroprusside and trimethaphan (Arfonad), used to maintain blood pressure in hypotensive patients, also induce severe platelet dysfunction.[172,173] This category is of particular importance because many patients deemed can-

Figure 4-10. Platelet Dysfunction in Immune Thrombocytopenia Purpura

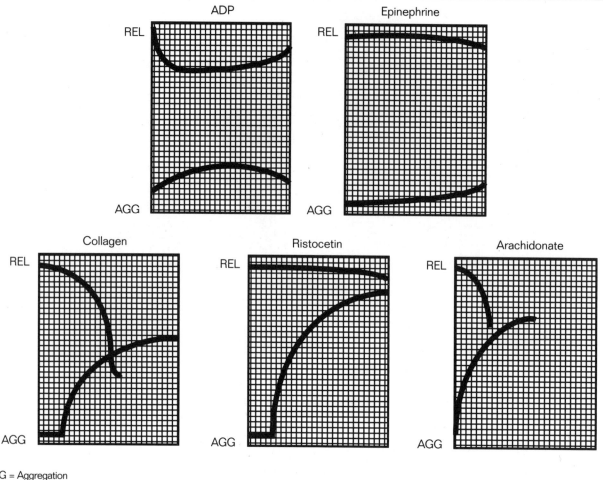

AGG = Aggregation
REL = Release Reaction

didates for cardiopulmonary bypass surgery will be taking one or several of these agents, such as papaverine, propranolol, theophylline, or a calcium-blocking agent. These patients may therefore have enhanced bleeding risk with bypass surgery due to a drug-induced platelet function defect.[174]

Antibiotics are also common inducers of platelet dysfunction. Most of the penicillin derivatives, including Nafcillin, ampicillin, carbenicillin, and ticarcillin, are capable of interfering with platelet function. This interference is most commonly seen with carbenicillin, which also commonly causes thrombocytopenia. Gentamicin is also capable of interfering with platelet function. Various anesthetics, including the local anesthetics, cocaine and procaine, as well as the volatile gaseous anesthetics, may interfere with platelet function and lead to clinically significant hemorrhage.

Miscellaneous drugs interfering with platelet function are the antihistamines, the most common offenders being Benadryl and Actifed, the dextrans, furosemide (Lasix), glycerol guaiacolate (the base of many common cough syrups), nitroprusside, and vincristine or vinblastine. Categories of common clinical drugs capable of causing a clini-

cally significant platelet function defect are listed in Table 4-8. The mechanism of action, where known, is also depicted. Table 4-9 lists common drugs containing aspirin.[175,176]

Laboratory Evaluation

The laboratory evaluation of platelet function defects, including older and newer methods available, are summarized in Table 4-10. Of the older manual methods, the platelet count is paramount to rule out thrombocytopenia in patients with petechiae and purpura, mucosal membrane bleeding, and other suggestive historical findings. The Duke bleeding time and nonstandardized Ivy bleeding time tests have been abandoned with availability of the newer standardized template bleeding time. Platelet aggregation to the aggregating agents ADP, epinephrine, serotonin, thrombin, and collagen have been generally available for longer than a decade.[177] In addition, numerous methodologies to assess platelet factor 3 release have been generally available for many years.[178,179]

The newer methods available to assess platelet function include the standardized template bleeding time,[94,180,181] the

Table 4-8. Drug-Induced Platelet Dysfunction

Cardiovascular/Respiratory
- Aminophylline***
- Clofibrate*
- Dibenzyline*
- Dicoumarol*****
- Dihydroergotamine*
- Dipyridamole***
- Heparin*****
- Hydralazine**
- Isuprel*
- Nitroglycerine****
- Nitroprusside*****
- Papaverine***
- Propanolol*
- Regitine*
- Reserpine*
- Theophylline***
- Varapamil**

Antibiotics
- Ampicillin*
- Aureomycin*****
- Carbenicillin*
- Furadantin*
- Gentamicin*
- Keflin*
- Moxalactam*
- Nafcillin*
- Piperacillin*
- Plaquenil*****
- Quinacrine**

Psychiatric
- Aventyl*
- Elavil*
- Norpramine*
- Sinequan*
- Stelazine*
- Thorazine*
- Tofranil*

Anesthetics
- Cocaine*
- Nupercaine*
- Procaine*
- Xylocaine*

Antiinflammatory
- Anturane**
- Aspirin**
- Colchicine******
- Ibuprofen**
- Indomethacin**
- Nalfon**
- Naprosyn**
- Phenylbutazone**
- Ponstel**

Diuretics
- Acetazolamide*****
- Ethacrynic acid*****
- Furosemide**

Miscellaneous
- Alcohol*
- Benedryl*
- Caffeine***
- Cyclosporin A**
- Dextran*
- Glycerol guaiacolate*****
- Hydroxyethyl starch*
- Hydrocortisone**
- Methylprednisolone**
- Periactin*****
- Phenergan*
- Sansert*****
- Tocoferol**
- Vinblastine******
- Vincristine******

* = interference with membrane or membrane receptors
** = interference with prostaglandin synthesis
*** = interference with phosphodiesterase
**** = interference with platelet cyclic-AMP
***** = unknown mechanism of action
****** = interference with thrombosthenin

Table 4-9. Common Drugs Containing Aspirin

- Alka seltzer
- Anacin
- Anahist
- APC
- APC with codeine
- APC with demerol
- ASA
- ASA compound
- ASA compound with codeine
- Aspergum
- Aspirin (USP)
- Aspirin - children's
- Bayer
- Bayer - children's
- Bayer timed-release
- Bufferin
- Calurin
- Cama inlay
- Cope
- Coricidin
- Coricidin "D"
- Coricidin demilets
- Coricidin medilets
- Darvon with ASA
- Darvon-N with ASA
- Darvon compound
- Dolene
- Dristan
- Ecotrin
- Empiral
- Empirin
- Empirin with codeine
- Emprazil
- Emprazil-C
- Equagesic
- Excedrin
- Excedrin PM
- Fiorinal
- Fiorinal with codeine
- Fizrin
- Four-way cold tablets
- Liquiprin
- Measurin
- Midol
- Norgesic
- PAC compound
- PAC compound with codeine
- Percodan
- Robaxisal
- Robaxisal-pH
- Sine-off
- St. Joseph's
- St. Joseph's for children
- Super-anahist
- Synalgos
- Synalgos-DC
- Triaminicin
- Vanquish

new aggregating agents ristocetin[182] and arachidonic acid,[183] and lumi-aggregation, which studies simultaneous platelet aggregation and ATP release.[184-186]

The aggregometer is a standardized spectrophotometer; platelet-rich plasma is added to a spectrophotometric well, and then various aggregating reagents are added.[187-189] One aggregating agent at a time is studied. As platelets aggregate, increasing amounts of light are able to pass through the spectrophotometric chamber. The change in light density (percent transmission) is then recorded on a strip recorder, giving rise to typical platelet aggregation patterns.[5,190] Figure

Table 4-10. Laboratory Evaluation of
Platelet Function

Older Methods
    Platelet count
    Duke bleeding time
    Ivy bleeding time
    Platelet aggregation
        ADP
        Epinephrine
        Collagen
        Serotonin
        Thrombin
    Platelet factor 3
    Clot retraction
    Prothrombin consumption

Newer Methods
    Template bleeding time
    Platelet aggregation
        Ristocetin
        Arachidonate
    Lumi-aggregation for release reaction
    Platelet factor 4
    Beta-thromboglobulin
    Thromboxane
    Cyclo-oxygenase

4-11 summarizes normal platelet aggregation patterns as seen on a standardized platelet aggregometer. The usual aggregating agents used are ADP, epinephrine, ristocetin, collagen, and arachidonic acid. Serotonin, or 5-hydroxytryptamine, was commonly used in the past but appears now to be an uncommonly used platelet aggregating reagent. Epinephrine is usually used at two doses (a final concentration of 2.5×10^{-5} [high-dose] and a final concentration of 2.5×10^{-6} [low-dose]). Similarly adenosine diphosphate (ADP) is characteristically used at two concentrations (2.0×10^{-5} [high-dose] and 2.5×10^{-6} [low-dose]). Collagen is used at a final concentration of 0.19 mg/mL; ristocetin is used at a final concentration of 1.5 mg/mL; and arachidonic acid is most often used at a final concentration of 0.5 mg/mL. The patterns depicted in Figure 4-11 are normal patterns elicited by the addition of each of these reagents, individually, to platelet-rich plasma in the aggregometer. A monophasic (all or none) curve is elicited with ADP (11A). The top of the curve represents platelet-rich plasma, and the bottom of the curve represents platelet-poor plasma after aggregation has occurred. A biphasic curve is usually elicited with epinephrine (11B). Ristocetin also usually induces a monophasic curve with the change in light density going from the very top, or platelet-rich plasma, to the very bottom, or platelet-poor plasma (11C). This is also true for arachidonic acid (11E).[191] Collagen characteristically demonstrates a lag phase, which is seen in the bottom of Figure 4-11 on the left-hand corner, followed by complete aggregation to platelet-poor plasma (11D). The slight curve seen with 5-

hydroxytryptamine is a normal serotonin-induced platelet aggregation curve (11F).

A much newer refinement of aggregation to assess platelet function is lumi-aggregation.[184-186,192,193] Figure 4-12 demonstrates a popular lumi-aggregation instrument. This instrument uses two wells: a photometric well and a fluorometric well. The use of firefly luciperase (ATP-ase) in the fluorometric well allows the measurement of simultaneous ATP release while measuring aggregation in the photometric well. Thus, aggregation and simultaneous ATP release can be studied with the use of this instrumentation. In our laboratory almost all aggregation or platelet work-ups are done exclusively with lumi-aggregation. The final concentrations of the aggregating agents are the same as those described for the aggregometer. The final concentration of luciperase (ATP-ase) used in the fluorometric well to assess the release reaction is 3.0 mg/mL. Figure 4-13 summarizes normal lumi-aggregation patterns generated by the aggregating reagents depicted. The aggregation curves are now read upside down as compared to the aggregation curves seen in Figure 4-11. The aggregating pattern is on the bottom (eg, on the bottom of the top left box in Figure 4-13 is the lag phase characteristically seen with collagen, going from platelet-rich plasma on the bottom to platelet-poor plasma on the top). Simultaneous ATP release is seen from top to bottom (13C). The right upper box demonstrates ATP release with epinephrine, the typical biphasic epinephrine curve going from platelet-rich plasma on the bottom to platelet-poor plasma at the end of the curve (13B). Ristocetin commonly causes only partial ATP release, usually about 35% (13D).[194] On the bottom right of Figure 4-13 is a normal lumi-aggregation pattern induced by ADP (13A). Thus, lumi-aggregation has added a significant new dimension to assessment of platelet function, allowing observation of simultaneous platelet release reaction and platelet aggregation.

Hyperactive Prethrombotic Platelets

"Large bizarre" platelets are commonly seen in hypercoagulable patients and in patients undergoing frank clinical or subclinical thrombotic episodes. Large platelets represent the young and presumably hemostatically more active platelets.[195,196] Therefore, in individuals undergoing thrombotic disorders manifest as increased fibrin deposition with the entrapment of platelets, one would expect concomitant consumption of platelets, a rapid platelet turnover and decreased platelet survival,[197,198] and a greater than usual number of young platelets, large platelets, or hemostatically more active platelets in the peripheral blood.[195,196] Thus, in a patient undergoing a thrombotic event, either subclinical or obvious, such as a deep venous thrombotic event, a pulmonary embolus, or acute arterial thromboembolus, an increase in the percentage of young or large platelets in the peripheral smear is expected in the presence of a normal bone marrow and absence of hypersplenism.[198,199] Platelet indices, including the

Figure 4-11. Normal Platelet Aggregation Patterns

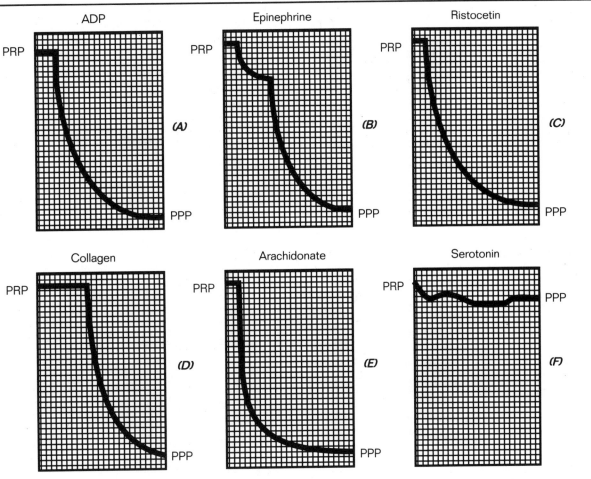

PRP = Platelet-Rich Plasma
PPP = Platelet-Poor Plasma

platelet crit, the platelet distribution width (PDW), and mean platelet volume (MPV) of platelets circulating in a patient, may be of significant diagnostic benefit and may be an important modality for assessing response to antiplatelet therapy in patients with hypercoagulability or thrombosis. These parameters are now readily available on numerous automated platelet particle counters.[200-202]

With the current trend of using antiplatelet agents as prophylaxis for thrombotic events, modalities to assess the efficacy of antiplatelet therapy are needed. Platelet indices and platelet size distributions may give a reasonable clinical indication of response to antiplatelet therapy.[203-205]

As platelets become activated, platelet factor 4, beta-thromboglobulin, and thromboxane A_2 are released. As platelets are consumed, subsequent to activation, large young platelets are anticipated in the peripheral blood. Thus, platelet activation is associated with elevated platelet factor 4, beta-thromboglobulin, the degradation product of thromboxane A_2, thromboxane B_2, and an increase in MPV. These parameters, in varying combinations, have been assessed in

a variety of prethrombotic and thrombotic conditions. In general, these parameters are elevated in deep vein thrombosis and pulmonary embolus[203,206] and in patients with unstable angina or acute myocardial infarction.[207-211] Some studies

Figure 4-12. Popular Lumi-Aggregation Instrument

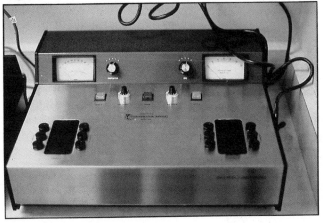

Figure 4-13. Normal Platelet Lumi-Aggregation Patterns

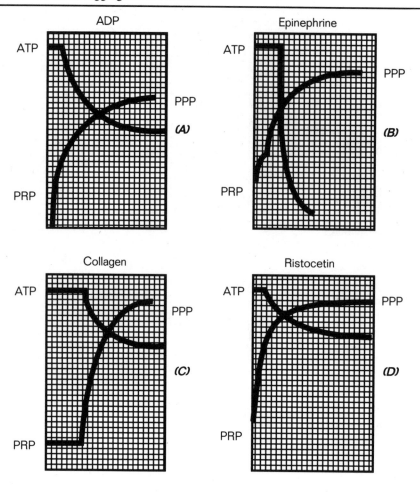

PRP = Platelet-Rich Plasma
PPP = Platelet-Poor Plasma
ATP = ATP Release

have shown these parameters to decrease with antithrombotic therapy. These molecular markers of platelet reactivity are also commonly noted to be elevated in patients with a variety of peripheral arterial diseases, including acute myocardial infarction, cerebrovascular thrombosis, transient cerebral ischemic attacks (TIAs), diabetic microangiopathy, and atherosclerotic peripheral vascular disease.[212-219] Disorders associated with a prethrombotic state commonly associated with arterial or venous thrombosis are also often noted to be accompanied by these elevated markers of platelet reactivity, including term delivery, pre-eclampsia, eclampsia, inflammatory bowel disease, early DIC, orthopedic surgery, and use of estrogens.[220-224] Available information suggests that these molecular markers of platelet reactivity, including platelet factor 4, beta-thromboglobulin, thromboxane derivatives, and MPV, may be useful clinical indices of early thrombotic or thromboembolic events. Some studies have clearly shown that correction of these parameters is associated with institution of effective antithrombotic therapy. Not-

ing decreases in platelet factor 4 levels or beta-thromboglobulin levels after the institution of antiplatelet therapy may also be indicative of clinical efficacy with respect to stopping or blunting increased fibrin deposition.[225-227] Some investigations, however, have failed to demonstrate decreases in platelet factor 4 or beta-thromboglobulin levels in patients with arterial occlusive disease being treated with antiplatelet drugs.[228]

Interestingly, a congenital platelet function defect leading to thrombosis, rather than hemorrhage, has recently been reported.[229] This defect is referred to as the Wein-Penzing defect and is characterized by a deficiency of the lipoxygenase metabolic pathway and concomitant compensatory increase in cyclo-oxygenase pathway products, including thromboxane, prostaglandin E_2, and prostaglandin D_2. Both patients described had precocious myocardial infarction.

Newer methods available to assess platelet hyperactivity and consumption, most of which are amenable to full automation, are summarized in Table 4-11 and consist of

Table 4-11. Evaluation of Hyperactive and Prethrombotic Platelets

---

Platelet factor 4
Beta-thromboglobulin
Thromboxane B$_2$
Mean platelet volume
Platelet crit ?

---

assessment of mean platelet volume and molecular markers of platelet reactivity. The diagnostic roles of these methods appear promising, but remain to be established.

Summary

Platelet function defects, especially the acquired forms, are common causes of hemorrhage, especially hemorrhage associated with trauma and surgical procedures. Although the hereditary platelet function defects are generally rare, hereditary storage pool disease is common enough to be suspected in an individual, usually a child, with characteristic historical and clinical findings. The acquired platelet function defects, especially those caused by drugs, are exceedingly common and should immediately be suspected in individuals who develop easy and spontaneous bruising, mild to moderate mucosal membrane hemorrhage, or unexplained bleeding associated with trauma, an invasive procedure, or general surgical procedure. Although the template bleeding time is useful as a screening test for platelet function, the recording of a normal template bleeding time, in association with a suggestive history, suggestive clinical findings, or in a patient with frank bleeding, is not reliable, and platelet aggregation or lumi-aggregation should immediately be performed in the appropriate clinical situations. The mainstay of therapy for essentially all of these defects, if bleeding is significant, is the liberal infusion of appropriate numbers of platelet concentrates. Of course, the acquired platelet function defects should also be managed by attempts to treat and/or control the underlying disease, if possible, and offending drugs or potentially offending drugs should promptly be discontinued.

References

1. Bick RL, E Shanbrom: A systematic approach to the diagnosis of bleeding disorders. Med Counterpoint 6:27, 1972.

2. Bick RL: A systematic approach to the diagnosis of bleeding disorders, ch 4. In: G Murano and RL Bick (Eds): Basic Concepts of Hemostasis and Thrombosis. CRC Press, Boca Raton, FL, 1980, p 81.

3. Bick RL: Vascular disorders associated with thrombohemorrhagic phenomena. Semin Thromb Hemost 5:167, 1979.

4. Kitchens CS: The purpuric disorders. Semin Thromb Hemost 10:173, 1984.

5. Bick RL: Platelet defects, ch 4. In: Disorders of Hemostasis and Thrombosis: A Practical Clinical Approach. Theime, Inc., New York, 1985, p 65.

6. Hirsh J: Laboratory diagnosis of thrombosis, ch 58. In: RW Coleman, J Hirsh, VJ Marder, E Salzman (Eds): Hemostasis and Thrombosis: Basic Principles and Clinical Practice. JB Lippincott, Philadelphia, 1982, p 789.

7. Meyer D, TS Zimmerman: von Willebrand's Disease, ch 6. In: RW Coleman, J Hirsh, VJ Marder, E Salzman (Eds): Hemostasis and Thrombosis: Basic Principles and Clinical Practice. JB Lippincott, Philadelphia, 1982, p 64.

8. Mieschner PA, J Graf: Drug-induced thrombocytopenia. Clin Haematol 9:505, 1980.

9. Bick RL, T Adams, WR Schmalhorst: Bleeding times, platelet adhesion, and aspirin. Am J Clin Pathol 65:65, 1976.

10. Mielke CH, MM Kaneshiro, LA Maer, SI Rappaport: The standardized normal ivy bleeding time and its prolongation by aspirin. Blood 34:204, 1969.

11. Bick RL: Vascular disorders associated with thrombohemorrhagic phenomenon, ch 3. In: Disorders of Hemostasis and Thrombosis: Principles of Clinical Practice. Thieme, Inc., New York, 1985, p 44.

12. Rodgers RP, J Levin: A critical reappraisal of the bleeding time. Semin Thromb Hemost 16:1, 1990.

13. Sienco. The Petechiometer: package insert. Sienco Inc., Morrison, CO, 1990.

14. Lusher JM, MI Barnhart: Congenital disorders affecting platelets. Semin Thromb Hemost 4:123, 1977.

15. Bernard J, JP Soulier: Sur une nouvelle variete dystrophic thrombocytaire hemorrhagipase congenitale. Semin des Hopitaux 24:3217, 1948.

16. White JG: Inherited abnormalities of the platelet membrane and secretory granules. Hum Pathol 18:123, 1987.

17. Bithel TC, SJ Parokh, RR Strong: Platelet function in the Bernard-Soulier Syndrome. Ann N Y Acad Sci 201:145, 1972.

18. Howard MA, RA Hutton, RM Hardisty: Hereditary giant platelet syndrome: a new disorder of platelet function. Br Med J 2:586, 1973.

19. Bick RL: Congenital coagulation factor defects and von Willebrand's disease, ch 5. In: Disorders of Hemostasis and Thrombosis: Principles of Clinical Practice. Thieme, Inc., New York, 1985, p 127.

20. Glanzmann E: Hereditare hamorrhagische thrombasthenic. Ein Beitrag zur Pathhologie der Blutplattchen. Jahresber Kinderheilkd 88:1, 1918.

21. Fonio A, J Schwendener: Die thrombocyten des menschlichen clutes. Huber, Bern, 1942.

22. Inceman S, V Tangun: Essential athrombia. Thromb Diath Haemorrh 33:278, 1975.

23. Cronberg S, IM Nilsson: Investigations in a family with thrombasthenia of moderately severe type with 16 affected family members. Scand J Haematol 5:17, 1968.

24. Caen JP, PA Castaldi, JC Leclerc, S Inceman, MJ Larrieu, M Probst, J Bernard: Congenital bleeding disorders with long bleeding time and normal platelet count, I: Glanzmann's thrombasthenia (report of 15 patients). Am J Med 41:4, 1966.

25. Caen JP: Glanzmann's thrombasthenia. Clin Haematol 1:383, 1972.

26. Bick RL: Pathophysiology of hemostasis and thrombosis. In: WA Sodeman, TM Sodeman (Eds): Pathologic Physiology: Mechanisms of Disease. WB Saunders, Philadelphia, 1985.

27. Holmsen H, HJ Weiss: Further evidence for a deficient storage pool of adenine nucleotides in platelets from some patients with thrombocytopathia: "storage pool disease." Blood 39:197, 1972.

28. Pareti FI, L Mannucci, A Capitanio, DCB Mills: Heterogeneity of storage pool deficiency. Thromb Haemost 38:3, 1977.

29. Grottum KA, T Hovig, H Holmsen, A Foss Abrahamsen, M Jeremic, M Seip: Wiskott-Aldrich Syndrome: qualitative platelet defects and short platelet survival. Br J Haematol 17:373, 1969.

30. Day HJ, H Holmsen: Platelet adenine nucleotide "storage pool deficiency" in thrombocytopenic absent radii syndrome. JAMA 221:1053, 1972.

31. Rendu F, J Breton-Gorius, G Trugnan, H Castro-Malispina, JM Andriev, G Bereziat, M Lebret, JP Caen: Studies on a new variant of the Hermansky-Pudlak Syndrome: qualitative ultrastructural bodies associated with a phospholipase A defect. Am J Hematol 4:387, 1978.

32. Buchanon GR, RI Handin: Platelet function in the Chédiak-Higashi syndrome. Blood 47:941, 1976.

33. Weiss HJ: Pathophysiology and detection of clinically significant platelet dysfunction. In: MG Baldini, S Ebbe (Eds): Platelets: Production, Function, Transfusion, and Storage. Grune and Stratton, New York, 1974, p 253.

34. Weiss HJ, BA Lages, LD Witte, KL Kaplan, DS Goodman, HL Nossel, HR Baumgartner: Storage pool disease: evidence for clinical and biochemical heterogeneity. Thromb Haemost 38:3, 1977.

35. Minkes MS, JN Joist, P Needleham: Arachidonic acid–induced platelet aggregation independent of ADP-release in a patient with a bleeding disorder due to platelet storage pool disease. Thromb Res 15:169, 1979.

36. Weiss HJ: Platelet aggregation, adhesion, and adenosine diphosphate release in thrombopathia (platelet factor 3 deficiency): a comparison with Glanzmann's thrombasthenia and von Willebrand's disease. Am J Med 43:570, 1967.

37. Stuart MJ: Inherited defects of platelet function. Semin Hematol 12:233, 1975.

38. Arkel YS: Evaluation of platelet aggregation in disorders of hemostasis. Med Clin North Am 60:881, 1976.

39. Weiss HJ, RP Ames: Ultrastructural findings in storage pool disease and aspirin-like defects of platelets. Am J Pathol 71:447, 1973.

40. Adashi E, M Farber, GW Mitchell: Congenital release thrombocytopathy. Pathophysiology and management. Obstet Gynecol 48:403, 1976.

41. Scheck R, H Rasche, W Queiber, H Burkhardt, W Calvo: Platelet dysfunction as a result of inhibition of a release (aspirin-like defect) in two identical twins. Dtsch Med Wochenschr 100:1842, 1975.

42. Weiss HJ, J Rogers: Thrombocytopathia due to abnormalities in platelet release reaction: studies on six unrelated patients. Blood 39:187, 1972.

43. Malmsten C, M Hamberg, J Svensson, B Samuelsson: Physiological role of an endoperoxide in human platelets: hemostatic defect due to platelet cyclo-oxygenase deficiency. Proc Natl Acad Sci 72:1446, 1975.

44. Horellou MH, T LeCompte, C LeCruber, F Fouque, M Chignard, J Conard, BB Vargaftig, F Drey, M Samama: Familial and constitutional bleeding disorder due to platelet cyclo-oxygenase deficiency. Am J Hematol 14:1, 1983.

45. Lagard M, PA Byron, BB Vargaftig, M Dechavanne: Impairment of platelet thromboxane A_2 generation and of the platelet release reaction in two patients with congenital deficiency of platelet cyclo-oxygenase. Br J Haematol 38:251, 1978.

46. Zucker S, H Meilke, JR Durocher, WH Crosby: Oozing and bruising due to abnormal platelet function. Ann Intern Med 76:725, 1971.

47. Lages B, HJ Weiss: Impairment of phosphatidylinositol metabolism in a patient with a bleeding disorder associated with defects of the initial platelet response. Thromb Haemost 59:175, 1988.

48. Rabiner SF: Uremic bleeding. Prog Hemost Thromb 1:233, 1972.

49. Lewis JH, MB Zucker, JH Ferguson: Bleeding tendency in uremia. Blood 11:1073, 1956.

50. Castaldi PA: Hemostasis and renal disease, ch 15. In: OD Ratnoff, CD Forbes (Eds): Disorders of Hemostasis. Grune and Stratton, Inc., New York, 1989, p 473.

51. Horowitz HI, DB Cohen, P Martinez, M Papayoanov: Defective ADP-induced platelet factor 3 activation in uremia. Blood 30:331, 1967.

52. Horowitz HI, IM Stein, DB Cohen, JG White: Further studies on the platelet-inhibiting effect of guanidino succinic acid and its role in uremic bleeding. Am J Med 49:339, 1970.

53. Rabiner SF, F Molinas: The role of phenol and phenolic acids on the thrombocytopathy and defective platelet aggregation of patients with renal failure. Am J Med 49:346, 1970.

54. Evans EP, GR Jones, AL Bloom: Abnormal breakdown of adenosine diphosphate in uraemic plasma and its possible relationship to defective platelet aggregation. Thromb Res 1:323, 1972.

55. Schondorf TH, D Hey: Platelet function tests in uraemia and under acetylsalicylic acid administration. Haemostasis 3:129, 1974.

56. Remuzzi G, M Livio, AE Cavenaghi, D Marchesi, G Mecca, MB Donati, G de Gaetano: Unbalanced prostaglandin synthesis and plasma factors in uraemic bleeding: a hypothesis. Thromb Res 13:531, 1978.

57. Kamoun P, D Kleinknecht, H Duerot, H Jerome: Platelet-serotonin in uraemia. Lancet 1:782, 1970.

58. Remuzzi G, AE Cavenaghi, G Mecca, MB Donati, G de Gaetano: Prostacyclin (PGI_2) and bleeding time in uremic patients. Thromb Res 11:919, 1977.

59. Albertazzi A, C Spisni, PF Palmieri: Nucleotide deficit and functional platelet alterations in patients on regular dialysis treatment. Life Support Systems 3:77, 1985.

60. Ware JA, BA Clark, M Smith: Abnormalities of cytoplasmic Ca++ in platelets from patients with uremia. Blood 73:172, 1989.

61. Escolar G, A Casa, E Bastidi: Uremic platelets have a functional defect affecting the interaction of von Willebrand factor with glycoprotein IIb-IIIa. Blood 76:1336, 1990.

62. Komarnicki M, T Twardowski: Platelet glycoprotein concentrations in patients with chronic uraemia. Folia Haematol 114:642, 1987.

63. Jubelirer SJ: Hemostatic abnormalities in renal disease. Am J Kidney Dis 5:219, 1985.

64. Rydzewski A, M Rowinski, M Mysiwiec: Shortening of bleeding time after intranasal administration of 1-deamino-8-arginine vasopressin to patients with chronic uremia. Folia Haematol 113:823, 1986.

65. Manucci PM: Desmopressin (DDAVP) for treatment of disorders of hemostasis. Prog Hemost Thromb 8:19, 1986.

66. Gotti E, G Mecca, C Valentino, E Cortinovis, T Bertanit, G Remuzzi: Renal biopsy in patients with acute renal failure and prolonged bleeding time: a preliminary report. Am J Kidney Dis 6:397, 1985.

67. Livio M, P Mannucci, G Vigano, G Mignardi, R Lombardi, G Mecca, G Remuzzi: Conjugated estrogens for the management of bleeding associated with renal failure. N Engl J Med 315:731, 1986.

68. Vigano GL, PM Mannucci, A Lattuada: Subcutaneous desmopressin (DDAVP) shortens the bleeding time in uremia. Am J Hematol 31:32, 1989.

69. Mannucci P: Desmopressin: a nontransfusional hemostatic agent. Ann Rev Med 41:55, 1990.

70. Vigaono G, F Gaspari, M Locatelli: Dose-effect and pharmokinetics of estrogens given to correct bleeding time in uremia. Kidney Int 34:853, 1988.

71. Harker LA: Acquired disorders of platelet function. Ann N Y Acad Sci 509:188, 1987.

72. Carvalho AC: Acquired platelet dysfunction in patients with uremia. Hematol Oncol Clin North Am 4:129, 1990.

73. Gordge MP, RW Faint, PB Rylance: Platelet function and the bleeding time in progressive renal failure. Thromb Haemost 60:83, 1988.

74. Lindsay RM, AV Moorthy, F Koens: Platelet function in dialyzed and non-dialyzed patients with chronic renal failure. Clin Nephrol 4:52, 1975.

75. Bick RL: Acquired circulating anticoagulants and defective hemostasis in malignant paraprotein disorders, ch 10. In: G Murano, RL Bick (Eds): Basic Concepts of Hemostasis and Thrombosis. CRC Press, Boca Raton, FL, 1980, p 205.

76. Bick RL: Alterations of hemostasis associated with malignancy: etiology, pathophysiology, diagnosis, and management. Semin Thromb Hemost 5:1, 1978.

77. Bick RL: Alterations of hemostasis in malignancy, ch 10. In: Disorders of Hemostasis and Thrombosis: Principles of Clinical Practice. Thieme, Inc., New York, 1985, p 262.

78. Lachner H: Hemostatic abnormalities associated with dysproteinemias. Semin Hematol 10:125, 1973.

79. Lisiewicz J: Plasma cell myeloma, ch 9. In: Hemorrhage in Leukemias. Polish Medical Publishers, Warsaw, 1976, p 153.

80. Adams T, L Schultz, L Goldberg: Platelet function abnormalities in myeloproliferative disorders. Scand J Haematol 13:215, 1974.

81. Tangun Y: Platelet aggregation and platelet factor 3 activity in myeloproliferative syndromes. Thromb Diath Haemorrh 25:241, 1971.

82. Bick RL: Alterations of hemostasis associated with malignancy, ch 11. In: G Murano, RL Bick (Eds): Basic Concepts of Hemostasis and Thrombosis. CRC Press, Boca Raton, FL, 1980, p 213.

83. Bick RL: Essential thrombocythemia. Check Sample Program. American Society of Clinical Pathologists, 1989.

84. Lofvenberg E, TK Nilsson: Qualitative platelet defects in chronic myeloproliferative disorders: evidence for reduced ATP secretion. Eur J Haematol 43:435, 1989.

85. Raman BK, EJ Van-Slyck, J Riddle: Platelet function and structure in myeloproliferative disease, myelodysplastic syndrome, and secondary thrombocytosis. Am J Clin Pathol 91:647, 1989.

86. Pfliegler G, Z Boda, M Udvardy: Platelet function studies in myeloproliferative disorders. Folia Haematol 113:655, 1986.

87. Bick RL: Alterations of hemostasis associated with surgery, cardiac surgery, organ transplantation and prosthetic devices, ch 12. In: OD Ratnoff, CD Forbes (Eds): Disorders of Hemostasis, ed 2. Grune and Stratton, New York, 1991, p 379.

88. Bick RL: Alterations of hemostasis associated with cardiopulmonary bypass: pathophysiology, prevention, diagnosis, and management. Semin Thromb Hemost 3:59, 1976.

89. Bick RL, WR Schmalhorst, NR Arbegast: Alterations of hemostasis associated with cardiopulmonary bypass. Thromb Res 8:285, 1976.

90. Bick RL: Alterations of hemostasis associated with surgery, cardiopulmonary bypass surgery, and prosthetic devices, ch 12. In: OD Ratnoff, CD Forbes (Eds): Disorders of Hemostasis. Grune and Stratton, New York, 1984, p 379.

91. Harker LA, TW Malpass, NE Bronson: Mechanisms of abnormal bleeding in patients undergoing cardiopulmonary bypass: acquired transient platelet dysfunction associated with selective alpha-granule release. Blood 56:824, 1980.

92. Rao AK, PN Walsh: Acquired qualitative platelet disorders. Clin Haematol 12:201, 1983.

93. Zahavi J: Acquired "storage pool disease" of platelets. Thromb Haemost 35:501, 1976.

94. Bick RL, SM Scates: Platelet function defects. Lab Med. In press.

95. Bick RL: The clinical significance of fibrinogen degradation products. Semin Thromb Hemost 8:302, 1982.

96. Bick RL: Primary fibrino(geno)lytic syndromes, ch 9. In: G Murano, RL Bick (Eds): Basic Concepts of Hemostasis and Thrombosis. CRC Press, Boca Raton, FL, 1980, p 181.

97. Kowalski E: Fibrinogen derivatives and their biological activities. Semin Hematol 5:45, 1968.

98. Bick RL: Disseminated intravascular coagulation and related syndromes: a clinical review. Semin Thromb Hemost 14:299, 1988.

99. Bick RL: Disseminated intravascular coagulation and related syndromes: etiology, pathophysiology, diagnosis, and management. Am J Hematol 5:265, 1978.

100. Bick RL: Disseminated intravascular coagulation, ch 2. In: RL Bick (Ed): Disseminated Intravascular Coagulation and Related Syndromes. CRC Press, Boca Raton, FL, 1983, p 31.

101. Bick RL: Syndromes associated with hyperfibrino(geno)lysis, ch 3. In: RL Bick (Ed): Disseminated Intravascular Coagulation and Related Syndromes. CRC Press, Boca Raton, FL, 1983, p 105.

102. Levine PH: A qualitative platelet defect in severe vitamin B_{12} deficiency: response, hyperresponse, and thrombosis after vitamin B_{12} therapy. Ann Intern Med 78:533, 1973.

103. Ingeberg S, E Stofferson: Platelet dysfunction in patients with vitamin B_{12} deficiency. Acta Haematol 61:75, 1979.

104. Triplett DA: Qualitative or functional defects of platelets, ch 5. In: DA Triplett (Ed): Platelet Function: Laboratory Evalua-

tion and Clinical Application. ASCP Press, Chicago, 1978, p 123.

105. Weiss HJ: Antiplatelet drugs: pharmacological aspects. In: Platelets: Pathophysiology and Antiplatelet Drug Therapy. Alan R Liss, New York, 1982, p 45.

106. Triplett DA: Appendix C: Miscellaneous lists and forms. In: DA Triplett (Ed): Platelet Function Evaluation: Laboratory Evaluation and Clinical Application. ASCP Press, Chicago, 1978, p 291.

107. Mills DCB, IA Robb, GCK Roberts: The release of nucleotides, 5-hydroxytryptamine and enzymes from blood platelets during aggregation. J Physiol 195:715, 1968.

108. Rysanek R, C Suehla, H Spankova, M Mlejnkova: The effect of tricyclic antidepressive drugs on adrenaline- and adenosine diphosphate–induced platelet aggregation. J Pharm Pharmacol 18:616, 1966.

109. Weiss HJ: Pharmacology of platelet inhibition. Prog Hemost Thromb 1:199, 1972.

110. Mills DCB, GCK Roberts: Membrane active drugs and the aggregation of human blood platelets. Nature 213:35, 1967.

111. Stacy RS: Uptake of 5-hydroxytryptamine by platelets. Br J Pharmacol 16:284, 1961.

112. O'Brien JR: Platelet aggregation, part I: some effects of the adenosine phosphates, thrombin and cocaine upon platelet adhesiveness. J Clin Pathol 15:446, 1962.

113. O'Brien JR: Some effects of adrenaline and anti-adrenaline compounds on platelets in vitro and in vivo. Nature 200:763, 1973.

114. Weksler BB, M Gillik, J Pink: Effect of propanolol on platelet function. Blood 49:185, 1977.

115. Natelson EA, CH Brown, MW Bradshaw: Influence of cephalosporin antibiotics on blood coagulation and platelet function. Antimicrob Agents Chemother 9:91, 1976.

116. Cazenave JP, MA Guccione, MA Packham, JF Mustard: Effects of cephalothin and penicillin G on platelet function in vitro. Br J Haematol 35:135, 1977.

117. Brown CN, EA Natelson, MW Bradshaw, TW Williams, CP Alfrey: The hemostatic defect produced by carbenicillin. N Engl J Med 291:265, 1974.

118. Brown CN, MW Bradshaw, EA Natelson, CP Alfrey, TW Williams: Defective platelet function following the administration of penicillin compounds. Blood 47:949, 1976.

119. O'Brien JRL: The adhesiveness of native platelets and its prevention. J Clin Pathol 14:140, 1961.

120. Seeman PM: Membrane stabilization of drugs: tranquilizers, steroids, and anesthetics. Int Rev Neurobiol 9:145, 1966.

121. Cowan DH: Effect of alcoholism on hemostasis. Semin Hematol 17:137, 1980.

122. Bygdeman S, I Johnson: Studies on the effect of adrenergic blocking agents on catecholamine-induced platelet aggregation and uptake of noradrenaline and 5-hydroxytryptamine. Acta Physiol Scand 75:129, 1969.

123. Born GVR, J Bricknell: The uptake of 5-hydroxytryptamine by blood platelets in the cold. J Physiol 147:153, 1959.

124. Mills DCB, GCK Roberts: Effects of adrenaline on human blood platelets. J Physiol 193:443, 1967.

125. White JG, ST Raynor: The effects of trifluoroperazine, and inhibitor of calmodulin on platelet function. Thromb Res 18:279, 1980.

126. Anderson ER, JG Foulkes, DV Godin: The effect of local anaesthetics and antiarrhythmic agents on the responses of rabbit platelets to ADP and thrombin. Thromb Haemost 45:81, 1981.

127. Rossie EC, NW Levin: Inhibition of primary ADP-induced platelet aggregation in normal subjects after administration of nitrofurantoin (Furadantin). Clin Invest 52:2457, 1973.

128. Alexander DP, ME Russo, DE Gohram, G Rothstein: Nafcillin-induced platelet dysfunction and bleeding. Antimicrob Agents Chemother 23:59, 1983.

129. Bang NU, SS Tessler, RO Heidenreich, CA Marks, LE Mattler: Effects of moxalactam on blood coagulation and platelet function. Rev Infect Dis 4:546, 1982.

130. Brown CN, EA Natelson, MW Bradshaw: A study of the effects of ticarcillin on blood coagulation and platelet function. Antimicrob Agents Chemother 7:652, 1975.

131. Ewald RA, JW Eichelberger, AA Young, HJ Weiss, WH Crosby: The effect of dextran on platelet factor 3. Transfusion 5:109, 1965.

132. Gollub S, C Shafer, A Squitieri: The bleeding tendency associated with plasma expanders. Surg Gynecol Obstet 124:1203, 1967.

133. Cohen LS: The pharmacology of acetylsalic acid. Semin Thromb Hemost 2:146, 1976.

134. Kocsis JJ, J Hernadovich, MJ Silver, JB Smith, C Ingerman: Duration of inhibition of platelet prostaglandin formation and aggregation by ingested aspirin or indomethacin. Prostaglandins 3:141, 1973.

135. Zucker MB, J Peterson: Effect of acetylsalicylic acid, other nonsteroidal anti-inflammatory agents, and dipyridamole on human blood platelets. J Lab Clin Med 76:66, 1970.

136. Nishizawa EE, DJ Wynalda: Inhibitory effect of ibuprofen (Motrin) on platelet function. Thromb Res 21:347, 1981.

137. Wiley JS, CN Chesterman, FJ Morgan, PA Castaldi: The effect of sulfinpyrazone on the aggregation and release reactions of human platelets. Thromb Res 14:23, 1979.

138. Rossie EC, NW Levin: Inhibition of ADP-induced platelet aggregation by furosemide. J Lab Clin Med 81:140, 1973.

139. Addonizio VP, CA Fisher, JF Strauss, LH Edmunds: Inhibition of human platelet function by verapamil. Thromb Res 28:545, 1982.

140. Burns TS, RN Saunders: Antiplatelet activity of hydralazine. Thromb Res 16:837, 1979.

141. Winocour PD, RL Kinlough-Rathbone, JF Mustard: The effect of the phospholipase inhibitor mepacrine on platelet release reaction, and fibrinogen binding to the platelet surface. Thromb Haemost 45:257, 1981.

142. O'Brien JR: Effect of anti-inflammatory agents on platelets. Lancet 1:894, 1968.

143. Steiner M, J Anastasi: Vitamin E: an inhibitor of the platelet release reaction. J Clin Invest 57:732, 1976.

144. Glass F, H Lippon, PJ Kadowitz: Effects of methylprednisolone and hydrocortisone on aggregation of rabbit platelets induced by arachidonic acid and other aggregating substances. Thromb Haemost 46:676, 1981.

145. Pierce CH, G Oshiro, M Nickerson: Effect of methylpredisone sodium succinate (MP) on platelet aggregation. Circulation 49(suppl III):289, 1974.

146. Neild GH, G Rocchi, L Imberti, F Fumagalli, Z Brown, G

Remuzzi, DG Williams: Effect of cyclosporin A on prostacyclin synthesis by vascular tree. Thromb Res 32:373, 1983.

147. Michel H, JP Caen, GVR Born: Relation between the inhibition of aggregation and the concentration of cAMP in human and rat platelets. Br J Haematol 33:27, 1976.

148. Rajah SM, MJ Crow, AF Perry, R Ahmad, DA Watson: The effects of dipyridamole on platelet function: correlation with blood levels in man. Br J Clin Pharmacol 4:129, 1979.

149. Ardlie NG, G Glew, BG Shultz, CJ Schwartz: Inhibition and reversal of platelet aggregation by methylxanthines. Thromb Diath Haemorrh 18:670, 1968.

150. Wolf SM, NR Shulman: Inhibition of platelet energy production and release reaction by PGE1, theophylline and cAMP. Biochem Biophys Res Commun 41:128, 1970.

151. Ball G, GG Brereton, M Fulwood, DM Ireland, P Yate: Effect of prostaglandin E, alone and in combination with theophylline or aspirin on collagen-induced platelet aggregation and on platelet nucleotides including adenosine 3':5'-cyclic monophosphate. Biochem J 120:709, 1970.

152. White JG: Effects of colchicine and vinca alkaloids on human platelets. I. Influence on platelet microtubules and contractile function. Am J Pathol 53:281, 1968.

153. Soppitt GD, JRA Mitchell: The effect of colchicine on human platelet behavior. J Atheroscler Res 10:247, 1969.

154. Zieve PD, HM Solomon: Effects of diuretics on the human platelet. Am J Physiol 215:650, 1968.

155. Murer EH, E Siojo: Inhibition of thrombin-induced secretion from platelets by chlortetracycline and its analogs. Thromb Haemost 47:62, 1982.

156. Carter AE, R Eban, RD Perrett: Prevention of postoperative deep venous thrombosis and pulmonary embolism. Br Med J 1:312, 1971.

157. Spooner M, OO Meyers: The effect of dicumerol (3.3-methylenebis) (4-hydroxy-coumarin) on platelet adhesiveness. Am J Physiol 142:279, 1944.

158. Saxon A, H Kattlove: Platelet inhibition by sodium nitroprusside, a smooth muscle inhibitor. Blood 47:957, 1976.

159. Rattazzi L, MN Haimov: Role of the platelet in the obliterative vascular transplant rejection phenomenon. Surg Forum 21:243, 1970.

160. Silverman JL, HA Wurzel: The effect of glyceryl guiacolate on platelet function and other coagulation factors in vivo. Am J Clin Pathol 51:35, 1969.

161. O'Brien JR, SM Shoobridge, WJ Finch: Comparison of the effect of heparin and citrate on platelet aggregation. J Clin Pathol 22:28, 1969.

162. Salzman EW, RD Rosenberg, HJ Smith, JN Lindon, L Favreau: Effect of heparin and heparin fractions on platelet aggregation. J Clin Invest 65:621, 1980.

163. Zucker MB: Effect of heparin on platelet function. Thromb Diath Haemorrh 33:63, 1975.

164. Wessler S, SN Gitel: Heparin: new concepts relevant to clinical use. Blood 53:525, 1979.

165. Schafer AJ, RW Alexander, RT Handin: Inhibition of platelet function by organic nitrate vasodilators. Blood 55:649, 1980.

166. Amezcua JL, M Parsons, S Moncada: Unstable metabolites of arachidonic acid, aspirin and the formation of the haemostatic plug. Thromb Res 13:477, 1978.

167. Altman R, A Scaziotta, JC Funes: Why single daily dose of aspirin may not prevent platelet aggregation. Thromb Res 51:259, 1988.

168. Weksler BB, SB Pett, D Alnoso, RC Richter, P Stelzer, V Subramanian, K Tack-Golman, WA Gay: Inhibition by aspirin of vascular and platelet prostaglandin synthesis in atherosclerotic patients. N Engl J Med 308:800, 1983.

169. Patrignani P, P Filabozzi, C Patrono: Selective cumulative inhibition of platelet thromboxane production by low-dose aspirin in healthy subjects. J Clin Invest 69:1366, 1982.

170. Preston FE, M Greaves, CA Jackson: Cumulative inhibitory effect of daily 40 mg aspirin on prostacyclin synthesis. Lancet 1:1211, 1981.

171. Yamauchi K, H Furui, N Taniguchi: Effects of diltiazem hydrochloride on cardiovascular response, platelet aggregation, and coagulation activity during exercise testing in systemic hypertension. Am J Cardiol 57:609, 1986.

172. Hines R, PG Barash: Infusion of sodium nitroprusside induces platelet dysfunction in vitro. Anesthesiology 70:611, 1989.

173. Hines R: Preservation of platelet function during trimethaphan infusion. Anesthesiology 72:834, 1990.

174. Bick RL, LF Fekete: Cardiopulmonary bypass hemorrhage: aggrevation by pre-op ingestion of antiplatelet agents. Vasc Surg 13:277, 1979.

175. Leist ER, JG Banwell: Products containing aspirin. N Engl J Med 291:710, 1974.

176. Selner JC: More aspirin-containing drugs. N Engl J Med 292:372, 1975.

177. Born GVR: Aggregation of blood platelets by adenosine diphosphate and its reversal. Nature 194:927, 1962.

178. Polasek T, F Duckert: Quantitative determination of platelet factor 3 activity. Thromb Diath Haemorrh 25:532, 1971.

179. Weiss HJ, JW Eichelberger: The detection of platelet defects in patients with mild bleeding disorders: use of quantitative assay for platelet factor 3. Am J Med 32:872, 1962.

180. Bick RL, T Adams, WR Schmalhorst: Bleeding times, platelet adhesion and aspirin. Am J Clin Pathol 65:65, 1976.

181. Rodgers RPC: Bleeding time tables: a tabular summary of pertinent literature. Semin Thromb Hemost 16:21, 1990.

182. Ruggeri ZM, TS Zimmerman: Platelets and von Willebrand disease. Semin Hematol 22:203, 1985.

183. Vericel E, M Croset, P Sedivy, P Courpron, M Dechavanne, M Lagarde: Platelets and aging I-arachidonate metabolism and antioxidant status. Thromb Res 49:331, 1988.

184. Feinman RD, MP Zabinski, J Lubowsky: Simultaneous measurement of aggregation and secretion. In: HJ Day, H Holmsen, MB Zucker (Eds): Platelet Function Testing. DHEW Publication (NIH) #78-1087, 1978, p 133.

185. Miller JL: Platelet function testing: an improved approach utilizing lumi-aggregation and an interactive computer. Am J Clin Pathol 81:471, 1984.

186. Feinman RD, J Lubowsky, I Charo, MP Zabinski: The lumi-aggregometer: a new instrument for simultaneous measurement of secretion and aggregation. J Lab Clin Med 90:125, 1977.

187. Adams GA: In vivo and in vitro platelet function testing. Plasma Ther Transfus Technol 3:265, 1982.

188. Henry RL: Platelet function. Semin Thromb Hemost 4:93, 1977.

189. Harms C: Laboratory evaluation of platelet function, ch 2. In: DA Triplett (Ed): Platelet Function: Laboratory Evaluation and Clinical Application. ASCP Press, Chicago, IL, 1978, p 35.

190. Packham MA, RL Kinlough-Rathbone, JF Mustard: Aggregation and agglutination. In: HJ Day, H Holmsen, MB Zucker (Eds): Platelet Function Testing. DHEW Publication (NIH) #78-1087, 1978, p 66.

191. Johnson GL, LA Leis, GHR Rao, JG White: Arachidonate-induced platelet aggregation in the dog. Thromb Res 14: 147, 1979.

192. Sweeney JD, JW Labuzetta, JE Fitzpatrick: The effect of the platelet count on the aggregation response and adenosine triphosphate release in an impedence lumi-aggregometer. Am J Clin Pathol 89:655, 1988.

193. Malmgren R: ATP secretion occurs as an initial response in collagen-induced platelet activation. Thromb Res 43: 445, 1986.

194. Hoyer L: von Willebrand's disease. Prog Hemost Thromb 3:231, 1976.

195. Karpatkin S, O Khan, M Freedman: Heterogeneity of platelet function: correlation with platelet volume. Am J Med 64:542, 1978.

196. Kraytman M: Platelet size in thrombocytopenias and thrombocytosis of various origin. Blood 41:587, 1973.

197. Harker LA: Platelet survival time: its measurement and use. Prog Hemost Thromb 4:321, 1978.

198. Karpatkin S, A Charmatz: Heterogeneity of human platelets, I: metabolic and kinetic evidence suggestive of young and old platelets. J Clin Invest 48:1073, 1969.

199. Penington DG, NLY Lee, AE Roxburgh, JR McGready: Platelet density and size: the interpretation of heterogeneity. Br J Haematol 34:365, 1976.

200. Roper-Drewinko P, B Drewinko, G Corrigan, D Johnston, KB McCredie, EJ Freireich: Standardization of platelet function tests. Am J Hematol 11:183, 1981.

201. Rowan RM, C Fraser, JH Gray: Comparison of channelyser and model S plus determined platelet size measurements. Clin Lab Haematol 3:165, 1981.

202. Corash L, B Shafter, D Weinberg, MB Steinfeld: Platelet sizing in whole blood total platelet populations. In: Day NJ, H Holmsen, MB Zucker (Eds): Platelet Function Testing. DHEW Publication (NIH) #78-1087, 1978, p 315.

203. Bick RL, BJ McClain: Platelet indices as markers of acute thrombosis and response to antithrombotic study. Thromb Haemost 50:153, 1983.

204. Weiss HJ: Antiplatelet drugs in clinical medicine, ch 4. In: Platelets: Pathophysiology and Antiplatelet Drug Therapy. Alan R Liss Inc, New York, 1982, p 75.

205. Renney JTG, EF O'Sullivan, PF Burke: Prevention of postoperative deep vein thrombosis with dipyridamole and aspirin. Br Med J 2:992, 1976.

206. Blanke H, G Praetorius, M Leschke: Significance of the thrombin-antithrombin III complex in the diagnosis of pulmonary embolus and deep venous thrombosis: a comparison with fibrinopeptide A, platelet factor 4 and beta-thromboglobulin. Klin Wochenschr 65:757, 1987.

207. Grande P, AM Grauholt, JK Madsen: Unstable angina pectoris: platelet behavior and prognosis in progressive angina and intermediate coronary sydrome. Circulation 81:16, 1990.

208. Rapold HJ, A Haeberli, H Kuemmerli: Fibrin formation and platelet activation in patients with myocardial infarction and normal coronary arteries. Eur Heart J 10:323, 1989.

209. von Reucker A, P Hufnagel, R Dickerhoff: Qualitative and quantitative changes in platelets after coronary artery bypass surgery may help identify thrombotic complications and infections. Klin Wochenschr 67:1042, 1989.

210. Dalby-Kristensen S, PC Milner, JF Martin: Bleeding time and platelet volume in acute myocardial infarction: a 2-year follow-up study. Thromb Haemost 59:353, 1988.

211. Erne P, J Wardle, K Sanders: Mean platelet volume and size distribution and their sensitivity to agonists in patients with coronary artery disease and congestive heart failure. Thromb Haemost 59:259, 1988.

212. Cortellaro M, E Cofrancesco, A Vicari: High heparin released platelet factor 4 in uncomplicated type 1 diabetes mellitus. Thromb Res 58:571, 1990.

213. Sinzinger H, I Virgolini, P Fitscha: Platelet kinetics in patients with atherosclerosis. Thromb Res 57:507, 1990.

214. Arusio E, C Lechi, P Pancera: Usefulness of several laboratory tests on prethrombotic status in arterial vascular pathology. Recenti Prog Med 80:18, 1989.

215. Tohgi H, H Suzuki, K Tamura: Platelet volume, aggregation, and adenosine triphosphate release in cerebral thrombosis. Stroke 22:17, 1991.

216. Catalano M, U Russo, S Belletti: Beta-TG and plasma catecholamines levels after sympathetic stimuli in hypertensives and patients with peripheral vascular disease. Thromb Haemost 63:383, 1990.

217. Wilson J, MA Orchard, AA Spencer: Anti-hypertensive drugs non-specifically reduce "spontaneous" activation of blood platelets. Thromb Haemost 62:776, 1989.

218. Uchiyama S, Y Tsutsumi, T Nagayama: Antiplatelet effects of combination therapy with low-dose aspirin and ticlopidine in cerebral ischemia. Rinsho Shinkeigaku 29:579, 1989.

219. Minar E, H Ehringer: Influence of acetylsalicylic acid (1.0 g/day) on platelet survival time, beta-thromboglobulin and platelet factor 4 in patients wih peripheral arterial occlusive disease. Thromb Res 45:791, 1987.

220. Gerbasi FR, S Bottoms, A Farag: Changes in hemostasis activity during delivery and the immediate postpartum period. Am J Obstet Gynecol 162:1158, 1990.

221. Rao AK, M Schapira, ML Clements: A prospective study of platelets and plasma proteolytic systems during the early stages of Rocky Mountain spotted fever. N Engl J Med 318:1021, 1988.

222. Gilabert J, A Estelles, J Anzar: Contribution of platelets to increased plasminogen activator inhibitor type 1 in severe preeclampsia. Thromb Haemost 63:361, 1990.

223. Hgevold HE, HH Mundal, N Norman: Platelet release reaction and plasma catecholamines during total hip replacement. Thromb Res 57:21, 1990.

224. Paramo JA, E Rocha: Deep vein thrombosis and related platelet changes after total hip replacement. Haemostasis 15:389, 1985.

225. Dumoulin-Lagrange M, C Capelle: Evaluation of automated platelet counters for the enumeration and sizing of platelets in the diagnosis and management of hemostatic problems. Semin Thromb Hemost 9:235, 1983.

226. Fareed J, JM Walenga, RL Bick, EJ Bermes, HL Messmore: Impact of automation on the quantitation of low molecular weight markers of hemostatic defects. Semin Thromb Hemost 9:355, 1983.

227. Fareed J, JM Walenga: Current trends in hemostatic testing. Semin Thromb Hemost 9:380, 1983.

228. Minar E, H Ehringer, M Jung, R Koppensteiner, A Stumpflen: Lack of influence of low-dose acetylsalicylic acid (100 mg daily) on platelet survival time, beta-thromboglobulin and platelet factor 4 in patients with peripheral arterial occlusive disease.Thromb Res 52:219, 1988.

229. Sinzinger H, J Kaliman, J O'Grady: Platelet lipoxygenase defect (Wien-Penzing Defect) in two patients with myocardial infarction. Am J Hematol 36:202, 1991.

Quantitative Platelet Defects

The common clinical findings of qualitative or quantitative platelet defects are petechiae and purpura, mild to moderate mucosal membrane bleeding, including bilateral epistaxis, gastrointestinal and genitourinary bleeding, and a history of easy and spontaneous bruising.[1] In addition, gingival bleeding with toothbrushing is a common clinical manifestation of platelet dysfunction or thrombocytopenia.[2] As was emphasized in chapters 2 and 3, gingival bleeding with toothbrushing can be normal if occurring occasionally, but if a patient relates gingival bleeding with toothbrushing frequently, then a platelet function defect, thrombocytopenia, or a vascular defect should be suspected. In platelet function defects or thrombocytopenia, petechiae and purpura are usually symmetrical (ie, found throughout the integumentary system, on the extremities as well as the torso). This is in distinction to the noting of dependent petechiae and purpura, which are more commonly associated with vascular disorders.[1] Clinical findings of platelet defects are summarized in Table 5-1.

Table 5-2 depicts traditional tests of platelet number and function, including older tests. New methodologies of assessing molecular markers of platelet reactivity and other modalities to assess platelet function were discussed in chapter 4. First, and extremely important in assessing platelets, is careful evaluation of a peripheral blood smear for a quantitative estimation of platelet number and evaluation of platelet morphology. This test is an often neglected simple modality performed in the hematology laboratory and certainly should be carefully evaluated in patients presenting with easy or spontaneous bruising and/or petechiae and purpura. Many clinical clues may be obtained from an evaluation of platelet morphology such the abnormal granularity in the gray platelet syndrome, the large platelets and borderline thrombocytopenia of Bernard-Soulier syndrome, or the many "large bizarre" platelets or young platelets indicative of rapid platelet turnover and decreased platelet survival. An examination of a peripheral blood smear may actually lead to the specific diagnosis accounting for petechiae and purpura or easy bruising (eg, an acute or chronic leukemia). In addition, a quantitative platelet count should always be performed. Only in the face of a normal platelet count can a platelet function defect be defined.[2] Platelet function defects were discussed in chapter 4.

Platelet defects are most easily divided into quantitative and qualitative types. The qualitative disorders, platelet function defects, are further divided into hereditary and acquired types and were discussed in chapter 4.

Quantitative defects are best divided into three categories: thrombocytopenia due to decreased production and metabolic/maturation defects, including the hereditary, congenital, and infantile thrombocytopenias associated with decreased platelet production, the acquired platelet production defects, and drug-induced nonimmune thrombocytopenias; acquired thrombocytopenia due to increased destruction, increased consumption, or peripheral loss; and thrombocytosis and thrombocythemia. Table 5-3 summarizes the quantitative platelet defects.

Thrombocytopenia

Pseudothrombocytopenia

Pseudothrombocytopenia is a laboratory artifact that may occur via several mechanisms and should be investigated thoroughly in the asymptomatic patient before embarking on an extensive and expensive evaluation for thrombocytopenia.[3]

Platelet autoagglutinins are usually IgG and/or IgM,[4] which may induce spontaneous autoagglutination of platelets, or, in some instances, IgG and IgM autoagglutination activity may be enhanced by the anticoagulant ethylenediaminetetraacetic acid (EDTA).[5] Additionally, adherence of platelets to granulocytes (platelet satellitism) may occur, which may be mediated by EDTA and/or platelet membrane IgG.[6,7] If unexplained thrombocytopenia is seen with an automated platelet counter, the peripheral blood smear should be carefully observed for platelet clumps (autoagglutination) or platelet satellitism. Pseudothrombocytopenia may also be noted in patients with a sig-

Table 5-1. Clinical Findings of Platelet Defects

Petechiae and purpura (usually symmetric)

Easy and spontaneous bruising

Gingival bleeding with toothbrushing

Mild to moderate mucosal membrane bleeding
    Gastrointestinal
    Genitourinary
    Bilateral epistaxis
    Pulmonary

nificantly expanded plasma volume, such as patients with marked fluid overload or patients with hyperviscosity syndromes. Pseudothrombocytopenia may also occur when a small platelet-trapping clot forms in the collection tube.[8] Instances of unexplained spontaneous platelet aggregation may occur, presumably from the presence of "hyperactive" or partially activated platelets that may aggregate in vivo or in vitro, giving rise to pseudothrombocytopenia. Unless pseudothrombocytopenia is suspected and investigated, an expensive and extensive examination of the patient may be unnecessarily instituted. Additionally, a misdiagnosis may be made, and inappropriate or unnecessary therapy may be rendered. Unnecessary splenectomy has been performed in patients with pseudothrombocytopenia suspected of having steroid-resistant immune thrombocytopenia purpura (ITP).[9] Although EDTA-induced clumping of platelets is the most common cause of pseudothrombocytopenia, other causes are listed in Table 5-4. When pseudothrombocytopenia is suspected, the platelets should be evaluated on a peripheral blood smear after blood collection in EDTA, and the platelet count should be repeated by finger-stick technique with an ammonium oxalate unipette and counting by phase microscopy.[8] Pretreating EDTA Vacutainers with 2.5 mL of acid citrate dextrose (ACD) or heparin has been noted to eradicate pseudothrombocytopenia.[10,11]

Decreased Platelet Production

Congenital and Neonatal Defects

Congenital and neonatal decreased platelet production defects are summarized in Table 5-5.

Table 5-2. Laboratory Assessment of Platelet Defects

Peripheral smear evaluation
Quantitative platelet count
Template bleeding time
Aspirin tolerance test
Petechiometer test (children and elderly)
Platelet aggregation and lumi-aggregation
Platelet factor 3 availability
Platelet factor 4 release
Serotonin release
Platelet-associated antibodies (direct and indirect)

Table 5-3. Types of Quantitative Platelet Defects

Thrombocytopenia
    Hereditary and congenital
    Decreased production
        Marrow defects
        Drug induced
        Infection
    Increased destruction
        Nonimmune
        Immune
        Drug induced
    Peripheral loss

Thrombocytosis

Thrombocythemia

Reactive platelets (prethrombotic?)

Fanconi's Syndrome

Fanconi's syndrome is a rare disorder inherited as an autosomal recessive trait that consists of congenital aplastic anemia with multiple congenital abnormalities.[12,13] The salient features are summarized in Table 5-6. Thrombocytopenia may precede the development of granulocytopenia and anemia, but macrocytic anemia is the most pronounced hematologic feature noted. Bone marrow hypoplasia is almost always seen. Other defects include hypermelanosis of the skin, microcephaly, dwarfism, strabismus, ocular blepharoptosis, nystagmus, hyperactive deep tendon reflexes, deafness, mental retardation, and numerous skeletal abnormalities.[14] Congenital heart disease may be present. The hematologic abnormalities usually occur after the age of 4 years and are usually present before the early teenage years. Splenectomy may increase the platelet count to nonbleeding levels. The most common cause of death in patients with Fanconi's syndrome is intracranial or gastrointestinal hemorrhage. Life-threatening hemorrhages should be treated with appropriate numbers of platelet transfusions. Single-donor platelets are preferable, since these patients are candidates for numerous platelet transfusions throughout their lifetimes. In some instances, a moderate response to the thrombocytopenia has been seen with androgens, but a rise in platelet count may require several months.

Tar Baby Syndrome

The Tar baby syndrome (thrombocytopenia and absent radii) is inherited as an autosomal recessive trait associated

Table 5-4. Causes of Pseudothrombocytopenia

EDTA-induced platelet autoagglutination
IgG- or IgM-induced platelet autoagglutination
Platelet satellitism
Expanded plasma volume
Collection tube clot formation
Spontaneous platelet aggregation (in vivo or in vitro)

Table 5-5. Causes of Congenital and Neonatal Decreased Platelet Production

Alport's syndrome

Bernard-Soulier syndrome

Congenital thrombopoietin deficiency

Fanconi's syndrome

Gray platelet syndrome

May-Hegglin anomaly

Tar baby syndrome

Wiskott-Aldrich syndrome

Congenital marrow infiltration
   Congenital leukemias
   Congenital reticuloendothelioses
   Congenital mucopolysaccharidoses
   Congenital granulomatous diseases

Maternal drug ingestion
   Ethanol
   Thiazides
   Tolbutamide
   Steroids (estrogen and progesterone)

Maternal infections
   Cytomegalovirus
   Hepatitis
   Rubella
   Varicella

Table 5-6. Fanconi's Syndrome

Clinical Findings
   Autosomal recessive
   Usually manifest after 4 years of age
   Petechiae and purpura
   Gastrointestinal hemorrhage
   Intracranial hemorrhage
   Hypermelanosis
   Microcephaly
   Mental retardation
   Hyperactive deep tendon reflexes
   Deafness
   Ocular blepharoptosis
   Skeletal deformities
   Dwarfism
   Congenital heart defects

Laboratory Findings
   Bone marrow hypoplasia
   Aplastic anemia
   Macrocytic anemia
   Granulocytopenia
   Thrombocytopenia

Therapy
   Platelet concentrates
   Androgens?

with severe thrombocytopenia caused by marked deficiency of marrow megakaryocytes.[15,16] Bilateral aplasia of the radii is the most common associated abnormality, but cardiac and renal abnormalities may also be present. The characteristic features are noted in Table 5-7. Infections with rubella have been incriminated in some instances.[17] More than 50% of patients die of intracranial hemorrhage before reaching 1 year of age.[15] Splenectomy or androgens usually do not correct thrombocytopenia, but a few responses have been noted.[18] The syndrome is differentiated from Fanconi's syndrome by the earlier onset and absence of granulocytopenia and anemia. When life-threatening bleeding occurs, platelet concentrates, preferably directed single-donor platelets, should be infused to control bleeding. Single-donor platelets are preferable since long-term platelet concentrate requirements can usually be anticipated.

Wiskott-Aldrich Syndrome

The Wiskott-Aldrich syndrome is a rare sex-linked recessive disorder characterized by severe eczema, increased susceptibility to infections, and severe thrombocytopenia[19,20] (Table 5-8). Circulating platelets are classically small and demonstrate a decreased mean platelet volume (MPV) when evaluated by electronic particle counters that have this capa-

bility.[21] Severe bleeding usually becomes manifest in the first 6 months of life, and then it may, like many other hereditary hemostasis defects, tend to improve. However, patients who survive bleeding episodes in their early childhood commonly die of overwhelming pyogenic infections or a malignancy, usually lymphoma.[19] Cellular and humoral immune defects are present,[22-24] and patients usually demonstrate decreased IgM levels with normal IgG and IgA levels. Steroids are usually not effective, even though some investigators have postulated that the thrombocytopenia of the Wiskott-Aldrich syndrome is due to IgG-induced immune mechanisms.[25,26] Splenectomy, however, has been successful in selected patients,[27] but this procedure places them at an

Table 5-7. Tar Baby Syndrome

Clinical Findings
   Autosomal recessive
   Petechiae and purpura
   Intracranial hemorrhage (50%)
   Absence of radii, bilaterally
   Congenital cardiac defects
   Congenital renal defects

Laboratory Findings
   Thrombocytopenia
   Deficiency of marrow megakaryocytes

Therapy
   Platelet concentrates

Table 5-8. Wiskott-Aldrich Syndrome

Clinical Findings
  Sex-linked recessive
  Severe thrombocytopenia
  Severe hemorrhage
  Bleeding improves with age
  Severe eczema
  Pyogenic infections

Laboratory Findings
  Severe thrombocytopenia
  Small platelets
  Decreased MPV
  Decreased IgM
  IgG and IgA usually normal
  Cellular immune defects
  Humoral immune defects

Therapy
  Platelet concentrates
  Splenectomy?

Table 5-10. Alport's Syndrome

Clinical Findings
  Autosomal dominant trait
  Microscopic or gross hematuria common
  Bleeding from other sites uncommon
  Deafness

Laboratory Findings
  Thrombocytopenia
  Increased MPV
  Platelet function defect
  Sclerosing glomerular lesions
  Interstitial nephritis

even greater risk of infection because of the already compromised cellular and humoral immune defects. Patients undergoing splenectomy for thrombocytopenia associated with Wiskott-Aldrich syndrome should either be given prophylactic antibiotic therapy or should be followed up carefully for observation, performance of rapid cultures, and institution of appropriate antibiotic therapy as soon as suggestive symptoms appear. Patients undergoing splenectomy should receive pneumococcal vaccine.[1]

Congenital Thrombopoietin Deficiency

Several cases of congenital thrombopoietin deficiency have been reported.[28,29] These cases are characterized by severe thrombocytopenia in the presence of adequate marrow megakaryocytes. Patients have not responded to steroids or splenectomy, but infusions of plasma or whole blood, pre-

sumably providing thrombopoietin, induce a rise in platelet counts. In the few cases reported, patients demonstrated a microangiopathic hemolytic anemia and features suggestive of hemolytic uremic syndrome. Thus, it may be disputed that some of these cases may indeed represent hemolytic-uremic syndrome or thrombotic thrombocytopenic purpura rather than congenital thrombopoietin deficiency.

May-Hegglin Anomaly

The May-Hegglin anomaly is inherited as an autosomal dominant trait and is extremely rare.[30] The disorder is characterized by giant platelets and a greatly increased MPV when platelet counts are performed by electronic particle counters.[31] Large Döhle's bodies are seen in peripheral and marrow granulocytes, and most patients have a mild neutropenia but no significant increased susceptibility to infection.[32] About 50% of patients have significant thrombocytopenia, but life-threatening hemorrhage is rare. However, some patients with severe thrombocytopenia do have significant hemorrhage. In those individuals who are significantly thrombocytopenic, marrow megakaryocytes are normal in number. The platelets of the May-Hegglin anomaly are not only enlarged, but many also display bizarre morphology and hypergranularity. The features of the May-Hegglin anomaly are listed in Table 5-9.

Table 5-9. May-Hegglin Anomaly

Clinical Findings
  Autosomal dominant trait
  Severe hemorrhage rare

Laboratory Findings
  Thrombocytopenia in 50%
  Giant platelets
  Increase MPV
  Bizarre morphology of platelets
  Hypergranularity of platelets
  Marrow megakaryocytes normal
  Dohle bodies in granulocytes

Therapy
  Platelet concentrates

Alport's Syndrome

Alport's syndrome is inherited as an autosomal dominant trait and is characterized clinically by proliferative and sclerosing glomerulonephritis, associated interstitial nephritis and fibrosis, and deafness.[33] Thrombocytopenia with an increased MPV is characteristically present, and, in addition, platelets harbor a poorly defined platelet function defect.[34,35] Clinical hemorrhage is usually manifest as microscopic or gross hematuria; however, severe nonrenal hemorrhage may also occur. Significant or life-threatening hemorrhage should be treated with, and usually responds to, the use of platelet concentrates. The features of Alport's syndrome are summarized in Table 5-10.

Table 5-11. Gray Platelet Syndrome

Clinical Findings
  Autosomal dominant trait
  Petechiae and purpura
  Ecchymoses
  Severe hemorrhage may occur

Laboratory Findings
  Thrombocytopenia
  Large gray platelets
  Increased MPV
  Platelets agranular or hypogranular
  Absence of alpha granules
    Decreased platelet factor 4
    Decreased beta-thromboglobulin
  Platelet nucleotides normal
  Platelet aggregation normal

Therapy
  Platelet concentrates
  Splenectomy

Gray Platelet Syndrome

The gray platelet syndrome is a rare disorder inherited as an autosomal dominant trait and characterized by large platelets and an increased MPV.[36] The platelets of the gray platelet syndrome are either markedly hypogranular or agranular.[37] The thrombocytopenia is usually pronounced, and severe hemorrhage may occur. The hypogranularity or agranularity is due to an absence or marked reduction of alpha granules. Although adenine nucleotide pools remain normal, the platelets lack beta-thromboglobulin and platelet factor 4.[38] Platelet function, however, as defined by aggregometry, is usually normal despite the absence of granularity and the large size of the platelets. If significant bleeding occurs, the thrombocytopenia can usually be normalized by splenectomy. If indicated, platelet concentrates should be used to control life-threatening hemorrhage.[1] The features of this syndrome are depicted in Table 5-11.

Bernard-Soulier Syndrome

Although the Bernard-Soulier syndrome was discussed in detail in chapter 4, it should be re-emphasized that this disorder is inherited as an autosomal recessive trait, platelets are markedly enlarged, a significantly elevated MPV is demonstrated, and shortened platelet survival may be seen. The degree of thrombocytopenia is moderate to severe. In some individuals, however, thrombocytopenia is periodic or absent. Since the Bernard-Soulier platelet classically does not aggregate to ristocetin, the disorder can be superficially confused with the von Willebrand's variant associated with thrombocytopenia unless platelet morphology is carefully examined and definitive laboratory assessment of von Willebrand's syndrome is performed. In patients with significant thrombocytopenia and Bernard-Soulier syndrome, splenectomy is usually not of benefit and not indicated.[1]

Other Congenital Defects

Reports of thrombocytopenia in von Willebrand's variant have been noted.[39] Von Willebrand's syndrome and its variants will be discussed in chapter 6. Hereditary thrombocytopenias of unclear pathophysiologic mechanisms have also been described, and several mechanisms of inheritance have been noted in these disorders.[31,40-44] These disorders may be inherited as an autosomal dominant trait, and those of autosomal dominant inheritance are divided into those with normal platelet survival and those with shortened platelet survival.[1] Rare hereditary thrombocytopenias of sex-linked inheritance, some with an associated elevation of IgA but without other characteristics of Alport's syndrome, have been described. Hereditary thrombocytopenia with autosomal recessive inheritance has also been described.[45] It may be impossible to distinguish many of these individuals from patients with immune thrombocytopenia purpura (ITP), especially if shortened platelet survival is documented.[1]

Congenital Marrow Infiltrative Disorders

The most common congenital marrow infiltrative processes leading to significant thrombocytopenia are the congenital leukemias and the congenital reticuloendothelioses. Thrombocytopenia with and without associated myeloid and erythroid depression occurs in children with numerous infiltrative disorders including leukemia, lymphoma, solid tumors, myelofibrosis, Gaucher's disease, Niemann-Pick disease, and the mucopolysaccharidoses.[46-48] Infiltrative thrombocytopenia may also be seen with granulomatous diseases. A leukoerythroblastic reaction noted on the peripheral blood smear may be seen in these clinical settings, and the noting of thrombocytopenia in association with teardrop red blood cells, nucleated red blood cells, marked anisocytosis and poikilocytosis, and polychromatophilia in some neonates and infants should suggest thrombocytopenia due to a marrow infiltrative process.

Maternal Disorders

Maternal ingestion of ethanol, thiazides, chlorpropamide, tolbutamide, or steroids, especially prednisone and estrogens, may lead to severe thrombocytopenia in the newborn.[49-54] In addition, if a pregnant woman ingests cytotoxic chemotherapeutic drugs that are capable of crossing the placenta, neonatal thrombocytopenia may result.

Maternal infections with cytomegalovirus, hepatitis, varicella, or rubella may lead to congenital thrombocytopenia in the newborn; additionally, recent maternal vaccinations (rubella or rubeola) may lead to neonatal thrombocytopenia.[55-57] Although these appear to be the most common, many other maternal viral infestations may also lead to congenital thrombocytopenia.[58]

Acquired Defects

Common causes of acquired platelet production defects are summarized in Table 5-12.

Table 5-12. Acquired Platelet Production Defects

Aplastic anemia

Isolated megakaryocyte aplasia (rare)

Marrow infiltrative diseases
  Leukemia
  Lymphoma
  Hodgkin's disease
  Metastatic carcinoma
  Myelofibrosis
  Myelosclerosis
  Gaucher's disease
  Niemann-Pick disease
  Mucopolysaccharidoses
  Infiltrative infections
    Coccidioidomycosis
    Tuberculosis
    Toxoplasmosis
    Histoplasmosis
    Various bacteria
    Various viruses

Drug-induced marrow suppression
  Cytotoxic chemotherapy
  Thiazides
  Ethanol
  Gold
  Anti-inflammatory drugs
  Tranquilizers
  Anticonvulsants

Cyclic thrombocytopenia

Renal failure

Myeloproliferative syndromes

Maturation/metabolic defects
  B_{12} deficiency
  Folate deficiency

Aplastic Anemia

Aplastic anemia is often associated with severe thrombocytopenia.[59] Thrombocytopenia may precede the myeloid and erythroid decreases by weeks to months in patients who are developing aplastic anemia, and early in the course of the disorder bone marrow examination may demonstrate only an absence of megakaryocytes.[60] Thrombocytopenia associated with aplastic anemia may lag many months behind the increase of myeloid and erythroid elements in recovering patients. In addition, many patients with aplastic anemia who eventually regenerate erythroid and/or myeloid elements may continue to demonstrate thrombocytopenia indefinitely. The symptoms of thrombocytopenia, primarily petechiae, purpura, and hemorrhage, may often lead the patient to the clinician and eventually to the diagnosis of aplastic anemia. Circulating platelets in thrombocytopenia associated with aplastic anemia are usually associated with a decreased mean platelet volume.[61]

Megakaryocytic Marrow Aplasia

Isolated selective megakaryocyte marrow aplasia is an extremely rare condition.[62] This finding may sometimes herald the future development of an autoimmune disorder (such as systemic lupus erythematosus) or a preleukemic state, or may represent a toxic effect from a drug, toxin, or infectious agent that was forgotten by the patient and not related to the clinician. If vacuolated megakaryocytes are noted on a bone marrow examination, however, a preleukemic state, a drug or toxin, or an infection should be strongly suspected, and the patient should be appropriately examined and followed up.[46-48] Patients with selective megakaryocytic marrow aplasia may have normal numbers of megakaryocytes; however, decreased megakaryocytes are more commonly noted. Those patients with normal numbers of megakaryocytes may be difficult, if not impossible, to distinguish from patients with immune thrombocytopenia purpura.

Myelophthisic Disorders

Decreased platelet production due to marrow infiltration (myelophthisis) may occur from chronic or acute leukemias, lymphomas, Hodgkin's disease, or metastatic carcinoma, the latter most commonly occurring from metastatic lung, breast, or prostatic primary.[63] Myelofibrosis and myelosclerosis may also present with selective peripheral thrombocytopenia. Marrow infiltration by Gaucher's disease, Niemann-Pick disease, mucopolysaccharidoses, disseminated tuberculosis, coccidioidomycosis, histoplasmosis, toxoplasmosis, brucellosis, and malaria may induce marrow myelophthisis and subsequent peripheral thrombocytopenia.[64-71]

Marrow Suppression

Thrombocytopenia due to marrow suppression from the administration of chemotherapy is usually not selective but is often seen in combination with granulocytopenia and, less commonly, anemia. The drug that is most likely to cause selective thrombocytopenia from interference with megakaryocyte production is cytosine arabinoside. Other drugs causing severe thrombocytopenia are nitrogen mustard, melphalan, busulfan, chlorambucil, the nitrosoureas, and vinblastine.[72] Intermediate degrees of marrow toxicity with associated megakaryocyte insult and resultant peripheral thrombocytopenia include cyclophosphamide, 5-fluorouracil, 6-mercaptopurine, methotrexate, procarbazine, and actinomycin D, assuming DIC does not occur with this last agent.[72] Mild degrees of megakaryocyte toxicity and peripheral thrombocytopenia are seen with vincristine, blenoxane, L-asparaginase, cis-platinum, and hormones, including diethylstilbesterol and prednisone.[72] Thrombocytopenia may also be induced by the anti-estrogen drug, tamoxifen, but this is uncommon. Estrogens may occasionally cause thrombocytopenia by decreased production; however, more commonly estrogens, estrogen derivatives, and decadron are not only associated with an increased risk of thrombosis and thromboembolism but may also cause thrombocytopenia by inducing in vivo or in vitro platelet aggregation after a blood

Table 5-13. Degree of Thrombocytopenia With Antineoplastic Chemotherapy

Mild Thrombocytopenia
  L-asparaginase
  Bleomycin
  Cis-platinum
  Vincristine
  Diethylstilbesterol
  Prednisone
  Tamoxifen

Moderate Thrombocytopenia
  Actinomycin D
  Cyclophosphamide
  5-Fluorouracil
  6-Mercaptopurine
  Methotrexate
  Procarbazine

Severe Thrombocytopenia
  Busulfan
  Chlorambucil
  Cytosine arabinoside
  Melphalan
  Nitrogen mustard
  Nitrosourea compounds
  Vinblastine

Table 5-14. Common Drugs Causing Decreased Platelet Production

Acetaminophen
Acetazolamide
Allopurinol
Amphotericin
Aspirin
Benzene
Chloramphenicol
Chlordiazepoxide
Chlorpromazine
Chlorpropamide
Chlorthalidone
Cimetidine
Colchicine
Diazepam
Diethylstilbestrol
Diphenylhydantoin
Estrogens
Ethanol
Furosemide
Gold
Indomethacin
Mephenytoin
Meprobamate
Oxyphenbutazone
Phenylbutazone
Prednisone
Primidone
Pyrimethamine
Quinacrine
Streptomycin
Sulfamethoxazole
Sulfisoxazole
Sulfonamides
Thiazides
Tolbutamide

sample has been drawn for platelet counting. Degrees of thrombocytopenia associated with chemohormonal therapy are summarized in Table 5-13.

Grades of thrombocytopenia associated with marrow (megakaryocyte) suppression have been developed by the division of Hematology Oncology at UCLA and consist of the following: Grade 0, platelets approximately 100 x 10^9/L (100,000/mm³); Grade 1, platelets 75 to 99 x 10^9/L (75,000 to 99,000/mm³); Grade 2, platelets 50 to 74.999 x 10^9/L (50,000 to 74,999/mm³); Grade 3, platelets 25 to 49.999 x 10^9/L (25,000 to 49,999/mm³); and Grade 4, platelets less than 25 x 10^9/L (25,000/mm³).[72] With initiation of radiation therapy, platelet suppression occurs after several days; however, megakaryocytes are less susceptible to radiation than myeloid and erythroid precursors. Radiation may also lead to rare, although often catastrophic, severe myelofibrosis and subsequent irreversible and severe thrombocytopenia.[73]

Many drugs and chemicals are capable of inducing severe and, uncommonly, irreversible thrombocytopenia by nonimmune marrow suppression/production mechanisms. The drug or chemical may act at the promegakaryocyte stem-cell stage directly on the megakaryocyte, or, more rarely, on the circulating platelet. Thiazide diuretics are the most common etiologic agents, but ethanol, nonsteroidal anti-inflammatory drugs (NSAIDs), tranquilizers, and anticonvulsants are also common offenders.[52,74-77] Unlike drug- and chemical-induced immune-mediated thrombocytopenia, the thrombocytopenia associated with drug- or chemical-induced marrow suppres-

sion is gradual in onset, requires weeks to several months to become manifest, and megakaryocytes are usually decreased rather than increased, as is commonly seen in immune-induced thrombocytopenia. When the offending drug is removed, the platelet count is slow to return to normal in comparison to drug-induced immune-mediated thrombocytopenia, wherein recovery is usually rapid. If the drug or chemical exposure is continued for a long period, however, irreversible thrombocytopenia and aplastic anemia may ensue. A list of the common drugs and chemicals causing thrombocytopenia by nonimmune marrow suppressive mechanisms is provided in Table 5-14.

Cyclic Thrombocytopenia

Cyclic thrombocytopenia of unclear mechanisms has been noted in women and older men.[78-80] The average cycle or nadir of thrombocytopenia is approximately 30 days. Thrombocytopenia may be severe enough that dangerous or life-threatening hemorrhage may occur. Splenectomy and

Table 5-15. Common Viruses Causing Decreased
Platelet Production

Adenoviruses
Cytomegalovirus
Enteroviruses
Epstein-Barr virus
Hepatitis virus
Herpes simplex virus
Herpes zoster virus
Human immunodeficiency virus
Mumps virus
Rubella
Rubeola
Variola

prednisone therapy have been without significant benefit, and thus, platelet transfusions, preferably directed single-donor platelets, remain the treatment of choice.[1]

Infections

Infections associated with decreased production of platelets include numerous viral, bacterial, and fungal agents. Disseminated tuberculosis, coccidioidomycosis, brucellosis, and toxoplasmosis have been previously discussed. Megakaryocytes provide an ideal cell for bacterial and viral invasion and replication, therefore interfering with platelet production.[81-83] When this occurs, morphologic changes in megakaryocytes are usually noted on marrow examination and commonly consist of cytoplasmic vacuolization and nuclear degeneration. Megakaryocytes may also be decreased in number. Viral invasion of megakaryocytes, with resultant viral replication, subsequent megakaryocyte degeneration, and associated decreased platelet production, occurs in measles, including individuals receiving live measles vaccinations, infectious mononucleosis, herpes simplex and herpes zoster, cytomegalovirus infection, and hepatitis.[31,84-88] Viruses known to be associated with thrombocytopenia due to marrow-suppressive mechanisms are summarized in Table 5-15. Bacterial infections, especially septicemia, are often associated with thrombocytopenia[89]; however, it is often difficult, if not impossible, to incriminate marrow suppression alone as the mechanism. In many instances, DIC secondary to sepsis may be involved, bacterial-platelet complexes may cause splenic removal of platelets (peripheral loss), and antibiotic use may also contribute to thrombocytopenia via several mechanisms. In gram-negative sepsis, endotoxin may induce platelet release and subsequent thrombocytopenia. Thus, in patients with bacterial infections, especially with septicemia, the often associated thrombocytopenia is usually a clinical summation of numerous pathophysiologic mechanisms. Since the mechanisms are unclear and often impossible to define clinically, significant or life-threatening hemorrhage is treated with 6 to 8 units of platelet concentrates every six to 12 hours depending on the site and severity of hemorrhage. In septicemia, especially if due to gram-negative organisms, the patient should first be given intravenous hydrocortisone succinate at 15 mg/kg intravenous push followed by 7 mg/kg intravenous push every six hours for at least 24 hours.[1] The platelets can be given after the first intravenous dose of hydrocortisone succinate, which will often blunt any immune-induced component of the septicemia-associated thrombocytopenia.

Miscellaneous Problems

Renal failure may be associated with defective platelet production, although often the precise mechanisms remain unclear. Other causes for thrombocytopenia in patients with renal disease include splenomegaly and associated hypersplenism, circulating immune complex–mediated thrombocytopenia, and sometimes other mechanisms that may be a direct consequence of the underlying disease leading to renal failure.[90,91] The platelet function defect seen in renal failure is a much more common cause of significant bleeding in patients with renal disease and azotemia than is thrombocytopenia. Effective treatment of the underlying disease process leading to renal failure or vigorous hemodialysis will usually partially correct both the quantitative and qualitative platelet defects seen in these patients.

Unexplained thrombocytopenia may herald the development of several of the myeloproliferative syndromes, especially paroxysmal nocturnal hemoglobinuria (PNH).[92] Thrombocytosis, however, may also be seen with many myeloproliferative disorders, including chronic myelogenous leukemia, essential thrombocythemia, and polycythemia rubra vera.[93,94] The primary exceptions are PNH and myelofibrosis with agnogenic myeloid metaplasia, in which significant thrombocytopenia is seen in 30% of individuals. Although defective platelets are produced in PNH,[95] the basic defect is a characteristic abnormality of red blood cells manifest as increased sensitivity to complement-mediated osmotic lysis, with activation by the primary or alternate (properdin) complement activation pathway. The disease is clearly a clonal stem-cell disorder, because not only erythrocytes and megakaryocytes but also granulocytes are defective. Thus, the presumably neoplastic clonal change occurs in a stem-cell precursor common to the erythroid, myeloid, and megakaryocytic maturation stages. Little is known of the megakaryocyte/platelet defect in PNH. Platelets, like red blood cells, demonstrate increased sensitivity to complement-mediated lysis and have decreased acetylcholinesterase activity and decreased or absent decay accelerating factor (DAF), a compound that degrades and inhibits C3 convertase (C4b,2a complex).[96] The noting of pancytopenia, a decreased leukocyte alkaline phosphatase score, and a history of hemoglobinuria should prompt an acid hemolysis and sucrose hemolysis test for PNH. Thrombocytopenic bleeding is best treated with appropriate platelet concentrates, but this may induce further platelet lysis if complement is infused with the small amount of plasma present in platelet concentrates.

Maturation/Metabolic Defects

Severe iron deficiency may be associated with either thrombocytosis or thrombocytopenia.[97] The mechanisms of decreased platelet production remain unclear but may be related to the need for iron by megakaryocytes for platelet production. Iron therapy will usually induce prompt correction of the thrombocytopenia or thrombocytosis. Significant bleeding and the need for platelet transfusions are extremely rare in severe iron-deficiency anemia.

Patients with severe vitamin B_{12} or folate deficiency may present with hemorrhage, usually petechiae and purpura, due to thrombocytopenia.[98,99] Thrombocytopenia may be severe and is usually due to ineffective megakaryopoiesis. Other mechanisms are also operative, including absence of megakaryocytes in the marrow and reduced platelet survival. The thrombocytopenia of severe folate or vitamin B_{12} deficiency usually corrects promptly with appropriate hematinic therapy.

Increased Consumption or Destruction

Neonatal Defects

Maternal ingestion of certain drugs or agents known to induce immune-mediated thrombocytopenia may induce immune-mediated thrombocytopenia in the newborn if these agents are capable of crossing the placenta. The maternal ingestion of quinine, quinidine, hydralazine, or selected antibiotics known to induce immune-mediated thrombocytopenia may induce congenital immune-mediated thrombocytopenia.[49-52,100,101] Thrombocytopenia in these neonates usually abates rapidly and only rarely does severe or fatal hemorrhage occur.

A more serious neonatal thrombocytopenia can arise from a maternal immune reaction to fetal platelet antigens that have been inherited from the father of the child.[102] Transplacental passage of the maternal antibody (usually an IgG) may create a severe thrombocytopenia in the neonate in utero.[103] This usually occurs when the mother has PLA[1]-negative platelets and the fetus has inherited PLA[1]-positive platelets from the father.[102,104] In other instances, anti-HLA antibodies have been incriminated.[104,105] Infants with this type of alloimmune neonatal thrombocytopenia may be covered with petechiae and purpura, may demonstrate more severe hemorrhage at the time of birth, or may appear normal at delivery and then manifest severe bleeding within the first week after birth. The thrombocytopenia usually abates within one month. Since approximately 30% of these individuals may die of central nervous system hemorrhage, cesarean sections have been advocated to avoid the trauma of childbirth if a prenatal diagnosis has been made.[55] Other successful modes of therapy have been the use of platelet transfusions, exchange transfusions, and steroids in the severely thrombocytopenic infant.[103,106,107] Prenatal administration of corticosteroids to the mother may also be of benefit. Splenectomy does not appear to be useful, as the disorder

Table 5-16. Common Causes of Increased Platelet Destruction/Consumption in the Neonate

Maternal drug ingestion
  Quinine
  Quinidine
  Hydralazine
  Antibiotics

Alloimmune neonatal thrombocytopenia

Neonatal infection
  Toxoplasmosis
  Syphilis
  Rubella
  Herpesvirus
  Cytomegalovirus

Maternal immune thrombocytopenia purpura (ITP)

Maternal pre-eclampsia

Maternal eclampsia

is self-limiting and the other modalities of therapy will usually control significant hemorrhage.

Neonatal infection with toxoplasmosis, rubella, cytomegalovirus, herpesvirus, or syphilis may cause an immune-mediated increased platelet destruction. However, the mechanisms remain poorly understood and poorly defined.[108,109]

Other causes of neonatal thrombocytopenia due to increased platelet consumption or destruction include neonatal thrombocytopenia in association with maternal immune thrombocytopenia purpura (ITP). In addition, neonatal thrombocytopenia may occur in women who are pre-eclamptic or develop frank toxemia of pregnancy.[110] This topic will be addressed in chapter 7. Infants of women with lupus erythematosus or other autoimmune diseases, especially if the woman has a lupus anticoagulant or anticardiolipin antibodies, may be born with immune-mediated thrombocytopenia. It is unclear if patients without autoimmune disease but with an anticardiolipin antibody give birth to thrombocytopenic neonates.[111] Causes of neonatal increased platelet consumption/destruction are summarized in Table 5-16.

Acquired Defects

Nonimmune Mechanisms

Hemolytic-Uremic Syndrome. Hemolytic-uremic syndrome (HUS) is a poorly understood platelet consumptive disease first described in 1955[112] that may be related to thrombotic thrombocytopenic purpura or disseminated intravascular coagulation with respect to pathophysiology. Unlike TTP or DIC, however, this disease is almost always organ specific with respect to endothelial damage and thrombus formation. The disorder may be seen in children or adults, but it is much more common in children.[113] Many of the clinical and laboratory findings seen in childhood and adult HUS are similar, but some striking differences are noted. The common clinical features are moderate to severe thrombocytopenia, a microangiopathic hemolytic anemia, renal failure, and hypertension, which may be severe.[114] In children, boys and girls are equally affected, but in adults, women develop the syndrome three times as commonly as men.[115,116] In childhood HUS a prodrome of a viral or bacterial febrile illness often associated with gastroenteritis or pneumonia is common.[117] Adult HUS, however, is almost never preceded by this prodrome but is often associated with complications of pregnancy, including pre-eclampsia, frank toxemia of pregnancy, obstetric accidents, or a seemingly normal postpartum state.[118] Adult HUS may also be associated with renal transplantation rejection or the use of oral contraceptives.[119,120] A typically fatal form of HUS has been noted to develop after bone marrow transplantation.[121-123]

Children and adults usually present with the usual clinical findings of anemia, petechiae, purpura, and, at times, more severe bleeding. Additionally, patients usually present with hematuria, renal failure, hypertension, and neurologic symptomatology. The neurologic symptoms may be mild, including slurred speech and dull mentation, or may be severe, including coma and frank seizures, but neurologic complaints are less common than in TTP or DIC. The neurologic symptoms may be due to renal failure and severe hypertension or to central nervous system (CNS) microvascular thrombosis or intracranial hemorrhage. A definite familial tendency has been noted in both children and adults with HUS, and some have suggested this to be due to an inherited deficiency of a plasma prostacyclin stimulating factor.[124] Tissue biopsy or autopsy examination usually reveals plateletlike and fibrinlike material in renal afferent arterioles and glomerular capillaries and in subendothelial spaces.[125,126] In some instances, especially fatal cases, these same findings may be noted systemically in multiple end organs.

Laboratory findings are those of a microangiopathic hemolytic anemia, schistocytes and thrombocytopenia with "large bizarre" platelets (young forms) usually obvious on a peripheral smear, and the usual findings of azotemia, hematuria, and proteinuria.[114,125] Coagulation abnormalities, besides thrombocytopenia, are usually limited to an almost universal elevation of FDPs. In occasional cases, however, typical laboratory findings of DIC may also be present.

Steroids, heparin, and antiplatelet agents are usually ineffective in childhood HUS[114]; however, the use of washed packed red blood cells, plasma exchange, and prompt dialysis have reduced the mortality to approximately 10%, and only 10% to 15% of surviving patients retain impaired renal function.[127] Unlike children, adults may respond to heparin or the use of antiplatelet agents (aspirin plus dipyridamole) in conjunction with dialysis, prompt control of hypertension, and infusion of washed packed red blood cells to control anemia.[127,128] Two other modes of therapy that deserve further investigation in adult HUS are plasma exchange and intravenous prostacyclin therapy.[129] In nine patients who

Table 5-17. Hemolytic-Uremic Syndrome

Clinical Findings
 Anemia
 Thrombocytopenia
 Petechiae and purpura
 Hypertension
 Renal failure
 Hematuria
 Neurologic findings
 Family history

Pediatric Differences
 More common than in adults
 Prodrome of fever/infection
 Female-to-male ratio of 1:1

Adult Differences
 Less common than in children
 Prodrome of:
  Eclampsia
  Obstetric accidents
  Oral contraceptive use
  Renal transplant rejection
  Normal postpartum state
 Female-to-male ratio of 3:1

Laboratory Findings
 Microangiopathic hemolytic anemia
 Schizocytes
 Thrombocytopenia
 Large "young" platelets
 Elevated fibrin(ogen) degradation products
 DIC-type laboratory findings are rare
 Hematuria
  Microscopic
  Gross
 Proteinuria
 Azotemia

developed HUS following bone marrow transplantation, the only one who survived was treated with plasma exchange.[123] The mortality in adults is much higher than in children and approaches 50% despite vigorous therapy. The clinical features and laboratory findings of hemolytic-uremic syndrome are listed in Table 5-17.

Other Renal Diseases. Renal transplant rejection may be preceded or accompanied by moderate to severe thrombocytopenia, microangiopathic hemolytic anemia, and elevated serum or urine FDPs.[130,131] The thrombocytopenia is thought to be caused by interactions between the platelets and damaged renal endothelium.[132] Findings of elevated FDPs and thrombocytopenia in renal transplant patients should prompt reinstitution or enhancement of immunosuppressive therapy, or, if clinically warranted, consideration of prompt retransplantation. Severe thrombocytopenia may also be seen in association with poststreptococcal glomerulonephritis, although the mechanisms are unclear, and it is not known if this is a platelet destructive process from platelet-renal vascular/glomerular interactions or from an immune complex–mediated platelet destructive process.[133] Additional coagulation changes associated with renal diseases will be discussed in chapter 8.

Thrombotic Thrombocytopenic Purpura. Thrombotic thrombocytopenic purpura (TTP) is a disorder in which the different theories regarding etiology, pathophysiology, diagnosis, and management are controversial and confusing.[134] Although the etiology remains unknown, case reports associate TTP with pregnancy, infections, autoimmune diseases, drugs, toxins, and insect bites. Since most of these associations come primarily from individual case reports, it is unclear if a true association between these events and TTP is of significance. Many case reports associate TTP with pregnancy, especially during the third trimester.[135] Thrombotic thrombocytopenic purpura has been associated with legionnaires' disease, meningiococcemia, *Mycoplasma pneumoniae*, and bacteroides.[136-139] Additionally, TTP has been associated with herpesvirus, influenza, coxsackievirus B, other viral infections, and after polio vaccination.[140-144] Thrombotic thrombocytopenic purpura has also been associated with the acquired immunodeficiency syndrome (AIDS) and the AIDS-related complex (ARC).[145-148] In general, however, the role of viral or other infections as an etiologic factor remains unclear in patients with TTP.[149] Since TTP is extremely rare and no single investigator or group of investigators often acquire any significant clinical experience with this disease, attempts to define the etiology, pathophysiology, diagnosis, or specific management remain difficult. Diagnostic criteria for TTP are so nonspecific that many proposed therapeutic modalities for true cases of TTP will appear to be ineffective when inappropriately applied to cases that simulate but do not represent TTP. Conversely, effective therapy may be looked on unfavorably when it does not correct a situation thought incorrectly to represent TTP.[134] Thrombotic thrombocytopenic purpura is difficult to distinguish from other similar conditions, especially the hemolytic-uremic syndrome and disseminated intravascular coagulation.[150-152] Table 5-18 summarizes conditions and diseases similar to TTP.

The universal finding in tissue sections taken from biopsies or autopsy examinations of patients with TTP includes the presence of microthrombi that segmentally involve small arterioles and capillaries with a notable absence of inflammation and are noted in virtually any and every organ system of the body.[153,154] Characteristically, intravascular hyaline microthrombi, absence of lysis at the periphery of microthrombi, and the absence of fibrinoid necrosis or vasculitis are noted. However, these are not pathognomonic lesions and can be found in tissue biopsy specimens of many of the conditions that simulate TTP.

The initial lesion of TTP is thought to be caused by some undetermined injury to discontinuous segments of the endothelium of small arteries and capillaries. This insult gives rise to a prethrombotic subendothelial deposit consist-

Table 5-18. Conditions Similar in Pathology to Thrombotic Thrombocytopenic Purpura

Autoimmune hemolytic anemia
Disseminated intravascular coagulation
Eclampsia
Evan's syndrome
Hemolytic-uremic syndrome
Malignant hypertension
Microangiopathic hemolytic anemia
Paroxysmal nocturnal hemoglobinuria
Pediatric respiratory distress syndrome
Polyarteritis nodosa
Rocky Mountain spotted fever
Systemic lupus erythematosus
Vasculitides

ing of platelets and fibrin.[155] These lesions are eventually replaced by hyaline microthrombi that may occlude the involved vascular segment.[156] If vasculitis or fibrinoid necrosis is noted, TTP can be excluded.[134] Kwaan and associates[157] have shown that injured endothelial cells in TTP, in contrast to normal endothelial cells, contain no plasminogen activator activity. However, patients with TTP with active disease retain plasminogen activator activity in uninvolved vascular segments. This finding is distinguished from the endothelial cells of vessels involved in DIC where plasminogen activator activity is uniformly present.[134] Interestingly, the only other condition noted with altered endothelial plasminogen activator activity is scleroderma.[158] Plasma levels of prostacyclin are also noted by some investigators to be decreased in TTP.[159] Thus, the hyaline microthrombi of thrombotic thrombocytopenic purpura may be the result of disseminated intravascular platelet aggregation occurring segmentally at the endothelial site.[160]

These findings have led to the general belief that the basic pathophysiology of TTP is an, as yet, unclear defect in platelet–endothelial cell interaction(s).[161] Plasma factors that activate platelets have now been described in patients with TTP; in particular a 37,000-d plasma protein, platelet activating protein (PAP),[162,163] has been noted in patients with TTP. Several authorities believe that the disappearance or absence of a normal plasma inhibitor to this PAP is the basic defect in TTP.[162,163] Of additional interest is the finding of abnormal von Willebrand factor, characterized by large multimers, in some patients with TTP.[164] One report failed to confirm this finding.[165] An additional study noted decreased free protein S in TTP.[166] Thus, several defects in plasma or endothelium are consistently noted in many patients with TTP, but it remains unclear exactly how these defects interact to precipitate an episode of TTP. Indeed, it is possible that some, or all, of these defects may even arise secondarily to an already established TTP syndrome. An additional possibility is that many etiologic defects may independently give rise to TTP (ie, TTP may be precipitated by any one of

Table 5-19. Summary of Plasma and Endothelial Defects in Thrombotic Thrombocytopenic Purpura

Absent/defective platelet-activating protein inhibitor
Abnormal von Willebrand's factor (large multimers)
Decreased free protein S
Decreased/defective prostacyclin
Decreased/defective plasminogen activator activity

Table 5-20. Thrombotic Thrombocytopenic Purpura

Pathologic Findings
    Microthrombi segmentally involve subendothelium, vessel lumen, precapillary arterioles, capillaries, and postcapillary veins
    Arteriocapillary aneurysmal dilatations
    Endothelial proliferation with a notable absence of inflammation or fibrinoid necrosis
    Microthrombi can be found in any organ system

Typical Signs and Symptoms
    Prodrome of fatigue, pallor, and nausea
    Petechiae, purpura, and ecchymoses
    Epistaxis
    Retinal hemorrhages
    Gastrointestinal bleeding
    Fever
    Jaundice
    Neurologic deficits
    Abdominal pain
    Hepatomegaly
    Splenomegaly

Typical Laboratory Findings
    Schizocytes
    Anemia
    Thrombocytopenia
    Reticulocytosis
    Hematuria
    Leukocytosis
    Elevated fibrin(ogen) degradation products
    DIC-type laboratory findings usually absent
    Coombs test usually negative
    Proteinuria
    Axotemia
    Indirect hyperbilirubinemia

Proposed Therapeutic Modalities
    Plasmapheresis
    Plasma transfusions
    Blood transfusions
    Exchange transfusions
    Splenectomy
    Platelet suppressant therapy
    Corticosteroids
    Heparin therapy
    Dextrans
    Urokinase
    Streptokinase
    Prostacyclin infusion

these defects independently). Table 5-19 summarizes the plasma and endothelial defects found in patients with TTP.

On rare instances, a DIC syndrome may develop in patients with TTP, but this is probably an independent event and serves only to complicate the course and clinical and laboratory findings of TTP.[167] The signs, symptoms, physical findings, pathologic findings, and typical laboratory findings of TTP are listed in Table 5-20. The pathophysiologic characteristics of DIC and TTP are different. For example, the fibrin seen in occlusive lesions is thought to be platelet-derived in TTP as opposed to thrombin-mediated in DIC. In addition, the lesion is pathogenically distinct and different from those produced in thrombin-mediated syndromes. As a consequence of the endothelial injury in the microcirculation, a disordered prostaglandin metabolism is anticipated in TTP,[168,169] which is manifest by potential absence of prostacyclin derivatives, such as 6-keto-PGF_1-alpha. In addition, thromboxane A_2 activity is usually increased as measured by the metabolic end-product thromboxane B_2.

The therapeutic approach originally advanced by Byrnes and Lian is compatible with these observations. The objective of plasma transfusion is the replacement of a missing platelet aggregation factor (PAP) inhibitor.[170] This factor is thought to be missing in TTP and present in normal plasma. Platelet inhibitors, including aspirin and dipyridamole, may have a significant ancillary role in the treatment of TTP as noted from clinical experience.[134]

Clinically, TTP has been defined in a variety of ways. As a triad, it consists of microangiopathic hemolytic anemia, thrombocytopenia, and fluctuating neurologic abnormalities.[134] When defined as a pentad or quintad, fever and renal abnormalities are added. Most patients with TTP (60%) are females between the ages of 10 and 40 years, with a peak incidence occurring in the third decade. Previously, 80% of patients died within two to three months of the onset of TTP. Almost always, evidence of hemorrhage, including petechiae, purpura, ecchymoses, retinal hemorrhage, gastrointestinal hemorrhage, and epistaxis, is present. The classic laboratory findings of DIC are usually absent in patients with TTP. Molecular marker profiles for the differential diagnosis between TTP and DIC are found in Table 5-21. When a patient fulfills the laboratory diagnostic findings of TTP and has some but not all of the laboratory features of DIC, TTP with additional complications should be diagnosed. Usually, normal or near normal levels of fibrinogen, no evidence of thrombin activity (as determined by the protamine sulfate

test or assays for fibrinopeptide A), no reduction of antithrombin III levels, or other evidence of concomitant DIC findings are present. The one consistent finding in TTP that is reminiscent of DIC and often confusing to clinicians is elevated FDP levels. When TTP is suspected, available assays for prostaglandin derivatives should be considered. The breakdown product of prostacyclin, 6-keto PGF_1-alpha, is often decreased, and the breakdown product of thrombox-

Table 5-21. Molecular Markers for the Differential Diagnosis of Disseminated Intravascular Coagulation and Thrombotic Thrombocytopenic Purpura

	DIC	TTP
6-Keto PGF-1-Alpha	Normal	Decreased
Plasminogen activator	Normal/increased	Decreased
B-beta 15-42 peptide	Increased	Normal
Fibrinopeptide A	Increased	Normal
Fibrinopeptide B	Increased	Normal

Table 5-22. Responses to Therapy in Thrombotic Thrombocytopenic Purpura

Therapy	Response
Corticosteroids	10%
Antiplatelet agents	50%
Splenectomy	50%
Whole blood exchange	50%
Plasma transfusion	65%
Plasma exchange	80%

ane A_2, thromboxane B_2, is often increased.[134] A schistocytosis is almost always present; however, this finding also is only suggestive and certainly not diagnostic.

Therapy for TTP was controversial and confusing for many years, because the pathophysiology remained unknown. Early therapeutic approaches were necessarily empiric and consisted of corticosteroids, antiplatelet agents, and splenectomy alone or with corticosteroids and antiplatelet agents. The overall response rate to high-dose corticosteroids, usually prednisone or an equivalent, is approximately 10%. The general response rate to antiplatelet agents alone, usually aspirin and dipyridamole, is about 50%, and the overall response rate to splenectomy alone or in combination with corticosteroids or antiplatelet agents is approximately 50%.[171] Because of disappointing response rates and the presumption of a plasma platelet aggregation factor (PAP) inhibitor deficiency, plasma transfusion, whole blood exchange, and, ultimately, the clear therapy of choice, high-dose plasma exchange, evolved. The rationale for plasma transfusion in TTP was to restore the missing "Byrnes-Lian" plasma factor and thus inhibit platelet aggregation.[134,170] Plasma transfusion is generally associated with a response rate of about 65%.[172] Exchange transfusions with whole blood are generally associated with a response rate of about 50%. Plasmapheresis/exchange, since it removed TTP plasma and replaced it with fresh plasma containing plasma aggregation inhibitor factor (PAP inhibitor), reduced the level of unopposed platelet aggregating factor in TTP plasma, and, therefore, became a rational approach.[173-175] Blood transfusions will hypothetically deliver to the patient with TTP quantities of the "Byrnes-Lian" factor but appear to be less effective than plasma exchange. Plasma exchange is generally started on a daily basis, and 50 to 60 mL/kg per day of plasma is exchanged. The total exchange volume may be adjusted appropriately depending on the rise in platelet count. Overall response rates with vigorous plasma exchange are approximately 80%.[176,177] The role of hemodialysis in TTP is minimal, since it does not supply significant amounts of plasma containing the proposed platelet aggregation inhibitor factor of "Byrnes-Lian" factor.

Numerous therapeutic modalities have been proposed for the treatment of thrombotic thrombocytopenia purpura

(Table 5-20). It appears, however, that Byrnes and associates originally proposed the most rational therapeutic approach to the patient with TTP, that of plasma infusion or plasma exchange, with large volume exchange now clearly being the treatment of choice.[17,178,179] The use of platelet suppressive therapy should be encouraged.[134,180,181] Plasma exchange or plasma infusion in conjunction with platelet suppressive therapy might enhance prostacyclin synthetase activity, should depress thromboxane synthetase activity, should increase intraplatelet cyclic AMP levels, and should inhibit platelet phosphodiesterase activity. Based on current theories of TTP pathophysiology, heparin does not have a rational therapeutic role since the occlusive lesions are mediated entirely by platelets and not by thrombin or DIC-type mechanisms.

If a complicating DIC process is coincidentally present in a patient with TTP, appropriate heparin therapy should be used to control the DIC. Urokinase or streptokinase may be useful as supplementary therapeutic modalities in lysing the platelet-derived fibrin component in the occluding microthrombi. However, the use of thrombolytic agents in TTP is not without significant hazard of hemorrhagic complications. In cases in which injury to endothelial cells is marginal and/or the duration of the occlusion is short, lysis and dislocation of the microthrombi may be of possible value. Since the lesions are variable in age and severity in numerous organ systems producing functionally deficient and physically absent endothelial cells at numerous points, massive tissue hemorrhage may be a potentially disastrous consequence of restoring patency to injured vessels with thrombolytic therapy. A new era of therapy in TTP may come about with the possible use of intravenous prostacyclin. Although prostacyclin has a very short half-life when infused, the beneficial effects of platelet suppression by this agent may be potentially desirous in patients with TTP.[182,183] Response rates to various forms of therapy are summarized in Table 5-22.

Thrombotic thrombocytopenic purpura remains a diagnostic and therapeutic challenge. If strict clinical and laboratory diagnostic features are applied, the syndrome can be distinguished from hemolytic-uremic syndrome as well as

Table 5-23. Common Reasons for Hypersplenism

Amyloidosis
Autoimmune disorders
    Systemic lupus erythematosus
    Rheumatoid arthritis
Gaucher's disease
Hemolytic anemias
Hodgkin's disease
Idiopathic splenomegaly
Infections
Inflammatory diseases
Leukemia
Lymphoma
Metastatic carcinoma
Multiple myeloma
Myeloproliferative syndromes
Niemann-Pick disease
Portal hypertension
Thalassemia
Waldenström's macroglobulinemia

DIC-related syndromes.[134,184] Therapeutic management is markedly different than that for DIC-type syndromes. The most effective therapy at present is plasma exchange, theoretically supplying the patient with TTP with platelet aggregation factor inhibitor (PAP inhibitor). The adjuvant use of platelet suppressive therapy in the form of aspirin and dipyridamole or the adjuvant use of corticosteroids, in association with plasma exchange, may also be beneficial. Of course, the majority of these patients also require meticulous intensive care support during the acute phase. Thorough and provocative reviews regarding the theory, etiology, pathophysiology, diagnosis, and management of TTP are available.[173,185-189]

Hypersplenism and Thrombocytopenia. Splenomegaly and associated hypersplenism can be of numerous origins and may cause pancytopenia and moderate to severe thrombocytopenia. Hypersplenism may occur without splenomegaly. The conditions commonly associated with hypersplenism are listed in Table 5-23. The mechanism of thrombocytopenia in hypersplenism is the pooling of a large percentage of the total body platelet population within the spleen.[190] Normally the spleen contains approximately one third of the total body platelet population at any given time.[191] Intravenous epinephrine causes a marked increase in platelet counts in hypersplenic patients but only a moderate increase in normal individuals, thus supporting the concept of splenic sequestration of platelets in hypersplenism.[192] In addition, large numbers of platelets can be extruded from an enlarged spleen removed during splenectomy.[193] Splenic pooling of platelets in hypersplenism appears to be brought on by the very slow passage of platelets through the spleen as a result of a percolating effect, causing platelets to take a tortuous and slow course through the splenic sinusoids, thus allowing prolonged contact and resultant cohesion between platelets and splenic macrophages and endothelial cells.[190] The noting of increased platelet counts following an infusion of epinephrine in the patient with hypersplenism may indicate that the patient will probably respond to splenectomy if the procedure is clinically indicated.[194]

The clinical manifestations of thrombocytopenia secondary to hypersplenism are usually related to the disorder causing the hypersplenism and/or splenomegaly.[190] Most individuals with hypersplenism have splenomegaly, but hypersplenism may occur in the presence of a normal-sized spleen. The most common cause of hypersplenism and associated thrombocytopenia is congestive splenomegaly due to portal hypertension secondary to chronic liver disease.[195] The degree of thrombocytopenia correlates reasonably well with the degree of splenic enlargement. Some patients, however, will have significant hypersplenism and thrombocytopenia despite no significant enlargement of spleen size.

The management of thrombocytopenia secondary to hypersplenism is dependent on the underlying disease process giving rise to hypersplenism. Splenectomy is rarely indicated, but when it is, the efficacy of splenectomy may be predicted by the presplenectomy infusion of epinephrine and the noting of significant elevation of the peripheral platelet count.[194] Portacaval shunting may be indicated in selected disease states, and radiation of the spleen is occasionally useful in patients who have splenomegaly and hypersplenism in association with leukemia, lymphoma, Hodgkin's disease, or other related disorders. Even though this is a nonimmune cause of thrombocytopenia, the use of steroids to blunt splenic reticuloendothelial function may also be useful if the patient has significant persistent thrombocytopenia. In addition, severe or life-threatening hemorrhage should immediately be treated with platelet concentrates.

Disseminated Intravascular Coagulation. Disseminated intravascular coagulation and related syndromes are almost uniformly associated with significant thrombocytopenia due to nonimmune consumption/destruction of platelets and will be discussed in detail in chapter 7.

Infections and Drugs Directly Toxic to Platelets. Thrombocytopenia is associated with numerous bacterial,[82,196] viral,[197] fungal,[68] and protozoan infections. The mechanisms are extremely complex, and the thrombocytopenia noted is often a clinical summation of many pathophysiologic events in patients with infections. Nonimmunologic mechanisms of thrombocytopenia in patients with infections may include direct platelet destruction by interaction of the infectious agent with platelets or megakaryocytes, in vivo platelet aggregation induced by bacteria or bacterial products, the development of infection-induced DIC with resultant consumption of platelets, the release of thromboxane A_2 by infectious agents or their products, or the interaction of platelets with endothelium that has sustained significant damage by the infectious agent.[68,82,196-198]

Thrombocytopenia often occurs early in the course of septicemia, and the noting of thrombocytopenia in a patient with a febrile illness should prompt early suspicion of the development of septicemia, especially due to meningococcus, other gram-negative organisms (particularly those producing endotoxin), or staphylococcal organisms.[199,200] The patient with a febrile illness and thrombocytopenia should be painstakingly examined for the possibility of subacute bacterial endocarditis.[200,201] Thrombocytopenia is seen much more commonly in gram-negative than in gram-positive septicemia.[199,200] Up to 60% of patients with sepsis will have some degree of thrombocytopenia.[1]

Thrombocytopenia may accompany infections with mumps, varicella, disseminated herpes, cytomegalovirus, hepatitis viruses, human immunodeficiency virus (HIV), and infectious mononucleosis.[31,84-88,202,203] Infections with toxoplasmosis, tuberculosis, histoplasmosis, coccidioidomycosis, brucellosis, diphtheria, typhoid fever, toxic shock syndrome, and Rocky Mountain spotted fever may be accompanied by severe thrombocytopenia.[64-68]

Thrombocytopenia associated with infections usually abates with control or resolution of the infectious process. If severe or life-threatening hemorrhage occurs or is thought to be impending, however, platelet concentrates should be readily used. If an immune complex is believed to be a component to the infection-associated thrombocytopenia, intravenous hydrocortisone succinate, dexamethasone, or oral prednisone should precede the use of platelet concentrates. Infections causing nonimmune-mediated thrombocytopenia are summarized in Table 5-24.

Drugs Toxic to Circulating Platelets. Selected drugs appear to be directly toxic to platelets causing increased platelet destruction by nonimmunologic mechanisms. The most common of these is ristocetin, an antibiotic that was removed from clinical use because it induced in vivo platelet aggregation/agglutination. The mechanism appears to be the ability of ristocetin to promote binding of factor VIII:vW to a platelet receptor.[204] Bleomycin sulfate and other selected chemotherapeutic agents may also cause direct injury to platelets.[205] In the case of bleomycin sulfate, it has been suggested that platelets are destroyed after interacting with endothelium previously damaged by this drug.[205] Heparin-induced thrombocytopenia may be a severe and life-threatening situation and will be discussed in chapter 14. Whether this is a direct toxic effect by heparin or an immune-mediated phenomenon remains controversial.[206]

Gold-induced thrombocytopenia occurs in many patients receiving gold therapy. The most serious side effect of gold therapy is aplastic anemia; however, thrombocytopenia is the single most common hematologic complication from gold therapy and occurs in approximately 3% of patients.[207] The exact mechanism is unclear, but the early onset of thrombocytopenia, decreased platelet survival, and normal or increased megakaryocytes in the marrow suggest that peripheral platelet destruction is operative in some cases.

Table 5-24. Common Infections Causing Nonimmune Thrombocytopenia

Brucellosis
Coccidioidomycosis
Cytomegalovirus
Diphtheria
Disseminated herpes
Hepatitis
Histoplasmosis
Infectious mononucleosis
Many gram-negative organisms
Meningococcus sp.
Mumps
Protozoan infections
Rocky Mountain spotted fever
Septicemia
Staphylococcus sp.
Subacute bacterial endocarditis
Toxic shock syndrome
Tuberculosis
Typhoid fever
Varicella

Treatment is immediate discontinuation of gold; other therapies of potential benefit are the use of chelating agents and prednisone.[208] Despite these therapeutic modalities, many patients remain persistently thrombocytopenic after discontinuation of gold. Protamine sulfate may be associated with rapid development of thrombocytopenia, but the effect is usually transient, often does not lead to serious or life-threatening hemorrhage, and is thought to be due to protamine-induced platelet sequestration in the liver.[209] Valproic acid has become popular as an anti-epileptic agent and is frequently associated with thrombocytopenia.[210] The mechanism is thought to be valproic acid interaction with platelets leading to increased peripheral destruction; however, immunologic mechanisms have been suggested. Drugs that are directly toxic to platelets and cause thrombocytopenia are summarized in Table 5-25.

Cardiovascular Disease and Thrombocytopenia. Mitral and aortic valvular diseases, especially secondary to rheumatic fever, have been associated with increased platelet consumption and destruction.[211,212] Mild thrombocy-

Table 5-25. Drugs Directly Toxic to Platelets Causing Thrombocytopenia

Bleomycin sulfate
Gold
Heparin (usually immunologic)
Protamine sulfate
Ristocetin
Valproic acid (immunologic)

Table 5-26. Disorders Associated With Nonimmune Increased Platelet Destruction/Consumption

Cardiovascular disorders
Cardiopulmonary bypass surgery
Disseminated intravascular coagulation
Drugs
Eclampsia
Hemodialysis
Hemolytic-uremic syndrome
Hypersplenism
Infections
Prosthetic devices
Renal diseases
Thrombotic thrombocytopenic purpura

Table 5-27. Common Causes of Immune-Mediated Increased Platelet Destruction/Consumption

Congenital and Neonatal
    Maternal drug ingestion
    Alloimmune neonatal thrombocytopenia
    Neonatal infection
    Maternal immune thrombocytopenia purpura

Acquired
    Acute immune thrombocytopenia purpura
    Chronic immune thrombocytopenia purpura
    Drug-induced immune thrombocytopenia
    Posttransfusion purpura

topenia frequently occurs in patients with severe aortic stenosis, but patients with mitral disease associated with left atrial thrombosis or peripheral vascular embolization may also have thrombocytopenia.[211,213-215] Thrombus formation and associated platelet consumption are common in patients with prosthetic valves. The frequency of platelet consumption is significantly lower in patients with tissue valves than with nontissue valves, but porcine valves are also associated with platelet consumption and thrombocytopenia.[213,216-219] Circulating platelet aggregates are seen in patients with severe coronary artery disease, and the presence of numerous circulating platelet aggregates may be associated with peripheral thrombocytopenia.[220-222]

Peripheral arterial disease, especially if associated with significant claudication, gangrene, or thromboembolism, is associated with increased platelet consumption and mild to severe thrombocytopenia.[223,224] Extensive deep venous thrombosis, especially involving the inferior vena cava, iliofemoral system, calf thrombosis, or extensive deep venous thrombosis associated with pulmonary embolism, may be associated with significant platelet consumption and resultant thrombocytopenia.[225,226] Thrombocytopenia is a frequent accompaniment of cardiopulmonary bypass surgery and will be discussed in chapter 9. Mechanisms of nonimmune-mediated increased consumption/destruction of platelets are summarized in Table 5-26.

Immune-Mediated Mechanisms

The common immune-mediated causes of thrombocytopenia are summarized in Table 5-27.

Acute ITP. Acute immune thrombocytopenia purpura (ITP), also referred to as idiopathic thrombocytopenia purpura, occurs primarily in children but may also be seen in adults.[227,228] In acute ITP a prodrome of an acute viral illness almost always occurs from one week to one month before the rapid onset of thrombocytopenia in about 80% of patients.[229] The most common viral illnesses noted to precede acute ITP are chickenpox, rubeola, rubella, or undefined, nonspecific upper respiratory tract infections.[227,230]

Acute ITP has also been noted following vaccination with live virus for measles, mumps, chickenpox, and smallpox.[227,228,230,231] In many children, spontaneous recovery will occur in several months. The mechanism thought to be responsible for the abrupt onset of thrombocytopenia is the binding of a viral-induced immune complex to platelets and megakaryocytes.[232] These platelets are thus removed by the reticuloendothelial system, primarily the spleen but also the liver and possibly the bone marrow. In addition, megakaryopoiesis is compromised because of immune complex binding. Since the disease usually occurs well after the viremia has abated, presumably the immune response against the initial virus later gives rise to an immune complex that then binds to platelet membrane Fc receptors.[232,233] Immune complexes isolated from patients with ITP will not bind to platelets of patients with Glanzmann's thrombasthenia, so the immune complexes may be directed toward Fc receptors on platelet membrane glycoproteins IIb or IIIa, which are missing from Glanzmann's platelets.[234] Significantly increased levels of platelet-associated IgG (PAIgG) are noted to be present in the vast majority of cases.[232] The noting that infusions of intravenous gamma globulin will block Fc receptors of phagocytic cells and subsequently reverse the thrombocytopenia provides some evidence that viral antigens may be absorbed onto the platelet membrane surface, followed by immune complex formation.[235,236]

Acute ITP usually occurs before the teenage years but may occur in adults. Clinical symptoms of petechiae, purpura, ecchymoses, and mucosal membrane bleeding from the gastrointestinal tract, genitourinary tract, gingivae, or epistaxis usually begin abruptly.[227-229,232] Hemorrhagic bullae may be noted on examination of the oral mucosa. Shotty adenopathy is usually found, but hepatosplenomegaly is found in fewer than 10% of patients with acute immune thrombocytopenia purpura. Recovery occurs in the vast majority of patients despite the mode of therapy used, if any. Recovery is usually within two months, but some patients may not recover for six to 12 months.[227-229,232,237] Very few patients have recurrences after recovery. Since a high spontaneous remission rate is noted in acute ITP, it is difficult to evaluate efficacy of any particular therapy, and indeed, sometimes no therapy is required in acute ITP unless severe hemorrhage occurs. The risk of significant hemorrhage is greatest at the onset and abates with initiation of corticosteroid therapy. This observation is attributed to a positive effect of corticosteroids on the vasculature or the improvement of capillary integrity by corticosteroids. Prednisone inhibits prostacyclin (PGI_2) synthesis by the endothelium, and the potential effect could be to favor less platelet inhibition and less vasodilatation, which might, therefore, account for increased capillary integrity. My usual approach is to start prednisone immediately at 2 mg/kg per day in twice daily dosages, each dose with 30 mL of a liquid antacid.[1] This regimen may abort a serious or life-threatening hemorrhage, including intracranial bleeding. Patients are also cautioned about restricted activity until the platelet count is greater than 50×10^9/L (50,000/mm³), and the patient and family are strictly cautioned regarding the use of any drug known to interfere with platelet function. Platelet transfusions are of minimal efficacy, as transfused donor platelets are also affected by the immune complex–containing recipient blood and are rapidly consumed by the reticuloendothelial system, primarily the spleen. Therefore, transfusion should only be used to abort intracranial or life-threatening hemorrhage. According to limited reports in the literature, therapeutic plasma exchange, infusions of fresh frozen plasma, vincristine, the use of danazol, and infusions of intravenous gamma globulin also are effective. These specific therapeutic modalities are more applicable to chronic ITP.[175,235,236,238]

Approximately 10% of children fail to respond to any mode of therapy. If no response is noted by six months, or if the child becomes unduly cushingoid or cannot tolerate other modes of therapy, splenectomy is usually recommended, followed by a slow taper of prednisone. The prednisone is decreased by 5 mg/day per week.[1] Children who fail to respond to these modalities in a reasonable period of time (six to 12 months) usually have no prodrome of a viral illness, have low levels of IgA, and are only moderately thrombocytopenic. These patients actually have chronic ITP. Only 60% of these individuals will have significant bleeding, which can be controlled with low to moderate doses of prednisone or azathioprine therapy. If splenectomy is performed in children with acute or chronic ITP, it should be accompanied by a pneumococcal vaccine.[1] The salient features of acute ITP are summarized in Table 5-28.

Chronic ITP. Chronic ITP usually occurs in adults with a female-to-male ratio of 3:1.[239] Although no prodrome of viral illness occurs in chronic ITP, this is also an immune complex–mediated disorder in which the immune complex attaches to platelets, leading to destruction by the spleen, bone marrow, or liver, in descending order of importance. Immune complex attachment to the megakaryocyte leading to ineffective platelet production is also operative in chronic ITP.[240-242] In addition, women with chronic ITP give birth to thrombocytopenic children in 50% to 80% of cases.[243,244]

Table 5-28. Acute Immune Thrombocytopenia Purpura

Clinical Findings
    Common in children, usually before 12 years of age
    Uncommon in adults
    Frequent prodrome of viral disease
    Spontaneous recovery common
    Abrupt onset of hemorrhage
        Petechiae and purpura
        Ecchymoses
        Epistaxis
        Gastrointestinal hemorrhage
        Genitourinary hemorrhage
    Shotty adenopathy common
    Less than 10% with hepatosplenomegaly
    Recurrence is very rare
    Associated platelet dysfunction in some

Therapy
    Prednisone, 2.0 mg/kg per day and slow taper
    Platelet concentrates (minimal efficacy)
    Minimal experience:
        Plasma exchange
        Infusion of fresh frozen plasma
        Intravenous gamma globulin
        In the 10% of patients who fail therapy, splenectomy is indicated

Although chronic (adult) ITP is not generally associated with any prodromal illness, increasing reports note an ITP-like syndrome occurring in patients with either HIV seropositivity or overt AIDS.[245-248]

Platelet-associated IgG (PAIgG) is elevated in 90% of patients, and results of serum tests for this antibody are positive in 50% of patients.[232,249] Any of the four classes of IgG may be the responsible agent, but IgG_1 has been the predominant type.[232,250-252] Both total platelet IgG, found primarily in platelet alpha granules, and surface-bound IgG are typically significantly increased in ITP. These are measured by two methods: total platelet IgG assay and the direct platelet-associated IgG assay.[253] Results of the indirect platelet-associated IgG test may be positive in about 50% of patients. This test measures serum antiplatelet antibody, most of which appears to be directed against platelet membrane glycoprotein complexes, usually the Ib/IX complex or the IIb/IIIa complex.[254,255] Both the total platelet IgG and surface-bound IgG have been correlated with initial platelet count and response to therapy.[256,257] It has been speculated that chronic ITP is a disorder of immunoregulation. Several studies have demonstrated decreased T-suppressor cell activity.[232,258] The often rapid rise in platelet counts and fall in PAIgG following splenectomy suggest the spleen to be both the primary site of platelet destruction as well as the major organ of pathologic immunoglobulin synthesis in chronic ITP. In those patients failing to respond to splenectomy, the IgG may originate from the bone marrow or possibly the liver. Like acute ITP, the Fc-receptor mechanism appears important. Platelet

Figure 5-1. Typical Marrow Findings in Immune Thrombocytopenic Purpura

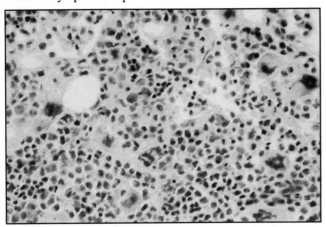

Figure 5-2. Typical Marrow Findings in Immune Thrombocytopenic Purpura

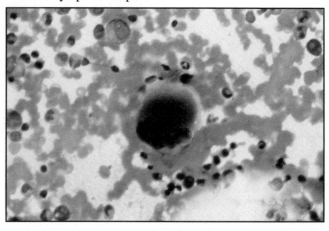

destruction in ITP may occur via splenic (or other reticuloendothelial) phagocytosis with or without complement activation.[232,249] The role of complement activation in platelet destruction remains unclear; however, the blockade of Fc-receptor activity will cause a rapid rise in the platelet count, according to the limited experience thus far noted.

Unlike acute ITP, chronic ITP usually begins insidiously, and a syndrome of easy and spontaneous bruising usually precedes other more serious hemorrhagic manifestations that eventually lead the patient to seek medical attention.[249] Epistaxis and gingival bleeding are common, and petechiae and ecchymoses are usually noted on examination. Petechiae and purpura of the oral mucosa are common; however, hemorrhagic bullae of the oral mucosa are only noted in severe cases. Mild splenomegaly is noted in approximately 30% of cases.[249,259] The finding of marked hepatosplenomegaly in association with thrombocytopenia should alert the clinician to consider a malignant lymphoreticular disorder, autoimmune disorder, carcinomatosis, or tuberculosis.

Bone marrow examination, like in acute ITP, usually reveals normal or increased megakaryocytes that have basophilic hypogranular cytoplasm and are without appreciable platelet budding.[46] Typical marrow findings of ITP are shown in Figures 5-1 and 5-2. These findings suggest a population of less mature megakaryocytes with premature platelet release, which is simply a response to peripheral thrombocytopenia. Examination of the peripheral blood smear reveals obvious thrombocytopenia with many large, young platelets.

The mainstay of therapy for chronic ITP is prednisone. My approach is to use prednisone at 2 mg/kg per day in twice daily dosages, each dose to be taken with 30 mL of liquid antacid.[1] Most patients (70%) will respond to this mode of therapy. Significant bleeding risk usually abates immediately after institution of prednisone therapy at these dosages. The cessation of bleeding risk is primarily due to the usual rapid rise in platelet count but may also be due to the decreased PGI_2 synthesis. After the platelet count has remained normal for one to two weeks, prednisone is tapered extremely slowly at 5 mg/kg per week. Those patients whose platelet count falls with steroid tapering may be considered steroid failures and are candidates for splenectomy. If the patient refuses splenectomy, other less satisfactory modes of therapy are available, including vinca alkaloids, danazol, azathioprine, cyclophosphamide, intravenous gamma globulin, and plasmapheresis/plasma exchange.

Of those patients subjected to splenectomy, about 70% will respond with respect to a reasonable platelet count, and 30% will fail to respond. Following splenectomy, steroid tapering should be extremely slow. My approach is to taper prednisone at 5 mg/kg per week following splenectomy. In those patients who require splenectomy, oral prednisone therapy is continued until the day before splenectomy. The night before splenectomy the patient is given long-acting dexamethasone acetate intramuscularly, and the morning of surgery the same dose (8 to 12 mg/kg) is repeated. In addition, just before splenectomy the patient is infused with 100 mg of hydrocortisone, and this dose is repeated the evening of the splenectomy. In addition, intramuscular dexamethasone acetate is continued twice daily until the patient is able to take oral medications, and then prednisone is reinstituted, and a very slow taper is begun. If this sequence of events is followed, clearly 70% of patients will respond satisfactorily to splenectomy without relapse.[1,260,261] Those patients who demonstrate a drop in their platelet count with steroid tapering following splenectomy may be considered splenectomy failures. In these individuals, long-term prednisone, azathioprine, or a combination of both will usually be needed to control significant thrombocytopenia. Many individuals, however, remain only borderline thrombocytopenic and will not usually have significant bleeding consequences. Plasma exchange and intravenous gamma globulin have been used with limited success in patients with chronic ITP, both presplenectomy and postsplenectomy, and more experience is needed with these modalities of therapy.[175,235,236,238,262-264] Intravenous gamma globulin is usually used at a total dosage of 2 g/kg for five days delivered as 400 mg/kg per day. Plasma exchange and plasmapheresis are most often used as 1

Figure 5-3. Platelet Dysfunction in Immune Thrombocytopenic Purpura

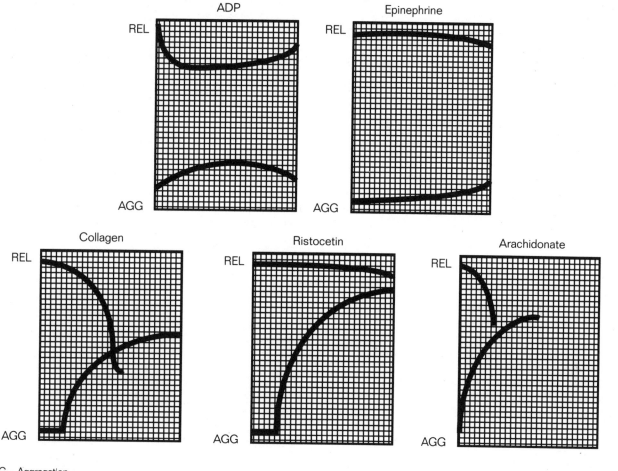

AGG = Aggregation
REL = Release Reaction

plasma volume per exchange at 40 to 80 mL/minute, repeated in 10 days and 20 days, if needed. An average of two exchanges are usually needed, and occasionally three are required. Exchange therapy is stopped or held when the platelet count consistently remains around 10 x 10⁹/L (100,000/mm³).[265,266] Danazol is given orally at a dosage of 200 mg three times a day, and slow tapering is attempted if a response occurs.[267,268] Vincristine is delivered as a 0.025-mg/kg intravenous push every one to three weeks,[269] and vinblastine is usually delivered as a 0.125-mg/kg intravenous push every one to three weeks.[270] The responses are often of short duration. The platelet count is unreliable as the sole predictor of bleeding propensity in chronic ITP. Many patients will not hemorrhage at a platelet count of less than 10 x 10⁹/L (10,000/mm³), whereas others may have severe hemorrhage (ie, intracranial) at platelet counts above 90 x 10⁹/L (90,000/mm³). The reason for this is an associated defect in platelet function in many, if not most, patients with chronic ITP. The defect is thought to arise from IgG coating the platelet membrane receptor(s). Thus, an acquired storage pool defect may be present, and in addition, abnor-

mal arachidonate metabolism may be present.[271,272] Patients with immune-mediated thrombocytopenia commonly have associated severe platelet dysfunction due to coating of the platelet membrane by immunoglobulin. Thus, assessment of bleeding in patients with immune-mediated thrombocytopenias, such as immune/idiopathic thrombocytopenia purpura (ITP), must be made by evaluation of not only the absolute platelet count but also associated platelet function. Figure 5-3 demonstrates platelet dysfunction in a patient with ITP.

As with acute ITP, the role of platelet transfusion is somewhat limited, because infused platelets are destroyed as rapidly as the patient's platelets. Platelet infusion should be reserved to abort serious, life-threatening, or intracranial hemorrhage. Some patients with chronic ITP may develop an autoimmune hemolytic anemia, and the combination is referred to as Evan's syndrome.[273-275] The characteristic features of chronic ITP are depicted in Table 5-29.

Drugs and Immune-Mediated Thrombocytopenia.
Drugs constitute a major cause of immune thrombocytopenia. Immune thrombocytopenia may be associated with a

Table 5-29. Chronic Immune Thrombocytopenic Purpura

Clinical Findings
    Common in adults
    Rare in children
    Female-to-male ratio of 3:1
    No prodrome of viral illness
    If maternal ITP, neonate has 50% to 80% chance of ITP at delivery
    PAIgG found in 90%
    Serum antibody found in 50%
    Insidious onset:
        Easy bruising
        Spontaneous bruising
        Epistaxis
        Gingival bleeding
        Petechiae and purpura
    Mild splenomegaly in 30%
    Platelet count may not predict bleeding (IgG- or IgM-induced platelet dysfunction)

Therapy
    Prednisone, 2.0 mg/kg per day given twice daily with 30 mL of liquid antacid
    70% of patients will respond; after platelet counts normalize for two weeks, slow prednisone taper at 5 mg/kg per week
    For steroid failures, splenectomy followed by slow prednisone taper is indicated; 70% will respond
    Splenectomy failure:
        Long-term prednisone
        Azathioprine
        Vincristine
        Intravenous gamma globulin
        Plasma exchange/infusion ?
        Combinations of these

Table 5-30. Drugs Causing Immune Thrombocytopenia

Common (Descending Order of Incidence)	Less Common
Gold	Allopurinol
Heparin	Antipyrine
Quinidine	Cephalexin
Quinine	Chlordiazepoxide
Sulfonamides	Chlorpheniramine
Indomethacin	Clonazepam
Arsenicals	Copper sulfate
Aspirin	Diazepam
Heroin	Disulfiram
Valproic acid	Gentamicin
Chlorthiazide	Imipramine
Chlorthalidone	Iopanoic acid
Furosemide	Levamisole
Rifampicin	Levodopa
Digitalis derivatives	Lidocaine
Diphenylhydantoin	Lincomycin
Para-amino salicylate	Meprobamate
Cimetidine	Methicillin
Acetaminophen	Nitroglycerin
Chlorpropamide	Novobiocin
Oxyphenbutazone	Paramethadione
Phenylbutazone	Penicillamine
Alpha methyl dopa	Pentamidine
Bleomycin sulfate	Phenytoin
Carbamazepine	Primidone
Acetazolamide	Prochlorperazine
Ampicillin	Propylthiouracil
Fenoprofen	Sodium salicylate
Isoniazid	Spironolactone
Mercurial diuretics	Streptomycin
Nitrofurantoin	Tetanus toxoid
Pertussis vaccine	Tetraethylammonium
Tolbutamide	Thioguanine
Trimethoprim	Thiouracil
Antazoline	Tobramycin
Barbiturates	
Cephalothins	
Clinoril	
Diazoxide	
Oxytetracycline	
Penicillin	
Procaine amide	

large number of drugs but is most commonly seen with quinidine, quinine, gold, heparin, sulfonamides, indomethacin, and thiazide diuretics.[276,277] Table 5-30 summarizes the drugs associated with immune-mediated thrombocytopenia most commonly in descending order of prevalence as well as the drugs causing immune-mediated thrombocytopenia less commonly.[259,276-292] The first incidence of drug-induced thrombocytopenia, which was noted after quinine ingestion, was reported in 1865.[293] Ackroyd was the first to study drug-induced thrombocytopenia carefully, and he demonstrated the immune-mediated nature of Sedormid-induced thrombocytopenia.[38,294,295] Subsequently, numerous studies have confirmed the immune nature of thrombocytopenia induced by quinine, quinidine, and sulfonamides.[259,276-278] Drug-induced immune thrombocytopenia is thought to occur by several postulated mechanisms. Ackroyd initially postulated that the drug became bound to the platelet membrane, and following this, antibody was formed against a platelet membrane–drug complex.[38,294,295] This mechanism is depicted in Figure 5-4. An alternate mecha-

nism, which appears to be operative for many drugs, is the so-called "innocent bystander" theory initially advanced by Shulman.[296-299] In this instance the drug interacts with an endogenous plasma protein or other endogenous plasma compound(s), and the antibody subsequently produced is directed against this drug–plasma protein complex. Thus, the drug is acting as a classic hapten. This resultant antibody plus drug/plasma protein (antigen) complex is then absorbed onto the platelet surface by Fc or C3 receptors. This mechanism appears operative in quinidine- and quinine-induced thrombocytopenia (Figure 5-5). In the case of quinidine- and

Figure 5-4. Drug-Induced Immune Thrombocytopenia: "Ackroyd" Mechanism

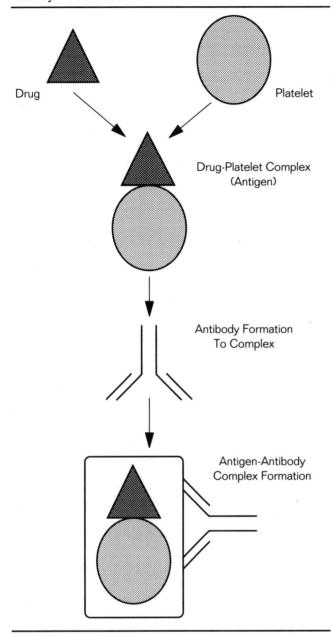

Figure 5-5. Drug-Induced Immune Thrombocytopenia: "Innocent Bystander" Mechanism

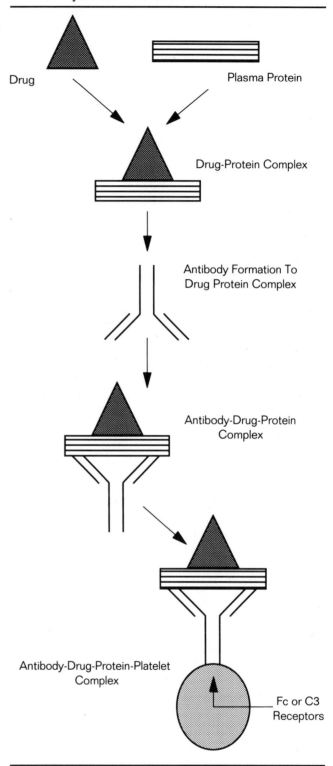

quinine-induced immune thrombocytopenia, the antibody complex appears to be heterogeneous and may react with platelet membrane glycoproteins Ib, IIb, IIIa, or IX.[300]

In most instances IgG antibody is produced in drug-induced immune thrombocytopenia; however, several cases of IgM-mediated thrombocytopenia have also been reported. Bernard-Soulier platelets, which are missing platelet membrane glycoproteins Ib and Is, do not agglutinate when incubated with drug plus serum from patients with immune-induced thrombocytopenia. This suggests that platelet glycoproteins Ib and Is are the receptors for some immune complex–mediated, drug-induced thrombocytopenia.[71,259,276]

Drug-induced immune thrombocytopenia usually appears with the rapid onset of petechiae and purpura and profound thrombocytopenia. The patient may have been ingesting the drug for only a short period or may have been taking the offending agent for months or, in some instances, years.

This is in contrast to nonimmune drug-induced thrombocytopenia, wherein the platelet count decreases very slowly and returns to normal only slowly after withdrawal of the offending drug. Although the integument is the most common site of hemorrhage, bleeding from other sites, including any mucosal membrane surface, may be seen. Catastrophic intracranial hemorrhage is uncommonly seen but is often the cause of death in fatal cases. The fatality rate of patients with drug-induced immune thrombocytopenia is approximately 5%. Many patients develop systemic symptomatology as well, consisting of fever, chills, headaches, generalized malaise, nausea, and emesis. Occasionally, severe abdominal cramping and generalized arthralgias may occur. Unlike nonimmune-mediated drug-induced thrombocytopenia, immune-mediated drug-induced thrombocytopenia usually, but not always, abates rapidly after removing the offending drug. The response is usually seen in three weeks to three months.

The diagnosis is made by noting the sudden onset of petechiae and purpura associated with thrombocytopenia in a patient ingesting one or more drugs. In this regard, taking a careful drug history is mandatory in thrombocytopenic patients, including a history for any compounds containing aspirin and any over-the-counter medications or home remedies that may contain quinine. Laboratory confirmation is best made by documenting the presence of platelet-associated IgG (PAIgG) plus the noting of control platelet agglutination when incubated with serum plus the offending drug. Numerous techniques for these tests have been devised and have recently been extensively reviewed.[232,276,277,301-307]

The mainstay of therapy for drug-induced immune thrombocytopenia consists of withdrawal of all suspected drugs, hospitalization of the patient if the platelet count is below 25×10^9/L (25,000/mm³), or, if significant hemorrhage is present, avoidance of any drug or compound known to interfere with platelet function and careful observation for suggestions of the potential for significant hemorrhage.[1] To help predict bleeding propensity, all stool specimens should be tested for blood, and a daily urinalysis sample should be collected and examined for red blood cells.[1] Steroids, in the form of oral prednisone or intravenous hydrocortisone succinate, may be of benefit in warding off life-threatening hemorrhage. This effect probably comes about via a beneficial effect on the vasculature, as previously discussed, rather than steroid-induced cessation or blunting of the immune mechanism. Patients who are suspected of developing a life-threatening hemorrhage, especially patients with intracranial bleeding, patients presenting with existing serious hemorrhage, or patients with platelet counts of less than 10×10^9/L (10,000/mm³) should be infused with platelet concentrates, directed single-donor platelets if feasible. Although infused platelets will demonstrate a shortened platelet life span, they usually are of benefit in achieving some degree of hemostasis (thus warding off fatal hemorrhage) and may be of benefit by complexing with the offending circulating immune complex (thus enhancing removal of the complex).

Table 5-31. Posttransfusion Purpura

Clinical Findings
  Occurs one week posttransfusion
  Most patients are PLA¹ negative
  Most patients are female previously sensitized by
    transfusion or pregnancy
  Sudden onset of petechiae, purpura, and ecchymoses
  Some patients have chills and fever at the time of
    transfusion
  Usually abates spontaneously in two weeks to two months

Laboratory Findings
  Thrombocytopenia usually severe
  Anti-PLA¹ antibody in most patients

Therapy
  Plasmapheresis/exchange
  Steroids?
  Platelets contraindicated

Posttransfusion Purpura. Posttransfusion purpura is a rare event and occurs approximately one week following transfusions in a patient who is PLA¹ negative.[308,309] The majority of the population (98%) is PLA¹ positive. Thus, the transfused patient who is PLA¹ negative has a high risk of receiving incompatible (PLA¹-positive) platelets.[308] The vast majority of cases are seen in women who are PLA¹ negative and have been previously sensitized by either transfusion or pregnancy.[310] A few cases have occurred in PLA¹-positive patients, and a few cases have also been noted in nonsensitized individuals, which suggests that in rare instances other platelet antibodies must be involved.[311] Patients with Glanzmann's thrombasthenia lack platelet glycoprotein IIb/IIIa and are PLA¹ negative.[312] Thus, it appears that the PLA¹ antigen site may be associated with platelet membrane glycoprotein IIIa or the IIb/IIIa complex. The clinical course is typically that of a sudden onset of petechiae, purpura, and mucosal membrane hemorrhage in association with thrombocytopenia occurring approximately one week following transfusions. Some patients demonstrate a mild transfusion reaction consisting of chills and fever at the time of the transfusion, but other patients have no such transfusion reaction when the offending transfusion is given approximately one week previous to the onset of signs or symptoms.[313] In most cases, anti-PLA¹ antibody can be easily demonstrated in the laboratory. In the majority of patients the thrombocytopenia will spontaneously abate in two weeks to two months, but in rare instances a protracted course occurs. Platelet transfusions should not be used, as further isoimmunization of the patient may occur.[224,313,314] Steroids are of questionable benefit but may ward off serious hemorrhage in some patients by the beneficial effect on the vasculature. If severe thrombocytopenia is present (platelet count less than 10×10^9/L [10,000/mm³]) or if significant hemorrhage is seen or suspected to be impending, the patient should be treated with plasmapheresis/exchange to remove the anti-

Table 5-32. Common Causes of Thrombocytosis

Acute infections (recovery phase)

Collagen vascular disorders

Chronic inflammatory/infectious diseases

Hemolytic anemias

Malignancy
  Lymphoma
  Hodgkin's disease
  Metastatic carcinoma

Myeloproliferative syndromes

Rebound phase of thrombocytopenia

Splenectomy

PLA[1] antibody.[1] This mode of therapy has almost always been successful and is the treatment of choice in high-risk patients. The features of posttransfusion purpura are summarized in Table 5-31.

Thrombocytosis and Thrombocythemia

Thrombocytosis refers to a benign secondary reactive increase in the platelet count. Thrombocytosis is usually associated with increased platelet production or interference with splenic pooling of platelets, such as postsplenectomy thrombocytosis, thrombocytosis following epinephrine infusion, or the use of large doses of steroids. Thrombocythemia, on the other hand, refers to a primary, uncontrolled (malignant) increase in megakaryocytes and platelet counts and may accompany any of the myeloproliferative syndromes, especially polycythemia vera and chronic myelogenous leukemia, or may represent a malignant transformation of the megakaryocyte or stem-cell precursor of the megakaryocyte. This latter myeloproliferative disorder is referred to as essential or primary thrombocythemia.

Thrombocytosis

Thrombocytosis is usually benign and asymptomatic and is commonly associated with acute or chronic inflammatory disorders, including collagen vascular disorders, recovery from acute infections, sarcoidosis, cirrhosis, tuberculosis, and other similar disorders.[315-319] Reactive thrombocytosis is commonly associated with acute hemorrhage, malignancy, hemolytic anemia, and severe iron deficiency.[320-323] A reactive thrombocytosis is often noted following treatment and subsequent recovery from a thrombocytopenic disorder (termed rebound thrombocytosis), such as immune thrombocytopenia purpura or drug-induced immune thrombocytopenia. Thrombocytosis usually occurs after splenectomy and may persist for several weeks or up to three months.[324] In thrombocytosis, platelets usually display normal morphologic features and usually function normally, which is in oppo-

sition to thrombocythemia where platelet morphology and platelet function are commonly abnormal. Reactive thrombocytosis is usually associated with normal results of tests of platelet function and reactivity, including platelet lumiaggregation or levels of platelet factor 4, beta-thromboglobulin, and thromboxane derivatives.

Patients with thrombocytosis are usually asymptomatic and require no therapy. Impaired hemostasis, manifest as increased risk of thrombosis or hemorrhage, is usually not associated with thrombocytosis. An increased risk of thrombosis is seen in two selected instances of reactive thrombocytosis. The first instance is postsplenectomy thrombocytosis in the presence of anemia of any etiology[315] and the second circumstance is thrombocytosis associated with severe iron deficiency.[325] In these selected instances, prophylactic anticoagulant therapy in the form of subcutaneous heparin or antiplatelet therapy in the form of aspirin plus dipyridamole is warranted. Additionally, the reactive thrombocytosis associated with iron-deficiency anemia will usually promptly cease within one week of initiating appropriate iron therapy. However, in the reactive thrombocytoses of other than these two etiologies, therapy is not indicated unless an actual thrombotic event occurs. Common causes of thrombocytosis are summarized in Table 5-32.

Reactive thrombocytosis is often associated with laboratory findings of hyperkalemia, hypercalcemia, and, occasionally, decreased pO_2 levels due to increased platelet consumption by the increased platelet population. In general, these laboratory findings can be considered to be occurring in vitro in the test tube collection system but not necessarily in the patient. In addition, increased markers of platelet release, platelet factor 4 and beta-thromboglobulin levels, are often increased, but template bleeding times and aggregation patterns typically remain normal.

Essential or Primary Thrombocythemia

Essential thrombocythemia is one of the myeloproliferative syndromes and is characterized by representing a disorder of uncontrolled megakaryocyte and platelet production, selected biochemical and bone marrow abnormalities, a sustained elevated platelet count with a peripheral platelet population composed of platelets demonstrating bizarre morphology, a clinical course commonly associated with hemorrhage and/or thrombosis, splenomegaly, and abnormal platelet function commonly leading to thrombohemorrhagic phenomena.[97,326-331] The disorder is clearly a clonal stem-cell disease, similar to the other myeloproliferative syndromes, as demonstrated by studies of female patients with essential thrombocythemia who demonstrate heterozygosity of glucose-6-phosphate dehydrogenase isoenzymes A and B. In these individuals the malignant platelet population will contain only one isoenzyme subspecies.[332] In addition, some individuals demonstrate the Philadelphia chromosome (c-*abl* oncogene).[333,334]

Essential thrombocythemia is the least common of the myeloproliferative syndromes and, like the others, may

Table 5-33. Essential Thrombocythemia

Diagnostic Criteria
    Platelet count approximately 1,000 x 10⁹/L
        (1,000,000/mm³)
    Normal red blood cell volume or hemoglobulin less than
        130 g/L (13 g/dL)
    No other cause for thrombocytosis
    Iron present in marrow, or one-month trial of iron increases
        hemoglobulin less than 10 g/L (1 g/dL)
    Absence of myelofibrosis
    Absence of Philadelphia chromosome (may no longer apply)

Clinical Findings
    Hemorrhage (60%)
    Thrombosis (20%)
    Hemorrhage and thrombosis (10%)
    Asymptomatic (20%)
    Mild splenomegaly
    Petechiae and purpura
    Large ecchymoses
    Bilateral epistaxis
    Mucosal membrane bleeding (especially gastrointestinal)
    Progression to AML (5%)
    Progression to CML (5%)
    Progression to myelofibrosis and myeloid metaplasia (5%)

Laboratory Findings
    Elevated LDH (90%)
    Elevated alkaline phosphatase (60%)
    Hyperuricemia (55%)
    Elevated muramidase (50%)
    Elevated or borderline leukocyte
    Alkaline phosphatase
    Mild leukocytosis
    Prolonged template bleeding time (50%)
    Abnormal platelet function (>90%)
    Hypercellular marrow with increased megakaryocytes with
        "bizarre" morphology
    Numerous platelet "lakes" in marrow

Therapy
    Hydroxyurea, busulfan, or alkeran
    Cytoreductive platelet pheresis
    Platelet suppressive drugs (combination)

Figure 5-6. Typical Marrow Findings in Essential Thrombocythemia

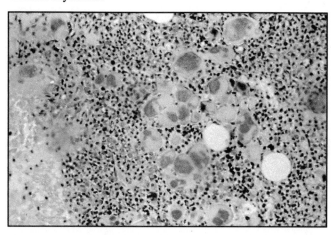

normal marrow iron stores and normal blood volume studies (red blood cell mass) in patients with essential thrombocythemia. To aid in distinguishing between these two disorders, the Polycythemia Vera Study Group has devised strict differential diagnostic criteria.[335,336] The diagnostic criteria and salient features of essential thrombocythemia are depicted in Table 5-33. The diagnosis of essential thrombocythemia is made by noting a platelet count approximating 1,000 x 10⁹/L (1,000,000/mm³) with no identifiable cause of thrombocytosis, a normal red blood cell mass, iron present in the bone marrow, or if absent a one-month trial of oral iron therapy resulting in a rise of the hemoglobin level of no more than 10 g/L (1 g/dL), an absence of collagen fibrosis on bone marrow biopsy, and, until recently, absence of the Philadelphia chromosome in bone marrow aspirates. This latter criterion may no longer apply, however, as several investigators have demonstrated the *c-abl* oncogene in patients with otherwise classic essential thrombocythemia.[333,334] In addition, the leukocyte alkaline phosphatase score is usually normal or elevated in patients with essential thrombocythemia, the vitamin B₁₂ binding protein is elevat-

Figure 5-7. Typical Marrow Findings in Essential Thrombocythemia

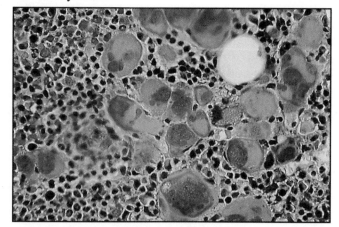

progress into a different and often more serious myelodysplastic disorder. Approximately 5% of patients will eventually develop acute myeloblastic leukemia, 5% will develop chronic myelogenous leukemia, 5% will develop myelofibrosis with agnogenic myeloid metaplasia, and approximately 5% will eventually be indistinguishable from polycythemia rubra vera.[97] In this latter instance it is likely that these patients actually had early quiescent polycythemia vera associated with thrombocythemia.

The diagnosis of essential thrombocythemia is one of exclusion. A reactive thrombocytosis is usually easy to exclude, but differentiation from polycythemia vera may be difficult. The primary differential points between essential thrombocythemia and polycythemia vera are the noting of

Figure 5-8. Platelet Function in Essential Thrombocythemia (Lumi-Aggregation)

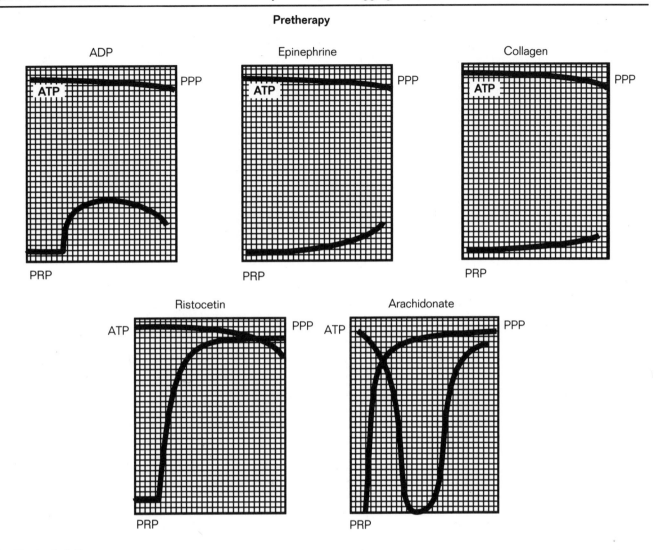

PRP = Platelet-Rich Plasma
PPP = Platelet-Poor Plasma
ATP = ATP Release

ed in 30% of patients, and other biochemical abnormalities are also commonly noted as is typical of other myeloproliferative syndromes.[329,337-339] Approximately 55% of patients will be hyperuricemic, 50% of patients will demonstrate elevated urine or serum lysozyme levels, almost all patients will demonstrate elevated lactate dehydrogenase (LDH) levels, and more than 80% will demonstrate elevated alkaline phosphatase levels.[329,337-340] Most patients (60%) will present with hemorrhage, approximately 20% of patients will present with thrombosis, 10% will present with hemorrhage and thrombosis, and approximately 20% of conditions are diagnosed in an asymptomatic state without thrombohemorrhagic phenomena yet becoming manifest.[337,338] Thrombotic events may involve the arterial or venous system, and peripheral arterial occlusion as well as peripheral venous occlusion, most commonly demonstrated in the lower

extremities, are common. The noting of erythema, cyanosis, or pregangrenous changes should immediately suggest the high probability of small vessel involvement and the necessity of definitive therapy.[97] The types of hemorrhage that can occur are highly varied. Most patients present with a history of easy and spontaneous bruising, and many have bilateral epistaxis. Bleeding from the gastrointestinal tract is extremely common, and patients may develop other types of mucosal membrane bleeding. Many patients may be noted to have petechiae and purpura, as well as large subcutaneous hematomas or bleeding into other organs.[97,329,337-340] A few instances can be associated with intra-articular bleeding.[341] Most patients (60%) will present with a mild leukocytosis usually with an increase in immature forms, which usually corrects promptly with myelosuppressive therapy. In addition, more than 50% of patients will have prolonged tem-

Figure 5-9. Platelet Function in Essential Thrombocythemia (Lumi-Aggregation)

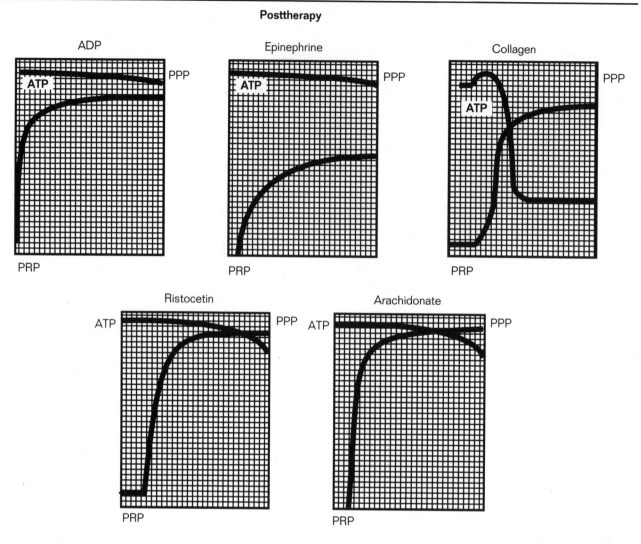

Posttherapy

PRP = Platelet-Rich Plasma
PPP = Platelet-Poor Plasma
ATP = ATP Release

plate bleeding times at presentation. The template bleeding time also tends to correct after myelosuppressive therapy.[329,337,338] The hyperuricemia, lysozyme levels, and LDH levels tend to correct with hydroxyurea therapy; however, the leukocyte alkaline phosphatase score usually does not change after myelosuppressive therapy.[329,337,338]

Platelet aggregation abnormalities are noted in the vast majority of patients: up to 100% of patients will demonstrate abnormalities to ADP, approximately 60% of patients will demonstrate abnormalities to epinephrine, 50% to collagen, 40% to arachidonic acid, and 30% to ristocetin-induced aggregation.[329,337,338] ATP release is also significantly abnormal in the vast majority of patients. ATP release induced by ADP and epinephrine is abnormal in 90% of patients, ATP release induced by collagen is abnormal in 30% of patients,

ATP release induced by arachidonic acid is abnormal in 80% of patients, and ATP release induced by ristocetin is abnormal in 70% of patients.[337,338] Aggregation may improve significantly after therapy with hydroxyurea and normalization of the platelet count; however, only moderate correction of release reaction abnormalities is noted following therapy with hydroxyurea.

Examination of the bone marrow in patients with essential thrombocythemia reveals the marrow to be typically hypercellular with a striking increase in megakaryocytes that are large, bizarre appearing, and often noted to be engulfing erythroid and myeloid precursors via active phagocytosis.[1,46] The megakaryocytes tend to be found in clusters. In addition, large islands of platelet aggregates are usually noted throughout the marrow smears.[329] Myeloid and erythroid hyperplasia are usually evident, and marrow iron stores are usually noted to be normal. The megakaryocyte volume is clearly increased as opposed to patients with chronic myelogenous leukemia who typically have decreased megakaryocytic volumes.[97] Evaluation of a peripheral smear will reveal a striking increase in platelets that are usually large and demonstrate bizarre morphology.[329] In addition, megakaryocyte fragments and large platelet aggregates are commonly noted on a peripheral smear.[329] The leukocytosis and the increase in immature forms is usually obvious. Typical marrow findings in essential thrombocythemia are shown in Figures 5-6 and 5-7.

The mainstay of therapy is to keep the platelet count below 700 x 10⁹/L (700,000 /mm³), because this usually eradicates the thrombotic or hemorrhagic complications of essential thrombocythemia.[329] Rapid lowering of the platelet count in the patient with hemorrhage, thrombosis, or in preparation for surgery can be easily accomplished by cytoreductive platelet pheresis. If the patient is asymptomatic, the platelet count can be effectively lowered by the use of numerous myelosuppressive agents including busulfan, phenylalanine mustard, and hydroxyurea. My choice of therapy is to use hydroxyurea at 15 to 20 mg/kg per day, which will usually result in prompt lowering of the platelet count.[329] This agent is chosen because it is not associated with prolonged pancytopenia and is not generally associated with mutagenicity when given over a long period. If the patient has sustained a thrombotic episode or if the platelet count is decreasing only very slowly, the addition of antiplatelet therapy in the form of aspirin and dipyridamole may be warranted until the platelet count is less than 700 x 10⁹/L (700,000/mm³). Once the platelet count is less than 700 x 10⁹/L (700,000/mm³), antiplatelet therapy is generally not warranted because thrombohemorrhagic manifestations usually cease at this level, and the template bleeding time is usually corrected, which appears to correlate reasonably well with clinical hemorrhage in this disorder. Most patients will require long-term myelosuppressive therapy, and my choice is, again, hydroxyurea given at a dose to maintain the platelet count at less than 700 x 10⁹/L (700,000/mm³). The choice of this agent over other myelosuppressive agents was previously discussed. Figures 5-8 and 5-9 depict platelet lumi-aggregation patterns in a patient both before and after therapy with hydroxyurea demonstrating significant but not total correction of platelet aggregation and platelet release abnormalities.

References

1. Bick RL: Platelet defects, ch 4. In: Disorders of Hemostasis and Thrombosis: Principles of Clinical Practice. Thieme, Inc., New York, 1985, p 65.

2. Bick RL: Clinical approach to the patient with hemorrhage, ch 2. In: Disorders of Hemostasis and Thrombosis: Principles of Clinical Practice. Thieme, Inc., New York, 1985, p 36.

3. Berkman N, Y Michaeli, J O'Gradey: EDTA-dependent pseudothrombocytopenia: a clinical study of 18 patients and review of the literature. Am J Hematol 36:195, 1991.

4. Veenhoven WA, GS Van Der Schans, W Huiges, HE Metting-Scherphuis, MR Halie, NO Nieweg: Pseudothrombocytopenia due to agglutinins. Am J Clin Pathol 72:1005, 1979.

5. Onder O, A Weinstein, CW Hoyer: Pseudothrombocytopenia caused by platelet agglutinins that are reactive in blood anticoagulated by chelating agents. Blood 56:177, 1980.

6. Zeigler Z: In vitro granulocyte-platelet rosette formation mediated by an IgG immunoglobulin. Haemostasis 3:282, 1974.

7. Kjeldsberg CR, J Swanson: Platelet satellitism. Blood 43:831, 1974.

8. Payne BA, RV Pierre: Pseudothrombocytopenia: a laboratory artifact with potentially serious consequences. Mayo Clin Proc 59:123, 1984.

9. Pegels JG, ECE Bruynes, CP Engelfriet, AEGR Von dem Borne: Pseudothrombocytopenia: an immunologic study on platelet antibodies dependent on ethylene diamine tetra-acetate. Blood 59:157, 1982.

10. Lombarts AJ, de Kieviet W: Recognition and prevention of pseudothrombocytopenia and concomitant pseudoleukocytosis. Am J Clin Pathol 89:634, 1988.

11. Payne BA: EDTA-induced pseudothrombocytopenia. Postgrad Med 77:75, 1985.

12. Babior BM: Folate and aplasia of bone marrow. N Engl J Med 298:506, 1978.

13. O'Neill EM, S Varadi: Neonatal aplastic anaemia and Fanconi's anaemia. Arch Dis Child 38:92, 1963.

14. Nilsson LR: Chronic pancytopenia with multiple congenital abnormalities. Acta Paediatr 49:518, 1960.

15. Hall JG, J Levin, JP Kuhn, E Jottenberg, KAP Van Berkum, V McKussik: Thrombocytopenia with absent radius (TAR). Medicine 48:411, 1969.

16. Edelberg SB, J Cohen, NJ Brandt: Congenital hypomegakaryocytic thrombocytopenia associated with bilateral absence of the radii: variation of the clinical picture. Hum Hered 27:147, 1977.

17. Berge T, F Brunnhage, LR Nisson: Congenital thrombocytopenia in rubella embryopathy. Acta Paediatr Scand 52:349, 1963.

18. Seip M: Hereditary hypoplastic thrombocytopenia. Acta Paediatr Scand 52:370, 1963.

19. Perry GS, BD Spector, LM Schuman, JS Mandel, VE Anderson, RB McHugh, MR Hanson, SM Fahlstrom, W Krivit, JH Kersey: The Wiskott-Aldrich syndrome in the United States and Canada (1892–1979). J Pediatr 97:72, 1980.

20. Aldrich RA, AG Steinberg, DC Campbell: Pedigree demonstrating a sex-linked recessive condition characterized by draining ears, ezcematoid dermatitis, and bloody diarrhea. Pediatrics 13:133, 1954.

21. Murphy S: Hereditary thrombocytopenia. Clin Haematol 1:359, 1972.

22. Ochs ND, SJ Slichter, LA Harker, WE Von Behrens, RA Clark, RJ Wedgwood: The Wiskott-Aldrich syndrome: studies of lymphocytes, granulocytes, and platelets. Blood 55:243, 1980.

23. Wolff JA: Wiskott-Aldrich syndrome: clinical, immunologic, and pathologic observations. J Pediatr 70:221, 1967.

24. Cooper MD, HP Chase, JT Lowman, W Krivit, RA Good: Wiskott-Aldrich syndrome: an immunologic deficiency disease involving the afferent limb of immunity. Am J Med 44:499, 1968.

25. Lum LG, DG Tubergen, L Corash, RM Blaese: Platelet-bound IgG in patients with the Wiskott-Aldrich syndrome. Cited by WE Hathaway, J Bonnar: Perinatal Coagulation. Grune and Stratton, New York, 1978.

26. Kelton JG, PB Neame, J Gouldie, J Hirsh: Elevated platelet-associated IgG in the thrombocytopenia of septicemia. N Engl J Med 300:760, 1979.

27. Lum LG, DG Tubergen, L Corash, RM Blaese: Splenectomy in the management of the thrombocytopenia of the Wiskott-Aldrich syndrome. N Engl J Med 302:892, 1980.

28. Schulman I, M Pierce, A Lukens, Z Cummimbhoy: Studies on thrombopoiesis, I: a factor in normal plasma required for platelet production; chronic thrombocytopenia due to its deficiency. Blood 16:943, 1960.

29. Lewis ML: Cyclic thrombocytopenia: a thrombopoietin deficiency? J Clin Pathol 27:242, 1974.

30. Godwin NA, AD Ginsburg: May-Hegglin anomaly: a defect in megakaryocyte fragmentation. Br J Haematol 26:117, 1974.

31. Gardner F, JD Bessman: Thrombocytopenia due to defective platelet production. Clin Haematol 12:23, 1983.

32. Brunning RD: Morphologic alterations in nucleated blood and marrow cells in genetic disorders. Hum Pathol 1:99, 1970.

33. Bernheim J, M Dechavanne, PA Bryon, M Lagarde, S Colon, N Pozet, J Traeger: Thrombocytopenia, macrothrombocytopathia, nephritis, and deafness. Am J Med 61:145, 1976.

34. Clare NM, MM Montiel, MD Lifschitz, GA Bannayan: Alport's syndrome associated with macrothrombopathic thrombocytopenia. Am J Clin Pathol 72:111, 1979.

35. Epstein CJ, MA Sahud, CF Piel, JR Goodman, MR Bernfield, JH Kushner, AR Ablin: Hereditary macrothrombocytopathia, nephritis, and deafness. Am J Med 52:299, 1972.

36. Raccuglia G: Gray platelet syndrome. A variety of qualitative platelet disorders. Am J Med 51:818, 1971.

37. Gerrard JM, DR Phillips, GHR Rao, EF Plow, DA Walz, R Ross, LA Harker, JG White: Biochemical studies of two patients with the gray platelet syndrome. J Clin Invest 66:102, 1980.

38. White JG: Ultrastructural studies of the gray platelet syndrome. Am J Pathol 95:445, 1979.

39. Takahashi N, R Nagayama, A Hattori, T Ihzumi, T Tsukada, A Shibata: von Willebrand disease associated with familial thrombocytopenia and increased ristocetin-induced platelet aggregation. Am J Hematol 10:89, 1981.

40. Murphy S, F Oski, L Nalman, CJ Lusch, S Goldberg, FN Gardner: Platelet size and kinetics in hereditary and acquired thrombocytopenia. N Engl J Med 286:499, 1972.

41. Kurstjens R, C Bolt, M Vossen, C Naanen: Familial thrombopathic thrombocytopenia. Br J Haematol 15:305, 1968.

42. Myllyla G, R Pelkonen, E Ikkala, J Apajalahti: Hereditary thrombocytopenia: report of three families. Scand J Haematol 4:441, 1967.

43. Sheth NK, TAJ Prankerd: Inherited thrombocytopenia with thrombasthenia. J Clin Pathol 21:154, 1968.

44. Von Behrens WE: Mediterranean macrothrombocytopenia. Blood 46:199, 1975.

45. Gutenberger J, CW Trygstad, ER Stiehm, JM Opitz, LG Thatcher, JMB Bloodworth, J Setzkorn: Familial thrombocytopenia, elevated serum IgA levels and renal disease. Am J Med 49:729, 1970.

46. Kass L: Bone Marrow Interpretation. JB Lippincott, Philadelphia, 1979, p 1.

47. Krause JR, RE Lee: Histiocytic infiltrates, ch 11. In: JR Krause (Ed): Bone Marrow Biopsy. Churchill Livingstone, New York, 1981, p 171.

48. Rywlin AM: Foreign cells, ch 10. In: Histopathology of the Bone Marrow. Little, Brown and Company, Boston, 1976, p 133.

49. Rodriquez S, S Leikin, MC Hiller: Neonatal thrombocytopenia associated with antepartum adminstration of thiazide drugs. N Engl J Med 270:881, 1964.

50. Pearson HA, S McIntosh: Neonatal thrombocytopenia. Clin Haematol 7:111, 1978.

51. Schiff D, JV Aranda, L Stern: Neonatal thrombocytopenia and congenital malformations associated with administration of tolbutamide to the mother. J Pediatr 77:457, 1970.

52. Pullen J: Drug-induced thrombocytopenias, ch 4. In: JM Lusher, MI Barnhart (Eds): Acquired Bleeding Disorders in Children: Platelet Abnormalities and Laboratory Methods. Masson Publishing, USA, New York, 1981, p 49.

53. Hathaway WE, J Bonnar: Bleeding disorders in the newborn infant, ch 5. In: Perinatal Coagulation. Grune and Stratton, New York, 1978, p 115.

54. Costello JM, FT Shannon: Drugs and children. N Z Med J 67:402, 1968.

55. Kelton JG, VS Blanchette, WE Wilson, P Powers, KRM Pai, SB Effer, RD Barr: Neonatal thrombocytopenia due to passive immunization. Prenatal diagnosis and distinction between maternal platelet alloantibodies and autoantibodies. N Engl J Med 302:1401, 1980.

56. Vossaugh P, J Leikin, G Avery, G Monif, T Sever: Neonatal thrombocytopenia in association with rubella. Acta Haematol 35:158, 1966.

57. Hanshaw HB: Congenital and acquired cytomegalovirus infection. Pediatr Clin North Am 13:279, 1966.

58. Baranski B, N Young: Hematologic consequences of viral infections. Hematol Oncol Clin North Am 1:167, 1987.

59. Gale RP, RE Champlin, S Feig, JH Fitchen: Aplastic anemia: biology and treatment. Ann Intern Med 95:477, 1981.

60. Lewis SM, EC Gordon-Smith: Aplastic and dysplastic anaemias, ch 31. In: RM Hardisty, DJ Weatherall (Eds): Blood and its disorders. Blackwell Scientific Publications, Oxford, 1982, p 1229.

61. Bessman JD, LJ Williams, PR Gilmer: Platelet size in health and hematologic disease. Am J Clin Pathol 78:150, 1982.

62. Stoll DB, S Blum, D Pasquale, S Murphy: Thrombocytopenia with decreased megakaryocytes: evaluation and prognosis. Ann Intern Med 198:170, 1981.

63. Nussbaum H, B Allen, AR Kagam, HA Gilbert, A Rao, P Chan: Management of bone metastases: multidisciplinary approach. Semin Oncol 4:93, 1977.

64. Chia YC, JJ Machin: Tuberculosis and severe thrombocytopenia. Br J Clin Pract 33:5, 1979.

65. Erb BD: Thrombocytopenic purpura accompanying brucellosis: a case report with demonstration of a granuloma in the bone marrow. J Tenn Med Assoc 59:876, 1966.

66. Diamant S, Z Spirer: Chronic thrombocytopenic purpura associated with toxoplasmosis. Br Med J 280:1505, 1980.

67. Skudowitz RB, J Katz, A Lurie, J Levin, J Metz: Mechanisms of thrombocytopenia in malignant tertian malaria. Br Med J 2:515, 1973.

68. Des Prez RM, S Steckley, RM Stroud, J Hawiger: Interaction of *Histoplasma capsulatum* with human platelets. J Infect Dis 142:32, 1980.

69. Volk BW, M Adachi, L Schneck: The pathology of the sphingolipidoses. Semin Hematol 9:317, 1972.

70. Brady RO: Biochemical and metabolic basis of familial sphingolipidoses. Semin Hematol 9:273, 1972.

71. Groover RV, EC Burke, N Gordon, WE Berdon: The genetic mucopolysaccharidoses. Semin Hematol 9:371, 1972.

72. Haskell CM: Principles of cancer chemotherapy, ch 4. In: CM Haskell (Ed): Cancer Treatment. WB Saunders, Philadelphia, 1990, p 21.

73. Fajardo LF: Hematopoietic tissue, ch 12. In: Pathology of Radiation Injury. Masson Publishing USA, New York, 1982, p 166.

74. Kutti J, A Weinfeld: The frequency of thrombocytopenia in patients with heart disease treated with oral diuretics. Acta Med Scand 183:245, 1968.

75. Cowan DH: Effect of alcoholism on hemostasis. Semin Hematol 17:137, 1980.

76. Chesterman CN, DG Penington: Platelet production and turnover: thrombocytopenia and thrombocytosis, ch 25. In: RM Hardisty, DJ Weatherall (Eds): Blood and Its Disorders. Blackwell Scientific Publications, Oxford, 1982, p 971.

77. Williams DM, RE Lynch, GE Cartwright: Drug-induced aplastic anemia. Semin Hematol 10:195, 1973.

78. Cohen T, DP Cooney: Cyclic thrombocytopenia: case report and review of the literature. Scand J Haematol 12:9, 1974.

79. Skoog WA, JS Lawrence, WS Adams: A metabolic study of a patient with idiopathic cyclical thrombocytopenic purpura. Blood 12:844, 1957.

80. Engstrom E, A Lundquist, N Soderström: Periodic thrombocytopenia or tidal platelet dysgenesis in a man. Scand J Haematol 3:290, 1966.

81. Clawson CC, JG White: Platelet interaction with bacteria: ultrastructure of congenital afibrinogenemic platelets. Am J Pathol 98:197, 1980.

82. Clawson CC, JG White, MC Nerzberg: Platelet interaction with bacteria: contrasting the role of fibrinogen and fibronectin. Am J Hematol 9:43, 1980.

83. Espinoza C, C Kuhn: Viral infection of megakaryocytes in varicella with purpura. Am J Clin Pathol 61:203, 1974.

84. Alter HJ, RT Scanlon, GP Schechter: Thrombocytopenic purpura following vaccination with attenuated measles virus. Am J Dis Child 115:111, 1968.

85. Osborn JE, NT Shahadi: Thrombocytopenia in murine cytomegalovirus infection. J Lab Clin Med 81:53, 1973.

86. Camitta BM, DG Nathan, EN Forman, R Parkman, JM Rappeport, TD Orellana: Posthepatic severe aplastic anemia: an indication for early bone marrow transplantation. Blood 43:473, 1974.

87. Chesney PJ, NT Shahidi: Acute viral-induced thrombocytopenia: a review of human disease, animal models, and in vitro studies. In: JM Lusher, MI Barnhart (Eds): Acquired Bleeding Disorders of Children. Masson Publishers USA, New York, 1981, p 65.

88. Carter RL: Platelet levels in infectious mononucleosis. Blood 25:817, 1965.

89. Cohen P, FH Gardner: Thrombocytopenia as a laboratory sign and complication of gram-negative bacteremic infection. Arch Intern Med 117:113, 1966.

90. Lewis JH, MB Zucker, JH Ferguson: Bleeding tendency in uremia. Blood 11:1073, 1956.

91. Rabiner SF: Uremic bleeding. Prog Hemost Thromb 1:233, 1972.

92. Hartmann RC, DE Jonkins: Paroxysmal nocturnal hemoglobinuria: current concepts of certain pathophysiological features. Blood 25:850, 1965.

93. Caranobe C, P Sie, C Nouvel, G Laurent, J Pris, B Boneu: Platelets in myeloproliferative disorders. Scand J Haematol 25:289, 1980.

94. Weinfeld A, I Branehog, J Kutti: Platelets in the myeloproliferative syndrome. Clin Haematol 4:373, 1975.

95. Aster HP, SE Enright: A platelet and granulocyte membrane defect in paroxysmal nocturnal hemoglobinuria: usefulness for the detection of platelet antibodies. J Clin Invest 48:1199, 1969.

96. Nicholson-Weller A: Deficiency of the complement regulatory protein, "deca-accelerating factor," on membranes of granulocytes, monocytes, and platelets in paroxysmal nocturnal hemoglobinuria. N Engl J Med 312:1091, 1985.

97. Murphy S: Thrombocytosis and thrombocythaemia. Clin Haematol 12:89, 1983.

98. Smith MD, DA Smith, M Fletcher: Hemorrhage associated with thrombocytopenia in megaloblastic anemia. Br Med J 1:982, 1962.

99. Levine PH: A qualitative platelet defect in severe vitamin B_{12} deficiency: response, hyperresponse, and thrombosis after vitamin B_{12} therapy. Ann Intern Med 78:533, 1973.

100. Mauer AM, W de Vaux, ME Lahey: Neonatal and maternal thrombocytopenic purpura due to quinine. Pediatrics 19:84, 1957.

101. Widerlov E, I Karlman, J Storsater: Hydralazine-induced neonatal thrombocytopenia. N Engl J Med 303:1235, 1980.

102. Pearson HA, NR Shulman, VJ Marder, TE Cone: Isoimmune neonatal thrombcytopenic purpura. Blood 23:154, 1964.

103. Shulman NR, VJ Marder, MC Hiller, EM Collier: Platelet and leukocyte isoantigens and their antibodies: serologic, physiologic and clinical studies. Prog Hematol 4:222, 1964.

104. von dem Borne AEG, EF van Leeurwen, LE von Riesz, CJ van Boxtel, CP Engelfriet: Neonatal alloimmune thrombocytopenia: detection and characterization of the responsible antibodies by the platelet immunofluorescence test. Blood 57:649, 1981.

105. von dem Borne AEGK, E von Reisz, FWA Verheugt, JW ten Cate, JG Kope, CP Engelfriet, LE Nijenhuis: Bak-a, a new platelet-specific antigen involved in neonatal alloimmune thrombocytopenia. Vox Sang 39:113, 1980.

106. Andrew M, RD Barr: Increased platelet destruction in infancy and childhood. Semin Thromb Hemost 8:248, 1982.

107. Mennuti M, RH Schwarz, F Gill: Obstetric management of isoimmune thrombocytopenia. Am J Obstet Gynecol 118:565, 1974.

108. Smith CH: The purpuras, ch 27. In: Blood Diseases of Infancy and Childhood. CV Mosby, St. Louis, 1972, p 760.

109. Whitaker JA, P Sartain, M Shahedy: Hematological aspects of congenital syphilis. J Pediatr 66:629, 1965.

110. Gibson B, D Hunter, PB Naeme, JG Kelton: Thrombocytopenia in preeclampsia and eclampsia. Semin Thromb Hemost 8:234, 1982.

111. Harris EN, JKH Chan, RA Asherson, VR Aber, AE Gharavi, GRV Hughes: Thrombosis, recurrent fetal loss, and thrombocytopenia. Arch Intern Med 146:2153, 1986.

112. Von Gasset C, E Gautier, A Steck, RE Siebenmann, R Oechslin: Hamolytisch-Uraemische syndrome: bilaterale nierenrindennekrosen bie akuten erworbenen hamolytischen anamien. Schweiz Med Wochenschr 85:905, 1955.

113. Harlan JM: Thrombocytopenia due to nonimmune platelet destruction. Clin Haematol 12:39, 1983.

114. Goldstein HN, J Churg, L Strauss, D Gribetz: Hemolytic-uremic syndrome. Nephron 23:263, 1979.

115. Mosgrave JE, YB Talwaker, NC Puri, RA Campbell, B Loggan: The hemolytic-uremic syndrome. Clin Pediatr 17:218, 1978.

116. Clarkson AR, JR Lawrence, R Meadowns, AE Seymour: The hemolytic-uremic syndrome in adults. Q J Med 39:227, 1970.

117. Ponticelli C, E Rivolta, E Imbasciati, E Rossi, PM Mannucci: Hemolytic uremic syndrome in adults. Arch Intern Med 140:353, 1980.

118. Schoolwerth AC, RS Sandler, S Klahr, JM Kissane: Nephrosclerosis postpartum and in women taking oral contraceptives: a report of two cases. Arch Intern Med 136:178, 1976.

119. Hauglustaine D, B Van Damme, Y Venrenteghem, P Michielsen: Recurrent hemolytic uremic syndrome during oral contraception. Clin Nephrol 15:148, 1981.

120. Folman R, GS Arbus, B Churchill, L Gaum, J Huber: Recurrence of the hemolytic-uremic syndrome in a $3^1/_2$ year old child 4 months after second renal transplantation. Clin Nephrol 10:121, 1978.

121. Arends MJ, DJ Harrison: Novel histopathologic findings in a surviving case of hemolytic uremic syndrome after bone marrow transplantation. Hum Pathol 20:89, 1989.

122. Marshall RJ, P Sweny: Haemolytic uremic syndrome in recipients of bone marrow transplants not treated with cyclosporine A. Histopathology 10:953, 1986.

123. Craig JIO, T Sheehan, K Bell: The hemolytic uremic syndrome and bone marrow transplantation. Br Med J 295:887, 1987.

124. Jurgensen KA, RS Pedersen: Familial deficiency of prostacyclin production stimulating factor in the hemolytic-uremic syndrome of childhood. Thromb Res 21:311, 1981.

125. Donckerwolcke RA, RH Kuijsten, HA Tiddens, JD Van Gool: Haemolytic uremic syndrome. Pediatrician 8:378, 1979.

126. Riella MC, CRP George, RO Hickman, GE Striker, SJ Slichter, L Harker, LJ Quadracci: Renal microangiopathy of the hemolytic-uremic syndrome. Nephron 17:188, 1976.

127. Brain MC, PB Neame: Thrombotic thrombocytopenic purpura and the hemolytic uremic syndrome. Semin Thromb Hemost 8:186, 1982.

128. G Remuzzi: Treatment of the hemolytic-uremic syndrome with plasma. Clin Nephrol 12:279, 1979.

129. Weksler BB: Prostacyclin. Prog Hemost Thromb 6:113, 1982.

130. Bick RL: Alterations of hemostasis associated with surgery, cardiovascular surgery, prosthetic devices and transplantation, ch 13. In: OD Ratnoff, CD Forbes (Eds): Disorders of Hemostasis, ed 2. WB Saunders, Philadelphia, 1991, p 382.

131. Pillay VKG, NA Kurtzman, JR Manaligod, O Jonasson: Selective thrombocytopenia due to localized microangiopathy of renal allografts. Lancet 2:988, 1973.

132. Lindsay RM, WF Clark: Platelet destruction in renal disease. Semin Thromb Hemost 8:138, 1982.

133. Kaplan BS, D Esseltine: Thrombocytopenia in patients with acute post-streptococcal glomerulonephritis. J Pediatr 93:974, 1978.

134. Nalbandian RM, RL Henry, RL Bick: Thrombotic thrombocytopenic purpura. Semin Thromb Hemost 5:216, 1979.

135. Weiner CP: Thrombotic microangiopathy in pregnancy and the postpartum period. Semin Hematol 24:119, 1987.

136. Riggs SA, NP Wray, CC Waddell, RD Rossen, F Gyorkey: Thrombotic thrombocytopenic purpura complicating legionnaires' disease. Arch Intern Med 142:2275, 1982.

137. Nussbaum M, W Dameshek: Transient hemolytic and thrombocytopenic episode (? acute transient thrombohemolytic thrombocytopenic purpura), with probable meningiococcemia. N Engl J Med 256:448, 1957.

138. Reynolds PM, JM Jackson, JAS Brine: Thrombotic thrombocytopenic purpura remission following splenectomy. Am J Med 61:439, 1976.

139. Shalev O, A Karni, A Kornberg, M Brezis: Thrombotic thrombocytopenic purpura associated with *Bacteroides* bacteremia. Arch Intern Med 141:692, 1981.

140. Myers TJ, CJ Wakem, ED Ball, SJ Tremont: Thrombotic thrombocytopenic purpura: combined treatment with plasmapheresis and antiplatelet agents. Ann Intern Med 92:149, 1980.

141. Brown RC, TE Blecher, EA French, PJ Toghill: Thrombotic thrombocytopenic purpura after influenza vaccination. Br Med J 2:303, 1973.

142. Berberich PR, SA Cuene, RL Chard: Thrombotic thrombocytopenic purpura: three cases with platelet and fibrinogen survival studies. J Pediatr 84:503, 1974.

143. Blecher TE, AB Raper: Early diagnosis of thrombotic microangiopathy by paraffin sections of aspirated bone marrow. Arch Dis Child 42:158, 1967.

144. Eisenstaedt RS, RW Coleman, VJ Marder: Thrombotic thrombocytopenic purpura, ch 63. In: RW Coleman, J Hirsh, VJ Marder, EW Salzman (Eds): Hemostasis and Thrombosis: Basic Principles and Clinical Practice. JB Lippincott, Philadelphia, 1987.

145. Nair JMG, R Bellevue, M Bertoni, H Dosik: Thrombotic thrombocytopenic purpura in patients with the acquired immunodeficiency syndrome (AIDS)– related complex. Ann Intern Med 109:209, 1988.

146. Oksenhendler E, P Bierling, F Ferchal, JP Clauvel, M Seligmann: Zidovudine for thrombocytopenic purpura related to human immunodeficiency virus (HIV) infection. Ann Intern Med 1210:365, 1989.

147. Leaf AN, LJ Laubenstein, B Raphael, H Hochster, L Baez, S Karpatkin: Thrombotic thrombocytopenic purpura assiciated with human immunodeficiency virus type 1 (HIV-1) infection. Ann Intern Med 109:194, 1988.

148. Botti AC, P Hyde, F DiPillo: Thrombotic thrombocytopenic purpura in a patient who subsequently developed the acquired immunodeficiency syndrome (AIDS). Ann Intern Med 109:242, 1988.

149. Kwann HC: Clinicopathologic features of thrombotic thrombocytopenic purpura. Semin Hematol 24:71, 1987.

150. Aster RH: TTP: new clues to the etiology of an enigmatic disease. N Engl J Med 297:1400, 1977.

151. Ligorsky RD: TTP: true or false. Am J Med 64:913, 1978.

152. Taub RN, F Rodriquez-Erdmann, W Dameshek: Intravascular coagulation, the Schwartzman reaction and the pathogenesis of TTP. Blood 24:775, 1964.

153. Craig DM, D Gitlin: The nature of the hyaline thrombi in thrombotic thrombocytopenic purpura. Am J Pathol 33:251, 1957.

154. Feldman JD, MR Mardiney, ER Unanue, H Cutting: The vascular pathology of thrombotic thrombocytopenic purpura: an immunohistochemical and ultrastructural study. Lab Invest 15:927, 1966.

155. Gore I: Disseminated arteriolar and capillary platelet thrombosis: a morphological study of its histogenesis. Am J Pathol 26:155, 1950.

156. Amorosi EL, JE Ultmann: Thrombotic thrombocytopenic purpura: report of 16 cases and review of the literature. Medicine 45:139, 1966.

157. Kwaan HC, RV Pierre, EV Potter, GE Gallo: The nature of vascular lesion in thrombotic thrombocytopenic purpura. Blood 28:986, 1966.

158. Furey NL, FR Schmid, HC Kwaan, HHR Friederici: Arterial thrombosis in scleroderma. Br J Dermatol 93:683, 1975.

159. Remuzzi G, G Mecca, M Livio, G DeGaetano, MB Donati, JD Pearson, JL Gordon: Prostacyclin generation by cultured endothelial cells in haemolytic uremic syndrome. Lancet 1:656, 1980.

160. Neame PB, J Hirsh, G Browman, J Denburg, TJ D'Souza, A Gallus, MC Brain: Thrombotic thrombocytopenic purpura: a syndrome of intravascular platelet consumption. Can Med Assoc J 114:1108, 1976.

161. Lian ECY: Pathogenesis of thrombotic thrombocytopenic purpura. Semin Hematol 24:82, 1987.

162. Lian EC, N Saravaj: Effects of platelet inhibitors on the platelet aggregation induced by plasma from patients with thrombotic thrombocytopenic purpura. Blood 58:354, 1981.

163. Siddiqui FA, ECY Lian: Novel platelet-agglutinating protein from thrombotic thrombocytopenic purpura plasma. J Clin Invest 76:1330, 1985.

164. Moake JL, CK Rudy, JH Troll, MJ Weinstein, NM Colannino, J Azocar, RH Seder, SL Hong, D Deykin: Unusually large plasma factor VIII:von Willebrand factor multimers in chronic relapsing thrombotic thrombocytopenic purpura. N Engl J Med 307:1432, 1982.

165. Lian ECY, FA Siddiqui: von Willebrand factor in thrombotic thrombocytopenic purpura. Blood 67:1524, 1986.

166. Takahashi H, W Tatewaki, T Nakamura, M Hanano, K Wada, A Shabita: Coagulation studies in thrombotic thrombocytopenic purpura, with special reference to von Willebrand factor and Protein S. Am J Hematol 30:14, 1989.

167. Bick RL: Disseminated intravascular coagulation and related syndromes: a clinical review. Semin Thromb Hemost 14:299, 1988.

168. Remuzzi G, EC Rossi, R Misiani, D Marchesi, G Mecca, G deGaetano, MB Donati: Prostacyclin and thrombotic microangiopathy. Semin Thromb Hemost 6:301, 1980.

169. Jemsbu CN, PJ Lewis, P Hilgard, GJ Mufti, J Hows, J Webster: Prostacyclin deficiency in thrombotic thrombocytopenic purpura. Lancet 2:748, 1979.

170. Byrnes JJ, ECY Lian: Recent therapeutic advances in thrombotic thrombocytopenic purpura. Semin Thromb Hemost 5:199, 1979.

171. Bukowski RM, JS Hewlett, RR Reimer, CW Groppe, JK Weick, RB Livingston: Therapy of thrombotic thrombocytopenic purpura: an overview. Semin Thromb Hemost 7:1, 1981.

172. Byrnes JJ: Plasma infusion in the treatment of thrombotic thrombocytopenic purpura. Semin Thromb Hemost 7:9, 1981.

173. Roggenenti P, G Remuzzi: Thrombotic thrombocytopenic purpura and related disorders. Hematol Oncol Clin North Am 4:219, 1990.

174. Bukowski RM, JW King, JS Hewlett: Plasmapheresis in the treatment of thrombotic thrombocytopenic purpura. Blood 50:413, 1977.

175. Gandolfo GM, A Afeltra, GM Ferri: Plasmapheresis for thrombocytopenia. Lancet 1:1095, 1978.

176. Shepard KV, RM Bukowski: The treatment of thrombotic thrombocytopenic purpura with exchange transfusions, plasma infusions, and plasma exchange. Semin Hematol 24:178, 1987.

177. Taft EG, ST Baldwin: Plasma exchange transfusion. Semin Thromb Hemost 7:15, 1981.

178. Bukowski RM: Thrombotic thrombocytopenic purpura: a review. Prog Hemost Thromb 6:287, 1982.

179. Myers TJ, CJ Wakem, ED Ball, SJ Tremont: Thrombotic thrombocytopenic purpura: combined treatment with plasmapheresis and antiplatelet agents. Ann Intern Med 92:149, 1980.

180. Amir J, S Krauss: Treatment of thrombotic thrombocytopenic purpura with antiplatelet drugs. Blood 42:27, 1973.

181. Amorosi EL, S Karpatkin: Antiplatelet treatment of thrombotic thrombocytopenic purpura. Ann Intern Med 86:102, 1977.

182. Remuzzi G, C Zola, EC Rossi: Prostacyclin in thrombotic microangiopathy. Semin Hematol 24:110, 1987.

183. Cocchetto DM, L Cook, AE Cato, JE Niedel: Rationale and proposal for use of prostacyclin in thrombotic thrombocytopenic purpura therapy. Semin Thromb Hemost 7:43, 1981.

184. Pisciotta AV, JI Gottschall: Clinical features of thrombotic thrombocytopenic purpura. Semin Thromb Hemost 6:330, 1980.

185. Mammen EF: The endothelial cell in health and disease from the coagulationists point of view. Semin Thromb Hemost 5:165, 1979.

186. Mammen EF: Thrombotic thrombocytopenic purpura, part 1. Semin Thromb Hemost 6:325, 1980.

187. Mammen EF: Thrombotic thrombocytopenic purpura, part 2. Semin Thromb Hemost 7:1, 1981.

188. Bennett J, J Kelton, C Linker: Acquired disorders of platelet function. Educational Program: American Society of Hematology 1986. Slack, Thorofare, 1986.

189. Kwann HC: Thrombotic microangiopathy, parts I and II. Semin Hematol 24:69, 1987.

190. Enriquez P, RS Neiman: The pathology of the spleen: a functional approach. ASCP Press, Chicago, 1976, p 1.

191. Aster RH: Pooling of platelets in the spleen: role in the pathogenesis of "hypersplenic" thrombocytopenia. J Clin Invest 45:645, 1964.

192. Libre EP, DN Cowan, SP Watkins, NR Schulman: Relationships between spleen, platelets, and Factor VIII levels. Blood 31:358, 1968.

193. Penny R, MC Rozenberg, BG Firkin: The splenic platelet pool. Blood 27:1, 1966.

194. Bick RL: Treatment of bleeding and thrombosis in the patient with cancer, ch 5. In: TF Nealon (Ed): Management of the Patient with Cancer. WB Saunders, Philadelphia, 1976, p 48.

195. Amir-Ahmadi H, RS McGray, F Martin, W Mitch, P Kantrowitz, N Zamcheck: Reassessment of massive upper gastrointestinal hemorrhage on the wards of the Boston City Hospital. Surg Clin North Am 49:715, 1969.

196. Hawiger J, A Hawiger, S Steckley, S Timmons, C Cheng: Membrane changes in human platelets induced by lipopolysaccharide endotoxin. Br J Haematol 35:285, 1977.

197. Terada N, M Baldini, S Ebbe, MA Madoff: Interaction of influenza virus with blood platelets. Blood 28:231, 1966.

198. Neame PB, JG Kelton, IR Walker, IU Stewart, HL Nossel, J Hirsh: Thrombocytopenia in septicemia: the role of disseminated intravascular coagulation. Blood 56:88, 1980.

199. Wilson JJ, PB Neame, JG Kelton: Infection-induced thrombocytopenia. Semin Thromb Hemost 8:217, 1982.

200. Baker WF: Clinical aspects of disseminated intravascular coagulation: a clinician's point of view. Semin Thromb Hemost 15:1, 1989.

201. Gould L, A Greisberg, GC Lewnew, R Roddy, S Werthamer: Right atrial myxoma associated with thrombocytopenia and bacterial endocarditis. N Y State J Med 78:2081, 1978.

202. Warkentin TE, JG Kelton: Heparin-induced thrombocytopenia. Prog Hemost Thromb 10:1, 1991.

203. Karpatkin S: HIV-1-related thrombocytopenia. Clin Hematol Oncol. 4:193, 1990.

204. Gangarosa EJ, TR Johnson, HS Ramos: Ristocetin-induced thrombocytopenia: site and mechanism of action. Arch Intern Med 105:83, 1960.

205. Hilgard H, DK Hossfeld: Transient bleomycin-induced thrombocytopenia: a clinical study. Eur J Cancer 14:1261, 1978.

206. Bell WR, RM Royall: Heparin-induced thrombocytopenia: a comparison of three heparin preparations. N Engl J Med 303:902, 1980.

207. Kay AGL: Myelotoxicity of gold. Br Med J 1:1266, 1976.

208. Stafford BT, WH Crosby: Late onset of gold-induced thrombocytopenia with a practical note on the injections of dimercaprol. JAMA 239:50, 1978.

209. Heyns A, MG Lotter, PN Badenhorst, H Kotze, FC Killian, C Herbst, OR van Reenen, PC Minnaar: Kinetics and in vivo redistribution of "indium-labelled" platelets after intravenous protamine sulfate. Thromb Haemost 44:65, 1980.

210. Cole AP: Transient thrombocytopenia in a child on sodium valproate. Dev Med Child Neurol 20:487, 1978.

211. Jacobson RJ, CE Rath, JK Perloff: Intravascular hemolysis and thrombocytopenia in left ventricular outflow obstruction. Br Heart J 35:849, 1973.

212. Szekely P: Systemic embolization and anticoagulant prophylaxis in rheumatic heart disease. Br Med J 1:1209, 1964.

213. Roberts WC, BH Bulkley, AG Morrow: Pathologic anatomy of cardiac valve replacement: a study of 224 necropsy patients. Prog Cardiovasc Dis 15:539, 1973.

214. Bick RL: Hemostasis defects associated with cardiac surgery, prosthetic devices, and other extracorporeal circuits. Semin Thromb Hemost 11:249, 1985.

215. Bick RL: Alterations of hemostasis associated with surgery, cardiac surgery, prosthetic devices and transplantation, ch 13. In: OD Ratnoff, CD Forbes (Eds): Disorders of Hemostasis. Grune and Stratton, New York, 1991, p 379.

216. Cavese PG, V Gallucci, M Morea, S Dalla Volta, G Fasoli, D Casarotto: Heart valve replacement with the Hancock bioprosthesis. Circulation 56(suppl 2):111, 1976.

217. Cohn LN, JK Koster, RBB Mee, JJ Collins: Long-term follow-up of the Hancock bioprosthetic valve. Circulation 60(suppl 1):87, 1978.

218. Malinovsky NN, VA Kozlov: Thrombosis and embolisms in heart valve prosthetics, ch 5. In: Anticoagulant and Thrombolytic Therapy in Surgery. CV Mosby, St. Louis, 1979, p 149.

219. Herzer R, JD Hill, WJ Kerth: Thromboembolic complications after mitral valve replacement with Hancock xenograft. J Thorac Cardiovasc Surg 75:651, 1978.

220. Wu KK, JC Hoak: A new method for the quantitative detection of platelet aggregates in patients with arterial insufficiency. Lancet 2:924, 1974.

221. Salem NH, J Kouts, BG Firkin: Circulating platelet aggregates in ischaemic heart disease and their correlation to platelet life scan. Thromb Res 17:707, 1980.

222. Lowe GDO, MM Reavy, RV Johnston, CD Forbes, CRM Prentice: Increased platelet aggregates in vascular and nonvascular illness. Correlation with plasma fibrinogen and effect of ancrod. Thromb Res 14:377, 1979.

223. Malinovsky NN, VA Kozlov: Acute arterial obstruction of aortic bifurcation and limb arteries, ch 4. In: Anticoagulant and Thrombolytic Therapy in Surgery. CV Mosby, St. Louis, 1979, p 79.

224. Duff GL, GC McMillan: Pathology of atherosclerosis. Am J Med 11:92, 1951.

225. Bick RL, BJ McClain: Deep venous thrombosis: a laboratory evaluation of 118 consecutive patients. Thromb Haemost 50:305, 1983.

226. Turpie AGG, AC de Boer, E Genton: Platelet consumption in cardiovascular disease. Semin Thromb Hemost 8:161, 1982.

227. Lusher JM, R Iyer: Idiopathic thrombocytopenic purpura in children. Semin Thromb Hemost 3:175, 1977.

228. McWilliams NB, HM Mauer: Acute idiopathic thrombocytopenic purpura in children. Am J Hematol 7:87, 1979.

229. Cohn J: Thrombocytopenia in childhood: an evaluation of 433 patients. Scand J Haematol 16:226, 1976.

230. McClure J: Idiopathic thrombocytopenic purpura in children: diagnosis and management. Pediatrics 55:68, 1975.

231. Carpentieri U, ME Naggard: Thrombocytopenia and viral diseases. Tex Med 71:81, 1975.

232. Kelton JG, S Gibbons: Autoimmune platelet destruction: idiopathic thrombocytopenic purpura. Semin Thromb Hemost 8:83, 1982.

233. Pfueller SL, LJ Cosgrove: Activation of human platelets in PRP via their Fc receptor by antigen-antibody complexes or immunoglobulin G: requirement for particle-bound fibrinogen. Thromb Res 20:97, 1980.

234. Klein CA, MA Blajchman: Alloantibodies and platelet destruction. Semin Thromb Hemost 8:105, 1982.

235. Imbach P, V d'Apuzzo, A Hirt, E Rossi, M Vest, S Barandun, C Baumgartner, A Morell, M Schoni, HP Wagner: High-dose intravenous gamma globulin for idiopathic thrombocytopenic purpura in childhood. Lancet 1:1228, 1981.

236. Carroll RR, WD Noyes, CS Kitchens: High-dose intravenous immunoglobulin therapy in patients with immune thrombocytopenic purpura. JAMA 249:1748, 1983.

237. Mueller-Eckhardt C: Idiopathic thrombocytopenic purpura (ITP): clinical and immunologic considerations. Semin Thromb Hemost 3:125, 1977.

238. Novak R, J Wilimas: Plasmapheresis in catastrophic complications of idiopathic thrombocytopenic purpura. J Pediatr 92:434, 1978.

239. Prankerd TAJ: Idiopathic thrombocytopenic purpura. Clin Haematol 1:327, 1972.

240. Harker LA: Thrombokinetics in idiopathic thrombocytopenic purpura. Br J Haemtol 19:95, 1970.

241. Yam LT, R McMillan, M Tauassoli, WH Crosby: Splenic hemopoiesis in idiopathic thrombocytopenic purpura. Am J Clin Pathol 62:830, 1974.

242. McMillan R, RL Longmire, R Xelenosky, RL Donnel, S Armstrong: Quantitation of platelet-binding IgG produced in vitro by spleens from patients with idiopathic thrombocytopenic purpura. N Engl J Med 291:812, 1974.

243. Epstein RD, EL Lozner, TS Cobbey, CS Davidson: Congenital thrombocytopenic purpura: purpura hemorrhagica in pregnancy and in the newborn. Am J Med 9:44, 1950.

244. Hathaway WE: The bleeding newborn. Semin Hematol 12:175, 1975.

245. Karpatkin S, MA Nardi, KB Hymes: Immunologic thrombocytopenia purpura after heterosexual transmission of human immunodeficiency virus (HIV). Ann Intern Med 109:190, 1988.

246. Beard J, GF Savage: High-dose intravenous immunoglobulin and splenectomy for the treatment of HIV-related immune thrombocytopenia in patients with severe hemophilia. Br J Haematol 68:303, 1988.

247. Abrams DI, DD Kiprov, JJ Goedert, MG Sarngadharan, RC Gallo, PA Volberding: Antibodies to human T-lymphotrophic virus type III and development of the acquired immunodeficiency syndrome in homosexual men presenting with immune thrombocytopenia. Ann Intern Med 104:47, 1986.

248. Ratner I: Human immunodeficiency virus–associated autoimmune thrombocytopenic purpura: a review. Am J Med 86:194, 1989.

249. McMillan R: Chronic idiopathic thrombocytopenic purpura. N Engl J Med 304:1135, 1981.

250. Bussel JB: Autoimmune thrombocytopenic purpura. Hematol Oncol Clin North Am 4:179, 1990.

251. George JN: Platelet IgG: measurement, interpretation, and clinical significance. Prog Hemost Thromb 10:97, 1991.

252. Arnott J, P Horsewood, JG Kelton: Measurement of platelet-associated IgG in animal models of immune and nonimmune thrombocytopenia. Blood 69:1294, 1987.

253. Buchanan GR: The nontreatment of childhood idiopathic thrombocytopenia purpura. Eur J Pediatr 146:107, 1987.

254. Beardsley DS: Platelet autoantigens. In: TJ Kunicki, JN George (Eds): Platelet Immunobiology: Molecular and Clinical Aspects. JB Lippincott, Philadelphia, 1989, p 121.

255. Imbach P, P Tani, A Kozlowska: Antiplatelet autoantibodies in children and adults with chronic ITP. Blood 74:400, 1989.

256. Cines DB, AD Schreiber: Immune thrombocytopenia: use of a Coomb's antiglobulin test to detect IgG and C3 on platelets. N Engl J Med 300:106, 1979.

257. Leporrier M, G Dighiero, M Auzemery: Detection and quantification of platelet-bound antibodies with immunoperoxidase. Br J Haematol 42:605, 1979.

258. Trent R, E Adams, C Erhardt, A Basten: Alterations in T-gamma-cells in patients with chronic idiopathic thrombocytopenic purpura. J Immunol 127:621, 1981.

259. McMillin R: Immune thrombocytopenia. Clin Haematol 12:69, 1983.

260. Siegel RS, JL Rae, S Barth, RE Coleman, RC Reba, R Kurlander WF Rosse: Platelet survival and turnover: important factors in predicting response to splenectomy in immune thrombocytopenic purpura. Am J Hematol 30:206, 1989.

261. Lacey JV, JA Penner: Management of idiopathic thrombocytopenic purpura in the adult. Semin Thromb Hemost 3:160, 1977.

262. Bussel JB, RP Kimberly, RD Inman, I Shulman, C Cunningham-Rundles, N Cheung, EM Smithwick, J O'Malley, S Barandun, MW Hilgartner: Intravenous gamma globulin treatment of chronic idiopathic thrombocytopenic purpura. Blood 62:480, 1983.

263. Fehr J, V Hofmann, U Kappeler: Transient reversal of thrombocytopenia in idiopathic thrombocytopenic purpura by high-dose intravenous gamma globulin. N Engl J Med 306:1254, 1982.

264. Nydegger UE: New aspects of immunoglobulin treatment for idiopathic thrombocytopenic purpura. Plasma Ther Trans Technol 9:83, 1988.

265. Blanchette VS, VA Hogan, NE McCombie: Intensive plasma exchange therapy in ten patients with idiopathic thrombocytopenic purpura. Transfusion 21:388, 1984.

266. Marder VJ, J Nusbacher, FW Anderson: One-year follow-up of plasma exchange therapy in 14 patients with idiopathic thrombocytopenic purpura. Transfusion 21:291, 1981.

267. Ahn YS, WJ Harrington, SR Simon, R Mylvaganam, LM Pall, AG So: Danazol for the treatment of idiopathic thrombocytopenic purpura. N Engl J Med 308:1396, 1983.

268. West SG, SC Johnson: Danazol for the treatment of refractory autoimmune thrombocytopenia in systemic lupus erythematosus. Ann Intern Med 108:703, 1988.

269. Ahn YS, WJ Harrington, RC Seelman, SC Eytel: Vincristine therapy of idiopathic and secondary thrombocytopenias. N Engl J Med 291:376, 1974.

270. Ahn YS, WJ Harrington, RR Mylvaganam: Slow infusion of vinca alkaloids in the treatment of idiopathic thrombocytopenic purpura. Ann Intern Med 100:192, 1984.

271. Weiss HJ, MH Rosove, BA Lages: Acquired storage pool deficiency with increased platelet-associated IgG: report of five cases. Am J Med 69:711, 1980.

272. Stuart MJ, JG Kelton, JB Allen: Abnormal platelet function and arachidonate metabolism in chronic idiopathic thrombocytopenic purpura. Blood 58:326, 1981.

273. Pui CN, J Wilimas, W Wang: Evan's syndrome in childhood. J Pediatr 97:754, 1980.

274. Pegels JG, FM Helmerhorst, EF van Leeuwen, C van dePlas-vanDalen, CP Engelfriet, AEGK von dem Borne: The Evans syndrome: characterization of the responsible autoantibodies. Br J Haematol 51:445, 1982.

275. Wang W, H Herrod, CH Pui, G Presbury, J Wilimas: Immunoregulatory abnormalities in Evan's syndrome. Am J Hematol 15:381, 1983.

276. Hackett T, JG Kelton, P Powers: Drug-induced platelet destruction. Semin Thromb Hemost 8:116, 1982.

277. Mieschner PA, J Graf: Drug-induced thrombocytopenia. Clin Haematol 9:505, 1980.

278. Mieschner PA: Drug-induced thrombocytopenia. Semin Hematol 10:311, 1973.

279. Levin J: Pathophysiology of drug-induced thrombocytopenia, ch 7. In: NV Dimitrov, JH Nodine (Eds): Drugs and Hematologic Reactions. Grune and Stratton, New York, 1974, p 87.

280. de Gruchy GC: Thrombocytopenia, ch 6. In: Drug-Induced Blood Disorders. Blackwell Scientific Publications, Oxford, 1975, p 118.

281. Karpatkin S: Drug-induced thrombocytopenia. Am J Med Sci 262:69, 1971.

282. Huguley CM, JW Lea, JA Butts: Adverse hematological reactions to drugs. Prog Haematol 5:105, 1966.

283. Horowitz HI, RL Nachman: Drug purpura. Semin Hematol 2:287, 1965.

284. Gynn TN, HI Messmore, IA Friedman: Drug-induced thrombocytopenia. Med Clin North Am 56:65, 1972.

285. Colombani J: Auto- and isoimmune thrombocytopenia. Semin Hematol 3:74, 1966.

286. Crosby WH, RM Kaufman: Drug-induced thrombocytopenia. Med Ann DC 33:199, 1964.

287. Doan CA, BA Bouronele, BK Wiseman: Idiopathic and secondary thrombocytopenic purpura: clinical study and evaluation of 381 cases over a period of 28 years. Ann Intern Med 53:861, 1960.

288. Bottiger LE, B Westerholm: Thrombocytopenia, II: drug-induced thrombocytopenia. Acta Med Scand 191:541, 1972.

289. Bettman JW: Drug hypersensitivity purpuras. Arch Intern Med 112:840, 1963.

290. Weintraub RM, L Pechet, B Alexander: Rapid diagnosis of drug-induced thrombocytopenic purpura. JAMA 180, 1962.

291. Mieschner PA, A Mieschner: Immunologic drug-induced blood dyscrasias. Klin Wochenschr 56:1, 1978.

292. Davidson C, SM Manohitharajah: Drug-induced platelet antibodies. Br Med J 3:545, 1973.

293. Vipan WH: Quinine as a cause of purpura. Lancet 2:37, 1865.

294. Ackroyd JF: The pathogenesis of thrombocytopenic purpura due to hypersensitivity to Sedormid (allyl-isopropyl-acetyl-carbamide). Clin Sci 8:249, 1949.

295. Ackroyd JF: The cause of thrombocytopenia in Sedormid purpura. Clin Sci 8:269, 1949.

296. Shulman NR: A mechanism of cell destruction in individuals sensitized to foreign antigens and the implications in autoimmunity. Ann Intern Med 60:506, 1964.

297. Shulman NR: Immunoreactions involving platelets, I: a steric and kinetic model for formation of a complex from a human antibody, quinidine as a heptene, and platelets, and for fixation of complement by the complex. J Exp Med 107:665, 1958.

298. Shulman NR: Immunoreactions involving platelets, III: quantitative aspects of platelet agglutination, inhibition of clot retraction and other reactions caused by the antibody of quinidine purpura. J Exp Med 107:697, 1958.

299. Shulman NR: Immunoreactions involving platelets, IV: studies on the pathogenesis of thrombocytopenia in drug purpura using test doses of quinidine in sensitized individuals; their implications in idiopathic thrombocytopenic purpura. J Exp Med 107:711, 1958.

300. Pfueller SL, RA Bilston, D Logan, JM Gibson, BG Firkin: Heterogeneity of drug-dependent platelet antigens and their antibodies in quinine- and quinidine-induced thrombocytopenia: involvement of glycoproteins Ib, IIb, IIIa and IX. Blood 72:1155, 1988.

301. Levine SJ, DB Brubaker: Detection of platelet antibodies using the platelet migration inhibition assay. Am J Clin Pathol 80:43, 1983.

302. Takahashi A, S Ohara, S Imaoka, J Kambayashi, G Kosaki: A simple and rapid method to detect platelet-associated IgG. Thromb Res 28:11, 1982.

303. Schiffer CA, V Young: Detection of platelet antibodies using a micro-enzyme-linked immunosorbent assay (ELISA). Blood 61:311, 1983.

304. Boisvert A, BR MacPherson: The detection of platelet antibodies using a modified platelet immunofluorescence test. Am J Clin Pathol 80:839, 1983.

305. Vizcaino GJ, M Diez-Ewald: Autoimmune thrombocytopenic purpura. Comparison of three different methods for the detection of platelet antibodies. Am J Hematol 14:279, 1983.

306. Murphy S: In search of a platelet Coombs test. N Engl J Med 309:490, 1983.

307. George JN: The origin and significance of platelet IgG. In: TJ Kunicki, JN George (Eds): Platelet Immunobiology: Molecular and Clinical Aspects. JB Lippincott, Philadelphia, 1989, p 305.

308. Seidenfeld AM, J Owen, MFX Glynn: Post-transfusion purpura cured by steroid therapy in a man. Can Med Assoc J 118:1285, 1978.

309. Kunicki YJ, DS Beardsley: The alloimmune thrombocytopenias: neonatal alloimmune thrombocytopenic purpura and post-transfusion purpura. Prog Hemost Thromb 9:203, 1989.

310. Zeigler Z, S Murphy, FH Gardner: Post-transfusion: a heterogeneous syndrome. Blood 45:529, 1975.

311. Vaughn-Neil EF, S Ardeman, G Bevan, AC Blakeman, WJ Jenkins: Post-transfusion purpura associated with unusual platelet antibody (Anti-PLB1). Br Med J 1:436, 1975.

312. Solum NO: Platelet membrane proteins. Semin Hematol 22:289, 1985.

313. Abramson N, PD Eisenberg, RH Aster: Post-transfusion purpura: immunologic aspects and therapy. N Engl J Med 291:1163, 1974.

314. Phadke KP, JP Isbister: Post-transfusion purpura. Med J Aust 1:430, 1980.

315. Hirsh J, JV Dacie: Persistent post-splenectomy thrombocytosis and thrombo-embolism: a consequence of continuing anaemia. Br J Haematol 12:14, 1966.

316. Bean RHD: Thrombocytosis in auto-immune diseases. Bibl Haematol 23:43, 1965.

317. Harker LA, CA Finch: Thrombokinetics in man. J Clin Invest 48:963, 1969.

318. Jellett LB, JA Bonnin: Platelet thromboplastic function in polycythaemia and thrombocythaemia. Aust Ann Med 15:15, 1966.

319. Marchasin S, RD Wallerstein, PM Aggeler: Variation of the platelet count in disease. Calif Med 101:95, 1964.

320. Desforges JF, FS Bigelow, TC Chalmers: The effects of massive gastrointestinal hemorrhage on hemostasis. J Lab Clin Med 43:501, 1954.

321. Schlosser LL, MA Kipp, FJ Wenzel: Thrombocytosis in iron-deficiency anemia. J Lab Clin Med 66:107, 1965.

322. Tranum BL, A Haut: Thrombocytosis: platelet kinetics in neoplasia. J Lab Clin Med 84:615, 1974.

323. Bick RL: Alterations of hemostasis in malignancy, ch 10. In: Disorders of Hemostasis and Thrombosis: Principles of Clinical Practice. Thieme, Inc., New York, 1985, p 262.

324. Lipson RL, ED Bayrd, CH Watkins: The postsplenectomy blood picture. Am J Clin Pathol 32:526, 1959.

325. Knizley H, WD Noyes: Iron deficiency anemia, papilledema, thrombocytosis and transient hemiparesis. Arch Intern Med 129:483, 1972.

326. Gunz FW: Hemorrhagic thrombocythemia: a critical review. Blood 15:706, 1960.

327. Silverstein MN: Primary or hemorrhagic thrombocythemia. Arch Intern Med 122:18, 1968.

328. Frick PG: Primary thrombocythemia: clinical, hematological, and chromosomal studies of 13 patients. Heluctica Med Acta 35:20, 1969.

329. Bick RL: Essential (primary) thrombocythemia. Check Sample #H-7. American Society of Clinical Pathologists, Chicago, 1989.

330. Schafer AI: Essential thrombocythemia. Prog Hemost Thromb 10:69, 1991.

331. Mitus AJ, AI Schafer: Thrombocytosis and thrombocythemia. Hematol Oncol Clin North Am 4:157, 1990.

332. Fialkow PJ, GB Faguet, RV Jacobson, K Vardya, S Murphy: Evidence that essential thrombocythemia is a clonal disorder with origin in a multipotent stem cell. Blood 58:916, 1981.

333. Stoll DB, P Peterson, R Exten, J Laszlo, AV Pisciotta, JT Ellis, P White, K Vaida, M Bozdech, S Murphy: Clinical presentation and natural history of patients with essential thrombocythemia and the Philadelphia chromosome. Am J Hematol 27:77, 1988.

334. Morris CM, PH Fitzgerald, PE Hollings, SA Archer, I Rosman, MEJ Beard: Essential thrombocythaemia and the Philadelphia chromosome. Br J Haematol 70:13, 1988.

335. Murphy S, DS Rosenthal, A Weinfeld: Essential thrombocythemia: response during first year of therapy with melphalan and radioactive phosphorus: a Polycythemia Vera Study Group report. Cancer Treatment Reports 66:35, 1982.

336. Berlin NI: Diagnosis and classification of the polycythemias. In: NI Berlin, ER Jaffe, PA Miescher (Eds): Polycythemia. Grune and Stratton, New York, 1975, p 5.

337. Bick RL: Essential (hemorrhagic) thrombocythemia: a clinical and laboratory study of 13 patients. Thromb Haemost 50:216, 1983.

338. Bick RL, WL Wilson: Essential (hemorrhagic) thrombocythemia: a clinical and laboratory study of 14 patients. Am J Clin Pathol 81:799, 1984.

339. Ozer FL, WE Traux, DC Miesch, WC Levin: Primary hemorrhagic thrombocythemia. Am J Med 28:807, 1960.

340. Hardisty RM, NH Wolfe: Haemorrhagic thrombocythaemia: a clinical and laboratory study. Br J Haematol 1:390, 1955.

341. Bick RL, M Lewis, TA Don Michael: Essential thrombocythemia presenting as intra-articular hemorrhage of the knee and thrombosis of the sino-atrial artery. Thromb Haemost 50:476, 1983.

C H A P T E R

6

Hereditary Coagulation Protein Defects

ereditary defects of the blood proteins leading to hemorrhagic disease and associated disease states are the topic of this chapter. Specific acquired inhibitors of isolated coagulation proteins leading to hemorrhage, thrombosis, and thromboembolus will be discussed in chapter 10. The clinical manifestations of coagulation factor disorders are different from those previously discussed for vascular or platelet defects (chapters 3, 4, and 5). Coagulation factor disorders are characterized by deep tissue bleeding, including intra-articular bleeding with resultant crippling hemarthrosis, deep intramuscular bleeding, and sometimes, intracranial bleeding that can be life threatening.[1] Patients with single or multiple coagulation factor defects have moderate to severe mucosal membrane hemorrhage; patients with vascular and platelet defects more commonly experience mild to moderate mucosal membrane hemorrhage.[2] Mucosal membrane hemorrhage may be gastrointestinal, genitourinary, intrapulmonary, or from paranasal sinuses or nasal mucosa. Patients develop large ecchymoses but not petechiae and purpura, except in von Willebrand's syndrome.[3] Petechiae and purpura are hallmark findings in vascular and platelet defects but are not generally found in coagulation protein defects except von Willebrand's disease, which is a blood protein defect manifest clinically as an endothelial-platelet interaction problem.[2] However, patients with coagulation protein defects may develop petechiae and purpura with other hemostasis compartment defects (eg, DIC or other multiple hemostatic compartment disorders).[1] The clinical findings and laboratory manifestations of coagulation factor disorders are summarized in Table 6-1.

Most clinically significant coagulation protein disorders are detected by global tests of coagulation, depending on conversion of fibrinogen to fibrin.[1-3] These include such tests as the prothrombin time, the activated partial thromboplastin time, thrombin time, Lee-White clotting time, activated clotting time (ACT), and whole blood clotting time. One or several of these are usually prolonged in clinically significant coagulation protein defects. The two exceptions are alpha-2-antiplasmin deficiency and factor XIII deficiency. The other screening tests of hemostasis, the platelet count, peripheral blood smear, and template bleeding time, are normal in patients with isolated coagulation protein problems. The specific diagnosis of the particular coagulation factor defect or defects present usually calls for specific quantitative factor assay, after demonstrating prolongation of one or several of these global tests.

The coagulation protein disorders are summarized in Table 6-2 and are categorized as hereditary or acquired. The hereditary disorders are usually single-factor defects, and acquired disorders usually involve multiple factors.

The hereditary coagulation protein disorders are summarized in Table 6-3. The afibrinogenemias, hypofibrinogenemias, and dysfibrinogenemias are rare. Hereditary dysfibrinogenemia, however, may be more common than generally appreciated, since this disorder has been recognized only recently. Isolated deficiencies of factors II, V, VII, or X are very rare, and isolated factor XII deficiency, Fletcher factor deficiency, and Fitzgerald factor deficiency are also rare. The hemophilias are not uncommon and account for about 1 in 8,000 to 10,000 male births in the United States, although regional and international differences are noted.[4]

Fibrinogen Defects

Hereditary abnormalities of fibrinogen are afibrinogenemia, hypofibrinogenemia, or dysfibrinogenemia. Dysfibrinogenemias are characterized by presence of a functionally abnormal protein. Although dysfibrinogenemias are the best characterized, dysfunctional or qualitative defects are also found in other blood protein defects. Congenital abnormalities of fibrinogen are summarized in Table 6-4. Fibrinogen abnormalities may be quantitative, such as afibrinogenemia and hypofibrinogenemia, or qualitative, such as dysfibrinogenemia. The quantitative defects are hypofibrinogenemia, involving heterozygous patients, and afibrinogenemia, involving

Table 6-1. Coagulation Protein Defects

Clinical Manifestations
    Deep tissue hemorrhage
        Intramuscular
        Intra-articular
        Intracranial
    Moderate to severe mucosal membrane hemorrhage
        Gastrointestinal
        Genitourinary
        Intrapulmonary
    Large subcutaneous hematomas
        No petechiae or purpura (except in von Willebrand's
            syndrome)

Laboratory Manifestations
    Prolongation of global tests dependent on the conversion of
        fibrinogen to fibrin
        Prothrombin time
        Partial thromboplastin time
        Thrombin time
        Lee-White clotting time
        Whole blood clotting time
        Activated clotting time
    Other screening tests normal
        Platelet count
        Template bleeding time (except in von Willebrand's
            syndrome)
        Peripheral blood smear
    Definitive diagnosis requires quantitative assays

homozygous patients. Hypofibrinogenemic patients have about 50% of normal fibrinogen levels, and afibrinogenemic patients have no fibrinogen. Some severely afibrinogenemic patients show small amounts of fibrinogen by immunologic techniques, usually about 0.05 to .1 g/L (5 to 10 mg/dL),[1] probably representing cross reactivity with a fibrinogenlike protein such as fibronectin. Quantitative defects of fibrinogen are usually inherited as autosomal recessive traits.[5]

Table 6-2. Classification of Coagulation Protein Defects

Hereditary Defects (usually monofactorial deficiency/dysfunction)
    Hemophilias
    von Willebrand's syndrome
    Deficiencies of II, VII, IX, or X (rare)
    Fibrinogen defects
    Other single factor defects (factors V, XI, XIII)
    Contact activation defects
    Kininogen defects
    Fibrinolytic defects

Acquired Defects (usually multifactorial deficiency/dysfunction)
    Disseminated intravascular coagulation syndromes
    Primary fibrinolytic syndromes
    Liver disease
    Renal disease
    Circulating anticoagulants
    Drug induced

Table 6-3. Hereditary Coagulation Factor Defects

Afibrinogenemia, hypofibrinogenemia, dysfibrinogenemia
Factor II defects
Factor V defects
Factor VII defects
Factor VIII:C defects (hemophilia A)
Factor VIII:vW defects (von Willebrand's syndrome)
Factor IX defects (hemophilia B)
Factor X defects
Factor XI defects
Factor XII defects (Hageman factor)
Factor XIII defects
Passovoy defect
Prekallikrein defects (Fletcher factor)
Kininogen defects (Williams, Fitzgerald, Reid, Flaujeac,
    Fujiwara factors)
Fibrinolytic system defects

Dysfibrinogenemias represent qualitative fibrinogen abnormalities, and patients may be homozygous or heterozygous. In homozygous patients, all fibrinogen is dysfunctional, and in heterozygous patients, 50% of circulating fibrinogen is dysfunctional. Qualitative defects are usually inherited as autosomal dominant traits.

Hypofibrinogenemic patients rarely have significant clinical bleeding, but some have a mild bleeding tendency, usually following surgery or trauma. Afibrinogenemic patients experience occasional spontaneous hemorrhage manifest as gastrointestinal blood loss, hematochezia, hematemesis, large hematomas, hypermenorrhagia, and gingival or other mucosal membrane bleeding.[6] Patients frequently have umbilical stump bleeding at birth. Intra-articular bleeding with resultant hemarthroses and occasional intracranial bleeding occur.[7] Clinical manifestations of congenital hypofibrinogenemia and afibrinogenemia are summarized in Table 6-5. The laboratory manifestations of hypofibrinogenemia and afibrinogenemia are summarized in Table 6-6. Global tests of coagulation, including the whole blood clotting time, recalcification time, activated partial thromboplastin time (APTT), prothrombin time (PT), and reptilase time are usually moderately prolonged in hypofibrinogenemic (heterozygous) patients.[6] These same global tests are usually markedly prolonged or infinite in afibrinogenemic (homozygous) patients.[6] When measuring fibrinogen concentration

Table 6-4. Hereditary Fibrinogen Defects

Quantitative Fibrinogen Defects
    Autosomal recessive inheritance
    Hypofibrinogenemia (heterozygous patients)
    Afibrinogenemia (homozygous patients)

Qualitative Fibrinogen Defects (Dysfibrinogenemias)
    Autosomal dominant inheritance
    50% fibrinogen defective (heterozygous patients)
    100% fibrinogen defective (homozygous patients)

Table 6-5. Clinical Manifestations of Quantitative Fibrinogen Defects

Hypofibrinogenemia
  Spontaneous hemorrhage is rare
  Some with a mild bleeding tendency
  May have severe bleeding with surgery or trauma

Afibrinogenemia
  Spontaneous hemorrhage may occur
  Gastrointestinal bleeding
  Subcutaneous hematomas
  Prolonged and excessive menstrual bleeding
  Common types of hemorrhage
    Umbilical stump bleeding
    Gingival bleeding
    Mucosal membrane bleeding
    Intra-articular bleeding
    Intracranial bleeding

by coagulation techniques, protein precipitation techniques, or immunologic assays, hypofibrinogenemic patients (heterozygotes) have fibrinogen levels of about 50%, but afibrinogenemic patients (homozygotes) show no detectable fibrinogen. Some afibrinogenemic patients appear to have trace levels of fibrinogen by immunologic techniques, which may represent cross reactivity with nonfibrinogen material, possibly fibronectin.

Patients with congenital dysfibrinogenemia often display no hemorrhagic diathesis, but some have a mild bleeding tendency and easy and spontaneous bruising.[6,8-10] Patients with dysfibrinogenemia may have severe bleeding following trauma or surgery, and women experience excessive menstrual flow. These findings are most common in homozygous patients in whom all fibrinogen is dysfunctional, but heterozygous patients have both normal functional fibrinogen (50%) and dysfunctional fibrinogen (50%) and are usually asymptomatic. Several types of congenital dysfibrino-

genemia have been associated with a thrombotic tendency, including fibrinogens Baltimore, Bergamo II, Chapel Hill, Charlottesville, Copenhagen, Dusard, Marburg, Naples, New York, Nijmegen, Oslo I, Paris II, and Wiesbaden,[11-23] which will be discussed in chapter 13. Clinical findings of congenital dysfibrinogenemia are summarized in Table 6-7. Laboratory evaluation reveals the global coagulation tests, the whole blood clotting time, recalcification time, activated clotting time (ACT), activated partial thromboplastin time, prothrombin time, reptilase time, and thrombin time to be normal or moderately prolonged in the heterozygous dysfibrinogenemic patients, as these patients have about 50% normal functioning fibrinogen and 50% dysfunctional fibrinogen. Homozygous dysfibrinogenemic patients have fibrinogen that is all dysfunctional, and infinite clotting times may result with most clotting tests. Laboratory findings of congenital dysfibrinogenemia are summarized in Table 6-8. When measuring fibrinogen concentration by clot-based techniques, the heterozygous dysfibrinogenemic patient has reduced levels, but the homozygous dysfibrinogenemic patient has no detectable fibrinogen by clotting technique. Protein precipitation methods for fibrinogen show both heterozygous or homozygous dysfibrinogenemic patients to have normal fibrinogen levels. Immunologic techniques also reveal normal levels in dysfibrinogenemic patients. Functional assays should always be used to make an initial diagnosis, followed by protein-based assays, which then show the quantitative or qualitative nature of the defect. This principle applies to all coagulation protein assays.

The congenital dysfibrinogenemias are listed in Table 6-9.[31-44] The dysfibrinogenemias are named after the city where the patient originated. Often in congenital dysfibrinogenemia, the precise molecular defect accounting for defective function is unknown. Most dysfibrinogenemias characterized have crucial amino acid substitutions, defects of fibrinopeptide A or B release, or abnormal carbohydrates.[6,8-10,24-28] Fibrinogen Detroit was the first congenital dysfibrinogenemia evaluated and defined. Dysfibrinogenemia Detroit

Table 6-6. Laboratory Manifestations of Quantitative Fibrinogen Defects

	Afibrinogenemia	Hypofibrinogenemia
Global Coagulation Tests		
Whole blood clotting time	Infinite	Prolonged
Partial thromboplastin time	Infinite	Prolonged
Prothrombin time	Infinite	Prolonged
Thrombin time	Infinite	Prolonged
Reptilase time	Infinite	Prolonged
Activated clotting time	Infinite	Prolonged
Fibrinogen concentration		
Coagulation tests	0%	Reduced
Precipitation tests	0%	Reduced
Immunologic tests	0%	Reduced
Other tests		
Template bleeding time	Borderline	Normal
Platelet function (aggregation)	Abnormal	Abnormal

Table 6-7. Laboratory Manifestations of Dysfibrinogenemia

	Homozygote	Heterozygote
Global coagulation tests		
Whole blood clotting time	Infinite	Prolonged
Prothrombin time	Infinite	Prolonged
Partial thromboplastin time	Infinite	Prolonged
Thrombin time	Infinite	Prolonged
Reptilase time	Infinite	Prolonged
Activated clotting time	Infinite	Prolonged
Fibrinogen concentration		
Coagulation tests	0%	Reduced
Precipitation tests	100%	100%
Immunologic tests	100%	100%
Other tests		
Template bleeding time	Normal	Normal
Platelet function (aggregation)	Normal	Normal

represents the second molecular defect leading to a clinically significant disease, the first being sickle cell anemia. Figure 6-1 depicts fibrinogen Detroit, showing the A-alpha, B-beta, and gamma chains and the amino acid sequence of fibrinopeptide A. Fibrinopeptide A has 16 amino acids; thrombin cleaves an arginine-glycine bond, the bond between arginine 16 and glycine 17. For this cleavage to happen, thrombin must attach to a thrombin binding site, three amino acids away at position 19. In fibrinogen Detroit the amino acid serine has been substituted for arginine at position 19, and thrombin binding cannot occur. No cleavage of the arginine-glycine bond between position 16 and 17 occurs. Fibrinopeptide A cannot be removed, and fibrinogen cannot be converted into fibrin monomer.[29,30] These patients have a hemorrhagic diathesis, since they are unable to make fibrin monomer and a subsequent fibrin clot.[6,9]

The differential diagnostic laboratory findings of quantitative and qualitative defects of fibrinogen are summarized in Table 6-10. Patient 1 is afibrinogenemic, showing absence of fibrinogen by clotting assay, absence of fibrinogen by protein precipitation, and absent to trace levels of fibrinogen by immunologic assay. Patient 2 is hypofibrinogenemic, having about 50% of normal fibrinogen levels. In this type of patient, clot-based techniques for fibrinogen determination demonstrate about 50% of normal fibrinogen

Table 6-8. Clinical Manifestations of Dysfibrinogenemia

Heterozygous patients
　Rarely have spontaneous hemorrhage
　May bleed with surgery or trauma

Homozygous patients
　Some are asymptomatic
　Some have spontaneous bleeding
　Easy bruising is common
　Severe bleeding with surgery or trauma
　Excessive menstrual bleeding common

levels, and protein precipitation or immunologic assays also show about 50% of normal fibrinogen levels. Patient 3 is homozygous and dysfibrinogenemic, and all fibrinogen is dysfunctional. Clot-based assays show absence of fibrinogen, and protein precipitation or immunologic assays reveal normal fibrinogen levels. Patient 4 is heterozygous and dysfibrinogenemic. The fibrinogen is 50% functional and 50% dysfunctional. Clot-based assays are prolonged, and about 50% of normal fibrinogen values are present, but protein precipitation and immunologic assays show normal fibrinogen levels.

The therapy for afibrinogenemia, hypofibrinogenemia, and dysfibrinogenemia is component replacement when severe bleeding happens or when extensive surgery is planned. The best therapeutic component for these patients is cryoprecipitate.[6] Bleeding is usually controlled easily by infusing enough cryoprecipitate, usually every three to five days, to maintain a clottable (functional) fibrinogen level of .75 to 1.0 g/L (75 to 100 mg/dL).

Factor II Defects

Congenital factor II (prothrombin) defects are very rare and are inherited as autosomal recessive traits.[45-50] Both quantitative and qualitative (dysfunctional) types have been described.[50] The quantitative defects are the hypoprothrombinemias and aprothrombinemias. These conditions are termed either cross-reacting material negative (CRM–), if factor II protein is absent, or cross-reacting material positive (CRM+), if dysfunctional factor II protein is present. This terminology is commonly used to distinguish quantitative and qualitative defects of coagulation factors. Qualitative defects of factor II are called dysprothrombinemias. The quantitative defects are more common than qualitative defects.[50] Since prothrombin defects are inherited as autosomal recessive traits, four subtypes are noted. In the quantita-

Table 6-9. Examples of Congenital Dysfibrinogenemias

Amsterdam	1971	Marseille	1980
Ashai	1989	Matika	1976
Baltimore	1964	Metz	1972
Bern	1978	Mexico	1978
Bergamo	1986	Milano	1986
Bethesda I	1970	Montreal I	1972
Bethesda II	1972	Montreal II	1975
Bethesda III	1979	Montreal III	1976
Bondy	1980	Munich	1980
Boulogne	1975	Nagoya	1979
Buenos Aires I	1975	Naifa	1981
Buenos Aires II	1978	Nancy	1971
Caracas I	1975	Naples I	1977
Caracas II	1977	Naples II	1979
Chapel Hill I	1975	Newark	1979
Chapel Hill II	1977	New Orleans	1977
Chapel Hill III	1983	New York I	1975
Charlottesville	1977	New York II	1979
Chicago	1981	Oklahoma	1970
Clermont-Ferrand	1975	Osaka I	1987
Cleveland I	1967	Osaka II	1988
Cleveland II	1973	Oslo I	1967
Copenhagen	1979	Oslo II	1977
Detroit	1968	Paris I	1963
Dusard	1984	Paris II	1968
Essen	1986	Paris III	1974
Frankfurt I	1979	Paris IV	1978
Frankfurt II	1979	Parma	1958
Freiberg	1979	Perugia	1986
Geneva	1972	Petoskey	1980
Giessen I	1972	Philadelphia	1974
Giessen II	1977	Pontoise	1978
Haifa	1989	Puerto Rico	1979
Hannover	1977	Quebec I	1978
Harva	1973	Quebec II	1978
Homberg	1979	Saint Louis	1968
Houston	1978	Saint Mande I	1976
Iowa City	1973	Saint Mande II	1976
Istanbul	1970	Seattle	1977
Kyoto I	1988	Tokyo	1975
Kyoto II	1989	Troyes	1972
Kyoto III	1990	Valencia	1974
Lille	1978	Vancouver	1963
Logrono	1979	Versailles	1979
London	1978	Vienna	1973
Los Angeles	1970	Vlissingen	1989
Louvain	1970	Wiesbaden I	1971
Manchester	1979	Wiesbaden II	1973
Manila	1974	Zurich I	1965
Marburg	1977	Zurich II	1970

Figure 6-1. Fibrinogen Detroit

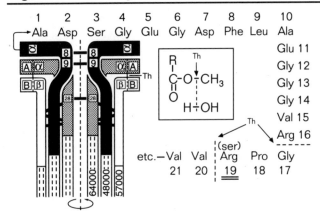

Courtesy of Dr. E. F. Mammen.

patients have no functionally normal prothrombin. As with fibrinogen defects, the quantitative and qualitative prothrombin defects can be precisely characterized by doing both functional and immunologic assays, although functional assays should always be done first.[51] In patients with quantitative defects, results of functional and immunologic assays will be concordant. In dysprothrombinemia, functional clotting-based assays show decreased or absent prothrombin levels, but immunologic assays show normal levels (discordant results). Several dysprothrombinemias have also been associated with a moderate quantitative defect (dysprothrombinemias Habana, Houston, Metz, Molise, and Quick).[52-56] Precise mechanisms accounting for dysfunctional prothrombins, where known, have been reviewed.[57] Like the dysfibrinogenemias and other qualitative coagulation protein defects and hemoglobinopathies, the dysprothrombinemias are named after the city where the family originated. The dysprothrombinemias are listed in Table 6-11.[53-56, 58-72] Clinically, homozygous patients can have severe spontaneous bleeding consisting of large hematomas, ecchymoses, and life-threatening mucosal membrane hemorrhage.[50] Heterozygous patients can have similar bleeding, which may become severe with surgery or trauma. The clinical manifestations and laboratory characteristics of prothrombin defects are summarized in Table 6-12. Once the diagnosis of a congenital factor II defect is made by functional assay, an immunologic assay may be done to differentiate between a qualitative or quantitative defect.[51] Patients with congenital factor II defects have a prolonged prothrombin time and activated partial thromboplastin time. The diagnosis is usually made after a specific factor II assay is done.

Treatment of patients with congenitally defective factor II is called for when clinically significant hemorrhage happens or surgery is planned. Prothrombin complex concentrates are the therapy of choice; however, plasma may also be used.[16] Functional factor II should be raised to about 50% of normal to stop hemorrhage or to afford surgical hemostasis in

tive prothrombin defects, heterozygous patients have about 50% of normal prothrombin levels and homozygous patients have very low or absent prothrombin. Similarly, patients with qualitative defects may be heterozygous or homozygous. Heterozygous patients have both functional (50%) and dysfunctional (50%) prothrombin, whereas homozygous

Table 6-10. Differential Diagnosis of Fibrinogen Defects

	Patient			
	1	2	3	4
Clotting tests	0%	50%	0%	50%
Precipitation tests	0%	50%	100%	100%
Immunologic tests	0%	50%	100%	100%
Diagnosis	Afibrinogenemia	Hypofibrinogenemia	Homozygous dysfibrinogenemia	Heterozygous dysfibrinogenemia

presurgical patients. The half-life of factor II is about three days, so infusions need not be frequent.[73]

Factor V Defects

Factor V deficiency was first described by Owren in 1947[74] and is extremely rare.[75-77] The defect is inherited as either an autosomal dominant or recessive trait.[78,79] Factor V deficiency has also been called parahemophilia.[74,76] Some cases of combined congenital factor VIII and V deficiency and combined factor V deficiency associated with von Willebrand's syndrome have occurred.[75,76,80] It has been suggested that combined factor V and factor VIII deficiency may represent congenital protein C inhibitor deficiency, although this remains to be clarified.[81-83] Most patients studied have had cross-reacting material–negative conditions or have an absence of factor V. Recently, however, several cases of dysfunctional factor V have been reported.[84-87] Another variant, called factor V Quebec, is characterized by moderately low levels of plasma factor V and extremely low levels of platelet alpha granule factor V.[88] Factor V deficiency associated with thrombosis has also been reported.[89] Clinical features of factor V defects are moderate to severe mucosal membrane bleeding, large hematomas, and large ecchymoses. Bleeding with surgery can be particularly severe, and spontaneous intra-articular bleeding episodes have been described. Heterozygous patients rarely have spontaneous bleeding, and propensity to hemorrhage correlates poorly with levels of circulating factor V.[90]

The laboratory diagnosis is suggested by noting prolongation of the prothrombin time and partial thromboplastin time. A specific diagnosis depends on a quantitative factor V assay. Patients are treated with infusions of fresh frozen plasma at 10 mL/kg or with cryoprecipitate.[90] The factor V levels should be kept above 30% for hemostasis, and since the half-life of factor V is around 24 hours, infusions need only be daily. The clinical and laboratory characteristics of congenital factor V deficiency are summarized in Table 6-13.

Table 6-11. Examples of Dysprothrombinemias

Barcelona	1971
Brussels	1974
Cardeza	1969
Clamart	1986
Denver	1980
Gainesville	1981
Habana	1983
Houston	1980
Madrid	1979
Mexico City	1987
Metz	1979
Molise	1978
Padua	1974
Parija	1986
Quick	1978
Salakta	1984
San Juan	1974
Segovia	1986
Tokushimi	1987

Table 6-12. Prothrombin Defects

Clinical Manifestations
  Homozygous patients
    Severe spontaneous hemorrhage at many sites
    Severe bleeding with surgery or trauma
    Large hematomas and ecchymoses
    Severe mucosal membrane bleeding
  Heterozygous patients
    Rare spontaneous hemorrhage
    Mild mucosal membrane hemorrhage
    Potentially severe bleeding with surgery or trauma
Therapy
    Level of factor II should be raised to 50%, or
      prothrombin complex concentrates every three days
    Fresh frozen plasma every three days

Laboratory manifestations
    Prolonged prothrombin time
    Prolonged partial thromboplastin time
    Normal thrombin time
    Normal template bleeding time
    Normal platelet function
    Definitive diagnosis usually requires quantitative factor II
      assay

Table 6-13. Factor V Defects

Clinical Manifestations
  Autosomal recessive
  Rare defect
  Severe mucosal membrane hemorrhage
  Large subcutaneous hematomas
  Spontaneous ecchymoses
  Severe bleeding with surgery or trauma
  Heterozygous patients often asymptomatic

Laboratory Manifestations
  Prolonged prothrombin time
  Prolonged partial thromboplastin time
  Normal thrombin time
  Normal template bleeding time
  Normal platelet function
  Definitive diagnosis requires a quantitative factor V assay

Therapy
  Fresh frozen plasma at 10 mL/kg daily
  Keep patient above 30% activity

Factor VII Defects

Factor VII deficiency is a rare, autosomal recessive trait.[5] Fewer than 200 cases of factor VII deficiency have been reported.[91-95] Both the absence (CRM–) form and dysfunctional (CRM+) form exist,[96-98] with the absence form being

Table 6-14. Factor VII Defects

Clinical Manifestations
  Autosomal recessive trait
  Rare defect
  Absence form and dysfunctional form
  Intra-articular bleeding
  Severe epistaxis
  Umbilical stump bleeding occasionally
  Mucosal membrane hemorrhage common
    Gastrointestinal
    Genitourinary
    Intrapulmonary
  Profuse bleeding with surgery or trauma
  Heterozygous patients rarely bleed spontaneously
  Heterozygous patients bleed with surgery or trauma

Laboratory Manifestations
  Prolonged prothrombin time
  Normal partial thromboplastin time
  Normal Russell's viper venom time
  Normal template bleeding time
  Normal platelet function (aggregation)
  Definitive diagnosis requires quantitative factor VII assay

Therapy
  Raise factor VII to greater than 30%
  Fresh frozen plasma
  Some prothrombin complex concentrates

Table 6-15. Examples of Dysfunctional Factor VII

Briet	1976
Croze	1982
Denson	1972
Girolami	1977
Girolami	1978
Girolami	1979
Goodnight	1971
Kernoff	1981
Mazzucconi	1977

more common. Curious variants of dysfunctional factor VII are called Padua I and II. Patients with factor VII Padua I have prolonged prothrombin times with rabbit brain thromboplastin but not ox-brain thromboplastin, and the opposite is seen in patients with factor VII Padua II.[99,100] The clinical features of factor VII defects are similar to other congenital single-factor defects and consist of intra-articular bleeding with hemarthroses, more common in male patients, severe epistaxis, and other mucosal membrane–type bleeding, including gastrointestinal, genitourinary, and intrapulmonary hemorrhage.[92] Patients may have significant life-threatening hemorrhage with surgery or trauma. Umbilical stump bleeding is also common. Spontaneous bleeding rarely happens in heterozygous patients unless trauma or surgery is undergone. The clinical and laboratory features of factor VII deficiency are summarized in Table 6-14. Examples of dysfunctional factor VII defects are noted in Table 6-15.[96,97,101-107]

The laboratory diagnosis depends on noting a prolonged prothrombin time (PT) and a normal partial thromboplastin time (PTT).[108] When this combination of abnormalities is noted, a factor VII assay should be performed.[108] The "Stypven time" (prothrombin time with Russell's viper venom) is usually normal.[1,92,109] The treatment of homozygous patients, when clinically significant hemorrhage occurs, is with prothrombin complex concentrates or plasma.[110] One available concentrate contains mainly factor VII and may be used.[111] If treating a patient with factor VII deficiency, the characteristics of available concentrates must be known. The factor VII levels should be maintained at 30% of normal. Infusions need to be frequent in bleeding or surgical patients, as the plasma half-life of factor VII is approximately four to six hours. Responses to DDAVP have also been noted.[112]

Factor VIII:C Defects

The hemophilias are more common than the congenital coagulation defects just discussed. The incidence of hemophilia is about 1 in 10,000 male births, although regional differences are observed.[113-116] Before addressing hemophilias and von Willebrand's disease, the properties and nomenclature of the factor VIII macromolecular com-

Figure 6-2. Factor VIII Macromolecular Complex

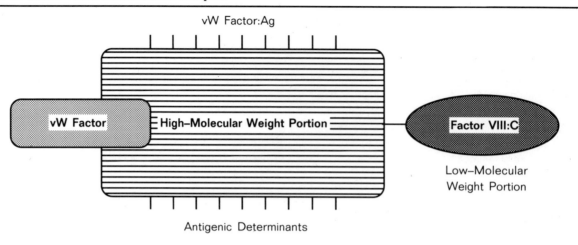

vW Factor = Factor VIII:vW = Ristocetin Cofactor
vW Factor:Ag = Factor VIII:RAg

plex will be summarized to avoid confusion and lend uniformity to the discussion. The factor VIII macromolecular complex is composed of three discrete portions and two discrete biologic activities.[117-123] The low–molecular weight part is responsible for procoagulant activity in the conversion of factor X to factor Xa (see chapter 1); this part is named factor VIII:C (for factor VIII:Coagulant activity). Factor VIII:C is measured in the PTT test system and the traditional PTT-derived factor VIII coagulant assay. With much difficulty, homologous nonprecipitating antibodies can be harvested against highly purified factor VIII:C, and these antibodies react with a moiety called factor VIII:CAg.[124] Generally, factor VIII:C and factor VIII:CAg levels parallel each other in normal patients and in most, but not all, hemophilic patients.[125] Factor VIII:C is made in the hepatocyte, like most other coagulation proteins.[126,127] A second discrete identifiable part of the factor VIII macromolecular complex is a high–molecular weight part, previously called factor VIII:RAg.[120,124] Heterologous precipitated antibodies, usually goat or rabbit, can easily be harvested against this part. The moiety with which these heterologous antibodies react was previously called factor VIII:RAg (factor VIII:Related Antigen), but the preferred terminology is vWF:Ag.[117,120,122-124] The third discrete part of the factor VIII macromolecular complex is an integral part of vWF:Ag, which contains the biologic activity responsible for normal platelet function, normal vascular function, and normal template bleeding times. This biologic activity (function) is called von Willebrand factor (factor VIII:vWF). Factor VIII:vWF is synonymous with the older ristocetin cofactor activity (factor VIII:RCo), but the term vWF is preferred. The factor VIII macromolecular complex and its components are shown in Figure 6-2.

Hemophilia A, called classic hemophilia, is inherited as a sex-linked recessive trait and is a deficiency or defect of fac-

tor VIII:C.[117] About 90% of patients have a deficiency of both factor VIII:C and factor VIII:CAg and have CRM– or factor VIII:C– defects. The remaining patients, about 10%, have missing factor VIII:C activity, normal factor VIII:CAg, and dysfunctional factor VIII:C, which is referred to as a CRM+ condition.[125] A contributory family history is elicited in 70% of hemophilic patients, and in about 30% the gene appears to arise spontaneously, representing a high mutation rate.[1] Patients with factor VIII:C– and factor VIII:C+ defects have similar clinical courses. Hemophilic patients typically experience hemorrhage, primarily manifest as deep tissue bleeding.[117,128] The types of bleeding are usually deep intramuscular bleeding, intra-articular bleeding with resultant joint fibrosis (called hemarthrosis), and potentially fatal intracranial bleeding.[117,128-131] Patients commonly have hematuria.[132] Particularly severe and potentially crippling bleeding can happen when hemorrhage into one of the closed muscular compartments of the extremities occurs, and this can lead to anterior or posterior compartment or compression syndrome leading to vascular or peripheral nerve compromise or later fibrotic tissue formation.[117,128,133]

The severity of bleeding in hemophilia A closely parallels circulating factor VIII:C. Patients with severe bleeding have 0% to 5% of circulating factor VIII:C levels or have circulating inhibitors to factor VIII:C.[117,128] These patients have severe spontaneous deep tissue bleeding episodes of the type previously described, and their conditions are usually diagnosed in early childhood, usually at circumcision or at the initiation of crawling when patients begin to show spontaneous bleeding into the knees or elbow joints.[1] Moderate hemophiliacs are those who have 5% to 10% of circulating factor VIII:C levels. These patients have some spontaneous bleeding episodes but may bleed profusely when subjected to surgery or trauma. Mild hemophiliacs are those who have 10% to 40% of circulating factor VIII:C levels.

Table 6-16. Hemophilia A

Clinical Manifestations
    Sex-linked recessive
    Absence of VIII:C in 90%
    Presence of dysfunctional VIII:C in 10%
    Deep tissue hemorrhage
        Intra-articular hemorrhage
        Intracranial hemorrhage
        Intramuscular hemorrhage
        Compartmental compression syndromes
    Clinical course parallels factor VIII:C level
        Severe, 0% to 5%, many spontaneous bleeds
        Moderate, 5% to 10%, some spontaneous bleeds
        Mild, 10% to 40%, rare spontaneous bleeds
    Severe bleeding with surgery or trauma
    Anti-VIII:C antibody in 10% (usually IgG-kappa)
    Hemophilia A accounts for 85% of hemophilic patients
    Most patients are male (sex-linked recessive)

Laboratory Manifestations
    Prolonged partial thromboplastin time
    Normal prothrombin time
    Normal template bleeding time
    Platelet dysfunction (aggregation) may be seen in very
        severe conditions

Table 6-17. Factor VIII:C Concentrate Dose in Hemophilia A

Units needed = desired level − initial level

Total units needed = units needed x 0.6 x body weight (kg)

Milliliters of concentrate needed = total units needed/units/mL in concentrate

Patients with mild hemophilia rarely have spontaneous bleeding but may have severe life-threatening bleeding with surgery or trauma. Severe hemophilia is usually clinically obvious and these patients are identified early in life, but mild hemophiliacs may not be identified until major surgical or traumatic bleeding occurs. For this reason, a sensitive activated partial thromboplastin time (APTT) and reliable associated reagents are of paramount importance when using this test as a presurgical screening procedure or when using it to evaluate a bleeding patient for potential hemophilia. Many studies have addressed the sensitivity and reliability of the activated partial thromboplastin time and associated reagents.[134-138] The key to a rapid diagnosis of hemophilia A is a prolonged PTT with a normal prothrombin time in a (usually) male child who has a contributory bleeding or family history. In this setting, the chances are about 85% that the child has factor VIII:C deficiency, and a quantitative factor VIII assay should be performed. If the results of this test are negative in this setting, a factor IX:C and, if warranted, a factor XI:C assay should be performed. The clinical features of hemophilia A are summarized in Table 6-16.

About 10% of patients with hemophilia A develop anti-VIII:C antibodies. These antibodies are most commonly IgG$_4$ kappa, but other IgG isotypes and IgM have also been noted.[117,139-143] The development of antibodies was first thought to be related to the source of factor VIII, with the commercially available factor VIII concentrates originally being incriminated. A large multicenter trial, however, suggested no correlation between the development of antibodies and the source of factor VIII exposure.[144] The anti-VIII:C

antibody is long-acting and may call for a long incubation in the PTT system for demonstration. The usual procedure is to incubate the APTT system for 15 minutes, 30 minutes, 45 minutes, and 60 minutes to prove the presence or absence of factor VIII:C antibody. Reliable screening and assay procedures have been published, and reagents are readily available.[141,145-148] Factor VIII:C antibodies are irreversible, and once the antibody combines with factor VIII:C, biologic activity is lost.

Therapy for hemophilia A is dependent on site and severity of hemorrhage. Mild bleeding can often be controlled with cold compresses, topical thrombin when necessary, bed rest, and other supportive measures.[16] Serious bleeding, including intra-articular bleeding, should be treated with factor VIII concentrates.[117,149-154] Factor VIII concentrates are more commonly used and are preferred over cryoprecipitate. Cryoprecipitate may have unreliable amounts of factor VIII:C. Large amounts of fibrinogen, potentially leading to renal damage, are infused with cryoprecipitate, and the response to factor VIII concentrate, unlike cryoprecipitate, is predictable. Generally, the infusion of 25 units/kg will give a 50% increase in activity in a patient with hemophilia A. A level of 50% of normal activity should readily achieve hemostasis in most instances.[117,152] A more precise formula for calculating a dose of factor VIII concentrate is given in Table 6-17. This method is preferred for nonemergent replacement (eg, preoperatively). The biologic half-life of infused factor VIII:C is between eight and 12 hours, and infusions, especially in surgical patients, patients undergoing physical therapy, or any patient needing several days or weeks of constant therapy, need to be adjusted appropriately, based on the formula given and frequent quantitative factor VIII:C assays. For some orthopedic procedures, cardiac procedures, and neurosurgical procedures, the factor VIII:C level should be maintained around 80% to 100% of normal.[117,149,152,155,156] When the patient does not show the expected postinfusion rise in factor VIII:C activity, an inhibitor should be strongly suspected and appropriate testing done. When factor VIII inhibitors are found, quantitative titers should be performed. Some patients with inhibitors require only supportive therapy, especially those with large ecchymoses unaccompanied by deep tissue bleeding.[157] When replacement therapy is clinically indicated, low-titer inhibitors can be overcome and treated with factor VIII concentrates.[158,159] In this instance, the inhibitor is quantitated, and an appropriate amount of factor VIII concentrate is given to neutralize the inhibitor exactly. Following this pro-

Table 6-18. Variants of Hemophilia B

Factor IX Protein	Ox-brain Thromboplastin Time	Term Used
CRM+	Normal	Hemophilia B+
CRM+	Long	Hemophilia B−$_M$
CRM−	Normal	Hemophilia B−
CRM−	Long	Hemophilia B−$_M$

Other CRM+ Variants: Factor IX Alabama, Cambridge, Deventer, Eindhoven, Kashihara, Lake Elsinore, Leyden (levels increase with age), Long Beach, Los Angeles, Nagoya, Niigata

Table 6-19. Hemophilia B

Clinical Manifestations
 Sex-linked recessive
 Absence of factor IX in 70% to 90%
 Presence of dysfunctional factor IX in 10% to 30%
 Deep tissue hemorrhage
  Intra-articular
  Intracranial
  Intramuscular
  Compartment compression syndromes
 Clinical course parallels factor IX level
  Severe, 0% to 5%, many spontaneous bleeds
  Moderate, 5% to 10%, occasional spontaneous bleeds
  Mild, 10% to 40%, rare spontaneous bleeds
 Severe bleeding with surgery or trauma
 Anti–factor IX antibody in 7% to 10% (usually IgG lambda)
 Hemophilia B accounts for 10% to 15% of hemophilic patients
 Most patients are male (sex-linked recessive)

Laboratory Manifestations
 Prolonged partial thromboplastin time
 Normal prothrombin time
 Normal template bleeding time
 Platelet dysfunction (aggregation) may be seen in very severe conditions

cedure it can be assumed the patient is at a 0% factor VIII:C level, and then an appropriate amount of concentrate is infused using the formula in Table 6-17 to give the desired factor VIII:C level. Both human and porcine factor VIII concentrates are available for this purpose.[160,161] Increased titers of antibodies are treated with activated prothrombin complex concentrates, and the response is generally, but not consistently, good.[162-165] Plasma exchange and extracorporeal inhibitor absorption with protein A columns have been used with some success.[166-168] DDAVP has also been attempted but without success.[169] Anti-VIII antibodies in hemophilic patients are generally not responsive to immunosuppressive therapy but are reasonably successful in nonhemophilic patients with autoantibodies.[140,170] Both factor VIII and factor IX concentrates are associated with a risk of hepatitis and HIV. This risk is lessened with heat-treated products and may be eradicated with newer genetically engineered products that are now being explored.[171,172] A major problem with factor IX concentrates is thrombogenicity, which will be discussed in the section dealing with hemophilia B. Some hemophilic patients are fortunate enough to be taking prophylactic "home therapy." In these individuals various dosage schedules have been devised by which the patient is infused with enough factor VIII concentrate to maintain factor VIII:C at a minimal or nonbleeding level. This type of therapy, however, is extremely expensive, only sometimes indicated, and may be associated with complications.

Methods of detecting carriers of hemophilia A and B have recently been described and are extremely accurate with new DNA cloning techniques.[173-177] The sampling of fetal blood in utero can be accomplished in high-risk carriers with these new techniques.

Factor IX Defects

Factor IX deficiency is also known as hemophilia B, Christmas disease, or PTC deficiency.[178-180] This disorder, like hemophilia A, is also inherited as a sex-linked recessive trait.[178] The clinical features are identical to those of hemophilia A: deep tissue bleeding, including intra-articular bleeding with hemarthroses, intramuscular bleeding,

intracranial bleeding, and potentially severe mucosal membrane hemorrhages.[178,181] The disease can be divided clinically into mild, moderate, or severe conditions.[178] Correlation between factor IX:C and severity of the disease is the same as that noted with factor VIII deficiency. Most patients (70% to 90%) have true deficiency in factor IX:C levels and have CRM− conditions. However, 10% to 30% of patients have CRM+ conditions.[178,182-184] As another variable, some patients with CRM+ have prolonged ox-brain thromboplastin times, whereas others have normal times.

Several variants of hemophilia B exist. One variant is hemophilia B Leyden; in this variant, the factor IX:C levels increase with age.[185] Other named variants are Chapel Hill, Alabama, Deventer, Kashihara, Zutphen, Eindhoven, Elsimore, Long Beach, Los Angeles, Nagoya, Cambridge, and Niigata.[178,186-201] Variants of hemophilia B are summarized in Table 6-18.

The clinical features of hemophilia B are summarized in Table 6-19. About 60% to 70% of patients have a contributory family history. Patients characteristically have a prolonged activated partial thromboplastin time and a normal prothrombin time.[178] The diagnosis is usually made when a patient with an appropriate history, family history, or appropriate bleeding history presents with a prolonged APTT, a normal prothrombin time, and a normal factor VIII:C assay. In this circumstance, the next logical assay to be done would be a factor IX assay. Management, such as that for hemophilia A, depends on the clinical significance of hemorrhage. Mild bleeding is best controlled by local supportive mea-

Table 6-20. Laboratory Modalities for Evaluation of Hemophilia

Prothrombin time

Partial thromboplastin time (activated)

Activated partial thromboplastin time–derived assays
    Factor VIII:C
    Factor IX
    Factor XI

Synthetic substrate-based assays
    Factor VIII:C
    Factor IX
    Factor XI

Factor VIII:RAg (vWF:Ag) assay

Factor VIII inhibitor assay

Factor IX inhibitor assay

External pathway–generated thrombin protime equivalent?

Internal pathway–generated thrombin APTT equivalent?

Table 6-21. Factor X Defects

Clinical Manifestations
    Autosomal recessive trait
    Absence form (CRM–) and dysfunctional form
        (CRM+) exist
    Factor X Friuli was first dysfunctional form
    Severe mucosal membrane hemorrhages are typical
    Umbilical stump bleeding is common
    Severe bleeding occurs with surgery or trauma

Laboratory Manifestations
    Prolonged partial thromboplastin time
    Prolonged prothrombin time
    Russell's viper venom time usually prolonged
    Normal template bleeding time
    Normal platelet function (aggregation)

Therapy
    Raise factor X level to 15% to 20%
    Fresh frozen plasma
    Prothrombin complex concentrates

sures, including cold compresses and, when appropriate, topical thrombin.[1] Severe bleeding or preparation for surgery is managed with prothrombin complex concentrates that contain factor IX.[178,202-206] The hazards of these concentrates are hepatitis, HIV, and thrombogenicity, including the initiation of DIC-type syndromes in recipients.[178,207-210] About 5% to 7% of patients with factor IX deficiency develop anti–factor IX antibodies.[178] The only proven therapy for this complication is to neutralize the antibody with prothrombin complex concentrate, followed by increasing the factor IX:C level to the desired range to achieve hemostasis. Like factor VIII antibodies, factor IX antibodies in patients with hemophilia B also respond poorly to immunosuppressive therapy.[140] New DNA techniques are available for detection of carriers.[211] Laboratory modalities for evaluating hemophilias are summarized in Table 6-20.

Factor X Defects

Factor X deficiency is a very rare disorder, with only approximately 50 families described.[1,212-215] The disorder is inherited as an autosomal recessive trait. Homozygous patients have very low factor X:C levels, and heterozygotes have approximately 50% of normal factor X:C activity. Both the absent form, factor X:C–, and dysfunctional form, factor X:C+, are known to exist.[212,216] The clinical features are similar for both forms.[1,212,217] Factor X Friuli was the first described, but factor X Roma, factor X San Antonio, and factor X Padua are more dysfunctional forms.[218-221] Patients with factor X deficiency are more prone to have severe mucosal membrane and skin hemorrhages and fewer deep tissue hemorrhages than those seen in the hemophilias.[212] Mucosal membrane hemorrhage can be from any site and is often severe in homozygous patients. Umbilical stump bleeding at birth is a particularly common early manifestation of factor X deficiency.[222]

The activated partial thromboplastin time and prothrombin time are markedly prolonged in homozygous patients and mildly prolonged or sometimes normal in heterozygous patients.[212] Since Russell's viper venom will activate factor X in vitro, this test is also usually prolonged.[212,223] The Russell viper venom time, however, may be normal in some patients with factor X:C+ defects.[218] These findings should prompt a quantitative factor X:C assay for definitive diagnosis. Since hemostasis can be achieved with 15% to 20% levels of factor X, management can often be achieved with plasma infusions.[212] Serious bleeding or the achieving of higher levels of factor X for surgery can be accomplished with prothrombin complex concentrates when the desired potential clinical benefits outweigh the potential hazards of thrombosis.[224] The clinical and laboratory findings of factor X defects are noted in Table 6-21.

Factor XI Defects

Factor XI deficiency is also called plasma thromboplastin antecedent (PTA) deficiency, Rosenthal's disease, or hemophilia C; these terms should be abandoned.[1,225] The disorder was first described by Rosenthal and coworkers in 1953.[226] Factor XI deficiency was first thought to be inherited as an autosomal dominant trait; however, more recent and thorough studies have revealed it to be inherited as an incomplete autosomal recessive trait.[225-227] Homozygous patients

Table 6-22. Factor XI Defects

Clinical Manifestations
Incomplete autosomal recessive trait
Highly variable clinical course
Most common in Ashkenazic Jews
Many other races also affected
Spontaneous mucosal membrane hemorrhage common
Spontaneous deep tissue hemorrhage rare
Severe bleeding may occur with surgery or trauma
Little correlation between bleeding and factor XI level
An individual course may change dramatically
Heterozygous patients rarely bleed
Oral mucosal bleeding frequent
Genitourinary tract bleeding frequent

Laboratory Manifestations
Bleeding history may be positive or negative
Prolonged partial thromboplastin time
Normal prothrombin time
Normal template bleeding time
Normal platelet function (aggregation)
Definitive diagnosis requires factor XI assay
Factor XI assay should be the first assay done in a female
child with prolonged partial thromboplastin time and
normal protime

have about 1% of normal factor XI levels, whereas heterozygous patients have about 50% of normal factor XI levels.[1,225,227] A high incidence occurs in Jewish patients of Russian descent (Ashkenazic Jews), and in this population homozygotes comprise approximately 0.2% of the population, and heterozygotes may comprise as much as 11%.[225,228,229] Many other ethnic groups are also affected. Most patients appear to have a true impaired factor XI synthesis defect, since few dysfunctional forms have yet been described.[230,231]

The clinical features are amazingly variable and sometimes confusing.[225,232] Homozygous patients have spontaneous bleeding from mucosal membranes, which may be serious; however, deep tissue bleeding, including intra-articular bleeding, is extremely rare. Up to 50% of homozygous patients may experience serious and life-threatening bleeding with surgery or trauma.[225,232,233] Bleeding from the oral mucosa or the genitourinary tract is a particular problem and has been ascribed to the enhanced fibrinolytic activity that may occur in these areas.[234,235] Most heterozygous patients have no bleeding, but a few patients may have spontaneous mucosal membrane hemorrhages, especially epistaxis, and some will have minor bleeding with surgery or trauma.[1] Homozygous patients may have no bleeding, minimal bleeding, or profuse bleeding.[225,232] In addition, the severity of bleeding does not correlate well with levels of circulating factor XI.[1] Patients may have a marked change in their clinical course. A nonbleeding patient or a patient with minimal bleeding may develop spontaneous or severe bleeding during the course of the disease. Alternatively, a frequently bleeding patient may become a nonbleeding patient. These changes in the clinical course often have no relationship to changes in circulating factor XI. Clinical manifestations and laboratory findings of factor XI deficiency are summarized in Table 6-22.

From the laboratory diagnostic standpoint, some patients present with a negative bleeding history, and some present with an appropriate positive bleeding history. Patients with factor XI deficiency will demonstrate a prolonged APTT and normal prothrombin time.[225,236] Unless the patient is a female, in which case a factor XI level should be considered immediately, the diagnosis is usually made by noting a typical personal or family history or significant bleeding and a prolonged PTT, a normal prothrombin time, normal factor VIII and factor IX levels, and a subsequent decreased level of factor XI.[225,237,238] Management is primarily the use of fresh frozen plasma infused at 10 mL/kg per day for significant bleeding episodes or in preparation for surgery.[1,225] The factor XI levels should be raised to 30% to 40% of normal to achieve hemostasis.[1]

Factor XII Defects

Congenital factor XII deficiency was first described by Ratnoff and Colopy in 1955.[240] Since then, more than 100 cases have been reported.[1,217,239] The name of the first patient studied by Ratnoff and Colopy was John Hageman, and the disorder is commonly called Hageman trait.[240] Usually, the disorder is inherited as an autosomal recessive trait, but instances of autosomal dominant inheritance have also been described.[217] Homozygous patients with the autosomal recessive variety have very low levels of factor XII; heterozygotes can have variable manifestations but tend to have approximately 50% of normal factor XII activity. The disorder is known to exist in the absence form, factor XII:C–, and the dysfunctional form, factor XII:C+ (CRM+).[241-243] However, the absence form appears more common than the dysfunctional variety.

Factor XII deficiency is usually found by chance when a screening PTT is done and noted to be markedly prolonged, often in a routine presurgical patient.[1,237,238] Since this is the manner in which many patients present, it is assumed and classically incorrectly taught that patients with factor XII deficiency have no bleeding diathesis. Some patients do have a mild bleeding tendency, and life-threatening bleeding can occur, although uncommonly.[240] Fatal hemorrhage has been reported.[244] Patients with factor XII deficiency have defective surface-mediated activation of fibrinolysis, and many patients who have died with factor XII deficiency have died of thrombosis or thromboembolism.[245-248] John Hageman, a railroad worker, died of a pulmonary embolus following hip fracture.[249] It appears that an inordinately large number of patients with factor XII deficiency have died of a myocardial infarction or pulmonary embolus and have an increased risk of deep vein thrombosis.[250] In addition, patients may have defects in neutrophil or macrophage chemotaxis.[251]

Table 6-23. Factor XII Defects

Clinical Manifestations
    Autosomal recessive trait in most patients
    Autosomal dominant trait in few patients
    Absence form (CRM–) and dysfunctional form
      (CRM+) exist
    Defect is often found by chance via prolonged PTT
    Many have a mild bleeding tendency
    Fatal bleeding has occurred
    Most have defective surface-mediated fibrinolytic activation
    High incidence of fatal thrombosis/thromboembolism

Laboratory Manifestations
    Markedly prolonged partial thromboplastin time
    Normal prothrombin time
    Normal template bleeding time
    Normal platelet function (aggregation)
    Definitive diagnosis requires factor XII assay

Therapy
    Plasma replacement for hemorrhage
    Anticoagulants for thrombosis/thromboembolus

Table 6-24. Prekallikrein Deficiency

Clinical Manifestations
    Autosomal recessive and dominant cases described
    Majority have absence of protein (CRM–)
    Some have dysfunctional protein (CRM+)
    No hemorrhagic tendency yet described
    Defective surface-mediated activation of fibrinolysis

Laboratory Manifestations
    Prolonged partial thromboplastin time
    Normal prothrombin time
    Normal template bleeding time
    Normal platelet function (aggregation)
    Definitive diagnosis requires prekallikrein assay

Correction of PTT with long incubation (10 minutes) is characteristic but should not be used as a diagnostic tool. The same findings may be seen in Passovoy defect.

The diagnosis is most commonly made by noting a prolonged PTT and normal prothrombin time in an asymptomatic patient, a patient with a mild hemorrhagic diathesis, or in a patient with thrombosis.[1,240] A definitive diagnosis requires specific quantitative factor XII assay by functional assay.[252] Since hemorrhage is rare, replacement therapy is generally not needed. In those exceptionally rare patients with significant hemorrhage, replacement should be with fresh frozen plasma. Although it is not known if prophylactic fibrinolytic enhancement therapy is indicated in patients with factor XII deficiency, perhaps more experience with this method will eventually dictate some type of prophylaxis for thrombosis, such as stanozolol enhancement of fibrinolysis. Certainly, when thrombosis or thromboembolism occurs it should be treated appropriately. Findings of factor XII defects are shown in Table 6-23.

Prekallikrein Defects

Prekallikrein deficiency was first noted by Hathaway in 1965, when children from a consanguineous marriage were involved in a fire.[253] After recuperation from burns, tonsillectomies were planned, and the preoperative PTT was markedly prolonged in four of 14 children. The defect was noted to correct with factor XII–deficient plasma, and the new disorder was called Fletcher trait, after the surname of the family.[253] The mode of inheritance is unclear or variable: some have described autosomal recessive characteristics while others have noted autosomal dominance.[254] Although most patients have a true deficiency (CRM–), several instances of a dysfunctional form (CRM+) have also been described.[255,256] Patients with prekallikrein deficiency have no bleeding ten-

dency, although these patients, like those with factor XII deficiency, also have defective activation of the fibrinolytic system.[257,258] The diagnosis is suggested when noting a markedly prolonged PTT and normal prothrombin and thrombin times in an asymptomatic individual, usually during presurgical screening procedures.[1,237,238,254] The diagnosis is made by doing a specific prekallikrein assay by clot-based or synthetic substrate–based techniques; both types of assays are readily available. A characteristic of prekallikrein deficiency is the correction of the partial thromboplastin time when incubating the PTT system for 10 minutes with kaolin, celite, silica, or ellagic acid.[253,259] This test should not be used for a diagnosis since the same phenomena can be noted with Passovoy deficiency, and an erroneous interpretation could lead to a missed diagnosis of Passovoy defect and a potential bleeding problem. The features of prekallikrein deficiency are summarized in Table 6-24.

Kininogen Defects

Deficiency of high–molecular weight kininogen is known by a variety of surnames, including the most common, Fitzgerald trait[260]; however, the defect is also known as Williams trait, Fleaujac trait, Fujiwara trait, and Reid trait.[261-264] The disorder is inherited as an autosomal recessive characteristic. Patients do not have a hemorrhagic tendency but do have abnormal surface-mediated activation of fibrinolysis as noted by a long euglobulin clot lysis time.[257] All patients studied thus far have a true deficiency of high–molecular weight kininogen. Fitzgerald and Reid traits represent a deficiency of high–molecular weight kininogen; however, Williams, Fleaujac, and Fujiwara traits represent a deficiency of both high–molecular weight and low–molecular weight kininogen. These last three forms of deficiency are also deficient in prekallikrein. The diagnosis is suspected by noting a prolonged PTT, normal prothrombin and thrombin times, and

Table 6-25. High–Molecular Weight Kininogen Deficiency

Clinical Manifestations
Autosomal recessive trait
No hemorrhagic tendency
Abnormal surface-mediated activation of fibrinolysis

Variety of Synonyms

Name	Deficiency
Fitzgerald trait	High–molecular weight kininogen only
Reid trait	High–molecular weight kininogen only
Williams trait	High– and low–molecular weight kininogen
Flaujeac trait	High– and low–molecular weight kininogen
Fujiwara trait	High– and low–molecular weight kininogen

Laboratory Manifestations
Prolonged partial thromboplastin time
Normal prothrombin time
Normal template bleeding time
Normal platelet function (aggregation)
Definitive diagnosis requires immunologic assay for high–molecular weight kininogen

Table 6-26. Passovoy Defect

Clinical Manifestations
Autosomal dominant trait
Moderate hemorrhagic tendency
Mucosal membrane bleeding is typical
Easy and spontaneous bruising is typical
Severe hemorrhage occurs with surgery or trauma

Laboratory Manifestations
Prolonged partial thromboplastin time
Normal prothrombin time
Normal thrombin time
Normal template bleeding time
Normal platelet function (aggregation)
PTT will shorten with long incubation times (10 minutes), and this disorder can be mistaken for prekallikrein deficiency

Therapy
Fresh frozen plasma for hemorrhage or preparation for surgery

noncorrecting of the PTT with prolonged incubation in an asymptomatic individual usually during a routine preoperative screening work-up.[1,237,238,254] A definitive diagnosis is made by immunologic assay for high–molecular weight kininogen.[254,265] Individuals with this defect are asymptomatic but have abnormal surface-activated fibrinolysis and defective neutrophil/macrophage chemotaxis. Abnormal inflammatory responses were noted in one individual.[260] The features of high–molecular weight kininogen deficiency are summarized in Table 6-25.

Passovoy Defect

Passovoy deficiency was first described by Hougie and associates in 1975.[266] The disorder appears to be inherited as an autosomal dominant trait. The molecular characteristics are unknown. Patients typically have a moderate bleeding tendency characterized by mucosal membrane bleeding, including epistaxis, easy and spontaneous bruising, and excessive menstrual flow.[1] Intra-articular bleeding is uncommon. Severe bleeding may happen with trauma or surgery. The PTT is moderately prolonged, and the prothrombin time and thrombin time are normal.[266-268] The partial thromboplastin time will shorten with incubation; and the disorder can be erroneously confused with prekallikrein deficiency.[267] Plasma infusions are used for traumatic or surgical hemorrhage. The features of Passovoy defect are noted in Table 6-26.

Alpha-2-Antiplasmin Defects

Alpha-2-antiplasmin deficiency is inherited as an autosomal recessive trait. Alpha-2-antiplasmin levels are less than 10% of normal in homozygous patients and about 50% of normal in heterozygous individuals.[269] Few dysfunctional forms have been noted, and most patients have parallel levels of biologic and immunologic alpha-2-antiplasmin.[270-276] Bleeding can be severe in homozygous patients and typically consists of mucosal membrane bleeding, with hematuria predominating, large subcutaneous hematomas, spontaneous bruising, and severe bleeding with trauma.[270-277] Intra-articular bleeding may occur. Results of laboratory tests are generally normal, except for low levels of alpha-2-antiplasmin.[1,269-272] Occasionally, elevated FDPs are seen. The therapies of choice are epsilon aminocaproic acid given at a dosage of 10 mg/kg orally or intravenously three times a day or tranexamic acid given at a dosage of 500 mg orally or intravenously two or three times a day.[269,274,278] The findings of antiplasmin deficiency are depicted in Table 6-27.

Factor XIII Defects

Congenital factor XIII deficiency has been described in more than 100 families and is inherited as an autosomal recessive trait, although originally thought to be sex linked.[279-281] A high incidence of consanguinity has been noted.[100,109] Factor XIII is a dimeric protein consisting of an alpha and beta chain, and the complex circulates as a dimer (A_2B_2).[281,282] Homozygous patients harbor defects of the alpha chain, which contains the activation site. Homozygotes may also have decreased levels of the beta chain, but patients have been described who have absent or normal beta chains. Heterozygotes generally have decreased alpha and beta chains. If immunologic techniques are used to assay factor XIII, anti–alpha chain and anti–beta chain antibodies must be used, and these techniques are available.[279,281-285] Conditions with decreased alpha and beta

Table 6-27. Antiplasmin Deficiency

Clinical Manifestations
  Autosomal recessive
  Most are CRM–
  Severe mucosal membrane hemorrhage
  Genitourinary tract bleeding is characteristic
  Large subcutaneous hematomas
  Easy and spontaneous bruising
  Severe bleeding with surgery or trauma
  Intra-articular bleeding has occurred

Laboratory Manifestations
  Normal prothrombin time
  Normal partial thromboplastin time
  Normal template bleeding time
  Normal platelet function (aggregation)
  Definitive diagnosis requires assay for alpha-2-antiplasmin

Therapy
  Epsilon aminocaproic acid, 10 mg/kg three times daily; or
    tranexamic acid, 500 mg twice daily or three times daily
    intravenously or orally

Table 6-28. Factor XIII Defects

Clinical Manifestations
  Autosomal recessive trait
  Most patients have absence of alpha chain (CRM–)
  Umbilical stump bleeding in 90%
  Delayed deep tissue hemorrhage is typical
    Intramuscular
    Intracranial
    Pseudotumors often develop
  Most common cause of death is intracranial bleeding
  Most homozygous men are sterile
  Most homozygous women have miscarriages
  Heterozygous patients are usually asymptomatic

Laboratory Manifestations
  Clot solubility in urea or monochloroacetic acid
  Clot solubility is a poor diagnostic tool
  Definitive diagnosis requires specific assay for factor XIII
    cross-linking activity

Therapy
  Fresh frozen plasma or cryoprecipitate every seven to
    10 days

chains are called type I and those with normal or near normal beta chains are type II.[286]

The clinical manifestations of factor XIII deficiency are characteristic, and the bleeding diathesis only occurs in homozygotes, as only 10% of normal factor XIII levels are necessary for normal fibrin monomer cross-linking to occur.[279-281] Most patients (90%) demonstrate delayed umbilical stump bleeding at birth, and this finding should immediately prompt a strong suspicion of factor XIII deficiency, or, less probably, afibrinogenemia, homozygous dysfibrinogenemia, or factor X deficiency, because only in these disorders is umbilical stump bleeding characteristic.[1,279,280,281] Patients with homozygous factor XIII deficiency also characteristically have significant deep tissue hemorrhages, especially into muscle and muscle compartments, which most commonly develop several days after minor trauma but may happen spontaneously.[280] Many patients develop later destruction of bone and pseudotumors, which are especially prominent in the thigh and gluteal areas.[280] The most common cause of death is intracranial hemorrhage, which occurs in factor XIII deficiency more commonly than in any of the other congenital coagulation protein defects. This bleeding is also commonly preceded by minor trauma occurring several days earlier.[279,280] Although deep tissue bleeding is common, intra-articular bleeding is rare. In addition, although patients have delayed posttraumatic bleeding, postsurgical bleeding is less commonly a problem. Most homozygous men are sterile, and a high incidence of spontaneous abortion is seen in homozygous women.[280] It has been suggested that factor XIII is not only involved in adequate wound healing, by possibly cross-linking collagen as well as fibrin, but it may also be necessary for normal implantation of a fertilized ovum into the uterine decidua.[280]

A screening test for the presence or absence of factor XIII consists of observing for clot solubility or insolubility in 5 mol/L urea or 1% monochloroacetic acid, two agents that will disrupt hydrophobic bonds but not the gamma glutamyl-lysine bonds created by factor XIIIa.[1,237,238,279] These solubility tests, however, are poor screening techniques because they are insensitive to levels slightly more than 1% of normal activity, and patients with a potential deficiency and bleeding can be missed.[279] More specific techniques are available, including assays for gamma-gamma dimer (cross-linked by factor XIII), radioactive amine incorporation tests, latex agglutination inhibition tests, or radioimmunoassay.[281,283,284] The therapy for factor XIII deficiency consists of infusion of fresh frozen plasma at 10 mL/kg every seven to 10 days.[1] Alternatively, cryoprecipitate can be used.[1] Adequate levels of factor XIII are also rendered to the surgical patient who may have received several units of whole blood. Characteristic findings of factor XIII defects are noted in Table 6-28.

von Willebrand's Disease

von Willebrand's syndrome was first reported by Eric von Willebrand in 1926.[287] This bleeding disorder was first noted in families living on the Åland island off the coast of Sweden in the Gulf of Bothnia; the islands are now called Ahvenanmaa. The original patients had a severe bleeding disorder that was autosomally inherited. In addition, a prolonged bleeding time, normal clot retraction, normal platelet counts, and a normal coagulation time were characteristic. These original patients, who were first labeled as "pseudohemophiliacs," were reexamined using a capillary "thrombometer" several years later by von Willebrand and Jurgens. This closer evaluation revealed prolonged thrombometer times, and patients were then labeled as having "constitutional thrombopathy."[288] The criteria for a diagnosis became the following: (1) a bleeding tendency, (2) autosomal inheritance, (3) a normal platelet count, (4) a long bleeding time, and (5) a normal whole blood clotting time. In 1953, Alexander and Goldstein,[289] Larrieu and Soulier,[290] and Quick and Hussey[291] simultaneously discovered a new characteristic of von Willebrand's syndrome: low factor VIII levels. This important discovery acted as a catalyst to launch investigations that have led subsequently to a more complete understanding of the biology of the factor VIII macromolecular complex, classic hemophilia, and von Willebrand's disease. In 1971, Zimmerman, Ratnoff, and Powell[292] developed an antibody to factor VIII and demonstrated the presence of an antigen, factor VIII:RAg (now called vWF:Ag), in normal and hemophilic plasma but not in von Willebrand's plasma. This discovery began the era of molecular biology of hemophilia, von Willebrand's disease, and factor VIII moieties and supplied a tool for the defining of von Willebrand types and the separately recognized portions and activities of the factor VIII macromolecular complex. A concept of the complex is depicted in Figure 6-2.[293-298] Factor VIII:C is a low–molecular weight part that is loosely complexed to a high–molecular weight portion now called vWF:Ag. Factor VIII:C, which is defective in classic hemophilia, is responsible for procoagulant activity, which is the biologic activity responsible for serving as a cofactor or determiner in the conversion of factor X to factor Xa.[296] This factor is probably synthesized in several cellular sites, but not the endothelium. Factor VIII:C has no other known biologic activity. Factor VIII:R, previously called factor VIII:RCo or ristocetin cofactor and now called vWF, is composed of vWF:Ag (to heterologous antibody) and von Willebrand factor, called vWF. von Willebrand factor is an integral part of the high–molecular weight portion and is the biologic activity that is necessary for normal bleeding times, normal platelet aggregation to ristocetin, normal platelet adhesion to subendothelial surfaces, and a normal platelet-endothelial interaction.[293-297,299] von Willebrand factor is a polymerized multimeric moiety and is synthesized in the endothelium of arteries and veins and in platelets and megakaryocytes.[293-302] It is thought that vWF may induce the synthesis or release of factor VIII:C, which accounts for a well-known phenomena in patients with von Willebrand's syndrome. When the patient with von Willebrand's syndrome is transfused with normal plasma, hemophilic plasma, or cryoprecipitate, a marked and sustained increase in factor VIII:C occurs.[293-295,303] The bleeding in von Willebrand's disease is reminiscent of a platelet-vascular problem and consists of purpura, easy and spontaneous bruising, hypermenorrhagia, mucosal membrane bleeding, including gastrointestinal and genitourinary hemorrhage, and bilateral epistaxis.[304] Bleeding, often in the form of bilateral epistaxis, and easy and spontaneous bruising can typically begin in early childhood, and this constellation of findings should prompt an early suspicion of von Willebrand's disease.

Table 6-29. von Willebrand's Syndrome

Clinical Manifestations
  Variable inheritance
  Easy and spontaneous bruising
  Petechiae and purpura
  Mucosal membrane hemorrhage
    Genitourinary
    Gastrointestinal
    Intrapulmonary
    Gingival bleeding
  Bilateral epistaxis in early childhood
  Deep tissue bleeding rare
  Hemorrhage may be severe with surgery or trauma

Therapy
  Cryoprecipitate, 1 to 3 bags per 10 kg of body weight
  Fresh frozen plasma to factor VIII:C greater than 75%
  Monitor template bleeding time (variable)
  DDAVP may be of benefit in selected types
  Inhibitors have been treated with intravenous
    immunoglobulin or protein A columns

Deep tissue bleeding and intra-articular bleeding are far less common than mucosal membrane bleeding. Hemorrhage, however, can be profuse with surgery or trauma. Clinical features of von Willebrand's syndrome are summarized in Table 6-29.

With the arrival of more sophisticated laboratory assessment, more and more subtypes of von Willebrand's syndrome are being recognized.[300,304-314] One study showed a high degree of variability in the laboratory features in any individual patient during a given period, which suggests that many patients who are categorized into one type based on a study at a single time may not be classified correctly.[315] The results of this study also suggest that if a patient has a history suggestive of von Willebrand's syndrome but does not meet the diagnostic laboratory criteria, the patient should be reexamined at another time. The laboratory assessment that has allowed for more clear classification of von Willebrand's disease subtypes is the analysis of vWF multimeric structure by agarose gel electrophoresis.[316,317] This analysis has led to further subclassification of common forms of von Willebrand's disease and to discovery of rare types only seen in one or a few families.[318,319] Only the common forms of von Willebrand's disease will be depicted in detail; excellent recent reviews are available for discussions of rare subtypes. Following are the currently accepted common types of von Willebrand's syndrome.

Type I

Heterozygous von Willebrand's type IA is inherited as an autosomal dominant trait and is characterized by concordant decreases in factor VIII:C, factor VIII:CAg, factor VIII:RCo (factor VIII:vW), and factor VIII:RAg. Multimer analysis of vWF reveals normal structure and distribution but is quantitatively reduced.[320] This type is a quantitative defect in the entire factor VIII macromolecular complex. Type IB is similar to type IA, except that vWF multimer analysis shows not only a quantitative decrease in total vWF but also a disproportionate decrease in the larger multimers.[321] Type IC is a rare form with similar features to type IA, except for the noting of structural abnormalities of multimers characterized by satellite bands around each multimer.[322]

Type II

Heterozygous von Willebrand's type II is subdivided into several forms depending on multimer analysis. Heterozygous von Willebrand's type IIA is inherited as an autosomal dominant trait and represents a dysfunction of vWF. There is absent or almost nonexistent vWF activity and discordance with levels of factor VIII:C, factor VIII:CAg, and vWF:Ag, all of which are usually much higher, often normal, than levels of vWF activity (ristocetin cofactor activity). This suggests a dysfunction of the complex instead of a quantitative defect. In this form of disease, it appears that depolymerization of the macromolecular complex occurs, with many monomeric fast forms circulating and absence of the large- and intermediate-sized multimers.[323,324] This type may represent an abnormality of polymerization ability of the complex. Heterozygous von Willebrand's type IIB is also usually inherited as an autosomal dominant trait, has the same discordant findings as seen in type IIA, and is often associated with thrombocytopenia.[325] Normal or near normal factor VIII:C, factor VIII:CAg, and vWF:Ag are present in this type. The two major differences from type IIA are that in this form enhanced platelet aggregability to ristocetin occurs (enhanced ristocetin cofactor activity)[326] and this form also appears to be associated with a defect in polymerization, because fewer of the monomeric forms and more of the polymerized forms circulating are typically seen in type IIA. In particular, decreased large multimeric forms in plasma but a normal vWF multimeric amount and distribution in platelets occur.[327] It has been suggested that the large plasma multimers are attached to platelets in this form of von Willebrand's disease, which explains the thrombocytopenia often seen in this type.[328] Types IIC through IIH are very rare subtypes described, based on characteristics of multimer analysis.[329-334]

Type III

Homozygous von Willebrand's disease, previously called type IS, is characterized by recessive inheritance, severe bleeding of the sites previously mentioned, and a high incidence of consanguinity.[335] The bleeding time is usually markedly prolonged. Activity of von Willebrand factor (ristocetin cofactor activity) is markedly decreased or absent, and vWF:Ag is markedly reduced or absent. Factor VIII:C and factor VIII:CAg are reduced but not as profoundly as vWF activity and vWF:Ag. Multimer analysis shows a marked decrease in all vWF.[336] About 10% of these patients may develop anti-vWF antibodies after exposure to exogenous sources of von Willebrand factor.[337]

Table 6-30. Common Forms of von Willebrand's Syndrome

Type I
  von Willebrand's syndrome type IA
    Autosomal dominant trait
    Concordant decreases in factor VIII:C, factor VIII:CAg, vW factor, vW factor:Ag
    vWF multimer analysis reveals decrease in normal structure and distribution
    A quantitative defect in entire factor VIII complex
  von Willebrand's syndrome type IB
    Same findings as in type IA but a disproportionate decrease in large vWF multimers

Type II
  von Willebrand's syndrome type IIA
    Autosomal dominant trait
    Discordant decreases in factor VIII:C (reduced), factor VIII:CAg (reduced), vW factor:Ag (reduced), vW factor (very reduced)
    Depolymerization of vWF complex with many monomeric "fast" forms
  von Willebrand's syndrome type IIB
    Autosomal dominant trait
    Discordant findings as in type IIA
    Factor VIII:C near normal
    vWF factor:Ag moderately reduced
    Enhanced platelet agglutination to ristocetin
    Depolymerization of vWF complex but fewer monomeric forms than IIA

Type III
  von Willebrand's syndrome type III/IS
    Severe hemorrhage of many sites
    High incidence of consanguinity
    Very prolonged template bleeding time
    Very reduced factor VIII:C
    Very reduced vWF (ristocetin cofactor)
    Very reduced vWF:Ag

Pseudo–von Willebrand's Disease

Platelet-type von Willebrand's disease is a platelet defect, not vWF, usually characterized by absence or dysfunction of platelet membrane glycoprotein Ib, the binding site for vWF activity.[338] Since it is a platelet function defect, the clinical features are similar to von Willebrand's syndrome. This disorder is characterized by large platelets and an increased MPV on electronic particle counters.[339] A diagnosis of this disorder is confirmed by not only noting the large platelets in the peripheral smear but by adding cryoprecipitate to the patient's platelet-rich plasma, which induces platelet aggregation. Aggregation will not occur in von Willebrand's disease.[340] The common types of von Willebrand's syndrome are characterized in Table 6-30.

Laboratory Tests

The laboratory diagnosis of von Willebrand's disease can be complex and complicated.[1,293,295,304,315] This complexity is

Table 6-31. Methods for the Evaluation of von Willebrand's Syndrome

Template bleeding time
Activated partial thromboplastin time
Factor VIII:C assay
von Willebrand's (ristocetin cofactor) assay
vW factor:Ag (factor VIII:RAg) assay
Agarose gel analysis of vWF multimers

further enhanced by the variability and changing of laboratory parameters in a given patient, including the past popularity of tests that are notoriously unreliable.[341-345] The ristocetin cofactor assay has replaced ristocetin-induced aggregation and is a sensitive test. The primary laboratory tests, however, are the factor VIII:C and vWF:Ag tests, ristocetin cofactor (vWF) activity, multimer analysis, and template bleeding time.[1,245,293,295,304,315,341] Laboratory tests for the diagnosis of von Willebrand's disease are shown in Table 6-31.

Therapy

The therapy of choice for patients with von Willebrand's syndrome is cryoprecipitate, which contains abundant levels of vWF.[1,295,304,341,345] The amount of cryoprecipitate currently used is variable, as is the amount of vWF present in cryoprecipitate. The response, by monitoring correction of the bleeding time, is also variable. The goal of therapy is to correct the bleeding time and factor VIII:C level to normal or near normal.[1] A general approach is to give 1 to 3 bags of cryoprecipitate per day per 10 kg of total body weight, depending on the site and severity of bleeding.[1] Presurgical patients should receive cryoprecipitate, preferably directed single-donor, the morning of the day of surgery. If cryoprecipitate is not available, infusions of fresh frozen plasma to raise the factor VIII:C level to 80% to 100% of normal or to normalize the bleeding time can be used, and this requires about 10 to 15 mL/kg per day.[1] The use of DDAVP has also been of benefit in maintaining hemostasis in patients with von Willebrand's syndrome, although the response depends on the type of von Willebrand's disease.[346-348] Patients with types IA and IB usually respond to DDAVP, patients with type IIA show variable responses, patients with type IIB may develop thrombocytopenia with DDAVP, and patients with other subtypes of type II usually do not respond. Patients with type III von Willebrand's syndrome do not respond to DDAVP. Patients with platelet von Willebrand's syndrome also do not respond to DDAVP, because they may develop thrombocytopenia with either DDAVP or cryoprecipitate. DDAVP may be effectively delivered by the intravenous, intranasal, or subcutaneous route, and the usual intravenous dose is 0.2 to 0.5 μg/kg diluted in 30 mL of normal saline. Infusions are delivered over 15 minutes every 24 to 48 hours.[349,350] DDAVP can sometimes be associated with enhanced hemorrhage, since it also releases endothelial plasminogen activator.[351] Because of this, the concomitant use of a fibrinolytic inhibitor, such as amino caproic acid or tranexamic acid, should be considered, especially if mucosal membrane bleeding is present.[352] Generally, factor VIII concentrates should not be used for von Willebrand's disease, because most contain little vWF activity. One apparent exception to this is a European preparation, Humate-P, which has been effective in controlling bleeding.[355] In all instances of replacement therapy, the constant threat of hepatitis and HIV infection must be considered, and directed single-donor products should be used whenever feasible. Both high-dose intravenous gamma globulin and protein A sepharose columns have been used for patients, especially with type III disease, who develop anti-vWF antibodies.[356,357] Table 6-32 compares and contrasts findings of hemophilia A and von Willebrand's syndrome.

Other Rare Defects

Other rare hereditary protein defects leading to a hemorrhagic disorder have also been described. An alpha-1-antitrypsin variant causing a severe life-long bleeding diathesis in a 10-year-old boy was described in 1978 by Lewis and coworkers.[358] The inhibitory action was similar to heparin but was not bound to barium citrate or inhibited by protamine. Evaluation of the inhibitor revealed it to be a dou-

Table 6-32. Comparison of von Willebrand's Syndrome and Hemophilia A

	von Willebrand's syndrome	Hemophilia A
Inheritance	Autosomal dominant	Sex-linked recessive
Bleeding time	Long	Normal
Factor VIII:C	Moderately decreased	Markedly decreased
vWF:Ag (VIII:RAg)	Decreased	Normal
vWF (ristocetin cofactor)	Decreased	Normal
Platelet adhesion	Abnormal	Normal
Clinical features	Mucosal bleeds, petechiae and purpura	Deep tissue bleeding

ble-banded alpha-1-antitrypsin, and the defect is called "antithrombin Pittsburgh." A similar case has been reported by Messmore and coworkers in Chicago.[359]

Congenital protein C inhibitor deficiency has been reported by both Marler and Griffin[82] and Giddings, Sugrue, and Bloom[81]; in both instances the patients were deficient in factor V and factor VIII:C. Four unrelated patients were studied by Marler and Griffin, but the clinical manifestations were not discussed.[82] Giddings, Sugrue, and Bloom reported another two cases of protein C inhibitor deficiency, and both were also associated with combined factor V and factor VIII:C deficiency.[81] In this report all patients examined who had only an isolated singular factor V or isolated factor VIII:C deficiency had normal protein C inhibitor activity. Because of these findings, it has been suggested that some earlier reported cases of combined factor V and factor VIII:C deficiency may, on reevaluation, be found to represent congenital protein C inhibitor deficiency. Combined congenital deficiencies have been reviewed.[360,361]

References

1. Bick RL: Congenital coagulation factor defects and von Willebrand's disease. In: Disorders of Hemostasis and Thrombosis: Principles of Clinical Practice. Thieme, Inc., New York, 1985, p 127.

2. Bick RL: Vascular disorders associated with thrombohemorrhagic phenomena, ch 3. In: Disorders of Hemostasis and Thrombosis: Principles of Clinical Practice. Theime, Inc., New York, 1985, p 44.

3. Bick RL: A systematic approach to the diagnosis of bleeding disorders, ch 4. In: G Murano, RL Bick (Eds): Basic Concepts of Hemostasis and Thrombosis. CRC Press, Boca Raton, FL, 1980, p 81.

4. National Heart, Lung, and Blood Institute Study to Evaluate the Supply-Demand Relationships for AHF and PTC Through 1980. DHEW, US Government Printing Office, 1977.

5. Mammen EF: Andere angeborene koaglopathien. In: Heene DL (Ed): Handbuch der Inneren Medizinink, vol 2. Springer, Heidelberg, 1985, p 353.

6. Mammen EF: Fibrinogen abnormalities. Semin Thromb Hemost 9:1, 1983.

7. Montgomery R, SE Natelson: Afibrinogenemia with cerebral hematoma. Am J Dis Child 131:555, 1977.

8. Menache D: Abnormal fibrinogens: a review. Thromb Diath Haemorrh 29:525, 1973.

9. Mammen EF: Congenital abnormalities of the fibrinogen molecule. Semin Thromb Hemost 1:184, 1974.

10. Morse EE: Fibrinogen and dysfibrinogenemia. Ann Clin Lab Sci 10:351, 1980.

11. Beck EA, JR Shainoff, A Vogel, DP Jackson: Functional evaluation of an inherited abnormal fibrinogen: fibrinogen "Baltimore." J Clin Invest 50:1874, 1971.

12. Reber P, M Furlan, A Hanschen: Three abnormal fibrinogen variants with the same amino acid substitution (gamma 275 Arg to His): fibrinogens Bergamo II, Essen and Parugia. Thromb Haemost 56:401, 1986.

13. Carrell N, DA Gabriel, PM Blatt, ME Carr, J McDonagh: Hereditary dysfibrinogenemia in a patient with thrombotic disease. Blood 62:439, 1983.

14. Laugen RH, TC Bithell: Fibrinogen Charlottesville: hereditary dysfibrinogenemia characterized by slow fibrinopeptide release and competitive inhibition of thrombin. Blood 50:273, 1977.

15. Sandbjerg-Hamsen M, I Clemmensen: An abnormal fibrinogen (Copenhagen) associated with severe thromboembolic disease, but with normal absorption of plasminogen. Thromb Haemost 42:137, 1979.

16. Lijnen HR, J Soria, C Soria: Dysfibrinogenemia (Fibrinogen Dusard) associated with impaired fibrin-enhanced plasminogen activation. Thromb Haemost 51:108, 1984.

17. Fuchs G, R Egbring, K Havemann: Fibrinogen Marburg: a new genetic variant of fibrinogen. Blut 34:107, 1977.

18. Quattrone A, M Colucci, MB Donati: Cerebral thrombosis in two young siblings with dysfibrinogenemia. Neurosci Lett 3:54, 1979.

19. Al-Mondhiry HAB, SB Bilezikian, HL Nossel: Fibrinogen "New York"—an abnormal fibrinogen associated with thromboembolism: functional evaluation. Blood 45:607, 1975.

20. Engesser L, J Koopman, G DeMunk: Fibrinogen Nijmegen: congenital dysfibrinogenemia associated with impaired t-PA mediated plasminogen activation and decreased binding of t-PA. Thromb Haemost 60:113, 1988.

21. Egeberg O: Inherited fibrinogen abnormality causing thrombophilia. Thromb Diath Haemorrh 17:176, 1967.

22. Samama M, J Soria, C Soria: Congenital and acquired dysfibrinogenemia. In: L Poller (Ed): Recent Advances in Blood Coagulation. Churchill Livingstone, London, 1977, p 313.

23. Winckelmann G: Kongenitale dysfibrinogenamie bericht uber eine neue familie (fibrinogen "Wiesbaden"). Thromb Diath Haemorrh 55:345, 1973.

24. Marder VJ: The functional defects of hereditary dysfibrinogens. Thromb Haemost 36:1, 1976.

25. Morse EE: The fibrinogenopathies. Ann Clin Lab Sci 8:234, 1978.

26. Ratnoff OD, WB Forman: Criteria for the differentiation of dysfibrinogenemic states. Semin Hematol 13:141, 1976.

27. Bithell TC: Hereditary dysfibrinogenemia. Clin Chem 31: 509, 1985.

28. Chung DA, A Ichinose: Hereditary disorders related to fibrinogen and Factor XIII, ch 85. In: CL Scriver, AL Beaudet, WS Sly, D Valle (Eds): The Metabolic Basis of Inherited Disease, ed 6. McGraw Hill, New York, 1989, p 2135.

29. Mammen EF, AS Prasad, MI Barnhart, CC Hu: Congenital dysfibrinogenemia: fibrinogen Detroit. J Clin Invest 48:235, 1969.

30. Blomback M, B Blomback, EF Mammen, AS Prasad: Fibrinogen Detroit: a molecular defect in the N-terminal disulfide knot of human fibrinogen? Nature 218:134, 1968.

31. Siebenlist KR, MW Mossesson, JP Di Orio: The polymerization of fibrin prepared from Fibrinogen Haifa (gamma 275 Arg-His). Thromb Haemost 62:875, 1989.

32. Yamazumi K, K Shimura, S Terukina: A gamma-methionine-310 to threonine substitution and consequent N-glycosylation at gamma asparagine-308 in a congenital dysfibrinogenemia associated with posttraumatic bleeding, fibrinogen Asahi. J Clin Invest 83:1590, 1989.

33. Terukina S, M Matsuda, H Hirata: Substitution of gamma ARG-275 by Cys in an abnormal fibrinogen, "Fibrinogen Osaka II." J Biol Chem 263:1357, 1988.

34. Bantia S, SM Mane, WR Bell: Fibrinogen Baltimore I: polymerization defect associated with a gamma 292 Gly-Val (GGL-GTC) mutation. Blood 11:2279, 1989.

35. Bantia S, WR Bell, CV Dang: Polymerization defect of Fibrinogen Baltimore III due to a gamma ASN-Ile mutation. Blood 75:1659, 1990.

36. Koopman J, F Haverkate, S Lord: A six-base deletion in the gamma chain gene of dysfibrinogen Vlissingen, coding for ASN 319 and Asp 320, resulting in defective interaction with calcium. Thromb Haemost 62:470, 1989.

37. Terukina S, K Yamazumi, K Okamoto: Fibrinogen Kyoto III: a congenital dysfibrinogen with a gamma aspartic acid 330 to tyrosine substitution manifesting impaired fibrin monomer polymerization. Blood 74:2681, 1990.

38. Reber P, M Furlan, M Kehl: Characterization of Fibrinogen Milano I: amino acid exchange gamma 330 Asp-Val impairs fibrin polymerization. Blood 67:1751, 1986.

39. Miyata T, K Furukawa, S Iwanaga: Fibrinogen Nagoya, a replacement of glutamine-329 by arginine in the gamma chain that impairs the polymerization of fibrin monomer. J Biochem (Tokyo) 105:10, 1989.

40. Denninger MH, M Jandrot-Perrus, J Elion: ADP-induced platelet aggregation depends on the conformation or availability of the terminal gamma chain sequence of fibrinogen. Study of the reactivity of Fibrinogen Paris I. Blood 70:558, 1987.

41. Yoshida N, S Terukina, M Okuma: Characterization of an apparently lower molecular weight gamma chain variant in fibrinogen Kyoto I. The replacement of gamma asparagine 308 by lysine which causes accelerated cleavage of fragment D1 by plasmin and the generation of a new plasmin cleavage site. J Biol Chem 263:1384, 1988.

42. Denninger MH, JS Finlayson, LA Reamer: Fibrinogen Lille. Thromb Res 13:453, 1978.

43. Thorson LI, H Stormorken, F Brosstad: A dysfibrinogenemia, Oslo I, acting as a more efficient cofactor in ADP stimulated platelet aggregation than normal fibrinogen. Thromb Haemost 50:202, 1983.

44. Liu CY, A Koehn, FJ Morgan: Characterization of Fibrinogen New York I: a dysfunctional fibrinogen with a deletion of B-Beta (9-17) corresponding exactly to exon 2 of the gene. J Biol Chem 260:4390, 1985.

45. Girolami A: The hereditary transmission of "true" hypoprothrombinemia. Br J Haematol 21:695, 1971.

46. Lusher JM, PM Blatt, JA Penner, LM Aledort, PH Levine, GC White, AI Warrier, DA Whitehurst: Autoplex versus proplex: a controlled, double-blind study of effectiveness in acute hemarthroses in hemophiliacs with inhibitors to Factor VIII. Blood 62:1135, 1983.

47. Gill F, SS Shapiro, E Schwartz: Severe congenital hypoprothrombinemia. J Pediatr 94:264, 1978.

48. Montgomery RR, A Otsuka, WE Hathaway: Hypoprothrombinemia: case report. Blood 51:299, 1978.

49. Pina-Cabral JM, B Justica: Congenital hypoprothrombinemia in a Portuguese family. Thromb Diath Haemorrh 30:451, 1973.

50. Mammen EF: Factor II abnormalities. Semin Thromb Hemost 9:13, 1983.

51. Bick RL: Clinical hemostasis practice: the major impact of laboratory automation. Semin Thromb Hemost 9:139, 1983.

52. Rubio R, D Almagro, A Cruz, JF Corral: Prothrombin Habana: a new dysfunctional molecule of human prothrombin associated with a true prothrombin deficiency. Br J Haematol 54:553, 1983.

53. Weinger RS, C Rudy, JL Moake: Prothrombin Houston: a dysprothrombin identifiable by crossed immunoelectrofocusing and abnormal Echis carcinatus venom activation. Blood 55:811, 1980.

54. Rabiet MJ, J Elion, D Labie: Prothrombin Metz: purification and characterization of a variant of human prothrombin. Thromb Haemost 42:57, 1979.

55. Girolami A, S Cocceri, G Palareti: Prothrombin Molise: a "new" congenital dysprothrombinemia, double heterozygosis with an abnormal prothrombin and "true" prothrombin deficiency. Blood 52:115, 1978.

56. Quick AJ, AV Pisciotta, CV Hussey: Congenital hypoprothrombinemic states. Arch Intern Med 95:2, 1955.

57. Mammen EF: Nature of inherited disorders. In: WA Seegers, DA Walz, (Eds): Prothrombin and Other Vitamin K Proteins, vol 1. CRC Press, Boca Raton, FL, 1986, p 115.

58. Giddings JC: Genetics and immunoanalysis in blood coagulation. Ellis Harwood Series in BioMedicine. Chichester, VCH, 1988.

59. Bezeaud A, L Drouet, C Soria: Prothrombin Salakta: an abnormal prothrombin characterized by a defect in the active site thrombin. Thromb Res 34:507, 1984.

60. Shapiro SS, J Martinez, RR Holburn: Congenital dysprothrombinemia: an inherited structure disorder of human prothrombin. J Clin Invest 48:2251, 1969.

61. Josso F, JM De Sanchez, JM Lavergne: Congenital abnormality of the prothrombin molecule (Factor II) in four siblings: Prothrombin Barcelona. Blood 38:9, 1971.

62. Shapiro SS, NI Maldonado, J Fradera: Prothrombin San Juan: a complex new dysprothrombinemia. J Clin Invest 53:73, 1974.

63. Girolami A, G Bareggi, A Burnetti: Prothrombin Padua: A "new" congenital dysprothrombinemia. J Lab Clin Med 84:654, 1974.

64. Kahn MJ, A Govaerts: Prothrombin Brussels: a new congenital defective protein. Thromb Res 5:141, 1974.

65. Bezeaud A, MC Guillin, F Olmeda: Prothrombin Madrid: a new familial abnormality of prothrombin. Thromb Res 16:47, 1979.

66. Montgomery RR, JJ Corrigan, S Clark: Prothrombin Denver: a new dysprothrombinemia. Circulation 62:279, 1980.

67. Smith LG, LA Coone, CS Kitchen: Prothrombin Gainesville: a dysprothrombinemia in a pair of identical twins. Am J Hematol 11:223, 1981.

68. Ruiz-Saez A, J Luengo, A Rodriquez: A new congenital dysprothrombinemia in an Indian family. Thromb Res 44:587, 1986.

69. Inomoto T, AS Whirakami, S Kawauchi: Prothrombin Tokushima: characterization of dysfunctional thrombin derived from a variant of human prothrombin. Blood 69:565, 1987.

70. Valls-de-Ruiz M, A Ruiz-Arguelles, GJ Ruiz-Arguelles: Prothrombin "Mexico City," an asymptomatic autosomal dominant prothrombin variant. Am J Hematol 24:229, 1987.

71. Rabie MJ, B Furie, B Furie: Molecular defect of Prothrombin Barcelona: substitution of cysteine for arginine at residue 273. J Biol Chem 261:15045, 1986.

72. Huisse MG, M Dreyfus, MC Guillin: Prothrombin Clamart: prothrombin variant with defective Arg 320-Ile cleavage by Factor Xa. Thromb Res 44:11, 1986.

73. Seegers WH: Purification of prothrombin and thrombin. Semin Thromb Hemost 7:199, 1981.

74. Owren PA: Parahemophilia, haemorrhagic diathesis due to absence of a previously unknown clotting factor. Lancet 1:446, 1947.

75. Terheggen HG: Faktor V: Mangel bei einem 8 monate alten Madchen. Monatsschr Kinderheilkd 119:627, 1971.

76. Seeler RA: Parahemophilia: factor V deficiency. Med Clin North Am 56:119, 1972.

77. Mitterstieler G, W Muller, W Geir: Congenital Factor V deficiency: a family study. Scand J Haematol 21:9, 1978.

78. Tracy PB, KG Mann: Abnormal formation of the prothrombinase complex: factor V deficiency and related disorders. Hum Pathol 18:162, 1987.

79. Barthels M, H Poliwada: Der kongenitale Factor-V-Mangel. Haemostaseologie 7:24, 1987.

80. Suzuki K, J Nishioka, S Hashimoto, T Kamiya, H Saito: Normal titer of functional and immunoreactive protein-C inhibitor in plasma of patients with congenital combined deficiency of Factor V and Factor VIII. Blood 62:1266, 1983.

81. Giddings JC, A Sugrue, AL Bloom: Quantitation of coagulant antigens and inhibition of activated Protein C in combined Factor V and VIII deficiency. Br J Haematol 52:495, 1982.

82. Marler RA, JH Griffin: Deficiency of protein C inhibitor in combined Factor V/VIII deficiency disease. J Clin Invest 66:1186, 1980.

83. Canfield WM, W Kisiel: Evidence of normal functional levels of activated protein C inhibitor in combined Factor V/VIII deficiency disease. J Clin Invest 70:260, 1982.

84. Chiu HC, E Whitaker, R Coleman: Heterogeneity of human Factor V deficiency: evidence for the existence of antigen-positive variants. J Clin Invest 72:493, 1983.

85. Miletich JP, DW Majerus, PW Majerus: Patients with congenital Factor V deficiency have decreased factor Xa binding sites on their platelets. J Clin Invest 62: 824, 1978.

86. Tracy PB, LL Eide, JW Bowie: Radioimmunoassay of Factor V in human platelets. Blood 60:59, 1982.

87. Chiu HC, E Whitaker, RW Coleman: Heterogeneity of human Factor V deficiency: evidence for the existence of an antigen-positive variance. J Clin Invest 72:493, 1983.

88. Tracy PB, AR Giles, KG Mann: Factor V Quebec: a bleeding diathesis associated with a qualitative Factor V deficiency. J Clin Invest 74:1221, 1984.

89. Manotti C, R Quintavalla, M Pina: Thromboembolic manifestations and congenital Factor V deficiency: a family study. Haemostasis 19:331, 1989.

90. Mammen EF: Factor V deficiency. Semin Thromb Hemost 9:17, 1983.

91. Alexander B, R Goldstein, R Landwehr: Congenital SPCA deficiency: a hitherto unrecognized coagulation defect with hemorrhage rectified by serum and serum fractions. J Clin Invest 30:596, 1952.

92. Mammen EF: Factor VII abnormalities. Semin Thromb Hemost 9:19, 1983.

93. Ragni MV, JH Lewis, JA Spero, V Hasiba: Factor VII deficiency. Am J Hematol 10:79, 1981.

94. Takamatsu J, K Hayashi, K Ogata, T Kamiya, K Koie: A family of congenital Factor VII deficiency. Rinsho Ketsueki 21:834, 1980.

95. Schricker KT: Congenital Factor VII deficiency. Med Klin 76:24, 1981.

96. Goodnight SH, DI Feinstein, B Osterud: Factor VII antibody-neutralizing material in hereditary and acquired Factor VII deficiency. Blood 38:1, 1971.

97. Denson KWE, J Conrad, M Samama: Genetic variants of Factor VII. Lancet 1:1234, 1972.

98. Mariani G, MG Mazzucconi: Factor VII congenital deficiency: clinical picture and classification of variants. Haemostasis 13:169, 1983.

99. Girolami A, F Fabris, R Zamon Dal Bo: Factor VII Padua: a congenital coagulation disorder due to an abnormal Factor VII with a peculiar activation problem. J Lab Clin Med 91:387, 1978.

100. Girolami A, G Cattorozzi, R Zamon Dal Bo: Factor VII Padua 2: another Factor VII abnormality with defective ox-brain thromboplastin activation and a complex hereditary pattern. Blood 54:46, 1979.

101. Briet E, A Loeliger, NH van Tilberg: Molecular variant of Factor VII. Haemostasis 35:289, 1976.

102. Croze M, CP Brizard: Factor VII Padua I: another case. Haemostasis 11:185, 1982.

103. Girolami A, G Falezza, G Petrassi: Factor VII Verona coagulation disorder: double heterozygosis with an abnormal Factor VII and heterozygous Factor VII deficiency. Blood 50:603, 1977.

104. Ragni MV, JH Lewis, JA Spero: Factor VII deficiency. Am J Hematol 10:79, 1981.

105. Triplett D, JT Brandt, MA McGann: Hereditary factor VII deficiency: heterogeneity defined by combined functional and immunochemical analysis. Blood 66:1284, 1985.

106. Kernoff LM, J Hughes, K Denson: Clinical and laboratory observations in congenital Factor VII deficiency. Thromb Haemost 46:1088, 1981.

107. Mazzucconi MG, F Mandelli, G Mariani: A CRM-positive variant of Factor VII deficiency and the detection of heterozygotes with the assay of Factor-like antigen. Br J Haematol 36:127, 1977.

108. Seligsohn U, B Osterud, SI Rapaport: Coupled amidolytic assay for Factor VII: its use with a clotting assay to determine the activity state of Factor VII. Blood 52:978, 1978.

109. Sirridge MS, Shannon R: Stypven (Russell's viper venom) time. In: Laboratory Evaluation of Hemostasis and Thrombosis, ed 3. Lea & Febiger, Philadelphia, 1983, p 156.

110. Roberts HR, PA Foster: Inherited disorders of prothrombin conversion, ch 11. In RJ Coleman, J Hirsh, V Marder (Eds): Hemostasis and Thrombosis. JB Lippincott, Philadelphia, 1987, p 162.

111. Diker G, E Bidwell, CR Rizza: The preparation and clinical use of a new concentrate containing factor IX, prothrombin, factor X and a separate concentrate containing factor VII. Br J Haematol 22:469, 1972.

112. Berrettini M, M De Cunto, G Agnelli: DDAVP increases Factor XII and VII activity in normal subjects and in patients with congenital FVII deficiency. Thromb Haemost 50:12, 1983.

113. Pilot Study of Hemophilia Treatment in the United States. National Heart and Lung Institute Blood Resource Pilot Studies, vol 3. DHEW, US Government Printing Office, 1972.

114. Larsson SA, IM Nilsson, M Blomback: Current status of Swedish hemophiliacs. Acta Med Scand 212:195, 1982.

115. Francis RB, C Kasper: Reproduction in hemophilia. JAMA 250:3192, 1983.

116. Ramgren O: A clinical and medico-social study of haemophilia in Sweden. Acta Med Scand 171:759, 1962.

117. Mammen EF: Factor VIII abnormalities. Semin Thromb Hemost 9:22, 1983.

118. Nilsson IM: Report of the working party on Factor VIII-related antigens. Thromb Haemost 39:511, 1978.

119. Hoyer LW: Immunologic properties of antihemophilic factor. Prog Hematol 8:191, 1973.

120. Hoyer LW: von Willebrand's disease. Prog Hemost Thromb 3:231, 1976.

121. Hirshgold EJ: Properties of Factor VIII (antihemophilic factor). Prog Hemost Thromb 2:99, 1974.

122. Gralnick H: von Willebrand's disease, ch 6. In: OD Ratnoff, CD Forbes (Eds): Disorders of Hemostasis. WB Saunders, Philadelphia, 1991, p 203.

123. Coller B: von Willebrand's disease, ch 6. In: OD Ratnoff, CD Forbes (Eds): Disorders of Hemostasis. Grune and Stratton, Orlando, FL, 1984, p 241.

124. Hoyer LW, RT Breckenridge: Immunologic properties of antihemophilic factor (AHF Factor VIII), II: properties of cross-reacting material. Blood 35:809, 1970.

125. Denson KWE, R Biggs, ME Haddon, R Borrett, K Cobb: Two types of hemophilia (A+ and A–): a study of 48 cases. Br J Haematol 17:163, 1969.

126. Hoyer LW: The Factor VIII complex: structure and function. Blood 58:1, 1981.

127. Wion KL, D Kelly, JA Summerfield: Distribution of factor VIII mRNA and antigen in liver and other tissues. Nature 317:726, 1985.

128. Veltkamp JJ: Clinical features of hemophilia, ch 23. In: KM Brinkhous, HC Hemker (Eds): Handbook of Hemophilia. Elsevier Publishing Co., New York, 1975, p 371.

129. Spiyack AR, LV Avioli: Orthopedic and medical treatment of patients with hemophilia. Arch Intern Med 143:1431, 1983.

130. Helske T, E Ikkala, G Myllyla, HR Nevanlinna, V Rasi: Joint involvement in patients with severe haemophilia A in 1957–59 and 1978–79. Br J Haematol 51:643, 1982.

131. Forbes CD, R Madhok: Genetic disorders of blood coagulation: clinical presentation and management, ch 5. In: OD Ratnoff, CD Forbes (Eds): Disorders of Hemostasis. WB Saunders, Philadelphia, 1991, p 141.

132. Singher LJ: Renal and urological complications of hemophilia, ch 24. In: KM Brinkhous, HC Hemker (Eds): Handbook of Hemophilia. Elsevier Publishing, New York, 1975, p 377.

133. Schreiber RR: Musculoskeletal system: radiologic findings, ch 22. In: KM Brinkhous, HC Hemker (Eds): Handbook of Hemophilia. Elsevier Publishing, New York, 1975, p 333.

134. Harper TA, K Chauhan: A collaborative study on the suitability of commercial, assayed plasmas for one-stage Factor VIII assays. Am J Clin Pathol 77:614, 1982.

135. Harper TA, EL Bailey, K Chauhan: Reliability of "standard" plasmas used by clinical laboratories for one-stage Factor VIII assays. Am J Clin Pathol 75:197, 1981.

136. Hoffmann JJML, PN Meulendijk: Comparison of reagents for determining the activated partial thromboplastin time. Thromb Haemost 39:640, 1978.

137. Elodi S, K Varadi, SR Hollan: Some sources of error in the one-stage assay of Factor VIII. Haemostasis 7:1, 1978.

138. Harms CS, DA Triplett, JA Koepke: Factor VIII (antihemophilic factor) assay results in the 1976 College of American Pathologists survey program. Am J Clin Pathol 70:560, 1978.

139. Hoyer LW, MS Gawryl, B de la Fuente: Immunochemical characterization of Factor VIII inhibitors. Prog Clin Biol Res 150:73, 1984.

140. Penner JA, PE Kelly: Management of patients with Factor VIII or IX inhibitors. Semin Thromb Hemost 1:386, 1975.

141. Weiss AE: Circulating inhibitors in hemophilia A and B: epidemiology and methods of detection, ch 42. In: KM Brinkhous, HC Hemker (Eds): Handbook of Hemophilia. Elsevier Publishing Co., 1975, p 629.

142. Glueck H, M Coots, M Benson: A unique Factor VIII:C monoclonal IgA (kappa) inhibitor in a patient with primary amyloidosis. Thromb Haemost 58:521, 1987.

143. Gralnick H, MA Flamm, CM Kessler: IgA inhibitor to factor VIII von Willebrand factor. Br J Haematol 59:149, 1985.

144. Biggs R: Jaundice and antibodies directed against Factors VIII and IX in patients treated for haemophilia or Christmas disease in the United Kingdom. Br J Haematol 26:313, 1974.

145. Noren I: Clinical application of a new assay of Factor VIII and Factor VIII inhibitors. Thromb Res 1:19, 1972.

146. Kasper CK, LM Aledort, RB Counts: A more uniform measurement of Factor VIII inhibitors. Thromb Diath Haemorrh 34:869, 1975.

147. Coots MC, HI Glueck, MA Miller: Agarose gel method: its usefulness in assaying Factor VIII inhibitors, evaluating treatment and suggesting a mechanism of action for factor IX concentrates. Br J Haematol 60:735, 1985.

148. Austin DEG, K Lechner, CR Rizza: A comparison of the Bethesda and new Oxford methods of Factor VIII antibody assay. Thromb Haemost 47:72, 1982.

149. Forbes CD: Clinical aspects of the hemophilias and their management, ch 5. In: OD Ratnoff, CD Forbes (Eds): Disorders of Hemostasis. Grune and Stratton, New York, 1984, p 177.

150. Webster WP, HR Roberts, GM Thelin: Clinical use of a new glycine-precipitated antihemophilic fraction. Am J Med Sci 250:643, 1965.

151. Abildgaard CF, JV Simone, JJ Corrigan, RA Seeler, G Edelstein, J Vanderheiden, I Schulman: Treatment of hemophilia with glycine-precipitated Factor VIII. N Engl J Med 275:471, 1966.

152. Rizza CR, P Jones: Management of patients with inherited blood coagulation defects. In: AL Bloom, DP Thomas (Eds): Haemostasis and Thrombosis. Churchill Livingstone, Edinburg, 1987, p 465.

153. Levin PH: Hemophilia and allied conditions. In: MC Brain (Ed): Current Therapy in Hematology Oncology. Marcel Decker, New York, 1983, p 147.

154. Aledort LM: The management of hemophilia: a perspective. Drug Ther 1:1, 1971.

155. Brockman SK, SN Aprill, FS Rabiner: Aortic valve replacement therapy in hemophilia: a case report. JAMA 222:660, 1972.

156. George JN, RT Breckenridge: The use of factor VIII and factor IX concentrates during surgery. JAMA 214:1673, 1970.

157. Lusher JM, S Shapiro, J Palascak: Hemophilia study group. Efficacy of prothrombin complex concentrates in hemophili-

acs with antibodies to Factor VIII: a multicenter therapeutic trial. N Engl J Med 303:421, 1980.

158. Shanbrom E: Rapid correction of AHF deficiency by antihemophilic factor–method four, with special reference to inhibitors. Bibl Haematol 34:52, 1970.

159. Kernoff PB, ND Thomas, PA Lilley: Clinical experience with polyelectrolyte-fractionated porcine Factor VIII in hemophiliacs with antibodies to Factor VIII. Blood 63:31, 1984.

160. Gatti L, PM Mannucci: Use of porcine factor VIII in the management of seventeen patients with factor VIII antibodies. Thromb Haemost 51:379, 1984.

161. Exner T, KA Rickard: Anamnestic response to high purity porcine AHF. Thromb Haemost 50:623, 1983.

162. Abildgaard CF, JA Penner, EJ Watson-Williams: Anti-inhibitor coagulant complex (Autoplex) for treatment of factor VIII inhibitors in hemophiliacs. Blood 56:978, 1980.

163. Aronstam A, DS McLellan, M Wassef: The use of an activated Factor IX complex (Autoplex) in the management of haemarthroses in haemophiliacs with antibodies to Factor VIII. Clin Lab Haematol 4:231, 1982.

164. Hilgartner MW, GL Knatterud: FEIBA Study Group. The use of factor eight inhibitor bypassing activity (FEIBA-Immuno) product for treatment of bleeding episodes in hemophiliacs with inhibitors. Blood 61:36, 1983.

165. Hutchinson RJ, JA Penner, RN Hensinger: Anti-inhibitor coagulant complex (Autoplex) in hemophilia inhibitor patients undergoing synovectomy. Pediatrics 71:631, 1983.

166. Apter B, V McCarthy, SS Shapiro: Successful preoperative apheresis of factor VIII antibody using factor VIII concentrate as a replacement fluid. J Clin Apheresis 3:140, 1986.

167. Lee H, D Tucker, JP Allain: Rapid isolation and purification of antibody to factor VIII by Protein A. Thromb Res 14:925, 1979.

168. Slocombe GW, AC Newland, MP Colvin: The role of intensive plasma exchange in the prevention and management of haemorrhage in patients with inhibitors to factor VIII. Br J Haematol 47:577, 1981.

169. Kesteven PJ, LJ Holland, AS Lawrie: Inhibitor to factor VIII in mild hemophilia. Thromb Haemost 52:50, 1984.

170. Nilsson IM, E Berntorp, O Zettervall: Tolerance induction in high-responding hemophiliacs with Factor VIII inhibitors by means of combined treatment with IgG, cyclophosphamide and Factor VIII. Thromb Haemost 58:519, 1987.

171. Kaufman RJ: Expression and characterization of Factor VIII produced in mammalian cells by recombinant DNA technology. In: Proceedings of Symposium on Biotechnology and the Promise of Pure Factor VIII. Proceedings of Baxter Healthcare Publications, Brussels, Belgium, 1989, p 119.

172. Roberts HR: Clinical trials of Factor VIII prepared by recombinant DNA techniques. In: Proceedings of Symposium on Biotechnology and the Promise of Pure Factor VIII. Proceedings of Baxter Healthcare Publications, Brussels, Belgium, 1989, p 147.

173. Klein HG, LM Aledort, BH Bouma, LW Hoyer, TS Zimmerman, DL de Mets: A cooperative study for the detection of the carrier state of classic hemophilia. N Engl J Med 296:959, 1977.

174. Ratnoff OD: The molecular basis of hereditary clotting disorders. Prog Hemost Thromb 1:39, 1972.

175. Ratnoff OD, PK Jones: The laboratory diagnosis of the carrier state for classic hemophilia. Ann Intern Med 86:521, 1977.

176. Thompson AR: Molecular biology of the hemophilias. Prog Hemost Thromb 10:175, 1991.

177. Gitschier J, B Levinson, AE Lehesjoki: Mosiacism and sporadic haemophilia: implications for carrier detection. Lancet 1:273, 1989.

178. Mammen EF: Factor IX abnormalities. Semin Thromb Hemost 9:28, 1983.

179. Aggeler PM, SG White, MB Glendening, EW Page, TB Leake, G Bates: Plasma thromboplastin component (PTC) deficiency: a new disease resembling hemophilia. Proc Soc Exp Biol Med 79:692, 1952.

180. Biggs R, AM Douglas, RA Macfarlane, JV Dacie, WR Pitney, C Merskey, JR O'Brien: Christmas disease: a condition previously mistaken for haemophilia. Br Med J 2:1378, 1952.

181. Ahlberg A: Haemophilia in Sweden: incidence, treatment and prophylaxis of arthropathy and other musculoskeletal manifestations of haemophilia A and B. Acta Orthop Scand 77:1, 1965.

182. Denson KWE, R Biggs, PM Mannucci: An investigation of three patients with Christmas Disease due to an abnormal type of Factor IX. J Clin Pathol 21:160, 1968.

183. Roberts HR, JE Grizzle, WD McLester: Genetic variants of hemophilia B: detection by means of a specific inhibitor. J Clin Invest 47:360, 1968.

184. Neal WR, DT Tayloe, AI Cederbaum, HR Roberts: Detection of genetic variants of hemophilia B with an immunosorbent technique. Br J Haematol 25:63, 1973.

185. Veltkamp JJ, J Meilof, HG Remmelts, D Vander Vlerg, EA Loeliger: Another genetic variant of haemophilia B: haemophilia B-Leyden. Scand J Haematol 7:82, 1970.

186. Brown PE, C Hougie, HR Roberts: The genetic heterogeneity of hemophilia B. N Engl J Med 283:61, 1970.

187. Hougie C, JJ Twomey: Hemophilia Bm: a new type of Factor IX deficiency. Lancet 1:698, 1967.

188. Kasper CK, B Osterud, JY Minami: Hemophilia B: characterization of genetic variants and detection of carriers. Blood 50:351, 1977.

189. Elodi S, E Puskas: Variants of haemophilia B. Thromb Diath Haemorrh 28:489, 1972.

190. Wang NS, SH Chen, AR Thompson: Point mutations in four hemophilia B patients from China. Thromb Haemost 64:302, 1990.

191. Chung KS, JC Goldsmith, HR Roberts: Purification and characterization of an abnormal Factor IX Alabama (IXAla). XVII Congress of the International Society of Haematology, Paris, 1978, p 859.

192. Noyes CM, MJ Griffith, HR Roberts: Identification of the molecular defect in Factor IX Chapel Hill: substitution of histamine for arginine at position 145. Proc Natl Acad Sci 80:4200, 1983.

193. Davis LM, RA McGraw, JL Ware: Factor IX Alabama: a point mutation in a clotting protein results in hemophilia B. Blood 69:140, 1987.

194. Sakai T, A Yoshioka, Y Yamamoto: Blood clotting Factor IX Kashihara: amino acid substitution of valine-182 by phenylalanine. J Biochem 105:756, 1989.

195. Bertina RM, IK van der Linden: Factor IX Zutphen: a genetic variant of blood coagulation factor IX with an abnormally high molecular weight. J Lab Clin Med 100:695, 1982.

196. Mertens K, R Capers, IR van der Linden: The functional defect of factor IX Eindhoven, a genetic variant of factor IX. Thromb Haemost 50:249, 1983.

197. Usharani P, BJ War-Cramer, CK Kasper: Characterization of three abnormal factor IX variants (BM Lake Elsinore, Long Beach and Los Angeles) of hemophilia B. Evidence for defects affecting catalytic sites. J Clin Invest 75:76, 1985.

198. Yoshioka A, Y Ohkuho, T Nishimura: Heterogeneity of Factor IX BM. Difference of cleavage sites by Factor IXa and Ca++ in Factor IX Kashihara, Factor IX Nagoya and Factor IX Niigata. Thromb Res 42:595, 1986.

199. Diuguid DL, MJ Rabiet, BC Furie: Molecular basis of hemophilia B: a defective enzyme due to an unprocessed propeptide is caused by a point mutation in the Factor IX precurser. Proc Natl Acad Sci 83:5803, 1986.

200. Hassan HJ, M Orlando, A Leonardi: Intragenic Factor IX restriction site polymorphism in hemophilia B variants. Blood 65:441, 1985.

201. Chung KS, DA Madar, JC Goldsmith, HS Kingdon, HR Roberts: Purification and characterization of an abnormal Factor IX (Christmas factor) molecule: Factor IX Chapel Hill. J Clin Invest 62:1078, 1978.

202. Tullis JL, M Melin, P Jurigian: Clinical use of human prothrombin complex concentrates. N Engl J Med 273:667, 1965.

203. Soulier JP, F Josso, M Steinbuch: The therapeutic use of fraction P.P.S.B. Bibl Haematol 29:1127, 1968.

204. Breen FA, JL Tullis: Prothrombin concentrates in treatment of Christmas disease and allied disorders. JAMA 208:1848, 1969.

205. Bidwell E, JM Booth, GW Dike: The preparation for therapeutic use of a concentrate of Factors IX containing also Factors II, VII and X. Br J Haematol 13:568, 1967.

206. Hermens WT: Dose calculation of human Factor VIII and Factor IX concentrates for infusion therapy. In: KM Brinkhous, HC Hemker (Eds): Handbook of Hemophilia. Elsevier, New York, 1975, p 569.

207. White GC, HR Roberts, HS Kingdon, RL Lundblad: Prothrombin complex concentrates: potentially thrombogenic materials and clues to the mechanism of thrombosis in vivo. Blood 49:159, 1977.

208. Blatt PM, RL Lundblad, HS Kingdon: Thrombogenic materials in prothrombin complex concentrates. Ann Intern Med 81:766, 1974.

209. Ratnoff OD: Prothrombin complex concentrates: a cautionary note. Ann Intern Med 81:852, 1974.

210. Hasegawa DK, JR Edson: Thrombocytopenia and hypofibrinogenemia following activated prothrombin complex concentrate therapy in a patient with hemophila A and factor VIII inhibitor. Prog Clin Biol Res 150:386, 1984.

211. Kitchens CS: Discordance in a pair of identical twin carriers of factor IX deficiency. Am J Hematol 24:225, 1987.

212. Mammen EF: Factor X abnormalities. Semin Thromb Hemost 9:31, 1983.

213. Mori K, H Sakai, N Nakano, S Suzuki, K Sugai, S Hisa, Y Goto: Congenital Factor X deficiency in Japan. Tohoko J Exp Med 133:1, 1981.

214. Telfer TP, KWE Denson, DR Wright: A "new" coagulation defect. Br J Haematol 2:308, 1956.

215. Hougie C, EM Barrow, JB Graham: Stuart clotting defect, I: segregation of an hereditary haemorrhagic state from the heterogeneous group heretofore called stable factor (SPCA) deficiency. J Clin Invest 36:485, 1957.

216. Denson DWE, A Lurie, F De Cataldo: The Factor X defect: recognition of abnormal forms of Factor X. Br J Haematol 18:317, 1970.

217. Seegers WH: Factor X (autoprothrombin III). Semin Thromb Hemost 7:233, 1981.

218. Girolami A, G Molaro, M Lazzarin, R Scarpa, A Brunetti: A "new" congenital haemorrhagic condition due to the presence of an abnormal Factor X (Factor X Friuli): study of large kindred. Br J Haematol 19:179, 1970.

219. Reddy SV, ZO Zhou, KJ Rao: Molecular characterization of Factor X San Antonio. Blood 74:1486, 1989.

220. De Stefano V, G Leone, R Ferrelli: Factor X Roma: a congenital factor X variant defective at different degrees in the intrinsic and extrinsic activation. Br J Haematol 69:387, 1988.

221. Girolami A, M Vicarioto, G Ruzza: Factor X Padua: a "new" congenital factor X abnormality with a defect only in the extrinsic system. Acta Haematol (Basel) 73:31, 1985.

222. Grosse KP, G Seiler, B Neidhardt, TH Schricker, M Kroehling: Kongenitaler faktor X-Mangel. Fallbericht und literaturubersicht. Monatsschr Kinderheilkd 127:285, 1979.

223. Bachmann F, F Duckert, F Koller: The Stuart-Prower factor assay and its clinical significance. Thromb Diath Haemorrh 2:24, 1958.

224. Tullis JL, M Melin: Management of Christmas disease and Stuart-Prower deficiency with a prothrombin-complex concentrate (Factors II, VII, IX, X). Bibl Haematol 29:1134, 1968.

225. Mammen EF: Factor XI deficiency. Semin Thromb Hemost 9:34, 1983.

226. Rosenthal RL, OH Dreskin, N Rosenthal: New hemophilia-like disease caused by deficiency of a third plasma thromboplastin factor. Proc Soc Exp Biol Med 82:171, 1953.

227. Rapaport SI, RR Proctor, MJ Patch, M Yettra: The mode of inheritance of PTA deficiency: evidence for the existence of major PTA deficiency and minor PTA deficiency. Blood 18:149, 1961.

228. Seligsohn U: High gene frequency of Factor XI (PTA) deficiency in Ashkenazi Jews. Blood 51:1223, 1978.

229. Seligsohn U, M Modan: Definition of the population at high risk of bleeding due to Factor XI deficiency in Ashkenazi Jews and the value of the activated partial thromboplastin time in its detection. Isreal J Med Sci 17:413, 1981.

230. Mannhalter C, P Hellstern, E Deutsch: Identification of a defective factor XI cross-reacting material in a factor XI deficiency patient. Blood 70:31, 1987.

231. Ragni MV, D Sinha, F Seaman: Comparison of bleeding tendency, factor XI coagulant activity, and factor XI antigen in 25 factor XI deficient kindreds. Blood 65:719, 1985.

232. Conrad FF, WL Breneman, DB Grisham: A clinical evaluation of plasma thromboplastin antecedent (PTA) deficiency. Ann Intern Med 62:885, 1965.

233. Rosenthal RL: Factor XI: general review. Bibl Haematol 23:1350, 1965.

234. Sidi A, U Seligsohn, P Jonas: Factor XI deficiency: detection and management during urological surgery. J Urol 119:528, 1978.

235. Megguier RJ: Fibrinolytic activity in human dental sockets after extractions. J Oral Surg 29:321, 1971.

236. Leiba H, B Ramot, M Many: Hereditary and coagulation studies in ten families with Factor XI (plasma thromboplastin antecedent) deficiency. Br J Haematol 11:654, 1965.

237. Frick PG: Relative incidence of anti-hemophilic globulin, plasma thromboplastin component (PTC) and plasma thromboplastin antecedent (PTC) deficiency. J Lab Clin Med 43:860, 1954.

238. Bick RL: Clinical approach to the patient with hemorrhage, ch 2. In: Disorders of Hemostasis and Thrombosis: Principles of Clinical Practice. Thieme, Inc., New York, 1985, p 36.

239. Meier HL, JV Pierce, RW Coleman: Activation and function of human Hageman Factor: the role of high molecular weight kininogen and prekallikrein. J Clin Invest 60:18, 1977.

240. Ratnoff OD, JE Colopy: A familial hemorrhagic trait associated with a deficiency of clot-promoting fraction of plasma. J Clin Invest 34:602, 1955.

241. Saito H, SJ Scialla: Isolation and properties of an abnormal Hageman factor (Factor XII) molecule in a cross-reacting material-positive Hageman trait plasma. J Clin Invest 68:1028, 1981.

242. Miyata T, SI Kawabata, S Iwanaga: Coagulation factor XII (Hageman factor) Washington, DC: inactive factor XIIa results from Cys-571-Ser substitution. Proc Natl Acad Sci 86:8319, 1989.

243. Saito H, JG Scott, HZ Movat, SJ Scialla: Molecular heterogeneity of Hageman trait (Factor XII deficiency). Evidence that two of 49 subjects are cross-reacting material positive (CRM+). J Lab Clin Med 94:256, 1979.

244. Kovalainen S, VV Myllyla, U Tolonen: Recurrent subarachnoid haemorrhages in patient with Hageman factor deficiency. Lancet 1:1035, 1979.

245. McPherson RA: Thromboembolism in Hageman trait. Am J Clin Pathol 68:420, 1977.

246. Azner J, A Fernandez Pavnon: Thromboembolic accidents in patients with congenital deficiency of Factor XII. Thromb Diath Haemorrh 31:525, 1974.

247. Hoak JC, LW Swanson, ED Warner, WE Connor: Myocardial infarction associated with severe Factor XII deficiency. Lancet 2:884, 1966.

248. Glueck HI, W Roehll: Myocardial infarction in a patient with a Hageman (Factor XII) defect. Ann Intern Med 64:390, 1966.

249. Ratnoff OD, RJ Busse, RP Sheon: The demise of John Hageman. N Engl J Med 279:760, 1968.

250. Goodnough LT, H Saito, OD Ratnoff: Thrombosis or myocardial infarction in congenital clotting factor abnormalities and chronic thrombocytopenias: a report of 21 patients and a review of 50 previously reported cases. Medicine 62:248, 1983.

251. Coleman RW, PY Wong: Participation of Hageman factor–dependent pathways in human disease states. Thromb Haemost 38:751, 1977.

252. Schmaier AH, M Silverberb, AP Kaplan: Contact activation and its abnormalities. In: RW Coleman, J Hirsh, VJ Marder, EW Salzman (Eds): Hemostasis and Thrombosis. JB Lippincott, Philadelphia, 1987, p 18.

253. Hathaway WE, LP Belhasen, HS Hathaway: Evidence for a new plasma thromboplastin factor, I: case report, coagulation studies, and physicochemical properties. Blood 26:521, 1965.

254. Mammen EF: Contact factor abnormalities. Semin Thromb Hemost 9:36, 1983.

255. Saito H, LT Goodnough, J Soria, C Soria, J Aznar, F Espana: Heterogeneity of human prekallikrein deficiency (Fletcher trait). Evidence that five of 18 cases are positive for cross-reacting material. N Engl J Med 305:910, 1981.

256. Bouma BN, DM Kerbiriou, J Baker: Characterization of a variant of prekallikrein, prekallikrein Long Beach, from a family with mixed cross-reacting material–positive and cross-reacting material–negative prekallikrein deficiency. J Clin Invest 78:170, 1986.

257. Sollo DG, A Saleem: Prekallikrein (Fletcher Factor) deficiency. Ann Clin Lab Sci 15:279, 1985.

258. Estelles A, J Aznar, F Espana: The absence of release of the plasminogen activator after venous occlusion in a Fletcher trait patient. Thromb Haemost 49:66, 1983.

259. Entes K, FM LaDuca, KD Tourbaf: Fletcher factor deficiency, source of variations of the activated partial thromboplastin time. Am J Clin Pathol 75:626, 1981.

260. Saito H, OD Ratnoff, R Waldmann: Fitzgerald trait: deficiency of a hitherto unrecognized agent, Fitzgerald factor, participating in surface-mediated reactions of clotting, fibrinolysis, generation of kinins, and the property of diluted plasma enhancing vascular permeability (PF/DIL). J Clin Invest 55:1082, 1975.

261. Coleman RW, A Bagdasarian, RC Talamo: Williams trait: human kininogen efficiency with diminished levels of plasminogen proactivator and prekallikrein associated with abnormalities of the Hageman factor–dependent pathways. J Clin Invest 56:1650, 1975.

262. Lacombe MJ, B Varet, JP Levy: A hitherto undescribed plasma factor acting at the contact phase of blood coagulation (Flaujeac factor): case report and coagulation studies. Blood 46:761, 1975.

263. Oh-Ishi S, A Ueno, Y Uchida: Abnormalities in the contact activation through Factor XII in Fujiwara trait: a deficiency in both high and low molecular weight kininogens with low level of prekallikrein. Tohoko J Exp Med 133:67, 1981.

264. Lutcher CL: Reid trait: a new expression of high molecular weight kininogen (HMW kininogen) deficiency. Clin Res 24:47, 1976.

265. Stormorken H, K Briseid, B Hellum: A new case of total kininogen deficiency. Thromb Res 60:457, 1990.

266. Hougie C, RA McPherson, L Aronson: Passovoy factor: a hitherto unrecognized factor necessary for haemostasis. Lancet 2:290, 1975.

267. Hougie C, RA McPherson, JE Brown: The Passovoy defect. Further characterization of a hereditary hemorrhagic diathesis. N Engl J Med 298:1045, 1978.

268. Jackson JM, LR Marshall, RP Herrmann: Passovoy factor deficiency in five western Australian kindreds. Pathology 13:517, 1981.

269. Mammen EF: Alpha-2-antiplasmin deficiency. Semin Thromb Hemost 9:52, 1983.

270. Aoki N, H Saito, T Kamiya: Congenital deficiency of alpha-2-plasmin inhibitor associated with severe hemorrhagic tendency. J Clin Invest 63:877, 1979.

271. Yoshioka A, H Kamitsuji, T Takase: Congenital deficiency of alpha-2-plasmin inhibitor in three sisters. Haemostasis 11:176, 1982.

272. Kluft C, E Vallenga, EJP Brommer: A familial hemorrhagic diathesis in a Dutch family: an inherited deficiency of alpha-2-antiplasmin. Blood 59:1169, 1982.

273. Miles LA, EF Plow, KJ Donnelly: A bleeding disorder due to deficiency of alpha-2-antiplasmin. Blood 59:1246, 1982.

274. Aoki N, Y Sakata, M Matsuda: Fibrinolytic states in a patient with congenital deficiency of alpha-2-plasmin inhibitor. Blood 55:483, 1980.

275. Bick RL, A Wheeler: Alpha-2-antiplasmin deficiency: a dysfunctional protein leading to hemorrhage in afflicted family members. Thromb Haemost 65:1261, 1991.

276. Nieuwenhuis HK, C Kluft, G Wijngaards: Alpha-2-antiplasmin Enshede: an autosomal recessive hemorrhagic disorder caused by a dysfunctional alpha-2-antiplasmin molecule. Thromb Haemost 50:170, 1983.

277. Marsh N: Fibrinolysis and disease, ch 6. In: Fibrinolysis. John Wiley and Sons, New York, 1981, p 125.

278. Koie K, T Kamiya, K Ogata: Alpha-2-plasmin inhibitor deficiency (Miyasato disease). Lancet 2:1334, 1978.

279. Mammen EF: Factor XIII deficiency. Semin Thromb Hemost 9:10, 1983.

280. Kitchens CS, TF Newcomb: Factor XIII. Medicine 58:413, 1979.

281. Lorand L, MS Losowsky, K Miloszewski: Human Factor XIII: fibrin-stabilizing factor. Prog Hemost Thromb 5:245, 1980.

282. McDonagh J: Structure and function of Factor XIII. In: RW Coleman, J Hirsh, VJ Marder, EW Salzman (Eds): Hemostasis and Thrombosis. JB Lippincott, Philadelphia, 1987, p 289.

283. Isreals ED, F Paraskevus, LG Isreals: Immunological studies of coagulation Factor XIII. J Clin Invest 52:2398, 1973.

284. Ikematsu S, RP McDonagh, HM Reisner: Immunochemical studies of human Factor XIII. Radioimmunoassay for the carrier subunit of the zymogen. J Lab Clin Med 97:662, 1981.

285. Girolami A, MG Capellato, AR Lazzaro: Type I and Type II disease in congenital factor XIII deficiency: a further demonstration of the correctness of the classification. Blut 53:411, 1986.

286. Girolami A, A Burul, MG Cappellato: A tentative classification of factor XIII deficiency in two groups. Acta Haematol (Basel) 58:318, 1977.

287. von Willebrand EA: Hereditar pseudohamofili. Finska Laeksaellsk Handl 68:87, 1926.

288. von Willebrand EA, R Jurgens: Veber ein neues vererbbares blutungsuebel: konstitutionelle. Dtsch Arch Klin Med 175:453, 1933.

289. Alexander B, R Goldstein: Dual hemostatic defect in pseudohemophilia. J Clin Invest 32:551, 1953.

290. Larrieu MJ, JP Soulier: Deficit en facteur anti-hemophilique A chez une fille associe a un trouble du saignement. Rev Haematol 8:361, 1953.

291. Quick AJ, CV Hussey: Hemophilic condition in the female. J Lab Clin Med 42:929, 1953.

292. Zimmerman TS, OD Ratnoff, AE Powell: Immunologic differentiation of classic hemophilia (Factor VIII deficiency) and von Willebrand's disease. J Clin Invest 50:244, 1971.

293. Zimmerman TS, ZM Ruggeri: von Willebrand's disease. Clin Haematol 12:175, 1983.

294. Titani K, S Kumar, K Takio: Amino acid sequence of human von Willebrand factor. Biochemistry 25:3171, 1986.

295. Loscalzo J, M Fisch, RI Handin: Solution studies of the quaternary structure and assembly of human von Willebrand factor. Biochemistry 24:4468, 1985.

296. Fowler WE, LJ Fretto, KK Hamilton: Substructure of human von Willebrand factor. J Clin Invest 76:1491, 1985.

297. Irwin JF: Factor VIII in von Willebrand's disease. Semin Thromb Hemost 2:85, 1975.

298. Ohmori K, LJ Fretto, RL Harrison: Electron microscopy of human factor VIII/von Willebrand glycoprotein: effect of reducing agents on structure and function. J Cell Biol 95:632, 1982.

299. Walsh RT: The platelet in von Willebrand's disease: interactions with ristocetin and Factor VIII. Semin Thromb Hemost 2:105, 1975.

300. Hoyer LW, CR Rizza, EGD Tuddenham: von Willebrand factor multimer patterns in von Willebrand's disease. Br J Haematol 55:493, 1983.

301. Piovella F, G Nalli, GD Malamani: The ultrastructural localization of Factor VIII-antigen in human platelets, megakaryocytes and endothelial cells utilizing a ferritin-labelled antibody. Br J Haematol 39:209, 1978.

302. Sultan Y, BN Bouma, S de Graaf: Factor VIII related antigen in platelets of von Willebrand's disease. Thromb Res 11:23, 1977.

303. Cornu P, MJ Larrieu, J Caen: Transfusion studies in von Willebrand's disease: effect on bleeding time and Factor VIII. Br J Haematol 9:189, 1963.

304. Bloom AL: The von Willebrand syndrome. Semin Hematol 17:215, 1980.

305. Firkin B, F Firkin, L Scott: von Willebrand's disease type B: a newly defined bleeding diathesis. Aust N Z J Med 3:225, 1973.

306. Peake IR, AL Bloom, JL Giddings: Inherited variants of Factor VIII-related protein in von Willebrand's disease. N Engl J Med 291:113, 1974.

307. McCarroll DR, ZM Ruggeri, RR Montgomery: Correlation between circulating levels of von Willebrand's antigen II and von Willebrand factor: discrimination between type I and type II von Willebrand's disease. J Lab Clin Med 103:704, 1984.

308. Bowie EJW, P Didisheim, JH Thompson: The spectrum of von Willebrand's disease. Thromb Diath Haemorrh 18:40, 1970.

309. Silwer J, IM Nilsson: On a Swedish family with 51 members affected by von Willebrand's disease. Acta Med Scand 175:627, 1964.

310. Mannucci PM: Spectrum of von Willebrand's disease: a study of 100 cases. Br J Haematol 35:101, 1977.

311. Shoai I, JM Lavergne, N Ardaillou: Heterogeneity of von Willebrand's disease: study of 40 Iranian cases. Br J Haematol 37:67, 1977.

312. Strauss HS, GE Bloom: von Willebrand's disease: use of a platelet adhesiveness test in diagnosis and family investigation. N Engl J Med 273:171, 1965.

313. Girma JP, N Ardaillou, D Meyer: Fluid-phase immunoradiometric assay for the detection of qualitative abnormalities of Factor VIII/von Willebrand factor in variants of von Willebrand's disease. J Lab Clin Med 93:296, 1975.

314. Weis JW, D Nelson: Factor VIII related antigen in variant von Willebrand's disease. Thromb Res 33:457, 1984.

315. Abildgaard CF, Z Suzuki, J Harrison: Serial studies in von Willebrand's disease: variability versus "variants." Blood 56:712, 1980.

316. Hoyer LW, JR Shainoff: Factor VIII-related protein circulates in normal human plasma as high molecular weight multimers. Blood 55:1056, 1980.

317. Ruggeri ZM, TS Zimmerman: Variant von Willebrand disease: characterization of two subtypes by analysis of multimeric composition of factor VIII/von Willebrand factor in plasma and platelets. J Clin Invest 65:1318, 1980.

318. Ruggeri ZM, TS Zimmerman: The complex multimeric composition of factor VIII/von Willebrand factor. Blood 57:1140, 1981.

319. Zimmerman TS, JA Dent, AB Federici: High resolution Na Dod SO-4 agarose electrophoresis identifies new molecular abnormalities in von Willebrand's disease. Clin Res 32:501, 1984.

320. Weiss WJ, G Pietu, R Rabinowitz: Heterogeneous abnormalities in the multimeric structure, antigenic properties, and plasma-platelet content of factor VIII/von Willebrand factor in subtypes of classic (type I) and variant (type II) von Willebrand disease. J Lab Clin Med 101:411, 1983.

321. Hoyer L, CR Rizza, EG Tuddenham: von Willebrand factor multimeric patterns in von Willebrand's disease. Br J Haematol 55:493, 1983.

322. Ciavarella G, N Caavarella, S Antoncecchi: High resolution analysis of von Willebrand factor multimeric composition defines a new variant of type I von Willebrand disease with aberrant structure but presence of all size multimers (type IC). Blood 66:1423, 1985.

323. Asakura A, J Harrison, E Gomperts: Type IIA von Willebrand disease with apparent recessive inheritance. Blood 69:1419, 1987.

324. Gralnick HR, SB Willaims, LP McKeown: In vitro correction of the abnormal multimeric structure of von Willebrand factor in Type IIa von Willebrand's disease. Proc Natl Acad Sci 82:5968, 1985.

325. Donner M, L Holmberg, IM Nilsson: Type IIb von Willebrand's disease with probable autosomal recessive inheritance and presenting as thrombocytopenia in infancy. Br J Haematol 66:349, 1987.

326. Federici AB, PM Mannucci, R Bader: Heterogeneity in type IIb von Willebrand's disease: two unrelated cases with no family history and mild abnormalities of ristocetin-induced interaction between von Willebrand factor and platelets. Am J Hematol 23:381, 1986.

327. Gralnick HR, SB Williams, LP McKeown: von Willebrand's disease with spontaneous platelet aggregation induced by abnormal plasma von Willebrand factor. J Clin Invest 76:1522, 1985.

328. Rick ME, SB Williams, RA Sacher: Thrombocytopenia associated with pregnancy in a patient with type IIB von Willebrand's disease. Blood 69:786, 1987.

329. Zimmerman TS, JA Dent, ZM Ruggeri: Subunit composition of plasma vWF; cleavage is present in normal individuals, increased in IIA and IIB vWd, but minimal in variants with aberrant structure of individual multimers (types IIC, IID, and IIE). J Clin Invest 77:947, 1986.

330. Ruggeri ZM, IM Nilsson, R Lombardi: Aberrant multimeric structure of von Willebrand factor in a new variant of von Willebrand's disease (type IIC). J Clin Invest 70:1124, 1982.

331. Mazurier,C, PM Mannucci, GA Parquet: Investigation of a case of subtype IIC von Willebrand disease: characterization of the variability of this subtype. Am J Hematol 22:301, 1986.

332. Batlle J, MF Lopez-Fernandez, A Fernandez-Villamore: Multimeric pattern discrepancy between platelet and plasma von Willebrand factor in type IIC von Willebrand disease. Am J Hematol 22:87, 1986.

333. Kinoshita S, J Harrison, J Lazerson: A new variant of dominant type II von Willebrand's disease with aberrant multimeric pattern of factor VIII-related antigen (type IID). Blood 63:1369, 1984.

334. Mannucci PM, R Lombardi, A Lattuada: High-resolution multimeric analysis identifies a new variant of type II von Willebrand's disease (type IIH) inherited in an autosomal recessive manner. Ric Clin Lab 16:237, 1986.

335. Zimmerman T, C Abildgaard, D Meyer: The factor VIII abnormality in severe von Willebrand's disease. N Engl J Med 301:1307, 1979.

336. Redaelli R, L Pezzetti, T Caimi: Severe von Willebrand's disease: SDS agarose multimer analysis. Haemostasis 17:278, 1987.

337. Mannucci PM, ZM Ruggeri, N Ciavarella: Precipitating antibodies to factor VIII/von Willebrand's factor in von Willebrand's disease: effects on replacement therapy. Blood 57:25, 1981.

338. Miller JL, A Castella: Platelet-type von Willebrand's disease: characterization of a new bleeding disorder. Blood 60:790, 1982.

339. Weiss HJ, D Meyer, R Rabinowitz: Pseudo-von Willebrand's disease: an intrinsic platelet defect with aggregation by unmodified human factor VIII/von Willebrand factor and enhanced adsorption of its high molecular weight multimers. N Engl J Med 306:326, 1982.

340. Miller JL, JM Kupinski, A Castella: von Willebrand factor binds to platelets and induces aggregation in platelet-type but not type IIB von Willebrand disease. J Clin Invest 72:1532, 1983.

341. Meyer D, TS Zimmerman: von Willebrand's disease, ch 6. In: RW Coleman, J Hirsh, VJ Marder, EW Salzman (Eds): Hemostasis and Thrombosis: Basic Principles and Clinical Practice. JB Lippincott, Philadelphia, 1982, p 64.

342. Turrito VT, HR Baumgartner: Platelet-surface interactions. In: In: RW Coleman, J Hirsh, VJ Marder, EW Salzman (Eds): Thrombosis and Hemostasis. JB Lippincott, Philadelphia, 1982, p 64.

343. Hirsh J: Laboratory diagnosis of thrombosis. In: RW Coleman, J Hirsh, VJ Marder, EW Salzman (Eds): Thrombosis and Hemostasis. JB Lippincott, Philadelphia, 1982, p 789.

344. Lowe GD: Laboratory evaluation of hypercoagulability. Clin Haematol 10:407, 1981.

345. Zimmerman TG, ZM Ruggeri: von Willebrand's disease. Clin Haematol 12:175, 1983.

346. Lundlam CA, IR Peake, N Allen, BL Davies, RA Furlong, AL Bloom: Factor VIII and fibrinolytic response to deamino-8-D-arginine vasopressin in normal subjects and dissociate response in some patients with haemophilia and von Willebrand's disease. Br J Haematol 45:499, 1980.

347. Schmitz-Huebner U, L Balleisen, P Arends: DDAVP-induced changes of Factor VIII-related activities and bleeding time in patients with von Willebrand's syndrome. Haemostasis 9:204, 1980.

348. Theiss W, G Schmidt: DDAVP in von Willebrand's disease: repeated administration and the behavior of the bleeding time. Thromb Res 13:1119, 1978.

349. Menon C, EW Berry, P Ockelford: Beneficial effect of DDAVP on bleeding time in von Willebrand's disease. Lancet 2:743, 1978.

350. Mannucci PM: Desmopressin: a nontransfusional form of treatment for congenital and acquired bleeding disorders. Blood 72:1449, 1988.

351. Lundlam CA, IR Peake, N Allen: Factor VIII and fibrinolytic response to deamino-8-d-arginine vasopressin in normal subjects and dissociate response in some patients with haemophilia and von Willebrand's disease. Br J Haematol 45:499, 1980.

352. Holmberg L, IM Nilsson: von Willebrand's disease. Clin Haematol 14:461, 1985.

353. Blatt PM, KM Brinkhous, HR Culp: Antihemophilic factor concentrate therapy in von Willebrand's disease: dissociation of bleeding time factor and ristocetin cofactor activities. JAMA 236:2270, 1976.

354. Green D, E Potter: Failure of AHF concentrate to control bleeding in von Willebrand's disease. Am J Med 60:357, 1976.

355. Fukui H, M Nashino, S Terada: Hemostatic effect of a heat-treated factor VIII concentrate (Humate-P) in von Willebrand's disease. Blut 56:171, 1988.

356. Uchlinger J, E Rose, LM Aledort: Successful treatment of an acquired von Willebrand's disease factor antibody by extracorporeal immunoadsorption. N Engl J Med 320:254, 1989.

357. Macik BG, DA Gabriel, GC White: The use of high-dose intravenous gamma-globulin in acquired von Willebrand's syndrome. Arch Pathol Lab Med 112:143, 1988.

358. Lewis JH, RM Iammarino, JA Spero: Antithrombin Pittsburgh: an alpha-1-antitrypsin variant causing hemorrhagic disease. Blood 51:129, 1978.

359. Messmore HL, Z Parvez, J Fareed: Isolation and partial characterization of a novel circulating antithrombin. Thromb Haemost 42:123, 1979.

360. Soff GA, J Levin: Familial multiple coagulation factor deficiencies, I: review of the literature. Semin Thromb Hemost 7:112, 1981.

361. Soff GA, J Levin: Familial multiple coagulation factor deficiencies, II: combined Factor VIII, IX and XI deficiency and combined Factor IX and XI deficiency. Semin Thromb Hemost 7:149, 1981.

Disseminated Intravascular Coagulation

Disseminated intravascular coagulation (DIC) is not an independent disease entity but rather is an intermediary mechanism of disease, usually seen in association with well-defined clinical disorders.[1-4] Disseminated intravascular coagulation serves as an intermediary mechanism of disease in many localized disease processes and, occasionally, remains organ specific. This catastrophic syndrome spans all areas of medicine and presents a broad clinical spectrum that is confusing to many physicians. The syndrome of DIC was called "consumptive coagulopathy" in early reports.[5,6] This is not a proper term, since little is consumed in DIC; most factors and plasma constituents are plasmin biodegraded. The terminology that followed this early descriptive phrase was "defibrination syndrome"[7,8]; however, a more proper term would be "defibrinogenation syndrome." The most common and contemporary terminology used is disseminated intravascular coagulation, which is a beneficial descriptive pathophysiologic term if one accepts that "coagulation" represents hemorrhage plus thrombosis.[1-4,9,10] Most consider DIC to be a systemic hemorrhagic syndrome, but this is only because hemorrhage is obvious and often impressive. What is less commonly appreciated is the formidable microvascular thrombosis and occasional large vessel thrombosis that also occur. The hemorrhage is often simple to contend with in patients with fulminant DIC. The small vessel and large vessel thrombosis with impairment of blood flow, ischemia, and associated end-organ damage usually leads to irreversible morbidity and mortality of patients. Disseminated intravascular coagulation is a syndrome associated with obvious hemorrhage but also with occult diffuse thrombosis, which is difficult to stop or reverse and leads to irreversible end-organ damage and death.

Fulminant DIC vs low-grade DIC and the attendant differences in clinical manifestations, laboratory findings, and treatment will be discussed. These distinctions are often pure, and often theoretic, clinical spectrums of a disease continuum; patients may present anywhere in this continuum and may lapse from one end of the spectrum into another.

Historical Perspectives

The first description of DIC comes from a lecture, "Factors in the Control of Bleeding," delivered by Walter H. Seegers, PhD, then professor and chair of the Department of Physiology at Wayne State University, to the Cincinnati Academy of Medicine on April 18, 1950.[11] In this lecture, Dr. Seegers gave special reference to newly found factor V. He postulated that "thromboplastin" may gain access to the maternal circulation and cause hemorrhagic problems. Several essential steps in developing this concept were discussed and served as the first logical, pathophysiologic thinking regarding DIC. Dr. Seegers noted that thromboplastin was present in many tissues and could initiate the blood clotting mechanism directly by activating prothrombin. When thromboplastin was deliberately placed in the circulation of animals, a variety of pathologic responses were obtained. Dr. Seegers recognized that in experimental animal models, mechanical trauma of the placenta released material that was probably thromboplastin, which induced a variety of pathologic changes in the animal.

A study of human patients revealed that many pathologic lesions corresponded to those produced by thromboplastin in animal models. Shortly before delivering this lecture, Seegers and his colleague, Charles L. Schneider, MD, had shown that amniotic fluid and placenta contained large amounts of thromboplastin. Seegers also noted that during observations in animal models the injection of thromboplastin caused complete cessation of blood flow in small vessels. When the animals were carefully examined, it was found that death was caused by characteristic intravascular thrombotic lesions and that thromboembolism was found throughout the pulmonary vascular tree. Furthermore, the central nervous system was damaged by perivascular hemorrhage, and liver necrosis was present. Seegers not only delivered the first description of DIC and offered a pathophysiologic mechanism but also recognized that hemorrhage plus thrombosis is the usual clinical result.

These observations were extended to several patients who were discussed in this early lecture, three of whom had eclampsia. Dr. Seegers described a case of complete placental abruption with nearly complete "defibrination" in the patient, which was shown by repeated laboratory assays for circulating fibrinogen. These studies were expanded and again reported at the Fourth American Congress on Obstetrics and Gynecology in 1951.[12] During this presentation, Drs. Seegers and Schneider focused attention on thromboplastin and reviewed the reasons thromboplastin might be responsible for a group of perplexing disorders of late pregnancy, including intracranial hemorrhagic diathesis of pregnancy and toxemia of pregnancy. The authors also recognized that thromboplastin led to an underlying disease process of intravascular coagulation, with thromboplastin presumably entering the blood stream. Although this material initiates the blood clotting mechanism or procoagulant system, it may be carried some distance and mixed with a variable volume of blood before fibrin starts to form in the microcirculation. This process of coagulation then results in a depletion of fibrinogen and a resultant extensive defibrination. Following this, blood was noted to be refractory to further injections of thromboplastin because of inadequate fibrinogen. They stated, "...by the same token, however, animals are subject to grave danger due to uncontrolled hemorrhage, for an important portion of the hemostatic mechanism has been depleted." They concluded by pointing out that the mechanism of thromboplastin introduction to the systemic maternal circulation needed to be considered a factor in several complications of late pregnancy and not simply as one type of complication, because the resultant foci of tissue destruction in different organs will cause differing clinical manifestations. During this same presentation, Drs. Seegers and Schneider documented and quantitated thromboplastin or procoagulant material that could be obtained from the placental, decidua, and amniotic fluid. They presented a hypothetical mechanism by which intravascular coagulation might happen because of this thromboplastin material. It was proposed that maternal blood within a retroplacental hematoma became admixed with material fragmented from or leached out of the torn uterine decidua within which the hematoma was enclosed. This mixture, rich in thromboplastin material from the decidua, could then enter the circulation by one path or another, with the likeliest path being into the maternal lake within the placenta. Once within the maternal lake, this admixture would be likely to be distributed throughout the maternal circulation. These are the first descriptions of clinical DIC.

In the same year, in the Harvey Lectures, Dr. Seegers further described decreases in factor V and fibrinogen during the hemorrhagic complications of pregnancy.[13] In 1952, this important work was further expanded and published in the *American Journal of Clinical Pathology*. The role of the accelerated conversion of prothrombin to thrombin leading to later defibrinogenation and hemorrhagic complications of pregnancy was incorporated and described.[14] In 1953, this original work was again extended to the clinical field and published in the *American Journal of Obstetrics and Gynecol-*

ogy in collaboration with Drs. Stevenson, Braden, Schneider, and Johnson.[15] In this classic report, Dr. Seegers and coworkers developed guidelines for early cesarean section to abort the hemorrhagic syndrome, which they called defibrination.

Major clinical extensions of this early observation were reported shortly thereafter by Drs. Ratnoff, Pritchard, and Colopy in an article published in the *New England Journal of Medicine* in 1955.[16,17] In this two-part article, many profound observations were described, including the following: the hemorrhagic syndromes of pregnancy including premature separation of the placenta, amniotic fluid embolism, the presence of a dead fetus in utero, and severe pre-eclampsia or frank toxemia of pregnancy; a generalized bleeding tendency may happen as a sequel to "criminal abortion"; the treatment of a patient with a hemorrhagic diathesis associated with premature separation of the placenta consisted, most importantly, of early evacuation of the uterus; if labor did not occur promptly, it was difficult to keep a patient out of shock; and if laboratory tests showed progressive hypofibrinogenemia, it was probably in the best interest of the patient to empty the uterus promptly by cesarean section. This was truly profound thinking for 1955. In the conclusion of this article, the authors recognized that more than simple hypofibrinogenemia accounted for the hemorrhagic syndromes associated with pregnancy: an "unexplained prolongation of the clotting time and associated severe thrombocytopenia" were present; multiple hemostatic defects were present. In addition, Ratnoff and coworkers were the first to note that in individuals with amniotic fluid embolism, hemorrhagic symptoms appeared, although the concentration of fibrinogen in the plasma did not seem to be sufficiently low to account adequately for ineffective hemostasis. This was the first description of a multifaceted defect that accounted for the hemorrhage of DIC.

Additional observations were that "...fibrinolysin was thought to be present," thus providing the first description of secondary activation of the fibrinolytic system and probably the essential cause of hemorrhage in these patients. This is the first report of septicemia associated with DIC. Two patients were described who had undergone attempts at self-induced abortion and then developed bacteremia with gram-negative coliform bacilli. In 1962, Drs. Ratnoff and Nebehay[18] described the severe changes in blood coagulation that may sometimes contribute to the bleeding tendency and shock in the Waterhouse-Friderichsen syndrome. A case of DIC associated with incoagulable blood with prolonged clotting and bleeding times, thrombocytopenia, and low levels of fibrinogen, factor V, and factor VII in a patient with Waterhouse-Friderichsen syndrome induced by infection with pneumococcus was also described. Following this, more reports of DIC began to appear in the literature, and finally, in the mid-1960s, DIC became a clinically accepted and easily recognized syndrome. We owe our basic understanding and appreciation of this syndrome to the astute clinical and laboratory observations of Drs. Seegers and Ratnoff and their coworkers. The reader is encouraged to scruti-

Table 7-1. Conditions Associated With Fulminant Disseminated Intravascular Coagulation

Obstetric accidents
    Amniotic fluid embolism
    Placental abruption
    Retained fetus syndrome
    Eclampsia
    Abortion (saline induced)

Intravascular hemolysis
    Hemolytic transfusion reactions
    Minor hemolysis
    Massive transfusions

Septicemia
    Gram negative (endotoxin)
    Gram positive (mucopolysaccharides)

Viremias
    Cytomegalovirus
    Hepatitis
    Varicella
    HIV

Disseminated malignancy

Leukemia
    Acute promyelocytic
    Acute myelomonocytic
    Many others

Burns

Crush injuries and tissue necrosis

Liver disease
    Obstructive jaundice
    Acute hepatic failure

Prosthetic devices
    LeVeen shunting and aortic balloon

Cardiac and peripheral vascular disorders

nize these early descriptions of DIC for a complete appreciation of the profound discoveries made by attentive biochemical observation and equally brilliant clinical observation.

Etiology of DIC

Fulminant

Disseminated intravascular coagulation is usually seen in association with well-defined clinical entities. Those clinical disorders and circumstances most commonly associated with fulminant DIC are summarized in Table 7-1.

Obstetric accidents are common events leading to DIC. Amniotic fluid embolism and associated DIC is the most catastrophic and common of the life-threatening obstetric accidents.[1-5,19,20] The syndrome of amniotic fluid embolism is manifest by the acute onset of respiratory failure, circulatory collapse, shock, and a most serious thrombohemorrhagic syndrome of DIC. The first attentive description of this syndrome was by Steiner and Lushbaugh in 1941.[21] In this landmark report, the authors described the clinical histories of eight obstetric patients and showed that these patients formed a distinct group with a unique pathophysiologic basis for the constellation of symptoms now associated with DIC. These eight cases came from 4,000 consecutive autopsies performed during 15 years, which represented an incidence of 0.2% of deaths in their series, and were among a total of 24,200 deliveries, which represented an incidence of 1 in 8,000 obstetric cases. These authors, when analyzing their data, were the first to show that amniotic fluid embolism was the most common cause of maternal death in the period between labor and the first nine hours postpartum. The common etiologic factor in this syndrome of amniotic fluid embolism is the entrance, by various proposed mechanisms and routes, of amniotic fluid into the systemic maternal circulation, followed by embolization of amniotic fluid and its contents to the lungs. Next, circulatory collapse and the development of DIC occur almost uniformly. The incidence of this catastrophic syndrome is between 1 per 8,000 and 1 per 30,000 births.[21,22] The syndrome is frequently fatal for both mother and child. Although the finding of amniotic fluid in maternal blood is not physiologic, amniotic fluid enters the systemic maternal circulation in rare instances without significant manifestations of this devastating syndrome.[23] In a 1970 study, the syndrome of amniotic fluid embolism represented 10% of all maternal deaths. A study in Sweden between 1965 and 1974 showed that the syndrome of amniotic fluid embolism accounted for 22% of all maternal deaths.[24,25] The risk factors associated with the development of amniotic fluid embolism include older age, multiparity, marked exaggeration of uterine contraction following rupture of the uterine membranes, markedly exaggerated uterine contraction resulting from the use of Oxytocin or other uterine-stimulatory agents, cesarean section, uterine rupture, high cervical lacerations, premature separation of the placenta, and intrauterine fetal death (Table 7-2).[21,26,27]

On rare occasions, the syndrome can happen late in pregnancy, but it most commonly occurs during labor in 80% of patients. The syndrome happens before labor begins and before rupture of the amniotic sac in only up to 20% of patients.[28,29] Within an hour of developing this syndrome, 25% of women will die; up to 80% of patients will die within the first nine hours.[30,31] The syndrome develops without premonitory warning in 10% of women, usually during delivery, as amniotic fluid enters the systemic maternal circulation during an apparently normal labor. Rapid onset of signs and symptoms of pulmonary failure and circulatory collapse generally occur, which is followed by systemic bleeding in at least 50% of women. Before the sudden maternal onset of fulminant respiratory failure and circulatory collapse, 50% of fetuses die or develop intrauterine distress.

The cause of amniotic fluid embolism is only partly understood, but the common etiologic event is entrance of amniotic

Table 7-2. Amniotic Fluid Embolism

Risk factors
    Older age
    Multiparity
    Physiologic intense uterine contractions
    Drug-induced intense uterine contractions
    Cesarean section
    Uterine rupture
    High cervical tear
    Premature placental separation
    Intrauterine fetal death
    80% of cases develop during labor
    20% may develop before or after labor

Incidence and statistics
    1 in 8,000 to 1 in 30,000 deliveries
    10% of all maternal deaths in U.S.
    22% of all maternal deaths in Sweden
    80% overall mortality
    25% will die within one hour
    50% fetal death or distress before symptoms

fluid into the systemic maternal circulation, which then causes extensive pulmonary microcirculatory occlusion and local pulmonary activation of the procoagulant system. In addition, systemic activation of the procoagulant system occurs. This happens in conjunction with intense induction of pulmonary fibrinolytic activity, presumably via release of pulmonary endothelial plasminogen activator in the lungs. Since this is a life-threatening and not uncommon syndrome, all clinicians involved with obstetrics and delivery should be familiar with its potential. When a patient presents with the risk factors depicted in Table 7-2 and suddenly develops respiratory distress, shock, and uncontrolled bleeding immediately preceding, during, or after delivery, DIC should be considered.

Amniotic fluid contains substantial cellular material including vernix caseosa, squamous epithelial cells, and other debris from the fetus.[21,32] The lipid content, cellular content, fetal debris, procoagulant activity, and viscosity of amniotic fluid all increase with the duration of pregnancy and are at a maximum at the time of delivery.[33,34] In most instances, the actual mechanisms and site of entry of amniotic fluid into the uterine and then into the systemic maternal circulation are unclear.

The diagnosis of amniotic fluid embolism should be strongly suspected when sudden development of acute respiratory failure occurs during an otherwise normal delivery. The acute respiratory failure occurs from occlusion of pulmonary vessels by amniotic fluid, intense vasoconstriction of pulmonary vessels, and then further occlusion by platelet-fibrin thrombi. This early event is usually followed by cardiogenic shock and systemic cardiovascular collapse. The usual clinical findings of acute pulmonary insufficiency are the sudden onset of tachypnea, dyspnea, and peripheral cyanosis resulting from the abrupt development of abnormal perfusion and diffusion. These findings are usually accom-

panied by acute cor pulmonale with resultant right-sided failure, later decreased filling of the left ventricle, and resultant low-output failure and peripheral end-organ hypoxia, ischemia, and metabolic acidosis. Abnormal diffusion capacity, metabolic acidosis, and elevated central venous pressure are also noted.

The approach to treatment of acute respiratory failure in these patients is straightforward and consists of immediate establishment of an airway, the use of oxygen, and the use of a mechanical ventilator if needed. Circulatory collapse must be managed immediately with the use of vasoconstrictive agents, usually dopamine. Other cardiovascular and respiratory modalities may also be needed. Circulatory collapse is further managed by vigorous volume replacement. Management of DIC should be via immediate use of heparin to stop further deposition of platelet-fibrin thrombi and the further generation of activated coagulation factors.

In instances of placental abruption, placental enzymes and tissues, including thromboplastinlike material, may be released into the uterine and then into the systemic maternal circulation, which, likewise, leads to activation of the coagulation system. In DIC associated with the retained fetus syndrome, the incidence of DIC approaches 50% if the woman retains a dead fetus in utero for more than five weeks. The first findings are usually those of a low-grade compensated DIC, which then amplifies into a more fulminant hemorrhagic-thrombotic DIC. In this instance necrotic fetal tissue, including enzymes derived from necrotic fetal tissue, is released into the uterine and then into the systemic maternal circulation and acts at diverse sites to activate the procoagulant system, triggering an episode of fulminant DIC.[1-5,35,36]

Intravascular hemolysis of any etiology is a common triggering event for DIC. A frank hemolytic transfusion reaction is unquestionably a triggering event for DIC; however, hemolysis of any etiology, even minimal, may provide a trigger for DIC. During hemolysis the release of red blood cell ADP or red blood cell membrane phospholipoprotein may activate the procoagulant system, and in clinical practice a combination of these may account for episodes of DIC associated with major or minor hemolysis.[1,3,37-41] An example is the use of multiple transfusions with banked whole blood over a short time. The use of 5 to 10 units of banked whole blood within a 24-hour period will provide a sufficient trigger for DIC via these mechanisms. Hemolysis resulting from a frank hemolytic transfusion reaction or even from a minor hemolytic reaction, with release of red blood cell ADP or red blood cell membrane phospholipoprotein, can provide a trigger for activation of the procoagulant system and a later episode of fulminant DIC.

Septicemia is often associated with DIC. An early organism to be associated with DIC was meningococcus.[42-44] Later, other gram-negative organisms were also noted to provide a triggering event for DIC.[45,46] The triggering mechanisms have been well described and include the initiation of coagulation by endotoxin: bacterial coat lipopolysaccharide.[47,48] Endotoxin can activate factor XII to factor XIIa, can induce a platelet release reaction, may cause endothelial sloughing with later activation of factor XII to factor XIIa or factor XI to factor XIa, or can initiate a release of granulocyte procoagulant materials. Any one of these events might independently trigger DIC. A clinical summation of several or all of these activation sequences is probably most commonly seen. Following these observations, many gram-positive organisms were also noted to be associated with DIC, and likewise, the mechanisms have been aptly described.[49,50] Bacterial coat mucopolysaccharides may demonstrate exactly the same activity as endotoxin, namely the activation of factor XII to factor XIIa, a platelet release reaction, endothelial sloughing, or the release of granulocyte procoagulant materials, any one of which may initiate DIC. As with gram-negative endotoxemia, however, a summation of several or all of these activation events is most probably seen clinically.[1-4]

Many viremias have been associated with DIC, and the most common are varicella, hepatitis, or cytomegalovirus infections.[51,52] Many other acute viremias may also induce DIC.[1-4] The exact triggering mechanisms are poorly documented, but the likeliest mechanisms are antigen-antibody–associated activation of factor XII, a platelet release reaction, or endothelial sloughing with subsequent exposure of subendothelial collagen and basement membrane.[53-55] Severe viral hepatitis and hepatic failure can lead to DIC. In addition, intrahepatic or extrahepatic cholestasis may be accompanied by fulminant DIC.[1-3]

Malignancy is often associated with DIC, and most individuals with disseminated solid malignancy will have at least laboratory evidence of DIC that may or may not become clinically manifest. Therefore, if one looks for laboratory evidence of DIC in patients with disseminated solid malignancy it is almost always found.[56-60] Malignancy may provide a trigger for initiation of DIC by many mechanisms. One such mechanism is simply neovascularization of tumor. The new vasculature is composed of abnormal endothelial lining that may activate the procoagulant system by several mechanisms.[61,62] In addition, solid tumors may release necrotic tumor tissue or tumor cell enzymes into the systemic circulation and activate the coagulation sequence.[60,63,64] Other mechanisms may also be operative in malignancy; for example, the sialic acid moiety of mucin in mucinous adenocarcinoma tissue is capable of the nonenzymatic activation of factor X to factor Xa that may then lead to a fulminant or low-grade compensated DIC, which may be manifest in the usual manner or as multiple or single thrombosis.[65,66]

It has long been debated whether prostatic carcinoma is associated with a primary hyperfibrino(geno)lytic syndrome or DIC. Rapaport and Chapman[69] have clearly shown that malignant prostatic tissue secretes enzyme-type materials that are capable of activating the coagulation system and are associated with the usual secondary fibrinolytic response, which represents a typical DIC syndrome.[67-69] In addition, these investigations have shown that malignant prostatic tissue may secrete materials that independently activate the fibrinolytic system, converting plasminogen to plasmin. In prostatic carci-

noma, patients develop a typical DIC syndrome with secondary fibrinolysis and a primary activation of the fibrinolytic system; thus, an overwhelming fibrinolytic response is seen. This accounts for the clinical observation that these patients more commonly present with hemorrhage instead of thrombosis. Studies at the Mayo Clinic have shown a direct correlation between laboratory findings of DIC before transurethral prostatectomy and the degree of postprostatectomy blood loss. These findings suggest that it is prudent to look for evidence of DIC, as defined by elevated levels of FDPs and circulating soluble fibrin monomer, since this may predict those patients who will bleed following surgery as well as the need for postoperative blood replacement.[70]

Pancreatic carcinoma has been classically associated with migratory thrombophlebitis, and the mechanisms have been carefully studied and described.[71,72] In this instance, the migratory thrombophlebitis is simply a clinical manifestation of DIC. The incidence of thrombophlebitis in carcinoma of the pancreas is much higher in patients with carcinoma of the body or tail of the pancreas as opposed to those with carcinoma in the head of the pancreas. When a carcinoma is present in the body or tail of the pancreas, minimal ductal obstruction is noted, and large amounts of trypsin are released into the systemic circulation. Trypsin, a serine protease, has activity much like thrombin or factor Xa and may activate the coagulation system, with a characteristic DIC-type syndrome emerging. The clinical manifestation is more commonly thrombosis instead of hemorrhage, as opposed to that seen in prostatic carcinoma.[1,2,60] Alternatively, if the carcinoma is found in the head of the pancreas, ductal obstruction is pronounced, only minimal trypsin release happens, and disseminated thromboses are much less commonly seen.[57,60] Many patients with disseminated solid malignancy show laboratory evidence of DIC. However, many patients never develop overt clinical manifestations of fulminant DIC, although a significant number may have clinical manifestations of a low-grade compensated DIC if it is suspected, looked for, and documented.

Patients with acute or chronic leukemias are candidates for DIC. The most common acute leukemia associated with DIC is acute hypergranular promyelocytic leukemia (FAB-M3). The mechanisms for this disorder have been carefully explored and described[73-78] and consist of the release of procoagulant material from granules of the progranulocyte. Furthermore, some authors[79-81] have shown that the use of heparin or miniheparin before the initiation of cytotoxic chemotherapy may ward off the development of DIC and significantly prolong survival. My experience has been that if a patient with acute promyelocytic leukemia does not present with findings of DIC, the patient will develop fulminant DIC when cytotoxic chemotherapy is started. This process is initiated by a large population cell "kill" with resultant release of granule procoagulant material into the systemic circulation, and subsequent DIC develops.[57,60] The next most common leukemia to be associated with fulminant DIC is acute myelomonocytic leukemia (FAB-M4).[1,82] However,

Table 7-3. Malignancies Commonly Associated With Disseminated Intravascular Coagulation

Gastrointestinal
Pancreas
Prostate
Lung
Breast
Ovary
Melanoma
Acute leukemia
Myeloma
Myeloproliferative syndromes

Table 7-4. Vascular Disorders/Defects Associated With Disseminated Intravascular Coagulation

Kasabach-Merritt syndrome
Hereditary hemorrhagic telangiectasia
Raynaud's syndrome
Leriche's syndrome
Vascular prostheses
Autoimmune disorders with vasculitis
Microangiopathic hemolytic anemia
Hemolytic-uremic syndrome
Thrombotic thrombocytopenic purpura (rare)
Malignant hypertension
Glomerulonephritis
Angiosarcoma
Arteriovenous fistulae

any acute leukemia or, less commonly, chronic leukemia may be associated with DIC and may significantly change the prognosis of patients.[56,57,60,75,76,82] Malignancies commonly associated with DIC are listed in Table 7-3.

Acidosis and, less commonly, alkalosis may also provide triggers for DIC.[1-4,83-85] In acidosis the triggering event is most probably endothelial sloughing with the attendant activation of factor XII to factor XIIa, factor XI to factor XIa, and/or platelet release with a subsequent activation of the procoagulant system. The mechanisms potentially operative in cases of alkalosis, however, are unclear.

Patients with extensive burns commonly develop DIC, and several mechanisms may be operative.[86,87] Microhemolysis with the attendant release of red blood cell membrane phospholipid or red blood cell ADP may provide the trigger.[1-3] In addition, necrotic burn tissue may be associated with the release of tissue materials or cellular enzymes into the systemic circulation, thus initiating a DIC-type process. Any patient with a large crush injury and attendant tissue necrosis may develop DIC by the release of tissue enzymes or phospholipoproteinlike materials into the systemic circulation.[84]

Selected vascular disorders and other miscellaneous types of disorders may also be associated with fulminant DIC, but these are more commonly associated with a chronic form of this syndrome,[88,89] specifically, the Kasabach-Merritt syndrome, the association of giant cavernous hemangiomas, and DIC.[90,91] Up to 25% of patients with giant cavernous hemangiomas will develop a chronic low-grade compensated DIC, which may or may not accelerate into a fulminant DIC. The progression into a fulminant DIC from a low-grade compensated DIC may happen with or without any particular identifiable reason. About 50% of patients with hereditary hemorrhagic telangiectasia will also have a low-grade DIC syndrome, and many of these individuals may develop a fulminant DIC process for unexplained reasons.[92,93] Individuals with small vessel disease, such as vasospastic phenomena, including Raynaud's syndrome or severe diabetic angiopathy, or angiopathy associated with autoimmune disorders, may also develop low-grade DIC, which may or may not become an acute process.[1-4,94] Vascular disorders associated with DIC are listed in Table 7-4. Many chronic inflammatory disorders, including sarcoidosis, Crohn's disease, and ulcerative colitis, may also be associated with compensated DIC.[1-3]

Selected prosthetic devices may provide a triggering event for DIC. Exposure of the blood to foreign surfaces is often linked with activation of the procoagulant system, and this may provide a major obstacle in the use of some prosthetic devices. The use of prosthetic devices has become extremely commonplace in the treatment of patients with vascular disease, cardiac disease, renal disease, angiographic studies, and ascites. The hemostatic complications that accompany the insertion of prosthetic devices include activation of coagulation factors, consumption of coagulation factors, other plasma proteins, platelets, and the generation of microthrombi that may or may not be of clinical consequence. In addition, thrombosis or thromboembolism may also give rise to serious life-threatening problems with prosthetic devices.[1-4,95] Intra-aortic balloon assistance is a widely used clinical maneuver to control postmyocardial infarction cardiogenic shock and to stabilize selected patients following bypass surgery. Activation of the coagulation system with an attendant low-grade DIC, which may become fulminant, may accompany the use of these devices.[95] LeVeen valve shunting for peritoneovenous shunting is a common palliative procedure for the treatment of intractable ascites associated with severe liver disease or malignancy. A generalized DIC-type syndrome is not infrequently seen with the use of the LeVeen shunt.[1,4,95] The removal of ascitic fluid at the time of valve implantation and the use of selected anticoagulants may abort DIC in these patients.[1-4] In an acute situation, simply placing the patient with a LeVeen shunt and DIC in a sitting position will usually stop the shunt function and at least temporarily abort the DIC process.[1] Hemostasis changes with prosthetic devices will be discussed in chapter 9.

Low Grade

Low-grade DIC is a compensated event and represents the pure end of a clinical spectrum that may not always represent reality.[96] The conditions most commonly associated

Table 7-5. Conditions Associated With Low-Grade Disseminated Intravascular Coagulation

Obstetric accidents
    Eclampsia
    Retained fetus syndrome
    Saline-induced abortion

Cardiovascular diseases
    Acute myocardial infarction
    Peripheral vascular disease
    Leriche's syndrome

Metastatic malignancy

Hematologic diseases
    Paroxysmal nocturnal hemoglobinuria
    Polycythemia vera
    Agnogenic myeloid metaplasia

Collagen vascular disorders
(especially if a microvascular component)

Renal disorders
    Glomerulonephritis
    Renal microangiopathies
    Hemolytic-uremic syndrome

Miscellaneous disorders
    Allergic vasculitis
    Sarcoidosis
    Amyloidosis
    Chronic inflammatory disorders
    Diabetes mellitus
    Hyperlipoproteinemias

with a low-grade DIC–type process are depicted in Table 7-5. Obstetric accidents are common causes of low-grade DIC. The retained fetus syndrome usually represents a fulminant DIC process. Many individuals with retained fetus syndrome may develop a low-grade DIC syndrome that then slowly amplifies into a more fulminant acute process.[97] Likewise, eclampsia represents the straightforward pathophysiology of DIC that often remains low grade and often is organ specific, remaining localized to the renal and placental microcirculation. In about 10% to 15% of women, however, the process may become systemic, acute, and fulminant.[98,99] Many patients enduring hypertonic saline-induced abortion develop a low-grade DIC–type process that sometimes becomes fulminant and at other times remains low grade and compensated until the abortion is finished.[100]

Cardiovascular diseases may likewise be associated with low-grade DIC, and occasionally patients with acute myocardial infarction may develop a low-grade compensated or alternatively an acute, fulminant DIC process.[1-4,101] The mechanisms are unclear but may simply be shock, hypoxia, and acidosis with resultant endothelial sloughing and/or activation of the contact activation system via stasis. Peripheral vascular diseases, such as giant cavernous hemangiomas, hereditary hemorrhagic telangiectasia, Leriche's syndrome,

and selected small vessel diseases, may lead to a low-grade compensated DIC process that may stay low-grade or may progress to a more acute phase.[1,102,103]

Most patients with disseminated malignancy have laboratory findings of a low-grade DIC–type process, although many of these individuals never develop specific clinical signs and symptoms of DIC. Pulmonary hemorrhage is a very early and prominent sign of low-grade DIC in patients with malignancy.[1-4,57,60,104] About 75% of patients with malignancy and low-grade DIC will eventually develop clinical evidence of this syndrome, and 25% will develop some type of noteworthy thrombotic event.[1-4,57,60] Many individuals with low-grade DIC and malignancy may show striking correction of both their clinical hemorrhage and thrombosis and laboratory findings of DIC when aggressive antineoplastic therapy is started.[105-107] Many hematologic disorders have been associated with DIC. Agnogenic myeloid metaplasia has been associated with DIC, and a substantial number of patients with polycythemia rubra vera have clinical and laboratory findings of an underlying low-grade compensated DIC process.[57,60,108,109] Thrombosis, or thromboembolus, has an increased tendency in patients with paroxysmal nocturnal hemoglobinuria, and this represents a DIC-type process that is clinically manifest primarily as thrombosis.[110,111]

Collagen vascular diseases may be associated with DIC, and any patient with a collagen vascular disorder, especially when associated with significant small vessel involvement, may develop DIC. This DIC, usually in a low-grade compensated form, may be seen in patients with severe rheumatoid arthritis, systemic lupus erythematosus, Sjögren's syndrome, dermatomyositis, and scleroderma. Again, this is most commonly seen when these disorders are associated with a serious microvascular component.[1-4,112]

Hemolytic-uremic syndrome, like eclampsia, shares similar pathophysiology to DIC. However, HUS often is organ specific and localized to the renal microcirculation.[113-115] In about 10% of individuals with HUS the syndrome becomes systemic.[113] When patients with HUS are examined, it is often clinically impossible to know whether the disease started as a primary insult to the renal vasculature and later activation of the coagulation system or whether a primary activation of the coagulation system initiated a localized or systemic DIC process that then induced local damage to the renal microcirculation secondary to fibrin deposition. No matter where the process started, the clinical manifestations may be similar. More importantly, when a patient with HUS is examined it is often impossible to know where the cycle was started.[113]

Innumerous assorted disorders have been associated with DIC, including the allergic vasculitides, such as Henoch-Schönlein purpura and the other allergic purpuras, sarcoidosis, amyloidosis, chronic ulcerative/inflammatory conditions, including Crohn's disease, AIDS, ulcerative colitis, and severe diabetes mellitus, especially when associated with a significant microvascular component.[1-4,116,117] In addition, a low-grade compensated DIC–type syndrome may occur in

Figure 7-1. Triggering Mechanisms for DIC

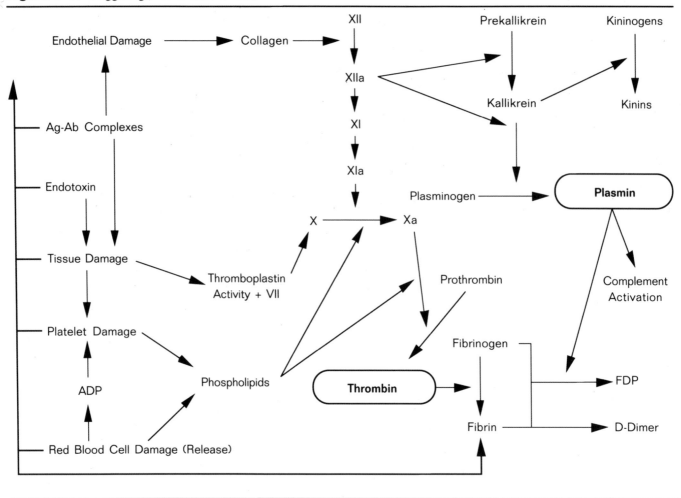

patients who have hyperlipoproteinemias types II and IV.[1,4] On rare occasions, patients may develop a low-grade DIC–type process in which no etiology can be found.[1-4]

Figure 7-1 illustrates how a broad spectrum of presumably unrelated pathophysiologic insults can give rise to the same common ultimate pathway, the syndrome of DIC. Many disorders are associated with endothelial damage, circulating antigen-antibody complex, endotoxemia, tissue damage of any type (with resultant release of tissue procoagulant materials or tissue procoagulant enzymes), platelet damage and release, or red blood cell damage.[118-121] When one of these insults happens, many potential activation pathways may ultimately give rise to systemically circulating plasmin plus systemically circulating thrombin. When these two enzymes are circulating systemically, DIC is the usual result.[121-124] Frequently, the pathways leading from the first pathophysiologic insult to the generation of systemic thrombin and plasmin are different. Despite the activation pathway, once triggered the resultant DIC-type pathophysiology stays the same.

Pathophysiology

The pathophysiology of DIC, once a triggering event has been provided, is summarized in Figure 7-2. After the coagulation system has been activated and both thrombin and plasmin are circulated systemically, the pathophysiology of DIC is similar in all disorders. When thrombin circulates systemically it behaves as it would locally and begins to cleave fibrinopeptides A and B from fibrinogen leaving behind fibrin monomer. Most of this fibrin monomer will polymerize into fibrin (clot) in the microcirculation, leading to microvascular and macrovascular thrombosis, interference with blood flow, peripheral ischemia, end-organ damage, and other attendant findings.[121,125-127] Because fibrin is deposited in the microcirculation, platelets become trapped, and the usual attendant thrombocytopenia, typical of DIC, follows.[113,128,129]

On the other side of the circle depicted in Figure 7-2, plasmin also circulates systemically, behaves as it normally would locally, and begins to cleave the carboxy-terminal

Figure 7-2. Pathophysiology of DIC

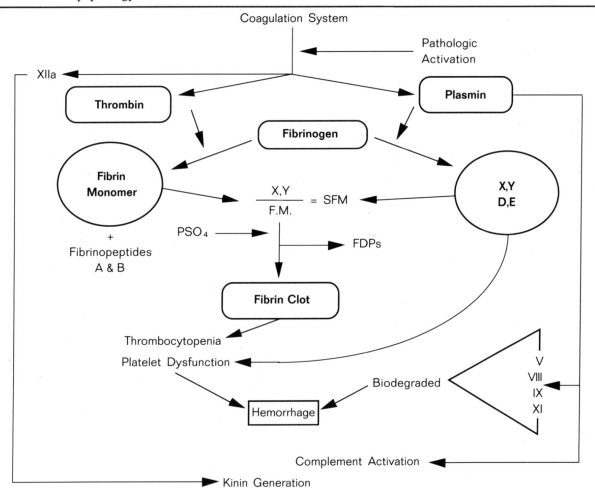

end of fibrinogen into FDPs systemically, creating the clinically recognized fragments X, Y, D, and E.[1,3,121,130-133] Plasmin also rapidly releases specific peptides, the B-beta 15-42 and related peptides that also serve as diagnostic molecular markers. Fibrin(ogen) degradation products may combine with circulating fibrin monomer before fibrin monomer has polymerized into fibrin. When these degradation products complex with fibrin monomer, fibrin monomer cannot polymerize, and therefore, it becomes solubilized. This complex of degradation products and fibrin monomer is called soluble fibrin monomer, which is a significant aid in the diagnosis of DIC. The presence of soluble fibrin monomer forms the basis of the paracoagulation reactions, the ethanol gelation test, or the protamine sulfate test.[134-137]

If protamine sulfate or ethanol is added to a citrated tube of plasma containing soluble fibrin monomer, the ethanol or protamine sulfate will clear the FDPs from fibrin monomer; fibrin monomer will complex with other fibrin monomer and polymerize; fibrin strands are formed in the test tube; and this is interpreted as a positive protamine sulfate or ethanol

gelation test.[1,3,138-140] Systemically circulating FDPs interfere with fibrin monomer polymerization, which further impairs hemostasis and leads to hemorrhage.[1-3] Another biologic activity of degradation products is that the later fragments have a high affinity for platelet membranes and coat their surfaces.[141] This often creates a clinically significant platelet function defect.[113,141-143] When examining a patient with DIC who has a reasonable platelet count and is only mildly to moderately thrombocytopenic, the clinician should not mistakenly harbor a false sense of security, because those platelets remaining in the circulation are usually dramatically dysfunctional and may lead to or contribute to clinically significant hemorrhage.

Plasmin, unlike thrombin, is a global proteolytic enzyme that has equal affinity for fibrinogen and fibrin.[144,145] In addition, plasmin also effectively biodegrades many clotting factors, including factor V, factor VIII, factor IX, factor XI, and other plasma proteins, including growth hormone, ACTH, insulin, and maybe many more.[121,146-149] As plasmin degrades cross-linked fibrin, specific FDPs appear in the circulation,

Figure 7-3. Selected "Pathocybernetics" in DIC

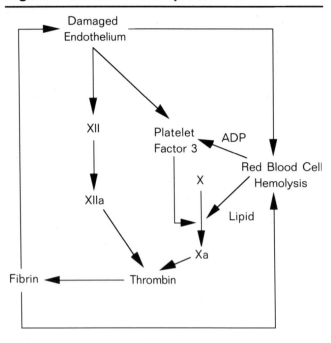

Furthermore, plasmin-induced lysis of many of these clotting factors leads to hemorrhage. By appreciating this circular type of pathophysiology, it is easy to appreciate why most patients with DIC endure hemorrhage plus thrombosis. Clinicians are repeatedly misguided by appreciating only the hemorrhage evolving in patients with DIC, since this is the most obvious physical finding observed during clinical assessment. Less often appreciated, but of equal or more importance, however, is the substantial extent of microvascular thrombosis and occasional large vessel thrombosis happening and leading to end-organ damage that may be extremely difficult to reverse. Microvascular thrombosis and later interference with blood flow and end-organ damage are usually not appreciated until laboratory parameters provide a clue to their presence (eg, impending renal failure, pulmonary failure, elevated muscle-derived enzymes, liver enzymes, bone enzymes, and severely compromised pulmonary function). Most patients with DIC are not only undergoing significant hemorrhage but also significant and often diffuse thrombosis.[1-4,121,158-161] Thrombosis is the more irreversible insult and more frequently leads to altered morbidity and mortality because of ischemic changes, end-organ damage, and potential death of the patient.[1-3]

Figure 7-3 represents selected pathocybernetic events in DIC. These events are depicted for illustrative purposes; only a few events in a DIC episode have been chosen. Many others could have been chosen to exemplify the all-important point that once a DIC process is started the cybernetic nature of the coagulation system and the DIC process itself are such that the process will continue to self-perpetuate until something is done medically to intervene with the procoagulant drive.[162] For example, if starting with a clinical insult resulting in damaged endothelium, damaged endothelium will convert factor XII to factor XIIa with the eventual generation of thrombin and the subsequent generation of fibrin. Deposition of fibrin on the endothelium will cause more damaged endothelium. Thus, a self-perpetuating cycle continues until stopped. In this selected instance the damaged endothelium will also lead to platelet release with eventual availability of platelet factor 3, thus leading to the conversion of factor X to factor Xa with the eventual generation of thrombin, more fibrin deposited on the endothelium, more endothelial damage, and more platelet release. The damaged endothelium will probably give rise to red blood cell hemolysis, as may the deposited fibrin, giving rise to release of red blood cell ADP, which causes more platelet release, more thrombin generation, further fibrin deposition, further endothelial damage, and further red blood cell hemolysis. Red blood cell hemolysis will release red blood cell membrane phospholipid, which may give rise to eventual factor Xa generation, thrombin generation, and fibrin deposition, which, likewise, is associated with more red blood cell hemolysis and damaged endothelium with attendant red blood cell hemolysis. The process is circular and self-perpetuating, and until something is done medically to intervene, the pathophysiologic process will continue.

including D-dimer. As plasmin circulates systemically, it often activates both C1 and C3 systemically with the attendant activation of the entire complement sequence leading to C8–C9 activation and subsequent cell and platelet lysis.[121,150-152] This process is significant clinically in DIC and related syndromes associated with circulating plasmin, because the attendant red blood cell lysis will release red blood cell ADP and red blood cell membrane phospholipid, supplying more procoagulant material. In addition, complement-induced platelet lysis not only causes further thrombocytopenia but also provides more platelet procoagulant material. Of additional clinical importance, activation of the complement system will increase vascular permeability, thus leading to hypotension and shock.[1-3]

Activation of the kinin system is also an important pathophysiologic event with serious clinical consequences in DIC and related syndromes. With early activation of the coagulation system, as commonly happens in DIC, factor XIIa is usually generated with the subsequent conversion of prekallikrein to kallikrein and later conversion of high–molecular weight kininogen into circulating kinins.[153-157] This activation also leads to kinin-induced increased vascular permeability, hypotension, and shock.[1]

As thrombin circulates systemically, the consequences are mainly thrombosis with deposition of fibrin monomer and polymerized (cross-linked) fibrin in the microcirculation and, occasionally, large vessels. Concomitantly, plasmin circulates systemically. This enzyme is primarily responsible for the hemorrhage seen in DIC because of the creation of FDPs and the interference of these degradation products with fibrin monomer polymerization and platelet function.

Table 7-6. Platelet Factor 3 Release in Disseminated Intravascular Coagulation

Exposed collagen (subendothelial)
Exposed basement membrane
Elevated epinephrine levels
Circulating antigen-antibody complexes
Complement activation
Endotoxin
Thrombin

Table 7-8. Clinical Manifestations of Factor XIIa Generation in Disseminated Intravascular Coagulation

Activation of fibrinolysis: biodegradation - hemorrhage
Kinin activation: vasodilatation - hypotension and shock
Complement activation: vascular changes, cell lysis and release, and platelet lysis and release

Table 7-6 lists the clinical situations that may give rise to platelet factor 3 release to begin or more importantly to perpetuate a DIC-type episode. The presence of subendothelial collagen, epinephrine, circulating antigen-antibody complexes, endotoxin, thrombin, or complement activation (possible through previous plasmin generation) will all cause a platelet factor 3 release and continue to augment a DIC process.[163-166] In addition, but less probable, any one of these may independently cause a platelet factor 3 release that may initiate instead of simply perpetuate a process of DIC. It is probable that the availability of platelet factor 3, by any of these potential mechanisms, is more important as an accelerating and self-perpetuating process than as a strictly etiologic singular mechanism in the initiation of DIC.[1-3]

Table 7-7 lists the consequences of endotoxemia in initiating DIC. Endotoxin (bacterial coat lipopolysaccharide) can induce a granulocyte release of procoagulant or coagulation activating enzymes, can directly convert factor XII to factor XIIa, may induce a platelet release reaction, and may cause endothelial sloughing with subsequent exposure of subendothelial collagen.[167-172] Any one of these insults may independently initiate an episode of fulminant DIC; however, a summation of several or all of these events is probably clinically seen in patients with endotoxemia and DIC.

Table 7-8 lists the clinical consequences of activating factor XII to factor XIIa in an episode of DIC. When factor XIIa is circulating, the fibrinolytic system may be activated via mechanisms previously discussed. Later, plasmin-induced biodegradation of many coagulation factors will occur, and the clinical manifestation will be hemorrhage. Secondly, the generation of factor XIIa may lead to kinin activation with attendant vasodilatation and the resultant clinical manifestations of hypotension and shock.[157,173-176] Thirdly, as factor XIIa circulates and activates the fibrinolytic system, the complement system will be imminently activated with cell lysis, vascular changes, and a platelet release reaction.[1,177,178] Platelet release will provide more coagulant material to self-perpetuate the intravascular clotting process; the vascular changes of complement activation are composed of increased vascular permeability, again leading to hypotension and shock.[1-4]

Table 7-9 signifies those clinical situations that may give rise to endothelial damage, endothelial sloughing with exposure of subendothelial collagen and subendothelial basement membrane, and the subsequent activation of factor XII to factor XIIa and possibly factor XI to factor XIa. These circumstances include viremias (presumably the mechanism is circulating antigen-antibody complex), heat stroke, patients with hyperacute renal allograft rejection, circulating antigen-antibody complexes of any origin, shock with attendant hypoxia and acidosis, endotoxemia, and, very importantly, ongoing DIC with subsequent vascular damage.[179-183] Many pathophysiologic events in DIC will cause substantial endothelial damage with endothelial sloughing, the exposure of subendothelial collagen and basement membrane, and subsequent activation of factor XII to factor XIIa and possibly factor XI to factor XIa, again self-perpetuating the DIC-type process.[121]

Clinical Findings

The general signs and symptoms of DIC can be endlessly variable and include fever, hypotension, acidosis, proteinuria, and hypoxia (Table 7-10).[1-4] These findings are largely ambiguous, may be found in many disorders, and are not specifically helpful from the diagnostic standpoint.

Table 7-7. Endotoxin and Induction of Disseminated Intravascular Coagulation

Granulocyte release
Activation of factor XII to XIIa
Platelet release
Endothelial damage

Table 7-9. Endothelial Damage and Induction of Disseminated Intravascular Coagulation

Viremia
Septicemia/bacteremia
Heat stroke
Renal graft rejection
Antigen-antibody complexes
Hypoxia
Acidosis
Shock
Endotoxemia
Ongoing disseminated intravascular coagulation

Table 7-10. Findings in Patients With Disseminated Intravascular Coagulation

General signs and symptoms
    Fever
    Hypotension
    Acidosis
    Hypoxia
    Proteinuria

Specific and suggestive findings
    Petechiae
    Purpura
    Hemorrhagic bullae
    Acryl cyanosis
    Gangrene
    Surgical wound bleeding
    Traumatic wound bleeding
    Venipuncture site bleeding
    Arterial line oozing
    Subcutaneous hematomas

Table 7-12. Typical Morphologic Findings in Disseminated Intravascular Coagulation

Peripheral smear changes
Hemorrhage in various organs
Thrombosis in various organ systems
Platelet-rich microthrombi, early (usually with vasoconstriction)
Fibrin monomer and fibrin oligomer, early
Fibrin-rich hyaline microthrombi, late
Pulmonary hyaline membranes

However, more specific signs found in patients with DIC that should immediately forewarn one to the possibility of DIC in the appropriate clinical settings consist of petechiae and purpura, found in the overwhelming majority of patients with DIC, hemorrhagic bullae, acryl cyanosis, and sometimes, frank gangrene (Table 7-10).[1-4,184-187] Additionally, wound bleeding, especially oozing from a surgical or traumatic wound, is an extremely prevalent finding in patients with DIC who have undergone surgery or trauma.[1-4] Oozing from venipuncture sites or intra-arterial lines is another common finding.[1-4] Large subcutaneous hematomas and deep tissue bleeding are also frequently seen.[1] The average patient with fulminant DIC usually bleeds from at least three unrelated sites.[1-4] For example, the patient may have petechiae and purpura, oozing from IV sites, and massive gastrointestinal blood loss. Sometimes, other types of bleeding may also occur in deep tissues, including intracranial bleeds and intramuscular hemorrhage with compartmental compression syndromes. Any combination of bleeding sites can be seen, and it is unclear why different individuals will bleed from differing sites. A remarkable volume of microvascular thrombosis and occasional large

vessel thrombosis may happen in DIC and may not be clinically obvious.[1-4,188,189]

Table 7-11 depicts the incidence of end-organ dysfunction in DIC. These findings represent microvascular thrombosis of tissues with resultant ischemia and hypoxia instead of end-organ hemorrhage. The organ systems having a high incidence of microvascular thrombosis associated with subsequent end-organ dysfunction include cardiac, pulmonary, renal, and central nervous system dysfunction.[1-4,190] Thrombotic thrombocytopenic purpura (TTP) is commonly associated with CNS dysfunction; however, this clinical finding can be observed just as commonly in fulminant DIC.[113,191]

The clinical findings of low-grade DIC are often significantly different from those in patients with fulminant DIC. Patients with low-grade DIC more commonly have bothersome bleeding and diffuse thromboses instead of acute fulminant life-threatening hemorrhage.[1-4,192] These patients have been appropriately described as having a compensated DIC.[193,194] An increased turnover and decreased survival of many components of the hemostasis system are usually noted, including the platelets, fibrinogen, factor V, and factor VIII. Because of this, most coagulation laboratory parameters are near normal or normal.[1-4,193,194]

Patients with low-grade DIC, however, almost uniformly have significantly elevated FDPs leading to impairment of fibrin monomer polymerization and a clinically significant platelet function defect resulting from the coating of platelet membranes by FDP.[113,141] Patients with low-grade DIC commonly present with findings of gingival bleeding, easy and spontaneous bruising, large cutaneous ecchymoses, and mild to moderate mucosal membrane bleeding often manifest as genitourinary or gastrointestinal hemorrhage. Patients may also present with diffuse or singular thromboses, which are taxing with respect to clinical management.

Morphologic Findings

Morphologic findings in DIC consist of characteristic but not pathognomonic peripheral smear findings and hemorrhage in any organ or combination of organs (Table 7-12).[1-4,195,196] Any organ may be associated with severe hemorrhage in patients with fulminant or low-grade DIC. Platelet-rich microthrombi are an early morphologic finding,[1,195,196] and

Table 7-11. End-Organ Dysfunction From Microthrombi in Patients With Disseminated Intravascular Coagulation

Organ system	Percentage involved
Skin	70%
Lungs	50%
Kidneys	50%
Pituitary	50%
Liver	35%
Adrenals	30%
Heart	20%

Table 7-13. Typical Peripheral Smear Alterations in Patients With Disseminated Intravascular Coagulation

Schistocytosis (red blood cell fragments)
Reticulocytosis
Polychromatophilia
Leukocytosis with mild shift
Thrombocytopenia
Large young platelets

Figure 7-4. Schistocytes

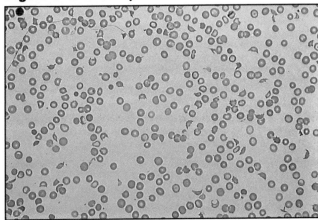

these are usually seen in association with intense vasoconstriction presumably resulting from compounds released from platelets, including thromboxanes, biogenic amines, adenine nucleotides, and kinins,[197] which are later replaced by hyaline-rich microthrombi.[195,196] Another early finding is that of fibrin monomer deposition, primarily in the reticuloendothelial system, which calls for special staining.[198] Later findings in patients with fulminant DIC are the typical fibrin-rich hyaline microthrombi thought to replace earlier deposited platelet-rich microthrombi and fibrin monomer deposits.[199,200]

Many patients with fulminant DIC develop typical pulmonary hyaline membranes that account, in part, for the significant degree of pulmonary dysfunction and hypoxemia seen in these patients.[201,202] Pure adult shock lung syndrome is probably an organ-specific DIC-type pathophysiology that usually stays localized to the pulmonary bed.[1-3] Peripheral smear changes typically seen in DIC are listed in Table 7-13. Schistocytes are red blood cell fragments, including typical so-called "Heilmeyer Helmet cells," which are seen in about 50% of individuals with fulminant DIC.[1-4,116,203-205] Schistocytes are shown in Figure 7-4. The mechanisms for the formation of schistocytes in fulminant DIC have been magnificently shown by Bull and associates, who described fibrin–red blood cell interactions.[206,207] The absence of schistocytes cannot be used to rule out a diagnosis of fulminant DIC, because they only occur in 50% of patients. Most patients with fulminant DIC will present with a mild reticulocytosis and a mild leukocytosis, usually associated with a mild to moderate shift to immature forms. Thrombocytopenia, which is usually present in most instances of fulminant DIC, is often obvious by examination of the peripheral blood smear.[208,209] Many so-called "large bizarre" platelets representing young platelets are usually seen on the peripheral smear in patients with DIC. This finding probably simply represents an increased population of young platelets resulting from increased platelet turnover and decreased platelet survival because of platelet entrapment in microthrombi.[1-4,113,210,211]

Platelet-rich microthrombi are early findings in patients with DIC and are often easily demonstrated in the pulmonary microcirculation where they are customarily seen in association with intense vasoconstriction resulting from vasoconstrictive compounds released from platelets. These platelet-rich microthrombi are later replaced by more typical hyaline-rich microthrombi.[195,196,212] Fibrin monomer may also be precipitated early in DIC, but this is uncommonly appreciated, since fibrin monomer is not shown with usual staining techniques but requires PAS staining following ethanol fixation of appropriate tissue. Fibrin monomer is most commonly precipitated in the reticuloendothelial system. The precipitation of fibrin monomer may cause severe end-organ damage due to both primary cellular/tissue damage and to microvascular occlusion. This precipitation will also induce impaired reticuloendothelial clearance of FDPs, activated clotting factors, and circulating soluble fibrin monomer.

Typical hyaline microthrombi occurring later in an episode of DIC and commonly accounting for significant end-organ damage is of three types: globular, intravascular, and pulmonary. Globular hyaline microthrombi may be seen on the peripheral blood smear and are composed of highly polymerized complexes of FDPs and many intermediates.[1,3,195,213] These microthrombi may be from 4 to 60 μm^3 in volume, may occur singly or in mass, and may be found on a peripheral smear stained with PAS. They are also seen intravascularly but rarely occlude the microcirculation.

Another type of hyaline microthrombus is the typical intravascular hyaline microthrombus so often seen by pathologists at postmortem examination in patients with DIC.[195,214,215] These microthrombi are not pathognomonic of DIC and may be seen in other related disorders including TTP.[113,191,216] These intravascular hyaline microthrombi are homogeneous, compact, intravascular hyaline structures oriented parallel to the blood flow and occasionally are noted to contain platelets or white blood cell fragments. They are easily seen by PAS staining, trichrome staining, tryptophan staining, and fluorescein-labeled antifibrinogen antiserum staining and are effortlessly seen by electron microscopy.[217-219]

Pulmonary hyaline membranes are highly polymerized complexes of FDPs and all types of intermediates.[220,221] They are usually seen to cover the alveolar epithelium with a preference for areas that have been denuded of epithelial cells. The interalveolar capillaries beneath these hyaline membranes typically exhibit abnormal vascular permeability with the circulation of endothelial cells, plasma protein precipitation between endothelial borders, and the formation of interstitial edema. Many patients with DIC develop pulmonary

Figure 7-5. Hyaline Membranes, Including Pulmonary Edema, in an Infant With DIC Secondary to Meningococcemia

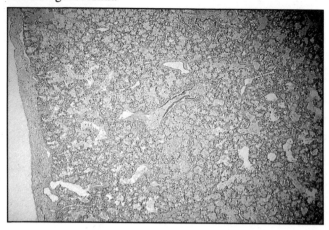

Table 7-14. Factors Leading to Precipitation of Microthrombi in Patients With Disseminated Intravascular Coagulation

Release of platelet factor 4 (antiheparin)

Granulocyte release (elastases, collagenases, etc)

Vasomotor reactions
    Elevated catecholamines
    Acidosis
    Elevated ACTH
    Glucocorticoid use

Impaired reticuloendothelial clearance
    Activated clotting factors
    Soluble fibrin monomer
    Fibrin(ogen) degradation products

Impaired fibrinolytic activity
    Plasminogen depletion
    Tissue plasminogen activator depletion
    Inhibitor elevation

hyaline membranes, which may account for significant pulmonary failure, abnormal arterial blood gases, and pulmonary function tests, including conspicuous altered diffusion capacity. So-called pure "adult shock-lung syndrome" shares similar pathophysiology with fulminant DIC, and in this instance, the pathophysiologic characteristics frequently stay localized to the pulmonary microcirculation instead of becoming a systemic process.[1-4,222,223] However, the pulmonary hyaline membranes of adult shock-lung syndrome and those seen in DIC are alike. For that matter the pulmonary hyaline membranes seen in pediatric respiratory distress syndrome are also composed of the same material: highly polymerized complexes of fibrinogen, fibrin, and FDPs. In this clinical situation the pathophysiology remains much the same as in systemic DIC. This phenomenon has been carefully studied by Ambrus and coworkers.[224-226] In the normal infant during normal delivery, a short period of hypoxia occurs, and concomitant with this is endothelial sloughing with the usual precipitation of fibrin, which is then removed by later activation of the fibrinolytic system. In patients with pediatric respiratory distress syndrome, however, this physiologic event may be altered. In infants born of diabetic mothers the same process occurs, with deposition of polymerized complexes of fibrinogen and fibrin. In these infants, however, elevated levels of alpha-2-macroglobulins inhibit the ability of the fibrinolytic system to degrade these deposits, and hence, a hyaline membrane results.[227] Similar pathophysiology exists in the premature infant. Hypoplasminogenemia and a hypoactive fibrinolytic system are present, and therefore, fibrinogen and fibrin deposition continues unchecked with no ability to resolve this deposition, and a pulmonary hyaline membrane results.[228,229] Comprehension of the pathophysiology in pediatric respiratory distress syndrome has led to the successful use of plasminogen concentrates in infants with this disorder. Figure 7-5 depicts hyaline membranes, including pulmonary edema, in an infant with DIC secondary to meningococcemia.

Disseminated intravascular coagulation is a process associated with hemorrhage and thrombosis, although thrombosis is less clinically evident and less commonly appreciated by the clinician until late in a course of DIC or until an autopsy is done. However, hemorrhage may often be successfully contended with in patients with DIC, whereas thrombosis in the microcirculation and macrocirculation often leads to end-organ damage with irreversible ischemic changes that may lead to death of a patient. Therefore, it is useful to examine those parameters that may accelerate or invoke precipitation of microthrombi and macrothrombi in patients with DIC. Identifiable precipitating causes for acceleration or induction of microthrombi are depicted in Table 7-14. Vasomotor reactions, including elevated catecholamines and progressive acidosis, are an important cause of acceleration or precipitation of thrombi in the circulation.[230,231] Glucocorticoids or ACTH elevation may contribute to the precipitation of microthrombi in patients with DIC, and cautious thought must accompany the use of steroids in these patients, although frequently steroid use is truly warranted.[232] Impaired reticuloendothelial clearance of FDPs, circulating soluble fibrin monomer, or activated coagulation factors (especially factor Xa or thrombin), resulting from fibrin monomer precipitation or use of steroids, could also conspicuously enhance the precipitation of microthrombi.[233] Impaired fibrinolytic system activation may lead to accelerated fibrin deposition throughout the circulation.[1-4,234,235] These mechanisms, including many interplays between these mechanisms, may lead to accelerated fibrin monomer precipitation in the microcirculation and macrocirculation with attendant end-organ damage that may be irreversible and lead to significant morbidity and mortality.[1-3] When examining a patient with DIC, these potential mechanisms and their interplays may be operative and should be kept in mind.

Laboratory Abnormalities

The laboratory findings of DIC may be highly variable, complex, and difficult to interpret unless the intricate pathophysiology of this disorder is clearly understood. The examination of patients with DIC, especially with respect to significant laboratory tests useful for aiding in a diagnosis and monitoring efficacy of therapy, are exceptionally bewildering and sometimes controversial. To further complicate the situation, many newer modalities have become available for assessing the patient with DIC, but the use of many of these modalities is, as yet, without enough experience to determine how clinically applicable they may be.[236-240]

The prothrombin time should be abnormal in the vast majority of patients with DIC for multiple reasons. First, the prothrombin time depends on the ultimate conversion of fibrinogen to fibrin. In DIC, hypofibrinogenemia, FDP interference with fibrin monomer polymerization, and thrombin interference with fibrin monomer polymerization are usually present. Plasmin-induced lysis of factors V and IX, to which the prothrombin time should be sensitive, is often present. In reality, the prothrombin time is prolonged in about 50% to 75% of patients with fulminant DIC, and in 25% of patients the prothrombin time is normal or supernormal. The reasons for this are several. If circulating activated clotting factor(s) is present, such as thrombin or factor Xa, this may accelerate the formation of thrombin and the subsequent conversion of fibrinogen to fibrin in the test system, giving a normal or supernormal result, although some coagulation factors to which the prothrombin time is sensitive may be extremely low. Early degradation products may be rapidly clottable by thrombin and may quickly "gel" the test system, giving a normal or supernormal prothrombin time.[1-3] Therefore, the prothrombin time is generally an unreliable and minimally useful test in patients with DIC.

The activated partial thromboplastin time (APTT) should be prolonged in fulminant DIC for multiple reasons. First, effective plasmin-induced biodegradation of many clotting factors to which the APTT is sensitive occurs, including factors V, VIII, IX, and XI. The PTT, like the prothrombin time, is sensitive to (prolonged by) fibrinogen levels less than 1 g/L (100 mg/dL). The prothrombin time or activated partial thromboplastin time begins to prolong at a fibrinogen level of about 1 g/L (100 mg/dL) or less. The APTT should at least theoretically be prolonged because of FDP inhibition of fibrin monomer polymerization. However, the APTT is prolonged in only 50% to 60% of individuals with fulminant DIC, and therefore, a normal PTT can certainly not be used to rule out a diagnosis of fulminant DIC. The reasons for a supernormal or normal PTT in 40% to 50% of patients are as follows: first, early degradation products may be rapidly thrombin-clottable and gel the test system, giving a supernormal result; second, and perhaps more common, circulating activated clotting factor is usually present in patients with fulminant DIC, and activated clotting factors, especially circulating factor Xa or circulating thrombin, may bypass the necessity of other clotting

factors being measured in the APTT system, leading to rapid conversion of fibrinogen to fibrin and a supernormal test result.[1-3] Like the prothrombin time, the APTT is of negligible usefulness in patients with DIC.

The thrombin or reptilase time is expected to be prolonged in patients with fulminant DIC. Both tests should be prolonged by the presence of circulating FDPs and interference with fibrin monomer polymerization and by the hypofibrinogenemia commonly present in fulminant DIC.[42,121,241-243] Both tests are generally prolonged in patients with DIC, and they may be normal or supernormal in isolated cases. Another bonus test that may be derived from either or both tests is to observe the resultant clot for absence or presence of clot lysis.[1-3] Since many small nonhospital laboratories do not have facilities for assessing the fibrinolytic system, this simple nonquantitative tool may provide significant clinical information. Instead of throwing away the thrombin time– or reptilase time–derived clot, the tube can be set aside for five to 10 minutes and observed for proof of clot dissolution. If the clot is not dissolving in 10 minutes, it may be assumed that plasmin circulating is not clinically significant. If the clot begins to lyse within this period, however, a clinically significant amount of plasmin is probably present.[1-3]

The platelet count is typically dramatically decreased in patients with fulminant DIC. The range, however, may be variable: as low as 2×10^9/L to 3×10^9/L (2,000/mm³ to 3,000/mm³) or greater than 100×10^9/L (100,000/mm³). In most patients with fulminant DIC, however, thrombocytopenia is customarily obvious by examination of a peripheral smear and averages approximately 60×10^9/L (60,000/mm³).[1-3]

In most tests of platelet function, including the template bleeding time, platelet aggregation, and platelet lumi-aggregation, results are abnormal in patients with DIC. This generally happens because of FDP coating of platelet membranes. Other potential reasons for platelet dysfunction include the partial release of platelet procoagulant materials. There is no reason for doing tests of platelet function in patients with fulminant DIC, because abnormal results will invariably be found and add little to the diagnosis. No typical aggregation or lumi-aggregation patterns are noted in DIC, and a wide variety of different types of aggregation and release defects may be seen in different patients.[113,236]

Coagulation factor assays will provide little, if any, clinically worthwhile information in patients with DIC. In most patients with fulminant DIC, systemically circulating activated clotting factors are present, especially factors Xa and IXa and thrombin.[244,245] Coagulation factor assays done by the standard APTT- or prothrombin time–derived laboratory techniques using deficient substrates will give uninterpretable and meaningless results in patients with DIC. For example, if a factor VIII:C assay was attempted in the presence of circulating factor Xa in a patient with DIC, a high level of factor VIII:C would be recorded, since factor Xa bypasses the necessity for factor VIII:C in the test system,[246-248] and a rapid conversion of fibrinogen to fibrin will be noted. A rapid time will be recorded on the typical standard curve,

Figure 7-6. Formation of FDPs

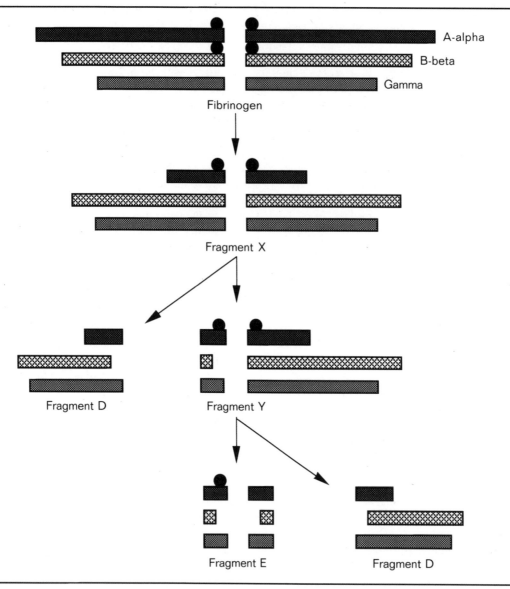

and this will be interpreted as a high factor VIII level when, in fact, no factor VIII:C may be present. Factor assays will give erroneous and meaningless results, are uninterpretable, and surely add little or nothing to the diagnosis in patients with DIC.[1-3]

Fibrin(ogen) degradation products are elevated in 85% to 100% of patients with fulminant DIC depending on the series reported.[1-3,141,236,249,250] It is a common misconception that elevated FDPs are diagnostic of DIC. These degradation products are only diagnostic of plasmin biodegradation of fibrinogen or fibrin, and therefore, FDPs are only indicative of the presence of plasmin.[141] Their method of formation is depicted in Figure 7-6. The possibility of false-negative results in some patients with DIC will be discussed subsequently.

The results of the protamine sulfate test or ethanol gelation test for circulating soluble fibrin monomer are almost always positive[134,251-254] in fulminant and low-grade DIC, and

this is a useful test. Like the FDP titer, however, it is not diagnostic, since both elevated FDPs and circulating soluble fibrin monomer can be noted in other clinical situations as well, including women using oral contraceptives, patients with pulmonary emboli, selected patients with myocardial infarction, patients with certain selected renal diseases, and patients with arterial or venous thrombotic or thromboembolic events.[255,256] On occasion, the protamine sulfate test or ethanol gelation test may be negative for reasons to be discussed. In these rare instances, after successful therapy, the test results may become positive for a short time and then revert to negative.[1-3] The protamine sulfate test as described by Kidder and associates[257] is the most sensitive and clinically applicable test for detecting circulating soluble fibrin.

The antithrombin III determination has become a key test for aiding in the diagnosis and monitoring of therapy in patients with fulminant and low-grade DIC.[258-260] In DIC, activated clotting factors (serine proteases) are overwhelmingly generated during the activation (triggering) process and during the ongoing intravascular coagulation event. When this happens, some circulating activating clotting factor is irreversibly complexed with antithrombin III, leading to considerable decreases of functional AT III in most patients with fulminant and low-grade DIC.[259,261-265] An AT III assay provides one of the few reliable modalities for monitoring efficacy of anticoagulant therapy in patients with DIC. Several studies have compared the clinical applicability of various AT III methodologies, and based on these studies synthetic substrate assays are obviously the method of choice.[266-268] Immunologic assays for AT III ignore biologic function, and their results may be normal or low. Antithrombin III complexing with a serine protease does not necessarily ensure that antigenic determinants, as measured by immunologic assays, will no longer be present.[141] Immunologic assays for AT III should not be used in patients with DIC.[1-3]

Increased platelet turnover and decreased platelet survival will usually be seen in patients with DIC[269,270]; however, since thrombocytopenia is often present, this method of following up patients may be of questionable significance, especially in severely thrombocytopenic patients. Regardless, simple methods for platelet sizing, using automated electronic counting techniques, may be useful in monitoring efficacy of therapy in patients with low-grade DIC if the platelet count is greater than 80×10^9/L (80,000/mm³).[271] Platelet factor 4 and beta-thromboglobulin levels are newer assay techniques that are markers of general platelet reactivity and release. Several reports have suggested that either of these two modalities may be exceptionally worthwhile in aiding in a diagnosis of DIC and in monitoring efficacy of therapy for blunting or termination of the intravascular clotting process.[271-276] Both assays are readily available for the clinical laboratory, and each has attendant advantages and disadvantages. Both platelet factor 4 and beta-thromboglobulin levels are elevated in the majority of patients with DIC. Neither of these modalities are diagnostic of DIC, however, since they may be elevated in a wide variety of intravascular coagulation disorders, including pulmonary emboli, acute myocardial infarction, deep venous thrombosis, and disorders associated with microvascular disease, such as diabetes and autoimmunity.[113,277,278] However, if the assays are elevated in the patient with DIC and then decrease after the institution of specific therapy, this may provide a useful sign that therapy has been successful in either blunting or stopping the intravascular clotting process.

Fibrinopeptide A is commonly elevated in patients with DIC and is an overall assessment of hemostasis, much like platelet factor 4 and beta-thromboglobulin levels. The presence of fibrinopeptide A is diagnostic of the presence of thrombin acting on fibrinogen. Fibrinopeptide A determinations may be of help in assessing efficacy of therapy, as has been suggested in several studies.[1-3,141,188,279-283] However, the determination of fibrinopeptide A is presently laborious for the routine clinical laboratory and is not diagnostic of DIC,

since it may be elevated in a wide variety of other microvascular or macrovascular thrombotic events. High fibrinopeptide A levels followed by decline with the institution of therapy may be a good prognostic sign for stopping or blunting the intravascular clotting process. A newer modality, also available by radioimmunoassay, is that of B-beta 15-42 and related peptide determinations.[284-286] The noting of elevated B-beta 15-42 and related peptide levels may, when done in conjunction with concomitant fibrinopeptide A levels, add greatly to the differential diagnosis of DIC vs primary lysis.[1] Plasmin will rapidly cleave B-beta peptides 1 through 118, 1 through 42, and 15 through 42 (after thrombin has cleaved fibrinopeptide B or amino acid sequence 1 through 14) from the B-beta chain of fibrinogen. The elevation of B-beta 15-42 and related peptides without the elevation of fibrinopeptide A is strong evidence for primary fibrinolysis, whereas the elevation of both fibrinopeptide A and B-beta 15-42 and related peptides is strong evidence for DIC. The formation of B-beta 15-42 and related peptides is summarized in Figure 7-7.

Fibrinolytic system assays are now readily available to the clinical laboratory and provide exceptionally useful information in patients with DIC. Typically decreased plasminogen levels and elevated circulating plasmin are present.[17,150,287] The presence or absence of a secondary fibrinolytic response is of clinical consequence for predicting potential microvascular thrombosis and resultant irreversible end-organ damage in patients. If activation of the fibrinolytic system is inadequate or absent, morbidity and mortality resulting from end-organ damage may be expected to be greater. Fibrinolytic system activation can be assessed by measuring plasminogen and plasmin levels by currently available synthetic substrate techniques.[236,288-292] In this regard, the euglobulin lysis time provides little or no clinically useful information for assessing the fibrinolytic system in clinical disorders, including DIC.[95,293,294] The preparation of a euglobulin fraction, by definition, destroys fibrinolytic inhibitors, and a positive result is of doubtful clinical significance and may simply represent an artifact. This test should not be used in clinical medicine.[95,236] The measurement of fibrinolytic inhibitors, including fast-acting alpha-2-antiplasmin[295-299] and slow-acting alpha-2-macroglobulin,[300-302] may also be of help in assessing the general fibrinolytic system in patients with DIC. If these two fibrinolytic system inhibitors are markedly elevated, the fibrinolytic response may be ineffective with resultant enhanced fibrin monomer precipitation, fibrin deposition, and microvascular and macrovascular thrombosis. Recently, assays for tissue (endothelial) plasminogen activator and tissue plasminogen activator inhibitor have become available. With experience, these determinations may become useful in patients with DIC.

Fibrinogen chromatography may provide a sensitive modality for assessing patients with DIC and may prove useful for aiding in a diagnosis and allowing detailed monitoring of efficacy of therapy in these patients.[303,304-309] Although this modality is usually only available in large centers specializing in thrombohemorrhagic disorders, it has

Figure 7-7. B-Beta 15-42 and Related Peptides

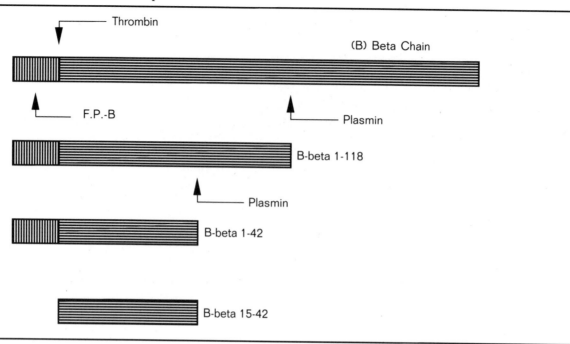

provided exceptionally impressive data and may ultimately become clinically applicable.

By understanding the pathophysiology of DIC, it is clear that hemostasis will be deranged, and results of most common laboratory tests of hemostasis will be dramatically abnormal.[1-4,121,310-312] Therefore, it is useful to establish which tests are of practical significance for providing a high degree of reliability and availability in assessing patients with DIC. Hospital laboratories must be equipped to offer assays that will quickly and reliably allow assessment of patients with DIC. If the laboratory cannot meet this need, the hospital is delivering substandard medical care in allowing admissions of patients with DIC or diseases associated with DIC.[1]

Tests useful for aiding in a diagnosis of DIC are depicted in Table 7-15. Tests routinely used by me for both aiding in a diagnosis of DIC and monitoring efficacy of therapy are noted with an asterisk.[1-4,243,244,313] Generally, I do not indulge in "DIC panels" and prefer to let the particular clinical situation, in combination with clinical judgment, mandate which laboratory tests shall be obtained both initially and after therapy. However, if a true DIC panel were devised, those tests marked with an asterisk would be the recommended contemporary tests for aiding in a diagnosis and monitoring efficacy of therapy, because they are readily available and reliable when evaluated concurrently. However, none of these tests are diagnostic of DIC, and as in all areas of clinical medicine, laboratory modalities must be evaluated in the appropriate clinical setting.[1-4] In addition, most of these laboratory tests are certainly not specific. The presence of soluble fibrin monomer is one of the more specific tests, but it is certainly not diagnostic. If circulating soluble fibrin mono-

mer is present, as detected by the protamine sulfate test or ethanol gelation test, this is strong evidence that thrombin and plasmin have circulated. Since fibrin monomer is created by the presence of thrombin, and fibrin monomer has to be solubilized by complexing with FDPs created by plasmin, this test determines the presence of both enzymes.

Table 7-15. Laboratory Evaluation of Fulminant Disseminated Intravascular Coagulation

Prolonged prothrombin time
Prolonged partial thromboplastin time
Prolonged thrombin time
Prolonged reptilase time
Low clotting factors by assay
Elevated fibrin(ogen) degradation products*
Positive protamine sulfate test*
Decreased antithrombin III*
Thrombocytopenia*
Schistocytosis*
Leukocytosis
Elevated platelet factor 4*
Elevated beta-thromboglobulin
Elevated fibrinopeptide A*
Elevated B-beta 15-42 and related peptides*
Low plasminogen levels*
Circulating plasmin*
Abnormal fibrinogen chromatograms
D-dimer by monoclonal antibody*
Prothrombin fragment 1.2 (F-1.2)?

* Most useful and reliable tests at present

Figure 7-8. The Formation of D-Dimer

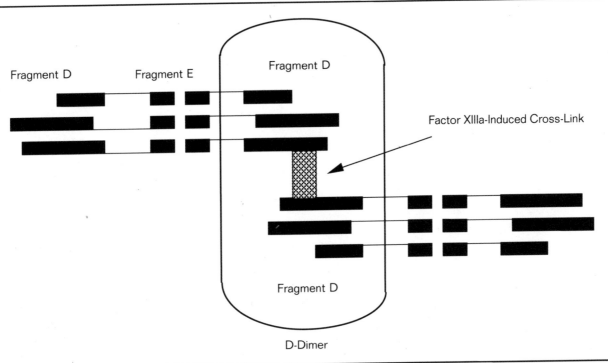

A newer, more specific, diagnostic test for the presence or absence of DIC is the D-dimer assay. D-Dimer is a neo-antigen formed when thrombin initiates the transition of fibrinogen to fibrin and activates factor XIII to cross-link the fibrin formed. This neo-antigen is formed as a result of plasmin digestion of cross-linked fibrin. [286,314] The D-dimer test is, therefore, specific for FDPs, whereas the formation of fibrinolytic degradation products, the X, Y, D and E fragments, may be either fibrinogen- or fibrin-derived, following plasmin digestion. Recently, monoclonal antibodies have been harvested against the D-dimer neo-antigen DD-3B6/22, and these are specific for cross-linked fibrin derivatives containing the D-dimer configuration. [315,316] The formation of D-dimer is depicted in Figure 7-8.

Following the harvesting of monoclonal antibodies, a latex agglutination procedure, using latex particle coated with anti–DD-3B6/22 antibody, has been developed into a commercially available test kit. Studies have shown the monoclonal antibody test, performed by enzyme immunoas-say, to be essentially equivalent to the latex agglutination assay, making the latex agglutination assay applicable for measuring D-dimer in plasma, resulting in a clinically applicable and easily performed test for patients with DIC. [317] I have used this assay as part of my laboratory's battery of DIC tests to assess efficacy of the D-dimer assay to diagnose suspected or documented DIC. [318] I have noted that in patients with documented DIC the D-dimer assay was abnormally elevated (greater than 200 μg/dL) in 93.2% of patients with the mean D-dimer level being 2,047 ng/dL; in those patients in whom DIC was ruled out the average D-dimer assay was only abnormal in 6% with the mean level being 541 ng/dL (Table 7-16).

The D-dimer assay is also of use in the diagnosis of deep venous thrombosis (DVT). The D-dimer level is abnormally elevated in 42% of patients with DVT, with the average level being 325 μg/dL. Based on our laboratory evaluation of the D-dimer assay done by latex agglutination technique, it is a highly useful assay for assessing the probability of

Table 7-16. D-Dimer Assay Results in Fulminant Disseminated Intravascular Coagulation

	DIC (N = 44)	No DIC (N = 17)	Deep venous thrombosis (N = 12)	Normal
D-Dimer	2047.0	541.0	325.0	< 200 ng/mL
AT-III	61.7	108.6	77.5	> 85% NHP
Fibrinopeptide A	24.4	22.8	6.4	< 9 ng/mL
FDP titer	221.6	23.5	23.5	< 40 μg/mL

DIC in appropriate clinical settings. Indeed, of the usual tests used in assessing patients with DIC, it appears to be the most reliable test with respect to probability of being abnormal in patients with confirmed DIC. Using my battery of DIC tests, in the appropriate clinical setting, the reliability of tests used, in descending order of reliability, are the D-dimer assay (abnormal in 93%), the antithrombin III level (abnormal in 89%), the fibrinopeptide A level (abnormal in 88%), and the FDP titer (usually abnormal in 75% of patients). Lane and coworkers have studied the D-dimer fragment in nine patients with DIC and found the levels to be elevated in eight of the nine.[319] Elms and coworkers have also done D-dimer assays in patients with DIC and found the levels to be elevated in all patients they studied.[320]

It seems reasonable to conclude that the D-dimer latex agglutination test, measuring the presence of the neo-antigen DD-3B6/22, is becoming a highly useful test that can easily be performed in a routine clinical laboratory and should be included in the armamentarium of tests used to confirm or rule out DIC. Since the D-dimer test is supplying the same information as both the FDP titer and the protamine sulfate or ethanol gelation test, it can easily replace both of these tests in the diagnostic work-up of a patient with suspected DIC, leading to cost effectiveness and enhanced diagnostic efficacy.[1,318]

Sometimes it appears that AT III, as an alpha-2-globulin, behaves as an acute-phase reactant and may be consumed (complexed) to normal or near normal levels in patients with disseminated malignancy and coexisting DIC.[56,57,60,322,323] In most other instances of fulminant or low-grade DIC, however, this serine protease inhibitor appears to be significantly and rapidly decreased. In addition, protein C, protein S, and fibronectin levels are decreased in patients with DIC, but their diagnostic efficacy and usefulness to monitor therapeutic efficacy remain to be established.[1,324,325] Figure 7-6 depicts fibrinogen and its degradation products, the X, Y, D, and E fragments. Fibrinogen is composed of A-alpha, B-beta, and gamma chains, and plasmin first digests along the carboxy-terminal of the A-alpha chain, giving rise to fragment X. Following this, asymmetric digestion by plasmin along the amino-terminal end of all three chains occurs, giving rise to a fragment Y and a fragment D. Next, fragment Y is further asymmetrically digested on the opposing amino-terminal portion, giving rise to another fragment D and a fragment E, or a so-called N-terminal disulfide knot.[1,141] Fragments X and Y still contain fibrinopeptides, and they are thrombin clottable. Understanding this process and the method of plasminogen-induced digestion allows an understanding regarding why, in selected instances in patients with fulminant or low-grade DIC, FDP titers may be negative. The currently available FDP determinations use latex particles that are "antifibrinogen," and since they are antifibrinogen, thrombin clot tubes are supplied to clot out fibrinogen so latex particles will not react with fibrinogen and erroneously measure fibrinogen instead of its degradation products.[1,141,326-328] However, fibrinogen and its degradation products have common antigenic determinants.[329] When

Table 7-17. Laboratory Evaluation of Low-Grade Disseminated Intravascular Coagulation

Platelet count	Usually normal/borderline
Fibrinogen	Normal or elevated
Factor VIII:C	Normal or elevated
Prothrombin time	Normal or fast
Activated partial thromboplastin time	Normal or fast
Schistocytes	Present in 90%
Fibrin(ogen) degradation products	Usually elevated
Protamine sulfate test	Usually positive
Fibrinopeptide A	Usually elevated
Plasminogen	Usually decreased
Plasmin	Usually present
D-dimer	Usually elevated
Platelet factor IV	Usually elevated

these thrombin clot tubes are used, not only is fibrinogen removed from the system but also fragments X and Y. For this reason, currently available FDP methods measure fragments D and E. In some instances of DIC a minimal secondary fibrinolytic response and minimal plasmin generation may occur, thus there may only be degradation to the X fragment stage or some intermediate between fibrin(ogen) and fragment X. In this instance, there may be nothing for the test to measure since fragment X and its intermediates may be removed from the test system by the thrombin clot tubes used. Alternatively, in instances of fulminant DIC where there is a massive secondary fibrinolytic activation and overwhelming amounts of plasmin circulating, degradation past the D and E stage may occur. Fragments D and E are the last degradation products retaining antigenic determinants capable of being detected by the currently available commercial FDP titer kits. Another problem is overwhelming release of granulocyte enzymes, collagenases, and elastases, which may degrade all available D and E fragments and again give false-negative FDP titers in patients with fulminant DIC.[330] Therefore, the presence of negative FDP titers cannot be used to rule out a diagnosis of fulminant or low-grade DIC. Despite these difficulties, FDP titers are almost always elevated in patients with DIC.

Typical laboratory findings of low-grade DIC are significantly different from those seen in fulminant DIC. Results of many usual tests of hemostasis are normal or near normal, and typical findings in low-grade DIC are depicted in Table 7-17. The platelet count is usually within normal limits or borderline in the patient with low-grade DIC. Most of these patients, however, develop decreased platelet survival and increased turnover of platelets resulting from platelet con-

Table 7-18. Average Laboratory Values in Fulminant Disseminated Intravascular Coagulation

	Pretherapy	Posttherapy
Prothrombin time	16.8 sec	13.6 sec
Activated partial thromboplastin time	55.8 sec	42.4 sec
Reptilase time	26.8 sec	18.8 sec
Thrombin time	23.8 sec	15.6 sec
FDP level	>40	>40
Platelets	64.6×10^9/L	204×10^9/L
Protamine sulfate	Positive	Positive
Fibrinogen	1. 29 g/L	2.21 g/L
Antithrombin III	57.8%	101.4%

Table 7-19. Reliability of Laboratory Tests in Fulminant Disseminated Intravascular Coagulation (Descending Order of Reliability)

	Pretherapy (% abnormal)	Posttherapy (% abnormal)
FDP level	100%	24%
Antithrombin III	97%	16%
Platelets	97%	34%
Protamine sulfate	92%	18%
Thrombin time	81%	32%
Fibrinogen	79%	16%
Prothrombin time	76%	58%
Activated partial thromboplastin time	63%	24%
Reptilase time	58%	8%

sumption, and this is often called a compensated state. Like the platelet count, fibrinogen levels are usually compensated, and increased turnover and decreased survival of fibrinogen and factor V, factor VIII, and other coagulation proteins are noted. Fibrinogen levels are usually normal or elevated. Fibrinogen levels may be significantly elevated in low-grade DIC, because fibrinogen may behave as an acute-phase reactant in many disorders associated with low-grade DIC, including malignancy, autoimmune disorders, and chronic inflammatory diseases. For similar reasons, factor VIII and factor V levels may be normal or elevated in patients with low-grade DIC. Like platelets and fibrinogen, increased turnover and decreased survival of factor VIII:C and factor V may be seen in patients with low-grade DIC. The prothrombin time is usually within normal limits or supernormal in patients with low-grade DIC. Likewise, the APTT is commonly within normal limits or is short (supernormal). Red blood cell fragments or schistocytes are present in almost all patients with low-grade DIC but are only present in 50% of patients with fulminant DIC. This is most probably because of the underlying disease processes giving rise to low-grade DIC, such as malignancy and related disorders. Fibrin(ogen) degradation products are almost always elevated in patients with low-grade DIC and are useful for aiding in a diagnosis. Elevation of these fragments accounts for much of the pathophysiologic characteristics and low-grade hemorrhage seen in patients with low-grade DIC because of the platelet dysfunction induced. Soluble fibrin monomer is commonly detected in patients with low-grade DIC and, like the FDP titer, can be a helpful and specific finding. Often, elevated levels of fibrinopeptide A, beta-thromboglobulin, platelet factor 4, and B-beta 15-42 and related peptides are noted in patients with low-grade DIC. The diagnostic efficacy of these tests remains unclear but appears promising. The use of these assays in monitoring efficacy of therapy is yet to be determined, but they may prove helpful. Circulating plasmin, associated with hypoplasminogenemia, is also a common finding in patients with low-grade DIC. In the appropriate clinical setting, the noting of elevated D-dimer, FDPs, a positive protamine sulfate test, elevated fibrinopeptide A, elevated B-beta 15-42 peptides, and hypoplasminogenemia are strongly suggestive of low-grade DIC.[1-3]

Table 7-18 demonstrates average laboratory values, using commonly available laboratory modalities, in a series of 48 patients with fulminant DIC.[331] Both average values for pretreatment and posttreatment are listed. Posttreatment values were derived four to six hours after delivering therapy that was considered to have stopped or significantly blunted the intravascular clotting process. Note that the prothrombin time and partial thromboplastin time were only borderline prolonged. In most patients, these two tests are corrected to well within normal limits following effective therapy. The average platelet count was 64.6×10^9/L (64,600/mm³) when making the diagnosis and 204×10^9/L (204,000/mm³) after the imparting of effective therapy. The average fibrinogen level was 1.29 g/L (129 mg/dL) before therapy and 2.21 g/L (221 mg/dL) after therapy. In this series of patients, the average biologic AT III level was 58% when making a diagnosis and well within the normal range four to six hours after delivering therapy that caused cessation or significant blunting of the intravascular clotting process.

Laboratory testing and the interpretation of laboratory results for aiding in a diagnosis and monitoring of therapy in patients with fulminant DIC are exceptionally bewildering and controversial, since very few series of patients have been described. The reliability of laboratory testing in patients with fulminant DIC is listed in Table 7-19.[331] In this series of patients, FDPs were elevated in 100% of patients when making a diagnosis but remained elevated in 25% of patients following effective therapy. Fibrin(ogen) degradation product determinations are of reasonable diagnostic value but are of

Table 7-20. Average Laboratory Values in Low-Grade Disseminated Intravascular Coagulation

Test	Pretherapy	Posttherapy
Prothrombin time	14.4 sec	12.6 sec
Activated partial thromboplastin time	43.9 sec	34.5 sec
Reptilase time	27.8 sec	18.2 sec
Thrombin time	17.7 sec	11.9 sec
FDP level	>40	>40
Platelet count	190 x 10⁹/L	254 x 10⁹/L
Protamine test	Positive	Positive
Fibrinogen level	2.31 g/L	3.33 g/L
Antithrombin level	83.9%	116.8%

Table 7-21. Reliability of Laboratory Tests in Low-Grade Disseminated Intravascular Coagulation

Test	Pretherapy (% abnormal)	Posttherapy (% abnormal)
FDP level	100%	50%
Protamine test	80%	20%
Prothrombin time	80%	30%
Antithrombin III	70%	10%
Reptilase time	70%	0%
Platelet count	50%	30%
Fibrinogen	30%	0%
Activated partial thromboplastin time	30%	10%
Thrombin time	30%	0%

only limited value for monitoring efficacy of therapy. The AT III level was decreased in 97% of patients when making a diagnosis and was only decreased in 16% of patients after delivering therapy that was thought to be successful at stopping the intravascular clotting process. The AT III level is useful both for aiding in a diagnosis and providing information regarding termination of the intravascular clotting process. The most dependable laboratory tests for aiding in a diagnosis of DIC and for monitoring efficacy of therapy in fulminant DIC are the D-dimer assay, the FDP titer, the AT III level, the platelet count, the presence of soluble fibrin monomer, and the finding of elevated fibrinopeptide A levels. The thrombin time, fibrinogen level, prothrombin time, PTT, and reptilase time all appear to be generally unreliable. In this series of patients, the PTT was only prolonged in 63% of patients when making a diagnosis of fulminant DIC, emphasizing that the APTT is not a credible test for aiding in a diagnosis of DIC or for monitoring therapy.

Table 7-20 summarizes average pretreatment and posttreatment values for commonly available laboratory modalities in a group of patients with low-grade DIC.[330,331] The prothrombin time and PTT are even less reliable as diagnostic aids in low-grade DIC. The fibrinogen level and platelet count are, likewise, less useful than in fulminant DIC. In low-grade DIC, the average fibrinogen level was 2.31 g/L (231 mg/dL) when making a diagnosis and 3.3 g/L (330 mg/dL) following therapy. The average platelet count was 190 x 10⁹/L (190,000/mm³) when making a diagnosis and increased to 254 x 10⁹/L (254,000/mm³) following therapy. The AT III level is also less reliable in diagnosing low-grade DIC; however, it appears to be almost as useful for monitoring efficacy of therapy as in fulminant DIC.

Table 7-21 depicts the percentage of patients demonstrating an abnormal laboratory test when making a diagnosis (pretherapy) and the percentage of those tests staying abnormal after it was clinically found that the intravascular clot-

ting process had been successfully suspended. The FDP titer was elevated in all patients and remained elevated in 50% of patients after therapy. Likewise, soluble fibrin monomer was present in 80% of patients with low-grade DIC but remained circulating in 20% of patients after successful therapy. The prothrombin time appears to be more useful in low-grade DIC than in fulminant DIC. The AT III level is of less diagnostic value, being decreased in only 70% of patients with low-grade DIC but remaining depressed in only 10% of patients after therapy, which suggests that it is a useful monitoring modality after therapy. The platelet count, fibrinogen level, APTT, and thrombin time are not useful diagnostic tests in low-grade DIC. The most reliable commonly available laboratory tests for aiding in a diagnosis and monitoring therapy in low-grade DIC are the D-dimer assay, the fibrinopeptide A assay, the FDP titer, the presence of soluble fibrin monomer, the prothrombin time, and the AT III determination.[243,244,331,332] The reptilase time, platelet count, fibrinogen level, APTT, and thrombin time are of negligible diagnostic reliability in low-grade DIC.[1-3]

Table 7-22 depicts the probability of pretreatment and posttreatment coagulation abnormalities in all forms of DIC. The noting of elevated D-dimer, elevated FDP levels, a depressed AT III level in conjunction with thrombocytopenia, and a positive protamine sulfate test or ethanol gelation test are the most reliable laboratory determinations for aiding in and confirming a diagnosis of DIC and for determining success of therapy.[243,244,330-332] Therefore, other traditionally used tests, including the prothrombin time, thrombin time, fibrinogen level, reptilase time, and partial thromboplastin time, are customarily unreliable as diagnostic or therapeutic indices. The D-dimer assay and the fibrinopeptide A assay are the most reliable newer tests available. The newest methods for evaluating DIC are totally automated, or at least automatable, and this may aid greatly in rendering rapid and

Table 7-22. Reliability of Laboratory Tests in Disseminated Intravascular Coagulation (Descending Order of Probability)

D-dimer
Antithrombin III
Fibrinopeptide A
Platelet factor 4
FDP
Platelet count
Protamine test
Thrombin time
Fibrinogen
Prothrombin time
Activated partial thromboplastin time
Reptilase time

Table 7-24. Molecular Markers Useful for the Differential Diagnosis of DIC vs Primary Lysis

Marker	DIC	Primary lysis
Fibrinopeptide A	Elevated	Normal
Fibrinopeptide B	Elevated	Normal
B-beta 15-42 peptide	Elevated	Normal
B-beta 1-42 peptide	Elevated	Elevated
B-beta 1-118 peptide	Elevated	Elevated
Platelet factor 4	Elevated	Normal
Beta-thromboglobulin	Elevated	Normal
D-dimer	Elevated	Normal
Fibronectin	Decreased	Normal

reliable laboratory data for diagnosis and monitoring efficacy of therapy in patients with DIC. Molecular marker profiling for DIC has become available and is fully automatable.[333-335] These molecular markers are not only useful for diagnosing DIC but are also worthwhile for providing a differential diagnosis of DIC vs primary fibrinolysis or DIC vs TTP. The differential diagnosis of DIC vs TTP by molecular marker profiling is depicted in Table 7-23. The differential diagnosis of DIC vs primary fibrinolysis by automated molecular marker profiling is summarized in Table 7-24. In uncommon instances of an extremely difficult differential diagnosis between DIC, TTP, or primary fibrinolysis, the use of these molecular markers may be exceptionally suitable.

Therapy for DIC

Fulminant

The treatment of fulminant and low-grade DIC is confusing to many and sometimes truly controversial.[336] Concomitant with this controversy and confusion is the global per-

Table 7-23. Molecular Markers Useful for the Differential Diagnosis of DIC vs TTP

Marker	DIC	TTP
6-keto-PGF-1-alpha	Normal	Decreased
Thromboxanes	Increased	Increased
Platelet factor 4	Increased	Increased
Beta-thromboglobulin	Increased	Increased
Plasminogen activator	Normal/increased	Decreased
B-beta 15-42 peptide	Increased	Normal
Fibrinopeptide A	Increased	Normal
Fibrinopeptide B	Increased	Normal

ception that therapy is often futile and that most patients succumb to the disease process. However, most published comments about therapy are based on fable instead of fact and frenzy instead of clinical judgment.[1-3] The reasons for this are because very few objective series of patients with DIC, with respect to therapy given, morbidity, mortality, and survival, have been published. Many argue vehemently opposing the use of heparin in fulminant or low-grade DIC despite the amazing lack of published case reports or series in the literature regarding the adverse effects of heparin in DIC.[337-339] Similarly, many advocate strongly the use of heparin in DIC, although a surprising void exists of published reports authenticating positive effects of heparin in patients with DIC.[340-342] If logical, aggressive, and sequential therapy is undertaken in the patient with DIC, morbidity and mortality are not as dismal as suspected.[243,244,331,336] Clinicians should synthesize judgment with respect to therapy formulated on experience and published series of patients and documentation instead of dogma and mythology. Hopefully, the future will offer more guidelines than are available now with respect to successes and failures with various forms of potential therapy.

My approach to therapy in fulminant DIC is somewhat vigorous and is summarized in Table 7-25. As a fundamental principle, therapy must be individualized for each patient depending on clinical findings and manifestations of the process. Individualization must be based on etiology of the DIC, age, hemodynamic status, site and severity of hemorrhage, site and severity of thrombosis, and other pertinent clinical factors. Although this approach is aggressive, it has been associated with a high survival rate (76%) and low morbidity in patients with classic fulminant DIC.[243,244,331] The essential therapeutic modality to be delivered to a patient with fulminant DIC is that of an aggressive but reasonable therapeutic approach to eliminate or treat the triggering disease process thought to be responsible for DIC.[243,244,331,336,343,344] Sometimes this is impossible; however, successful therapy to remove or blunt the triggering event

Table 7-25. Logical and Sequential Therapy for Fulminant Disseminated Intravascular Coagulation

Individualize therapy
    Site(s) and severity of hemorrhage
    Site(s) and severity of thrombosis
    Precipitating disease state
    Hemodynamic status
    Age
    Other clinical considerations

Treat or remove the triggering process
    Evacuate uterus
    Antibiotics
    Control shock
    Volume replacement
    Maintain blood pressure
    Steroids?
    Antineoplastic therapy
    Other indicated therapy

Stop intravascular clotting process
    Subcutaneous calcium heparin
    Intravenous heparin?
    Antiplatelet agents
    Antithrombin concentrate

Component therapy as indicated
    Platelet concentrates
    Packed red blood cells (washed)
    Antithrombin concentrate
    Fresh frozen plasma
    Prothrombin complex
    Cryoprecipitate

Inhibit residual fibrino(geno)lysis
    Aminocaproic acid
    Tranexamic acid

may sometimes stop or at least significantly blunt the intravascular clotting process. If endeavors are not made to treat the triggering event and triggering pathophysiology, subsequent attempts at anticoagulant therapy, including heparin, will rarely, if ever, alleviate the disseminated intravascular clotting process.[1-4,336] Attempts to treat the underlying disease process do provide a reasonable chance of the patient responding to therapy designed to stop the intravascular clotting process.

Sometimes it is impossible or unlikely that the underlying disease pathophysiology can be alleviated. Frequently the removal of the triggering pathophysiology will stop the disease process, and the classic example of this is an obstetric accident. More commonly, however, therapy for the underlying process will at least blunt the process enough so the patient may respond to anticoagulant therapy. Sometimes this therapy will stop the intravascular clotting process, and another common situation where this happens is septicemia. The successful treatment of septicemia will blunt the process in many patients, giving them the opportunity to respond to anticoagulant therapy. Sometimes treatment of septicemia

and alleviating the triggering pathophysiology will stop the intravascular clotting process. In cases of obstetric accidents of any type, except amniotic fluid embolism, anticoagulant therapy, especially heparin, is rarely required. Simply evacuating the uterus, or in rare instances hysterectomy, will typically rapidly stop the intravascular clotting process.[345,346] Although it is often difficult to convince the obstetrician/gynecologist to take a hemorrhaging hypofibrinogenemic patient to the operating room, the results are rewarding when this is accomplished. The results are usually immediate and dramatic.[1-3] In septicemia, specific antibiotic therapy, alleviation of shock, volume replacement, the potential use of steroids, and other specific therapy to maintain hemodynamics, will often cause significant blunting of the intravascular clotting process and on some occasions may stop the DIC process. Each case must be evaluated on its own merits depending on the clinical situation and what the clinician determines to be the dominant triggering event. However, the crucial point is that an attempt to treat the triggering event is the essential therapeutic modality that must be administered to the patient with DIC.

Most patients, except those with DIC secondary to obstetric accidents or massive liver failure, will next usually require anticoagulant therapy of some form. The use of subcutaneous low-dose heparin appears to be highly effective in DIC and has been my choice of anticoagulant therapy for the last 10 years.[243,244,331] Anticoagulant therapy is indicated to stop or blunt the triggering pathophysiologic event if the patient continues to bleed or clot significantly for about four hours after the initiation of therapy. This time period is somewhat empiric and depends on the sites and severity of bleeding. When the patient continues to bleed in this situation, subcutaneous calcium heparin is given at 80 to 100 units/kg every four to six hours as the clinical situation, site and severity of bleeding and thrombosis, and patient size dictate. Low-dose subcutaneous heparin appears to be as effective or possibly more effective than larger doses of intravenous heparin in fulminant DIC.[192,243,244,347,348] With this approach one often notes cessation of AT III consumption, lowering of FDP levels, increases in fibrinogen levels, and slow or rapid correction of other abnormal laboratory modalities of fulminant DIC in three to four hours, followed shortly by blunting or cessation of clinically significant hemorrhage and thrombosis.

The use of subcutaneous low-dose heparin, instead of intravenous heparin, appears reasonable for several reasons: (1) if the patient does not respond, larger doses of heparin can always be administered if thought appropriate; (2) unlike fears with larger intravenous doses of heparin, low-dose subcutaneous heparin therapy is associated with minimal chances of increasing the risk of hemorrhage; and (3) most importantly, the use of low-dose subcutaneous heparin has been as efficacious as large-dose heparin therapy and is associated with a high patient survival rate when used with other therapeutic modalities.[1-3] Because of current understanding of the heparin/AT III/serine protease/thrombin/fibrinogen axis, low-dose subcutaneous heparin, from a theoretic standpoint and in published reports, is thought to be equal or more effective than larger intravenous doses of USP heparin.[192,347,348]

Other anticoagulant modalities available, depending on the clinician's experience, are intravenous heparin, the use of combination antiplatelet agents, or the use of AT III concentrates. Those clinicians using intravenous heparin therapy for fulminant DIC usually deliver between 20,000 and 30,000 units per 24 hours by constant infusion, and this may be associated with significant blunting or cessation of the intravascular clotting process. Combination antiplatelet agents are far less effective in fulminant DIC but on occasion may be called for as the specific clinical situation dictates. Fulminant DIC has been successfully treated with AT III concentrates in small groups of patients, and preliminary experience would suggest these to be effective for fulminant DIC.[1-3,259,349-351] From a theoretic standpoint, AT III concentrates should be highly effective in treating fulminant DIC. With respect to heparin, it is my opinion that subcutaneous heparin, or heparin in any dose, is contraindicated in patients with fulminant DIC and central nervous system insults of any type, patients with DIC associated with fulminant liver failure, and in most instances of obstetric accidents.[1-3] About 75% of patients will respond to these two sequential therapeutic steps.

If patients continue to bleed after beginning reasonable attempts to treat the triggering pathophysiology thought to be responsible for DIC and after starting anticoagulant therapy, however, the most probable cause of continued bleeding is component depletion. In this instance, the precise components missing and clinically thought to be contributing to hemorrhage should be defined and given. The delivery of certain components is associated with attendant hazards in patients with ongoing DIC, and as a general guideline, only concentrates and components void of fibrinogen and other clotting factors should be delivered to a patient with ongoing DIC, ongoing DIC being manifest by continued severe depression of the AT III level. If, however, the AT III level, or other specific monitoring modality that the clinician chooses to use, returns to normal and is associated with a potential response, it can be assumed the intravascular clotting process has been controlled, and in this instance any component or concentrate thought necessary can safely be given. Generally, the only components generally safe in patients with an active uncontrolled DIC process are washed packed red blood cells, platelet concentrates, AT III concentrates, and nonclotting protein containing volume expanders, such as plasma protein fraction, albumin, and hydroxyethyl starch. If a patient continues to bleed after successful anticoagulant therapy and cessation of the DIC process, as manifest by correcting AT III levels, then any component thought depleted to the point of contributing, with a high degree of probability, to continued hemorrhage is safe to give to the patient.

However, components containing clotting factors and/or fibrinogen are, generally, not safe in patients with ongoing DIC, and the use of fresh frozen plasma and fresh whole blood may be associated with enhanced hemorrhage and thrombosis in a patient with active DIC to whom these components are unwisely delivered.[243,244,352] Not only has this been seen clinically but would be expected from a theoretic standpoint by understanding the pathophysiology of DIC. If whole blood, fresh frozen plasma, or cryoprecipitate is given to a patient with ongoing intravascular coagulation, it is to be expected that plasmin will readily biodegrade most, if not all, of the coagulation factors supplied.[352] This event in itself may not be particularly harmful but is surely not helpful.[1] Of more significance is that these components contain fibrinogen and are associated with a great potential for creation of even higher levels of FDPs that will further impair hemostasis by interference with fibrin monomer polymerization, further impair already compromised platelet function, and will lead to enhanced microvascular deposition and subsequent thrombocytopenia.[141,352] A reasonable approach is to assess the patient after anticoagulant therapy and continued bleeding. If the AT III level, or other selected monitoring modality, has returned to normal or near normal, any component thought significantly depleted and likely to be contributing to continued hemorrhage is reasonable to use. Alternatively, if the patient continues to bleed after anticoagulant therapy has been delivered and the AT III level and other modalities used to monitor the patient remain abnormal, it is highly probable in this situation that the intravascular clotting process has not been controlled and continues. In this instance the component(s) should be restricted to washed packed red blood cells, platelets, volume expanders, and AT III.[1-3] By adhering to these three sequential aggressive steps, greater than 95% of patients will stop hemorrhaging if they are going to survive.

In those rare instances where bleeding continues afer these three sequential steps are instituted, the next step in the therapy of fulminant DIC is to consider inhibition of the fibrinolytic system. This step is rarely needed and is only necessary in about 3% of patients. In some rare instances, although the intravascular coagulation process has been alleviated, the patient may continue to bleed because, for unexplained reasons, secondary fibrinolysis has continued with the concomitant biodegradation of the usual plasma protein targets of plasmin. In this rare instance, which is necessary in less than 3% to 5% of all patients with fulminant DIC, antifibrinolytic therapy may be indicated. However, antifibrinolytic therapy should never be delivered to patients with ongoing DIC, because these patients desperately need the fibrinolytic system to keep the microcirculation as clear of microthrombi as possible.[1-3] Antifibrinolytic therapy should never be delivered unless the other sequential steps have been resorted to and it has been well documented from the laboratory and clinical standpoint that the intravascular coagulation process has been terminated by noting correction of biologic AT III levels or other modalities used by the clinician to monitor the event. Antifibrinolytic therapy should never be used unless the cessation of DIC and the

Table 7-26. Pretherapy and Posttherapy Antithrombin III Values in Acute Disseminated Intravascular Coagulation (38 Patients)

	Pretherapy	Posttherapy	Normal
	66.3% ± 27	115.0% ± 30.2	85% –116%
Percentage of patients abnormal	89%	19%	

presence of significant amounts of circulating plasmin are documented by laboratory modalities. In those rare instances where antifibrinolytic therapy is indicated, epsilon amino-caproic acid is given as an initial 5- to 10-g slow intravenous push followed by 2 to 4 g per hour for 24 hours or until bleeding stops. This agent should be used with great caution as it may cause ventricular arrhythmias, severe hypotension, and severe hypokalemia.[353-356] Epsilon aminocaproic acid or any fibrinolytic inhibitor used in a patient with ongoing DIC may cause enhanced precipitation of fibrin in the microcirculation and macrocirculation and often lead to fatal disseminated thrombosis.[1-3] Tranexamic acid has recently become available as a potent antifibrinolytic agent, although as of yet no significant experience has been reported with this agent in DIC.

Table 7-26 depicts a series of patients with fulminant DIC to show how AT III levels may be used as an aid in the diagnosis and may be used to monitor potential efficacy of therapy.[243,244,357] The biologic AT III levels are significantly depressed when making a diagnosis. When noting a patient with fulminant or low-grade DIC and normal or high AT III levels, underlying disseminated malignancy should be searched for and considered.[57,60] In almost all individuals receiving successful therapy, however, an associated rapid return to normal or near normal biologic AT III levels is noted. Even in those instances when the AT III levels are normal or elevated, as in association with malignancy, the delivery of effective therapy is frequently associated with

further increases in AT III levels. When the AT III level is noted to increase to normal or near normal levels after the delivery of therapy, it can be assumed with reasonable certainty that the intravascular coagulation process has undergone cessation or significant blunting. More clinical experience may demonstrate that drastic dropping of previously elevated fibrinopeptide A levels, beta-thromboglobulin levels, or platelet factor 4 levels may be of equal efficacy in assessing response to therapeutic manipulation in patients with DIC. Table 7-27 depicts a patient with fulminant DIC treated with miniheparin.[244] The pretherapy and posttherapy laboratory values are listed. Within four hours the laboratory modalities were generally corrected, which was associated with termination of clinical hemorrhage. Table 7-28 shows a patient treated with an investigational AT III concentrate, and the patient not only stopped bleeding and thrombosing but also survived the DIC process with minimal morbidity.[349]

Low Grade

Therapy for low-grade DIC is approached much differently than that for fulminant DIC, and an outline is summarized in Table 7-29. Most patients with low-grade DIC do not have life-threatening hemorrhage but have bothersome hemorrhage that is often associated with diffuse superficial or deep venous thrombosis and thromboembolus.[194,358] As with fulminant DIC, the essential therapy for a patient with low-grade DIC is treatment for the underlying disease process, which will frequently produce cessation of the intravascular clotting

Table 7-27. Low-Dose Heparin Therapy in Disseminated Intravascular Coagulation (Typical Response)

Test	Pretherapy	Posttherapy (4 hours)	Posttherapy (8 hours)
Fibrinogen	.68 g/L	1.04 g/L	4.5 g/L
Platelets	48 x 10⁹/L	270 x 10⁹/L	270 x 10⁹/L
Thrombin time	22 sec	22 sec	20 sec
Reptilase time	20 sec	16 sec	24 sec
Prothrombin time	16 sec	14.8 sec	12 sec
Activated partial thromboplastin time	48 sec	36 sec	36 sec
FDP titer	> 40	> 40	< 10
Protamine test	Positive	Positive	Negative
Antithrombin III level	60%	76%	185%

Table 7-28. Antithrombin III Concentrate Therapy in Disseminated Intravascular Coagulation (Typical Response)

Test	Pretherapy	Posttherapy (12 hours)	Posttherapy (24 hours)
Fibrinogen	.3 g/L	1.1 g/L	1.5 g/L
Platelets	62×10^9/L	90×10^9/L	128×10^9/L
Thrombin time	30 sec	18 sec	16 sec
Reptilase time	38 sec	18 sec	18 sec
Prothrombin time	18 sec	13 sec	12 sec
Activated partial thromboplastin time	62 sec	59 sec	38 sec
FDP level	> 40	> 10	< 10
Protamine test	Positive	Positive	Negative
Antithrombin III level	48%	102%	115%

process and alleviation of hemorrhage and thrombosis. If treatment for the triggering disease process thought responsible for the intravascular coagulation process does not stop the event, at least it will often greatly blunt the process so that bothersome bleeding or thrombosis ceases being a clinical problem. If this first step is vigorously attempted and hemorrhage, thrombosis, and/or thromboembolus continue, then anticoagulant therapy is indicated. However, since patients with low-grade DIC usually do not have life-threatening hemorrhage, anticoagulant therapy need not be vigorous in many instances. Vigorous anticoagulant therapy may be contraindicated in selected instances of malignancy, especially those with intracranial metastases.[359,360]

Combination antiplatelet therapy is frequently successful in stopping a low-grade DIC process if attempts to treat the triggering pathophysiology have also been initiated. A combination of two antiplatelet agents, with independent mechanisms of action, are often needed. Commonly, a combination of acetylsalicylic acid, 600 mg orally twice daily to be taken with 30 mL of liquid antacid plus dipyridamole 50 to 75 mg orally four times daily will stop a low-grade intravascular coagulation process within 24 to 30 hours, shown by

generalized correction of laboratory parameters and the cessation of bleeding and/or thrombosis. Alternatively, the use of sulfinpyrazone, 200 mg orally twice daily to be taken with 30 mL of liquid antacid plus dipyridamole 50 mg orally four times a day may be used.[361,362] Both acetylsalicylic acid and sulfinpyrazone are cyclo-oxygenase inhibitors leading to a decreased synthesis of thromboxane A_2, and it is often without avail to use both agents in combination since they both have the same mechanism of action.[363] Dipyridamole, however, is an inhibitor of phosphodiesterase, leading to increased concentrations of intraplatelet cyclic AMP.[117] Therefore, the ideal combination is acetylsalicylic acid plus dipyridamole or sulfinpyrazone plus dipyridamole. Miniheparin, or intravenous heparin, is rarely indicated in patients

Table 7-30. Therapy for Disseminated Intravascular Coagulation in Malignancy

Treat the malignancy (trigger)
    Surgery as indicated
    Radiation as indicated
    Chemotherapy, hormonal therapy as indicated

Stop intravascular clotting process
    Antiplatelet agents
    Low-dose heparin*
    Intravenous heparin*
    Warfarins**

Component therapy as indicated
    Platelet concentrates
    Packed red blood cells (washed)
    Fresh frozen plasma
    Antithrombin III concentrate

Inhibit residual fibrinolysis
    Rarely needed or indicated

Individualize therapy as indicated

* Hazardous with central nervous system metastases
** Usually ineffective

Table 7-29. Sequential Therapy for Low-Grade Disseminated Intravascular Coagulation

Therapy for the triggering disease process
    Any therapy clinically indicated

Anticoagulant therapy when indicated
    Antiplatelet agents
    Low-dose calcium heparin
    No warfarins

Component therapy
    Only rarely indicated or necessary

Inhibit fibrinolysis
    Almost never indicated

Individualize therapy as indicated

Table 7-31. Conditions Similar to Disseminated Intravascular Coagulation

Pediatric respiratory distress syndrome
Adult "shock lung" syndrome
Hemolytic-uremic syndrome
Malignant hypertension
Pre-eclampsia or frank eclampsia
Glomerulonephritis
Collagen vascular disorders
Circulating immune complex diseases
Serum sickness
Cavernous hemangiomas
Hemangio(endothelio)sarcoma
Traumatic arteriovenous fistulae
Vasculitis
Rocky Mountain spotted fever
Mycoplasma infections
"Waring blender" syndrome
Thrombotic thrombocytopenic purpura

with low-grade DIC. However, low-dose subcutaneous calcium heparin therapy should be considered in patients with low-grade DIC that appears to be evolving into a more subacute or fulminant DIC process or who are developing active thrombotic or thromboembolic problems. Replacement therapy is rarely, if ever, indicated in the patient with low-grade DIC unless the patient demonstrates component depletion from other triggering mechanisms, such as the patient with low-grade DIC and malignancy who also demonstrates thrombocytopenia because of cytotoxic therapy, bone marrow replacement, hypersplenism, or other mechanisms. Inhibition of the fibrinolytic system with epsilon aminocaproic acid or tranexamic acid is also rarely, if ever, indicated in low-grade DIC.

Malignancy

Successful therapy for DIC in the patient with malignancy represents a major clinical challenge and is summarized in Table 7-30. Effective therapy is multiphasic and must be approached in a sequential and logical manner if the process is to be controlled. The first and essential modality is to treat the malignancy itself since this is providing the trigger(s) for intravascular coagulation.[57,60,336] Therapy may be surgical, radiotherapeutic, or chemotherapeutic as the clinical situation warrants. Treatment of the specific tumor is often associated with cessation or significant improvement in DIC, and until attempts at antineoplastics are instituted, therapy for bleeding or thrombosis is often unsuccessful.[56,57,60,244,359] A classic example of response to antineoplastics is seen in patients with prostatic carcinoma.[364,365] These individuals will often show a marked improvement of their hemorrhagic, thrombotic, or thromboembolic problems with the institution of diethylstilbesterol therapy or cytotoxic chemotherapy as clinically indicated. This phenomenon may also be noted in other tumors when antineoplastic therapy is started. The

use of antiplatelet agents, especially as aspirin plus dipyridamole, has been associated with correction of altered laboratory tests suggestive of DIC, including normalization of fibrinogen and platelet survival in patients with malignancy and low-grade DIC. Patients with malignancy are also notoriously resistant to anticoagulant therapy with respect to stopping minor to moderate bleeding and major thrombotic and thromboembolic episodes, all of which are commonly caused by low-grade DIC.[1-4,56,57,60,359]

Summary

Considerable attention has been devoted to interrelationships between current concepts of the etiology, pathophysiology, diagnosis, and management of fulminant and low-grade DIC that have remained confusing. Only by clearly understanding these pathophysiologic interrelationships can the clinician and laboratorian appreciate the divergent and wide spectrum of often confusing clinical and laboratory findings in patients with DIC. Many therapeutic decisions to be made in these patients are controversial and will remain so until more series of patients are published concerning specific therapeutic modalities and survival patterns. Many syndromes that are organ specific share common pathophysiology with DIC but are typically identified as an independent disease entity, such as hemolytic-uremic syndrome, adult shock lung syndrome, eclampsia, and many other isolated organ-specific disorders. Many of these similar disorders, some systemic and some organ specific or multiorgan specific, are listed in Table 7-31.

References

1. Bick RL: Disseminated intravascular coagulation and related syndromes: a clinical review. Semin Thromb Hemost 14:299, 1988.

2. Bick RL: Disseminated intravascular coagulation, ch 2. In: Disseminated Intravascular Coagulation. CRC Press, Boca Raton, FL, 1983, p 31.

3. Bick RL: Disseminated intravascular coagulation and related sydromes, ch 6. In: Disorders of Hemostasis and Thrombosis: Principles of Clinical Practice. Thieme, Inc., New York, 1985, p 157.

4. Baker WF: Clinical aspects of disseminated intravascular coagulation: a clinician's point of view. Semin Thromb Hemost 15:1, 1989.

5. Lasch HG, DL Henne, K Huth, W Sandritter: Pathophysiology, clinical manifestations, and therapy of consumptive coagulopathy. Am J Cardiol 20:381, 1967.

6. Rodriquez-Erdman F: Bleeding due to increased intravascular blood coagulation: hemorrhagic syndromes caused by consumption of blood-clotting factors (consumption coagulopathies). N Engl J Med 273:1370, 1965.

7. Dubber AHC, GP McNicol, AS Douglas: Acquired hypofibrinogenemia: the "defibrination syndrome." A study of seven patients. Scott Med J 12:138, 1967.

8. Mersky C, AJ Johnson, GJ Kleiner, H Wohl: The defibrination syndrome: clinical features and laboratory diagnosis. Br J Haematol 13:528, 1967.

9. Bick RL: Hypercoagulability and thrombosis. In: G Murano, RL Bick (Eds): Basic Concepts of Hemostasis and Thrombosis. CRC Press, Boca Raton, FL, 1980, p 237.

10. Bick RL: Hypercoagulability and thrombosis, ch 12. In: Disorders of Hemostasis and Thrombosis: Principles of Clinical Practice. Theime, Inc., New York, 1985, p 294.

11. Seegers WH: Factors in the control of bleeding. Cincinnati J Med 31:395, 1950.

12. Seegers WH, CL Schneider: The nature of the blood coagulation mechanism and its relationship to some unsolved problems in obstetrics and gynecology. Trans Int and 4th Am Cong Obstet Gynecol 61A:469, 1951.

13. Seegers WH. Coagulation of the blood. Harvey Lecture Series XLVII, 180, 1952.

14. Johnson JF, WH Seegers, RG Braden: Plasma AC-globulin changes in placenta abruptio. Am J Clin Pathol 22:322, 1952.

15. Stevenson CS, RG Braden, CL Schneider, JF Johnson, WH Seegers: Am J Obstet Gynecol 65:88, 1953.

16. Ratnoff OD, JA Pritchard, JA Colopy: Hemorrhagic states during pregnancy: I. N Engl J Med 253:63, 1955.

17. Ratnoff OD, JA Pritchard, JA Colopy: Hemorrhagic states during pregnancy: II. N Engl J Med 253:97, 1955.

18. Ratnoff OD, WG Nebehay: Multiple coagulative defects in a patient with the Waterhouse-Friderichsen syndrome. Ann Intern Med 56:627, 1962.

19. Cohen E, CA Ballard: Consumptive coagulopathy associated with intra-amniotic saline instillation and the effect of Oxytocin. Obstet Gynecol 43:300, 1974.

20. Malofiejew M: Kallikrein-like activity in human myometrium, placenta, and amniotic fluid. Biochem Pharmacol 22:123, 1973.

21. Steiner PE, CC Lushbaugh: Maternal pulmonary embolism by amniotic fluid as a cause of shock and unexplained deaths in obstetrics. JAMA 117:1245, 1941.

22. Sperry K: Amniotic fluid embolism: to understand an enigma. JAMA 225:2183, 1986.

23. Graeff N, W Kuhn: The amniotic infection syndrome. In: Coagulation Disorders in Obstetrics. WB Saunders, Philadelphia, 1980, p 91.

24. Fiana S: Maternal mortality in Sweden: 1955–74. Acta Obstet Gynecol Scand 57:129, 1978.

25. Peterson EP, HB Taylor: Amniotic fluid embolism: an analysis of 40 cases. Obstet Gynecol 35:787, 1970.

26. Aguillon A, T Andrus, A Grayson, GJ Race: Amniotic fluid embolism: a review. Obstet Gynecol Surv 17:619, 1962.

27. Cortney LD: Amniotic fluid embolism. Obstet Gynecol Surv 29:169, 1974.

28. Morgan M: Amniotic fluid embolism. Anesthesia 34:20, 1979.

29. Price T, VV Baker, RL Cefalo: Amniotic fluid embolism: three case reports with a review of the literature. Obstet Gynecol Surv 40:462, 1985.

30. Albrechtsen OK: Hemorrhagic disorders following amniotic fluid embolism. Clin Obstet Gynecol 7:361, 1964.

31. Russel WS, WH Jones: Amniotic fluid embolism: a review of the sydrome with a report of 4 cases. Obstet Gynecol 26:476, 1965.

32. Atwood HD: The histological diagnosis of amniotic fluid embolism. J Pathol Bacteriol 76:211, 1958.

33. Yaffe H, A Eldor, E Hornshtein, E Sadovsky: Thromboplastic activity in amniotic fluid during pregnancy. Obstet Gynecol 50:454, 1977.

34. Yaffe H, E Hay-am, E Sadovsky: Thromboplastic activity of amniotic fluid in term and postmature gestations. Obstet Gynecol 57:490, 1981.

35. Hafter R, H Graeff: Molecular aspects of defibrination in a reptilase-treated case of "dead-fetus syndrome." Thromb Res 7:391, 1975.

36. Steichele DF: Consumptive coagulopathy in obstetrics and gynecology: Thromb Diath Haemorrh (suppl) 36:177, 1969.

37. Egeberg O: Blood coagulation and intravascular hemolysis. Scand J Clin Lab Invest 14:217, 1962.

38. Krevins JR, DP Jackson, CL Cowley, RC Hartman: The nature of the hemorrhagic disorder accompanying hemolytic transfusion reactions in man. Blood 12:834, 1957.

39. Langdell RD, EM Hedgpeth: A study of the role of hemolysis in the hemostatic defect of transfusion reactions. Thromb Diath Haemorrh 3:566, 1959.

40. Quick AJ, JG Georgatsos, CV Hussey: The clotting activity of human erythrocytes: theoretic and clinical implications. Am J Med 228:207, 1954.

41. Surgenor DM: Erythrocytes and blood coagulation. Thromb Diath Haemorrh 32:247, 1974.

42. Abildgaard CF, JJ Corrigan, RA Seeler, JV Simone, I Schulman: Meningiococcemia associated with intravascular coagulation. Pediatrics 40:78, 1967.

43. McGehee WG, SI Rapaport, PF Hjort: Intravascular coagulation in fulminant meningiococcaemia. Ann Intern Med 67:250, 1967.

44. Winkelstein A, CL Songster, TS Caras: Fulminant meningiococcemia and disseminated intravascular coagulation. Arch Intern Med 124:55, 1969.

45. Corrigan JJ: Changes in the blood coagulation system associated with septicemia. N Engl J Med 279:851, 1968.

46. Yoshikawa T, R Tanaka, LB Guze: Infection and disseminated intravascular coagulation. Medicine (Baltimore) 50:237, 1971.

47. Cline MJ, KL Melmon, WC Davis, HE Williams: Mechanism of endotoxin interaction with leukocytes. Br J Haematol 15:539, 1968.

48. McKay DG, SS Shapiro: Alterations in the blood coagulation system induced by bacterial endotoxin I: in vitro (generalized Schwartzman reaction). J Exp Med 107:353, 1958.

49. Cronberg S, P Skansberg, K Nivenios-Larsson: Disseminated intravascular coagulation in septicemia caused by beta-hemolytic streptococci. Thromb Res 3:405, 1973.

50. Rubenberg WL, LR Baker, JA McBride, JA Sevitt, WL Brain: Intravascular coagulation in a case of *Clostridium perfringens* septicemia: treatment by exchange transfusion and heparin. Br Med J 3:271, 1967.

51. Gagel C, M Linder, G Mueller-Berghous, H Lasch: Virus infection and blood coagulation. Thromb Diath Haemorrh 23:1, 1970.

52. McKay DG, W Margaretten: Disseminated intravascular coagulation in virus diseases. Arch Intern Med 120:129, 1967.

53. Niewiarwski S, E Bandowski, I Rogowicka: Studies in the absorption and activation of Hageman Factor (Factor XII) by collagen and elastin. Thromb Diath Haemorrh 24:387, 1965.

54. Robbins JE, CA Stetson: An effect of antibody-antigen interaction in blood coagulation. J Exp Med 109:1, 1959.

55. Salmon SJ, PH Lambert, J Louis: Pathogenesis of the intravascular coagulation syndrome induced by immunological reactions. Thromb Diath Haemorrh 45:161, 1971.

56. Bick RL: Alterations of hemostasis associated with malignancy. In: G Murano, RL Bick (Eds): Basic Concepts of Hemostasis and Thrombosis. CRC Press, Boca Raton, FL, 1980, p 213.

57. Bick RL: Alterations of hemostasis associated with malignancy: etiology, pathophysiology, diagnosis, and management. Semin Thromb Hemost 5:1, 1978.

58. Coleman RW, RN Rubin: Disseminated intravascular coagulation due to malignancy. Semin Oncol 17:172, 1990.

59. Luzzato G, AI Schafer: The prethrombotic state in cancer. Semin Oncol 17:147, 1990.

60. Bick RL: Alterations of hemostasis in malignancy, ch 10. In: Disorders of Hemostasis and Thrombosis: Principles of Clinical Practice. Theime, Inc., New York, 1985, p 262.

61. Folkman J: Tumor angiogenesis: therapeutic implications. N Engl J Med 285:1182, 1971.

62. Folkman J, RS Coltran: Relation of capillary proliferation to tumor growth. In: GW Richter (Ed): International Review of Experimental Pathology, vol 16. Williams & Wilkins, Baltimore, 1976, p 16.

63. Semeraro N, MB Donati: Pathways of blood clotting initiation by cancer cells. In: MB Donati, JF Davidson, S Garattini (Eds): Malignancy and the Hemostatic System. Raven Press, New York, 1981, p 65.

64. Levine M, J Hirsh: The diagnosis and treatment of thrombosis in the patient with cancer. Semin Oncol 17:160, 1990.

65. Pineo GF, E Regoeczi, MW Haton, ML Brain: The activation of coagulation by extracts of mucin: a possible pathway of intravascular coagulation accompanying adenocarcinoma. J Lab Clin Med 82:255, 1976.

66. Pineo GF, MC Brain, AS Gallus, J Hirsch, MW Hatton, E Regoeczi: Tumors, mucus production, and hypercoagulability. Ann N Y Acad Sci 230:262, 1974.

67. Dobbs RM, JA Barber, JW Weigel, JE Bergin: Clotting predisposition in carcinoma of the prostate. J Urol 123:706, 1980.

68. Pergament ML, WR Swaim, CE Blackard: Disseminated intravascular coagulation in the urologic patient. J Urol 116:1, 1976.

69. Rapaport SI, CG Chapman: Coexistent hypercoagulability and hypofibrinogenemia in a patient with prostatic carcinoma. Am J Med 27:144, 1959.

70. Mertins BF, LF Greene, EJW Bowie, LR Elueback, CA Owen: Fibrinolytic split products and ethanol gelation test in pre-operative evaluation of patients with prostatic disease. Mayo Clin Proc 49:642, 1974.

71. Gore I: Thrombin and pancreatic carcinoma. Am J Pathol 29:1093, 1953.

72. Jacobson RJ, SF Sandler, CE Rath: Systemic amyloidosis associated with microangiopathic hemolytic anemia and Factor X (Stuart Factor) deficiency. S Afr Med J 46:1634, 1972.

73. Gralnick HR, HK Tan: Acute promyelocytic leukemia: a model for understanding the role of the malignant cell in hemostasis. Hum Pathol 5:661, 1974.

74. Gralnick HR: Cancer cell procoagulant activity. In: MB Donati, JF Davidson, S Garattini (Eds): Raven Press, New York, 1981, p 57.

75. Lisiewicz J: Mechanisms of hemorrhage in leukemias. Semin Thromb Hemost 4:241, 1978.

76. Lisiewicz J: Acute leukemias, ch 2. In: Hemorrhage in Leukemias. Polish Medical Publishers, Warsaw, 1976, p 51.

77. Rand JJ, WE Moloney, HS Sise: Coagulation defects in acute promyelocytic leukemia. Arch Intern Med 123:39, 1969.

78. Lisiewicz J: Disseminated intravascular coagulation in acute leukemia. Semin Thromb Hemost 14:339, 1988.

79. Bennett RM; H Rappaport (Ed): Proceedings of a Tutorial in Hematopathology. University of Chicago Press, Chicago, 1980.

80. Gralnick HR, J Bagley, E Abrell: Heparin treatment for the hemorrhagic diathesis of acute promyelocytic leukemia. Am J Med 52:167, 1974.

81. Bick RL, WF Baker: Disseminated intravascular coagulation: a review. Hematol Pathol 6:1, 1992.

82. Perry S: Coagulation defects in leukemia. J Lab Clin Med 50:229, 1957.

83. Beller FK: Experimental animal models for the production of disseminated intravascular coagulation. In: N Bang, FK Beller, E Deutsch, EF Mammen (Eds): Thrombosis and Bleeding Disorders. Academic Press, New York, 1971, p 514.

84. McKay DG: Progress in disseminated intravascular coagulation. Calif Med 111:186, 1969.

85. Mersky C: Defibrination syndrome. In: R Biggs (Ed): Human Blood Coagulation. Blackwell Scientific, London, 1976, p 492.

86. Holder LA, LL Malin, CL Fox: Hypercoagulability after thermal injuries. Surgery 54:316, 1963.

87. Saliba MJ, WL Demsey, JL Kruggel: Large burns in humans: treatment with heparin. JAMA 225:261, 1973.

88. Bick RL: Vascular disorders associated with thrombohemorrhagic phenomena. Semin Thromb Hemost 5:167, 1979.

89. Bick RL: Hereditary hemorrhagic telangiectasia and disseminated intravascular coagulation: a new clinical syndrome. In: DA Walz, LE McCoy (Eds): Contributions to Hemostasis. Ann N Y Acad Sci 370:851, 1981.

90. Inceman S, Y Tangun: Chronic defibrination syndrome due to a giant hemangioma associated with microangiopathic hemolytic anemia. Am J Med 46:997, 1969.

91. Kasabach HH, KK Merritt: Capillary hemangioma with extensive purpura: report of a case. Am J Dis Child 59:1063, 1940.

92. Bick RL: Vascular disorders. In: G Murano, RL Bick (Eds): Basic Concepts of Hemostasis and Thrombosis. CRC Press, Boca Raton, FL, 1980, p 89.

93. Bick RL: Hereditary hemorrhagic telangiectasia and disseminated intravascular coagulation: a new clinical syndrome. Vasc Surg 15:394, 1981.

94. Kaxmier FJ, P Didisheim, VK Fairbanks, J Ludwig, WS Payne, EJW Bowie: Intravascular coagulation and arterial disease. Thromb Diath Haemorrh (suppl) 36:295, 1969.

95. Bick RL: Alterations of hemostasis associated with surgery, cardiopulmonary bypass surgery, and prosthetic devices, ch 12. In: OD Ratnoff, C Forbes (Eds): Disorders of Hemostasis. WB Saunders, Philadelphia, 1991.

96. Owen CA, H Oels, EJW Bowie, P Didisheim, JH Thompson: Chronic intravascular coagulation syndrome. Thromb Diath Haemorrh (suppl) 36:197, 1969.

97. Pritchard A, G Cunningham, MA Mason: Coagulation changes in eclampsia: their frequency and pathogenesis. Am J Obstet Gynecol 124:855, 1970.

98. Bonnar J, GP McNicol, AS Douglas: Coagulation and fibrinolytic systems in pre-eclampsia and eclampsia. Br Med J 1:12, 1971.

99. Roberts JM, WJ May: Consumption coagulopathy in severe pre-eclampsia. Obstet Gynecol 48:163, 1976.

100. Spivack JL, DB Sprangler, WR Bell: Defibrination after intra-amniotic injection of hypertonic saline. N Engl J Med 287:321, 1972.

101. Owen CA, EJW Bowie: Chronic intravascular coagulation fibrinolysis (ICF) syndromes (DIC). Semin Thromb Hemost 3:268, 1977.

102. Collins GJ, RL Heymann, R Zajtchuk: Hypercoagulability in patients with peripheral vascular disease. Am J Surg 130:2, 1975.

103. Schnetzer GW, JA Penner: Chronic intravascular coagulation syndrome associated with atherosclerotic aortic aneurysm. South Med J 66:264, 1973.

104. Rohner RF, JT Prior, JH Sipple: Mucinous malignancies, venous thrombosis, and terminal endocarditis with emboli: a syndrome. Cancer (Philadelphia) 19:1805, 1966.

105. Patterson WP, QS Ringenberg: The pathophysiology of thrombosis in cancer. Semin Oncol 17:40, 1990.

106. Davis RB, A Theologides, BJ Kennedy: Comparative studies of blood coagulation and platelet aggregation in patients with cancer and nonmalignant disease. Ann Intern Med 71:67, 1969.

107. Slickter SJ, LA Harker: Hemostasis in malignancy. Ann N Y Acad Sci 230:252, 1974.

108. DeVries WI, MAJ Braat-van Straaten, E Muller, M Wettermark: Antiplasmin deficiency in polycythaemia: a form of thrombopathy. Thromb Diath Haemorrh 6:445, 1961.

109. Silverstein MH: Agnogenic myeloid metaplasia. Publishing Sciences Group, Action, MA, 1975, p 10.

110. Hartman RC, DE Jenkins: Paroxysmal nocturnal hemoglobinuria: current concepts of certain pathophysiological features. Blood 25:850, 1965.

111. McKay DG: Disseminated intravascular coagulation: an intermediary mechanism of disease. Harper and Row, New York, 1965.

112. Ryan TJ: Coagulation and fibrinolysis. In: TJ Ryan (Ed): Microvascular Injury. WB Saunders, Philadelphia, 1976, p 221.

113. Bick RL: Platelet defects, ch 4. In: Disorders of Hemostasis and Thrombosis: Principles of Clinical Practice. Thieme, Inc., New York, 1985, p 65.

114. Katz J, S Krawitz, PV Sachs, SE Levin, P Thompson, J Levin, J Metz: Platelet, erythrocytes, and fibrinogen kinetics in the hemolytic-uremic syndrome of infancy. J Pediatr 83:739, 1973.

115. Kisker CT, R Rush: Detection of intravascular coagulation. J Clin Invest 50:2235, 1971.

116. Heyes H, W Kohle, B Slijerpcevic: The appearance of schistocytes in the peripheral blood in correlation to degree of disseminated intravascular coagulation. Haemostasis 5:66, 1976.

117. Henry RL: Platelet function in hemostasis. In: G Murano, RL Bick (Eds): Basic Concepts of Hemostasis and Thrombosis. CRC Press, Boca Raton, FL, 1980, p 17.

118. Backman F: The paradoxes of disseminated intravascular coagulation. Hosp Pract 6:113, 1971.

119. Deykin D: The clinical challenge of disseminated intravascular coagulation. N Engl J Med 283:636, 1970.

120. Muller-Berghous G, HG Lasch: Microcirculatory disturbances induced by generalized intravascular coagulation. In: GVR Born (Ed): Handbook of Experimental Pharmacology. Springer Verlag, Berlin, 1975, p 429.

121. Muller-Berghous G: Pathophysiologic and biochemical events in disseminated intravascular coagulation: dysregulation of procoagulant and anticoagulant pathways. Semin Thromb Hemost 15:58, 1989.

122. Flute PT: Intravascular coagulation. Postgrad Med J 48:346, 1972.

123. Haragawa N, N Watanabe, H Nagata, M Murao: Analysis of the disappearance curve of labeled fibrinogen at the time of hypofibrinogenemia in rabbits with acute or chronic intravascular coagulation. Thromb Haemost 50:49, 1976.

124. Heyes H, P Hilgard, W Theiss: Induction of disseminated intravascular coagulation by endotoxin and saline loading in rats, I: the influence on fibrinogen turnover and plasma parameters. Thromb Res 7:37, 1975.

125. McKay DG, D Gitlin, JM Graig: Immunochemical demonstration of fibrin in the generalized Schwartzman reaction. Arch Pathol 67:270, 1969.

126. McKay DG, W Margaretten, I Csavossy: An electron microscope study of the effects of bacterial endotoxin on the blood-vascular system. Lab Invest 15:1815, 1966.

127. Muller-Berghous G, L Roka, HG Lasch: Induction of glomerular microclot formation of fibrin monomer infusion. Thromb Diath Haemorrh 29:375, 1973.

128. Lee D, D Brown, L Baker, D Littlejohns, D Roberts: Hematological complications of chlorate poisoning. Br Med J 2:31, 1970.

129. Owen CA, EJW Bowie, HA Cooper: Turnover of fibrinogen and platelets in dogs undergoing induced intravascular coagulation. Thromb Res 2:251, 1973.

130. Latallo ZS: Products of fibrin(ogen) proteolysis. Thromb Diath Haemorrh (suppl) 24:145, 1973.

131. Marder VJ, HR Shulman, WR Carroll: High molecular weight derivatives of human fibrinogen produced by plasmin, I: physico-chemical and immunological characterization. J Biol Chem 244:2111, 1969.

132. Marder VJ, AZ Budzynski, HL James: High molecular weight derivatives of human fibrinogen produced by plasmin, III: their NH_2-terminal amino acids and comparison of the "NH_2-terminal amino disulfide knot." J Biol Chem 247:4775, 1972.

133. Plow EF, C Hougie, TS Edgington: Immunochemical and molecular investigations of fibrinogen cleavage fragments. In: L Plooer (Ed): Recent Advances in Thrombosis. Churchill Livingstone, London, 1973, p 203.

134. Bang NU, M Chang: Soluble fibrin complexes. Semin Thromb Hemost 1:91, 1974.

135. Fletcher AP, N Alkjaersig, S Fisher, S Sherry: The proteolysis of fibrinogen by plasmin: the identification of thrombin-clottable fibrinogen derivatives which polymerize abnormally. J Lab Clin Med 68:780, 1966.

136. Jacobson E, B Ly, P Kieulf: Incorporation of fibrinogen with soluble fibrin complexes. Thromb Res 4:499, 1974.

137. Shainoff JR, IH Page: Significance of cryoprofibrin in fibrinogen-fibrin conversion. J Exp Med 116:687, 1962.

138. Breen FA, JZ Tullis: Ethanol gelation, a rapid screening test for intravascular coagulation. Ann Intern Med 69:1197, 1968.

139. Derechin M, S Szuchet: Gelation phenomena in degraded fibrinogen and fibrin. Arch Biochem Biophys 87:100, 1960.

140. Gurewich V, E Hutchinson: Detection of intravascular coagulation by protamine sulfate and ethanol gelation tests. Thromb Res 2:539, 1973.

141. Bick RL: The clinical significance of fibrinogen degradation products. Semin Thromb Hemost 8:302, 1982.

142. Kopec M, Z Wegrzynowiczy, A Budzynski, Z Latallo, B Lipinski, E Kowalski: Interaction of fibrinogen degradation products with platelets. Exp Biol Med 3:73, 1968.

143. Niewiarowski S, E Regoeczi, G Stewart, A Senyi, J Mustard: Platelet interaction with polymerizing fibrin. J Clin Invest 51:685, 1972.

144. Pechet L: Fibrinolysis. N Engl J Med 273:96, 1965.

145. Sharp AA: Pathological fibrinolysis. Br Med Bull 20:240, 1964.

146. Chesterman CN: The fibrinolytic system and haemostasis. Thromb Diath Haemorrh 34:308, 1975.

147. Donaldson V: Effect of plasmin in vitro on clotting factors in plasma. J Lab Clin Med 56:644, 1960.

148. Nilsson IM: Local fibrinolysis as a mechanism for haemorrhage. Thromb Diath Haemorrh 34:623, 1975.

149. Stormorken H: Relation of the fibrinolytic to other biological systems. Thromb Diath Haemorrh 34:378, 1975.

150. Ratnoff OD, GB Haff: The conversion of Cils to C1' esterase by plasmin and trypsin. J Exp Med 125:337, 1961.

151. Schreiber AD, KF Austen: Interrelationships of the fibrinolytic, coagulation, kinin generation, and complement systems. Semin Hematol 6:593, 1973.

152. Ward PA: A plasmin split fragment of C-3 as a new chemotactic factor. J Exp Med 126:189, 1967.

153. Kaplan A, H Meier, R Mandel: The Hageman factor dependent pathways of coagulation, fibrinolysis, and kinin generation. Semin Thromb Hemost 3:6, 1976.

154. Sherry S: The kallikrein system: a basic defense mechanism. Hosp Pract 5:75, 1970.

155. Ulevich R, C Cochran, S Revak, D Morrison, A Johnson: The structural and enzymatic properties of the Hageman Factor-activated pathways. In: E Reich, D Rifkin, E Shaw (Eds): Proteases and Biological Control. Cold Spring Harbor Symposium, Cold Spring Harbor, NY, 1975, p 85.

156. Webster ME: Human plasma kallikrein, its activation and pathological role. Fed Proc Fed Am Soc Exp Biol 27:84, 1968.

157. Murano G: "The Hageman Connection": interrelationships between complement, kinins, and coagulation. Am J Hematol 4:409, 1978.

158. Beller FK, W Theiss: Fibrin derivatives, plasma hemoglobin and glomerular fibrin deposition in experimental intravascular coagulation. Thromb Diath Haemorrh 29:363, 1973.

159. McKay DG, MM Linder, VK Cruse: Mechanisms of thrombosis of the microcirculation. Am J Pathol 63:231, 1971.

160. Penick GD, HR Roberts, WP Webster, KM Brinkhous: Hemorrhagic states secondary to intravascular clotting. Arch Pathol 66:708, 1958.

161. Penick GD, HR Roberts: Intravascular clotting: focal and systemic. Int Rev Exp Pathol 3:269, 1964.

162. Seegers WH: Use and regulation of blood clotting mechanisms. In: WH Seegers (Ed): Blood Clotting Enzymology. Academic Press, New York, 1971, p 1.

163. Brown DL, PJ Lachmann: The behavior of complement and platelets in lethal endotoxin shock in rabbits. Int Arch Allergy Appl Immunol 45:193, 1973.

164. Davey MG, EF Luscher: Release reactions of human platelets induced by thrombin and other agents. Biochem Biophys Acta 165:490, 1968.

165. Des Prez RM, HI Horowitz, EW Hook: Effects of bacterial endotoxin on rabbit platelets, I: platelet aggregation and release of platelet factors in vitro. J Exp Med 114:857, 1961.

166. Evenson SA, M Jeremic: Platelets and the triggering mechanism of intravascular coagulation. Br J Haematol 19:33, 1970.

167. Apitz K: A study of the generalized Schwartzman phenomenon. J Immunol 29:255, 1935.

168. Hjort PF, SI Rapaport: The Schwartzman reaction: pathogenetic mechanism and clinical manifestations. Annu Rev Med 16:135, 1965.

169. McKay DG, W Margaretten, I Csavossy: An electron microscopic study of endotoxin shock in rhesus monkeys. Surg Gynecol Obstet 125:825, 1967.

170. Muller-Berghous G, M Hocke: Effect of endotoxin on the formation of microthrombi from circulating fibrin monomer complexes in the absence of thrombin generation. Thromb Res 1:541, 1972.

171. Shen SM, SI Rapaport, DI Feinstein: Intravascular clotting after endotoxin in rabbits with impaired intrinsic clotting produced by a factor VIII antibody. Blood 42:523, 1973.

172. Wong TC: A study on the generalized Schwartzman reaction in pregnant rats induced by bacterial endotoxin. Am J Obstet Gynecol 84:786, 1962.

173. Coleman RW, M Shapira, CF Scott: Regulation of the formation and inhibition of human plasma kallikrein. In: DA Walz, LE McCoy (Eds): Contributions to Hemostasis. Ann N Y Acad Sci 370:261, 1981.

174. Kaplan AP, M Silverberg, JT Dunn, G Miller: Mechanisms for Hageman Factor activation and role of HMW kininogen as a coagulation cofactor. In: DA Walz, LE McCoy (Eds): Contributions in Hemostasis. Ann N Y Acad Sci 370:253, 1981.

175. Kaplan AP: The Hageman Factor dependent pathways of human plasma. Microvasc Res 8:97, 1974.

176. Stormorken H: Interrelationships between the coagulation, the fibrinolytic, and the kallikrein-kinin systems. In: GG Neri-Sernari, CRM Prentice (Eds): Haemostasis and Thrombosis. Academic Press, London, 1979, p 203.

177. Henson PM: The adherence of leukocytes and platelets induced by fixed IgG antibody or complement. Immunology 16:107, 1969.

178. Henson PM: Complement-dependent platelet and polymorphonuclear leukocyte reactions. Transplant Proc 6:27, 1963.

179. Dennis LH, BE Reisberg, J Crosbie, D Crozier, ME Conrad: The original haemorrhagic fever: yellow fever. Br J Haematol 17:455, 1969.

180. Heene D, G Hoffmann-Fezer, R Hoffmann, E Weiss, G Muller-Berghous, HG Lasch: Coagulation disorders in acute hog cholera. Beitr Pathol 144:259, 1931.

181. Sohal RS, SC Sun, HL Colcolough, GE Burch: Heat stroke: an electron microscopic study of endothelial cell damage and disseminated intravascular coagulation. Arch Intern Med 122:43, 1968.

182. Starzl TE, NJ Boehmig, N Amemiya, CB Wilson, FJ Dixon, GR Giles, KM Simpson, CG Halgrimson: Clotting changes including disseminated intravascular coagulation during rapid renal-allograft rejection. N Engl J Med 283:383, 1970.

183. Wilner GD, HL Nossell, EI Leroy: Activation of Hageman factor by collagen. J Clin Invest 47:2608, 1968.

184. Lerner RG: The defibrination syndrome. Med Clin North Am 60:871, 1976.

185. McKay DG: Tissue damage in disseminated intravascular coagulation: mechanisms of localization of thrombi in the microcirculation. Thromb Diath Haemorrh (suppl) 36:67, 1969.

186. Pitner W: Disseminated intravascular coagulation. Semin Hematol 8:65, 1971.

187. Robboy SJ, RW Coleman, JD Minna: Pathology of disseminated intravascular coagulation (DIC): analysis of 26 cases. Hum Pathol 3:327, 1972.

188. Mombelli G, A Roux, AW Haelberli, PW Straub: Comparison of 125-I fibrinogen kinetics and fibrinopeptide A in patients with disseminated neoplasia. Thromb Haemost 46:9, 1981.

189. Sandritter W, NG Lasch: Pathologic aspects of shock. Arch Exp Pathol 3:86, 1967.

190. Muller-Berghous G: Pathophysiology of generalized intravascular coagulation. Semin Thromb Hemost 3:209, 1977.

191. Nalbandian RM, RL Henry, RL Bick: Thrombotic thrombocytopenic purpura. Semin Thromb Hemost 5:216, 1979.

192. Bentley PG, VV Kakkar, MF Scully, IR MacGregor, P Webb, P Chan, H Jones: An objective study of alternative methods of heparin administration. Thromb Res 18:177, 1980.

193. Cooper HA, EJW Bowie, P Didisheim: Paradoxic changes in platelets and fibrinogen in chronically induced intravascular coagulation. Mayo Clin Proc 46:521, 1971.

194. Owen CA, EJW Bowie: Chronic intravascular syndromes. Mayo Clinical Proc 49:673, 1974.

195. Bleyl U: Morphologic diagnosis of disseminated intravascular coagulation: histologic, histochemical, and electron-microscopic studies. Semin Thromb Hemost 3:247, 1977.

196. Skjorten F: Hyaline microthrombi in an autopsy material: a quantitative study with discussion of the relationship to small vessel thrombosis. Acta Pathol Microbiol Scand 76:361, 1969.

197. Morris JA, RW Smith, NS Assali: Hemodynamic action of vaso-pressor and vaso-depressor agents in endotoxin shock. Am J Obstet Gynecol 91:491, 1965.

198. Bleyl U, W Kuhn, H Graeff: Reticulo-endotheliale clearance intravascaler. Fibrinmonere in der milz. Thromb Diath Haemorrh 22:87, 1969.

199. Boyd JF: Disseminated fibrin-thromboembolism among neonates dying within 48 hours of birth. Arch Dis Child 42:401, 1967.

200. Lendrum AC, DC Fraser, W Slidders, R Henderson: Studies on the character and staining of fibrin. J Clin Pathol 15:401, 1962.

201. Bleyl U, CM Busing, B Kremplen: Pulmonale hyaline membranen und perinataler kreislaufschock. Virchows Arch Pathol Anat Physiol 348:187, 1969.

202. Busing CM, U Bleyl, G Dohnert: Pulmonary hyaline membranes in the rabbit after thrombin infusion. Fourth International Congress of Haemostasis, Vienna, 1973.

203. Baker LR, ML Rubenberg, JV Dacie, MC Brain: Fibrinogen catabolism in microangiopathic hemolytic anemia. Br J Haematol 14:617, 1968.

204. Bull B, IN Kuhn: The production of schistocytes by fibrin strands (a scanning electron microscope study). Blood 35:104, 1970.

205. Bull B, MC Brain: Experimental models of microangiopathic hemolytic anemia. Proc R Soc Med 61:1134, 1968.

206. Bull B, M Rubenberg, J Dacie, MC Brain: Microangiopathic hemolytic anemia: mechanisms of red-cell fragmentation. Br J Haematol 14:643, 1968.

207. Rubenberg M, E Regoeczi, B Bull, J Dacie, MC Brain: Microangiopathic hemolytic anemia: the experimental production of hemolysis and red-cell fragmentation by defibrination in vivo. Br J Haematol 74:627, 1968.

208. Harker L, S Slichter: Platelet and fibrinogen consumption in man. N Engl J Med 287:999, 1972.

209. Slaastad RA, NC Godal: Coagulation profile and ethanol gelation test with special reference to components consumed during coagulation. Scand J Haematol 16:25, 1976.

210. Karpatkin S, Q Khan, M Freedman: Heterogeneity of platelet function correction with platelet volume. Am J Med 64:542, 1978.

211. Karpatkin S: Heterogeneity of human platelets, VI: correlation of platelet function with platelet volume. Blood 51:307, 1978.

212. Eckhardt T, G Muller-Berghous: The role of blood platelets in the precipitation of soluble fibrin endotoxin. Scand J Haematol 14:181, 1975.

213. Skjorten F: Bilateral renal cortical necrosis and the generalized Schwartzman reaction. Acta Pathol Microbiol Scand 65:405, 1964.

214. Brozovic M: Acquired disorders of blood coagulation. In: A Bloom, DP Thomas (Eds): Hemostasis and Thrombosis. Churchill Livingstone, New York, 1981, p 411.

215. Muller-Berghous G, HG Lasch: Consumption of Hageman factor activity in the generalized Schwartzman reaction induced by liquoid: its prevention by inhibition of Hageman factor activation. Thromb Diath Haemorrh 23:386, 1970.

216. Mustard JF, MA Packham, RL Kinlough-Rathbone: Mechanisms in thrombosis. In: AL Bloom, DP Thomas (Eds): Hemostasis and Thrombosis. Churchill Livingstone, New York, 1981, p 503.

217. Blaisdell FW, RJ Stallone: The mechanism of pulmonary damage following traumatic shock. Surg Gynecol Obstet 130:15, 1970.

218. Gitlin D, JM Graig: The nature of the hyaline membrane in asphyxia of the newborn. Pediatrics 17:64, 1956.

219. Van Breeman VL, HB Heustein, PD Bruns: Pulmonary hyaline membranes studied with the electron microscope. Am J Pathol 33:769, 1957.

220. Martin AM, HB Soloway, RL Simmons: Pathologic anatomy of the lungs following shock and trauma. J Trauma 8:687, 1968.

221. Soloway HB, Y Castillo, AM Martin: Adult hyaline membrane disease. Ann Surg 168:937, 1968.

222. Hardaway RM: Acute respiratory distress syndrome and disseminated intravascular coagulation. South Med J 71:596, 1978.

223. Killough J: Protective mechanisms of the lungs: pulmonary diseases, pleural diseases. In: WA Sodeman, TM Sodeman (Eds): Mechanisms of Disease. WB Saunders, Philadelphia, 1979, p 459.

224. Ambrus CM, TS Choi, DH Weintraub, B Eisonberg, HP Staub, NG Courey, RJ Foote, D Goperlund, RV Moesch, M Ray, I Bross, OS Jung, IB Mink, JL Ambrus: Studies on the prevention of respiratory distress syndrome of infants due to hyaline membrane disease with plasminogen. Semin Thromb Hemost 2:42, 1975.

225. Ambrus CM, DH Weintraub, D Dunphy, JE Dowd, JW Pickren, KR Niswander, JL Ambrus: Studies on hyaline membrane disease, I: the fibrinolysis system in pathogenesis and therapy. Pediatrics 32:10, 1963.

226. Ambrus CM, JW Pickren, DH Weintraub, KR Niswander, JL Ambrus, D Rodbard, JL Levy: Studies on hyaline membrane disease: oxygen-induced hyaline membrane disease in guinea pigs. Biol Neonates 12:246, 1968.

227. Ambrus CM, JL Ambrus, DH Weintraub, RJ Foote, NG Courey, KR Niswander: Thrombolytic therapy in hyaline membrane disease. Thromb Diath Haemorrh (suppl) 47:269, 1971.

228. Cohen MM, DH Weintraub, AM Lilienfeld: The relationship of pulmonary hyaline membrane to certain factors in pregnancy and delivery. Pediatrics 26:42, 1960.

229. Weintraub DH, JL Ambrus, CM Ambrus: Studies on hyaline membrane disease: diagnostic and prognostic problems. Pediatrics 38:244, 1966.

230. Hardaway RM: Syndromes of Disseminated Intravascular Coagulation With Special Reference to Shock and Hemorrhage. Charles C Thomas, Springfield, IL, 1966.

231. Muller-Berghous G, B Mann: Precipitation of ancrod-induced soluble fibrin by aprotinin and norepinephrine. Thromb Res 2:305, 1973.

232. Latour JG, JB Prejean, W Margaretten: Corticosteroids and the generalized Schwartzman reaction: mechanisms of sensitization in the rabbit. Am J Pathol 65:189, 1971.

233. Lee L: Reticuloendothelial clearance of circulating fibrin in the pathogenesis of the generalized Schwartzman reaction. J Exp Med 115:1065, 1962.

234. McKay DG, G Muller-Berghous: Therapeutic implications of disseminated intravascular coagulation. Am J Cardiol 20:392, 1967.

235. Hardaway R: Disseminated intravascular coagulation in shock. Thromb Diath Haemorrh (suppl) 36:159, 1967.

236. Bick RL: Clinical hemostasis practice: the major impact of laboratory automation. Semin Thromb Hemost 9:139, 1983.

237. Fareed J, HL Messmore, EW Bermes: New perspectives in coagulation testing. Clin Chem 26:1380, 1980.

238. Fareed J: New methods in hemostatic testing. In: J Fareed, HL Messmore, J Fenton, KM Brinkhous (Eds): Perspectives in Hemostasis. Pergamon Press, New York, 1981, p 310.

239. Messmore HL, J Fareed, J Kniffin, G Squillacia, J Walenga: Synthetic substrate assays of the coagulation enzymes and their inhibitors. Comparison with clotting and immunologic method for clinical and experimental usage. In: DA Walz, LE McCoy (Eds): Contributions to Hemostasis. Ann N Y Acad Sci 370:785, 1981.

240. Messmore HL: Automation in coagulation testing: clinical applications. Semin Thromb Hemost 9:335, 1983.

241. Bick RL: Disseminated intravascular coagulation: pathophysiology and diagnosis. Pract Cardiol 7:145, 1981.

242. Bick RL: Clinical significance of fibrino(geno)lytic degradation product (FDP) testing. Lab Lore 9:683, 1981.

243. Bick RL: Disseminated intravascular coagulation. In: J Fareed, HL Messmore, J Fenton, KM Brinkhous (Eds): Perspectives in Hemostasis. Pergamon Press, New York, 1981, p 121.

244. Bick RL: Disseminated intravascular coagulation and related syndromes. In: G Murano, RL Bick (Eds): Basic Concepts of Hemostasis and Thrombosis. CRC Press, Boca Raton, FL, 1980, p 163.

245. Bick RL: Pathophysiology of disseminated intravascular coagulation. In: Clinical Significance of FDP Testing. Health Sciences Consortium Press, Chapel Hill, 1981.

246. Kurcznski EM, JA Penner: Activated prothrombin concentrate for patients with Factor VIII inhibitors. N Engl J Med 291:164, 1974.

247. Penner JA, PE Kelly: Management of patients with Factor VIII or IX inhibitors. Semin Thromb Hemost 1:386, 1975.

248. Seegers WH, E Marceniak: Autoprothrombin C in irregular blood clotting. Thromb Diath Haemorrh 8:81, 1962.

249. Marder VJ, M Matchett, S Sherry: Detection of serum fibrinogen and fibrin degradation products: comparison of six techniques using purified products and application in clinical studies. Am J Med 51:71, 1971.

250. Myers AR, KJ Bloch, RW Coleman: A comparative study of four methods for detecting fibrinogen degradation products in patients with various diseases. N Engl J Med 283:663, 1970.

251. Gurewich V, B Lipinsky, I Lipinska: A comparative study of precipitation and paracoagulation by protamine sulfate and ethanol gelation tests. Thromb Res 2:539, 1973.

252. Hedner U, IM Nilsson: Parallel determinations of FDP and fibrin monomers with various methods. Thromb Diath Haemorrh 28:268, 1972.

253. Phillips L, V Skrodelis: Intravascular coagulation in obstetric complications: fibrin monomer and fibrin split products. In: GG Neri-Sernari, CRM Prentice (Eds): Hemostasis and Thrombosis. Academic Press, New York, 1979, p 551.

254. Zirlinsky A, R Aitman, J Rouvier: Comparison between a modified ethanol gelation test and protamine sulfate test: experimental studies. Thromb Haemost 36:165, 1976.

255. Pindyck J, NC Lichtman, SG Kohl: Cryofibrinogenemia in women using oral contraceptives. Lancet 1:51, 1970.

256. Sonnabend D, D Cooper, P Fiddes, R Penny: Fibrin degradation products in thromboembolic disease. Pathology 4:47, 1972.

257. Kidder WR, LJ Logan, SI Rapaport, MJ Patch: The plasma protamine paracoagulation test: clinical and laboratory evaluation. Am J Clin Pathol 58:675, 1972.

258. Bick RL: ML Dukes, WL Wilson, L Fekete: Antithrombin III (AT-III) as a diagnostic aid in disseminated intravascular coagulation. Thromb Res 10:721, 1977.

259. Bick RL: Clinical relevance of antithrombin III. Semin Thromb Hemost 8:276, 1982.

260. Huseby RM, RE Smith: Synthetic oligopeptide substrates: their diagnostic application in blood coagulation, fibrinolysis, and other pathological states. Semin Thromb Hemost 6:173, 1980.

261. Abildgaard U, K Graven, HC Godal: Assay of progressive antithrombin in plasma. Thromb Diath Haemorrh 24:224, 1970.

262. Bick RL, I Kovacs, LF Fekete: A new two-stage functional assay for antithrombin-III: clinical and laboratory evaluation. Thromb Res 8:745, 1976.

263. Harpel PC, RD Rosenberg: Alpha-2-macroglobulin and antithrombin-heparin cofactor: modulators of hemostasis and inflammatory reactions. Prog Hemost Thromb 3:145, 1976.

264. Odegard OR, M Lie, U Abildgaard: Heparin cofactor activity measured with an amidolytic method. Thromb Res 6:287, 1975.

265. Seegers WH: Antithrombin III: theory and clinical applications. Am J Clin Pathol 69:367, 1968.

266. Bick RL, BJ McClain: A clinical comparison of chromogenic, fluorometric, and natural (fibrinogen) substrates for determination of antithrombin-III. Thromb Haemost 46:364, 1981.

267. Bishop RC, PM Hudson, G Mitchell, SP Pochron: Use of fluorogenic substrates for the assay of antithrombin III and heparin. Ann N Y Acad Sci 370:720, 1981.

268. Fareed J, HL Messmore, JM Walenga, EW Bermes, RL Bick: Laboratory evaluation of antithrombin III: a critical overview of currently available methods for antithrombin III measurements. Semin Thromb Hemost 8:288, 1982.

269. Kraytman M: Platelet size in thrombocytopenias and thrombocytosis of various origin. Blood 41:587, 1973.

270. Zieve PM, J Levin: Disseminated intravascular coagulation. In: PD Zieve, J Levin (Eds): Disorders of Hemostasis. WB Saunders, Philadelphia, 1976, p 71.

271. Bick RL, BJ McClain: Sequential platelet size distribution profiling for assessing platelet survival and response to antiplatelet drugs. Blood 58:230, 1981.

272. Farrel RJ, MJ Duffy, GJ Duffy: Elevated plasma beta-thromboglobulin in patients with malignancy. Thromb Haemost 42:143, 1979.

273. Lundham CA, JD Cash: B-thromboglobulin: a new tool for the diagnosis of hypercoagulability. In: GG Neri-Sernari, CRM Prentice (Eds): Hemostasis and Thrombosis. Academic Press, London, 1979, p 159.

274. Matsuda T, T Seki, M Ogawara, R Miura, M Yokouchi, M Murakami: Comparison between plasma levels of B-thromboglobulin and platelet factor 4 in various diseases. Thromb Haemost 42:288, 1979.

275. Zahavi J, VV Kakkar: B-thromboglobulin: a specific marker of in vivo platelet release reaction. Thromb Haemost 44:23, 1980.

276. Zieman M, I Friedrich, HK Beddin: Activated platelets and platelet function in traumatic septic and haemorrhagic preshock conditions. Thromb Haemost 42:410, 1979.

277. Lundham CA, N Allen, RB Bradford, R Dowdle, N Bentley, AL Bloom: B-thromboglobulin and platelet survival in patients with rheumatic diseases and prosthetic heart valves and their treatment with sulfinpyrazone. Thromb Haemost 42:329, 1979.

278. Niewiarowski S, J Guzzo, AK Rav, I Berman, P James: Increased levels of low-affinity platelet factor 4 in plasma and urine of patients with chronic renal failure. Thromb Haemost 42:416, 1979.

279. Budzynski AZ, VJ Marder: Determination of human fibrinopeptide A by radioimmunoassay in purified systems and in the blood. Thromb Diath Haemorrh 34:709, 1975.

280. Cronlund M, J Hardin, J Burton, L Lee, I Haber, KJ Bloch: Fibrinopeptide A in plasma of normal subjects and patients with disseminated intravascular coagulation and systemic lupus erythematosis. J Clin Invest 58:142, 1976.

281. Douglas JT, M Shah, GDO Lowe, CRM Prentice: Fibrinopeptide-A and Beta-thromboglobulin levels in pre-eclampsia and hypertensive pregnancy. Thromb Haemost 46:8, 1981.

282. Kockum C: Radioimmunoasay of fibrinopeptide-A: clinical applications. Thromb Res 8:225, 1976.

283. Nossel HL, M Ti, KL Kaplan, K Spandonis, T Soland, VD Butler: The generation of fibrinopeptide-A in clinical blood samples: evidence for thrombin activity. J Clin Invest 58:1136, 1976.

284. Fareed J, RL Bick, J Walenga, HL Messmore, EW Bermes: Clinical and experimental studies using a modified radioimmunoassay for B-beta 15-42 related peptides. Thromb Haemost 50:300, 1983.

285. Fareed J, RL Bick, G Squillaci, J Walenga, HL Messmore, EW Bermes: Clinical and experimental utilization of a modified radioimmunoassay for B-beta 15-42 related peptides. Clin Chem 29:1161, 1983.

286. Plow EF, TS Edgington: Surface markers of fibrinogen and its physiologic derivatives related by antibody probes. Semin Thromb Hemost 8:36, 1982.

287. Johnson AJ, C Mersky: Diagnosis of diffuse intravascular clotting: its relation to secondary fibrinolysis and treatment with heparin. Thromb Diath Haemorrh (suppl) 20:161, 1966.

288. Clavin SA, JL Bobbitt, RT Shuman, EL Smithwick: Use of peptidyl-4-methoxy-2-naphthylamides to assay plasmin. Anal Biochem 80:355, 1977.

289. Gaffney PJ, RD Philo: A commentary of new methodology in haemostasis using chromogenic substrates. In: J Fareed, JL Messmore, J Fenton, KM Brinkhous (Eds): Perspectives in Hemostasis. Pergamon Press, New York, 1981, p 405.

290. Latallo ZS, E Teisseyre, S Lopaciuk: Evaluation of a fibrinolytic profile of plasma using chromogenic substrates. In: MF Scully, VV Kakkar (Eds): Chromogenic Peptide Substrates. Churchill Livingstone, London, 1979, p 262.

291. Soria CS, M Samama: A plasminogen assay using a chromogenic synthetic substrate: results from clinical work and from studies of thrombolysis. In: JF Davidson, RM Rowan, MM Samama, PC Desnoyers (Eds): Progress in Chemical Fibrinolysis and Thrombolysis. Raven Press, New York, 1978, p 337.

292. Triplett DA, C Harms, L Hermelin, RM Huseby, GA Mitchell, SP Pochron: Clinical studies of the use of fluorogenic substrate assay method for the determination of plasminogen. Thromb Haemost 42:50, 1979.

293. Kowalski E, M Kopec, S Niewiarowski: An evaluation of the euglobulin method for the determination of fibrinolysis. J Clin Pathol 12:215, 1959.

294. Menon IS: A study of the possible correlation of euglobulin lysis time and dilute blood clot lysis time in the determination of fibrinolytic activity. Lab Pract 17:334, 1968.

295. Collen D, F DeCock, M Verstraete: Immunological distinction between anti-plasmin and alpha-1-anti-trypsin. Thromb Res 7:245, 1975.

296. Collen P: Identification and some properties of a new fast-acting plasmin inhibitor in human plasma. Eur J Biochem 69:209, 1976.

297. Edy J, D Collen, M Verstraete: Quantitation of the plasma protease inhibitor antiplasmin with the chromogenic substrate (S-2251). In: JF Davidson, RM Rowan, MM Samama, PC Desnoyers (Eds): Chemical Fibrinolysis and Thrombolysis. Raven Press, New York, 1978, p 315.

298. Gyzander E, P Friberger, H Myrwold, H Noppa, R Olsson, AC Teger-Nilsson, L Walmo: Antiplasmin determination by means of the plasmin specific substrate S-2251: methodology studies and some clinical applications. In: I Witt (Ed): New Methods for the Analysis of Coagulation Using Chromogenic Substrates. Waltor deGruyter, Berlin, 1977, p 229.

299. Teger-Nilsson AC, E Gryzander, U Hedner, H Myrwold, H Noppa, R Olsson, L Walmo: Antiplasmin and other natural inhibitors of fibrinolysis in clinical material. In: FJ Davidson, RM Rowan, MM Samama, PC Desnoyers (Eds): Progress in

Chemical Fibrinolysis and Thrombolysis. Raven Press, New York, 1978, p 327.

300. Harpel PC, MW Mosesson, NR Cooper: Studies on the structure and function of 2-macroglobulin and C1 inactivator. In: E Reich, DB Rifkin, E Shaw (Eds): Proteases and Biological Control. Cold Spring Harbor Symposium, Cold Spring Harbor, NY, 1975, p 387.

301. Murano G: Plasma protein function in hemostasis. In: G Murano, RL Bick (Eds): Basic Concepts of Hemostasis and Thrombosis. CRC Press, Boca Raton, FL, 1980, p 43.

302. Parvez Z, R Moncada: Immunological vs functional methods for the evaluation of serine protease inhibitors. In: J Fareed, HL Messmore, J Fenton, KM Brinkhous (Eds): Perspectives in Hemostasis. Pergamon Press, New York, 1981, p 355.

303. Alkjaersig N, L Roy, AP Fletcher: Analysis of gel exclusion chromatographic data by plasma fibrinogen chromatography. Thromb Res 3:525, 1973.

304. Marder VJ, SE Martin, CW Francis, RW Coleman: Consumptive thrombohemorrhagic disorders, ch 63. In: AW Coleman, J Hirsh, VJ Marder, EW Salzman (Eds): Hemostasis and Thrombosis. JB Lippincott, Philadelphia, 1987, p 975.

305. Takahashi S, Y Hoguchi, T Kitagawa: Analysis of urinary and circulating FDP subfragments and subunits: application of the Western blot technique. Acta Paediatr Jpn 31:127, 1989.

306. Arneson H: Characterization of fibrinogen and fibrin degradation products by isoelectric focusing in polyacrylamide gel. Thromb Res 4:861, 1974.

307. Fletcher AP, N Alkjaersig: Blood hypercoagulability, intravascular coagulation, and thrombosis: new diagnostic concepts. Thromb Diath Haemorrh (suppl) 45:389, 1974.

308. Fletcher AP, N Alkjaersig: Gel chromatography of fibrinogen in the diagnosis of prethrombotic states. In: GG Neri-Sernari, CRM Prentice (Eds): Hemostasis and Thrombosis. Academic Press, London, 1979, p 113.

309. Neri-Sernari GG, GF Gensini, R Abbate: High molecular weight fibrinogen complexes in the assessment of hypercoagulability. In: GG Neri-Sernari, CRM Prentice (Eds): Hemostasis and Thrombosis. Academic Press, London, 1979, p 123.

310. Kwaan HC: Disseminated intravascular coagulation. Med Clin North Am 56:177, 1972.

311. Maki M, K Sasaki, S Sata: Methods for differential diagnosis of consumptive coagulopathy. Tohoku J Exp Med 99:347, 1969.

312. Simpson JG, AL Stalker: The concept of disseminated intravascular coagulation. Clin Haematol 2:189, 1973.

313. Bick RL: Disseminated intravascular coagulation and related syndromes, II. Pract Cardiol 7:152, 1981.

314. Francis CW, VJ Marder: A molecular model of plasmic degradation of cross-linked fibrin. Semin Thromb Hemost 8:25, 1982.

315. Matsumoto T, Y Nishijima, Y Teramura, K Fujino, M Hibino, M Hirata: Monoclonal antibodies to fibrinogen-fibrin degradation products which contain D-domain. Thromb Res 38:279, 1985.

316. Rylatt DB, AS Blake, LE Cottis, DA Massingham, WA Fletcher, PP Masci, AN Whitaker, M Elms, I Bunce, AJ Weber, D Wyatt, PG Bundesen: An immunoassay for human D-dimer using monoclonal antibodies. Thromb Res 31:767, 1983.

317. Elms MJ, IH Bunce, PG Bundesen, DB Rylatt, AJ Webber, PP Masci, AN Whitaker: Rapid detection of cross-linked fibrin degradation products in plasma using monoclonal antibody-coated latex particles. Am J Clin Pathol 85:360, 1986.

318. Bick RL, W Baker: Diagnostic efficacy of the D-dimer assay in DIC and related disorders (D-dimer assay). Blood 68:329, 1986.

319. Lane DA, FE Preston, ME Van Ross, VV Kakkar: Characterization of serum fibrinogen and fibrin fragments produced during disseminated intravascular coagulation. Br J Haematol 40:609, 1978.

320. Elms MJ, IH Bunce, PG Bundesen, DB Rylatt, AJ Webber, PP Masci, AN Whitaker: Measurement of cross-linked fibrin degradation products: an immunoassay using monoclonal antibodies. Thromb Haemost 50:591, 1983.

321. Bick RL, I Kovacs, LF Fekete: A two-stage functional assay for antithrombin III: clinical and laboratory evaluation. Thromb Res 8:745, 1976.

322. Bick RL: Acquired circulating anticoagulants and defective hemostasis in malignant paraprotein disorders. In: G Murano, RL Bick (Eds): Basic Concepts of Hemostasis and Thrombosis. CRC Press, Boca Raton, FL, 1980, p 205.

323. Bick RL: Malignancy's effect on hemostasis: complex questions finding answers. Diagn Dialog 2:1, 1980.

324. Esmon CT: Protein C: biochemistry, physiology, and clinical implications. Blood 62:1155, 1983.

325. Griffin JH: Clinical studies of protein C. Semin Thromb Hemost 10:162, 1984.

326. Fibrin(ogen) Degradation Products (FDP) Detection Set. A Product of the Data-Fi System, Product Circular. American Dade Corporation, Miami, September 1980, p 1.

327. Murakami M: A new method of fibrinolysis measurement. Acta Haematol Jpn 28:341, 1965.

328. Wellcome FDP Kit. In: Detection of fibrinogen degradation products and fibrinogen. Burroughs Wellcome Company, Research Triangle Park, North Carolina, 1977, p 39.

329. Murano G: The molecular structure of fibrinogen. Semin Thromb Hemost 1:1, 1974.

330. Bick RL: Disseminated intravascular coagulation and related syndromes. Am J Hematol 5:265, 1978.

331. Bick RL: Disseminated intravascular coagulation: a clinical laboratory study of 48 patients. In: D Walz, L McCoy (Eds): Contributions to Hemostasis. Ann N Y Acad Sci 370:843, 1981.

332. Bick RL: Disseminated intravascular coagulation: clinical laboratory correlations. Am J Clin Pathol 77:244, 1982.

333. Bick RL, J Fareed, G Squillaci, J Walenga, EW Bermes, HL Messmore: Molecular markers of hemostatic processes: implications in diagnostic and therapeutic management of thrombotic and hemorrhagic disorders. Fed Proc 42:1031, 1983.

334. Bick RL, J Fareed, J Walenga, EW Bermes: Automation in coagulation testing. Clin Chem 29:1196, 1983.

335. Fareed J, J Walenga, RL Bick, EW Bermes, HL Messmore: Impact of automation on the quantitation of low molecular weight markers of hemostatic defects. Semin Thromb Hemost 9:355, 1983.

336. Feinstein DI: Treatment of disseminated intravascular coagulation. Semin Thromb Hemost 14:351, 1988.

337. Heene DL: Blood coagulation mechanism and endotoxins: hemostatic defect in septic shock. In: B Urbaschek (Ed): Gram-Negative Bacterial Infections and Mode of Endotoxin Actions. Springer-Verlag, Vienna, 1975, p 367.

338. Leroy J, JD Lamagnere, C Mercier: La Coagulopathic de consommation au cours des purpuras fulminans et son traitement (10 observations). Semin Hosp Paris 50:843, 1974.

339. Lo SS, WH Hitzig, PG Frick: Clinical experience with anticoagulant therapy in the management of disseminated intravascular coagulation in children. Acta Haematol 45:1, 1971.

340. Corrigan JJ, CM Jordan: Heparin therapy in septicemia with disseminated intravascular coagulation. Effect on mortality and correction of hemostatic defects. N Engl J Med 283:778, 1970.

341. Good RA, L Thomas: Studies on the generalized Schwartzman reaction: prevention of the local and generalized Schwartzman reactions with heparin. J Exp Med 97:871, 1953.

342. Heene DL: Disseminated intravascular coagulation: evaluation of therapeutic approaches. Semin Thromb Hemost 3:291, 1977.

343. Al-Mondhiry H: Disseminated intravascular coagulation: experience in a major cancer center. Thromb Diath Haemorrh 34:181, 1975.

344. Minna JD, S Robboy, RW Coleman: Clinical aproach to a patient with suspected DIC. In: JD Minna, S Robboy, RW Coleman (Eds): Disseminated Intravascular Coagulation. Charles C Thomas, Springfield, IL, 1974, p 167.

345. Bonnar J: Blood coagulation and fibrinolysis in obstetrics. Clin Hematol 2:213, 1973.

346. Kuhn W, H Graeft: Gerinnungsstorungen in der Geburtshilfe. Theime Verlag, Stuttgart, 1977, p 90.

347. Bick RL: Monitoring heparin therapy. Diagn Dialog 1:1, 1979.

348. Jaques LB: The premises involved in the clinical use of heparin. Semin Thromb Hemost 4:275, 1978.

349. Bick RL, LF Fekete, WL Wilson: Treatment of disseminated intravascular coagulation with antithrombin III. Transactions of the American Society of Hematology, 1976, p 167.

350. Kakkar VV: The clinical use of antithrombin III. Thromb Haemost 42:265, 1979.

351. Thaler E, K Lechner: Antithrombin III deficiency and thromboembolism. Clin Haematol 10:369, 1981.

352. Bick RL, WR Schmalhorst, LF Fekete: Disseminated intravascular coagulation and blood component therapy. Transfusion (Philadelphia) 16:361, 1976.

353. Gralnick HR, P Greipp: Thrombosis with epsilon-aminocaproic acid therapy. Am J Clin Pathol 56:151, 1971.

354. McNicol GP, AS Douglas: Thrombolytic therapy and fibrinolytic inhibitors. In: Human Blood Coagulation, Haemostasis, and Thrombosis. Oxford Press, London, 1972, p 393.

355. Naeye RL: Thrombolytic state after hemorrhagic diathesis, possible complications of therapy with epsilon-amino-caproic acid. Blood 19:694, 1962.

356. Ratnoff OD: Epsilon aminocaproic acid: a dangerous weapon. N Engl J Med 280:1124, 1969.

357. Bick RL, MB Bick, LF Fekete: Antithrombin III patterns in disseminated intravascular coagulation. Am J Clin Pathol 73:577, 1980.

358. Edwards EA: Migrating thrombophlebitis associated with carcinoma. N Engl J Med 240:1031, 1949.

359. Bick RL: Treatment of bleeding and thrombosis in the patient with cancer. In: T Nealon (Ed): Management of the Patient with Cancer. WB Saunders, Philadelphia, 1976, p 48.

360. Goodnight SH: Bleeding and intravascular clotting in malignancy: a review. Ann N Y Acad Sci 230:271, 1974.

361. Harker LA, J Hirsh, M Gent, E Yenton: Critical evaluation of platelet inhibiting drugs in thrombotic disease. Prog Hematol 9:229, 1975.

362. Weiss HJ: The pharmacology of platelet inhibition. Prog Hemost Thromb 1:199, 1972.

363. Nalbandian RM, RL Henry: Platelet-endothelial cell interactions: metabolic maps of structures and actions of prostaglandins, prostacyclin, thromboxane, and cyclic AMP. Semin Thromb Hemost 5:87, 1978.

364. Brown RC, DC Campbell, JH Thompson: Increased fibrinolysis with malignant disease. Arch Intern Med 109:129, 1962.

365. Omar JB, H Saxena, HS Mitel: Fibrinolytic activity in malignant diseases. J Assoc Physicians India 19:293, 1971.

Hemostasis in Liver and Renal Disease

Alterations of hemostasis in patients with liver disease and renal disease are multifaceted and involve not only multiple coagulation proteins and protein systems but usually also multiple hemostatic compartments, including the platelets and vasculature. These types of defects are the topic of this chapter.

Liver Disease

Patients with acute and chronic liver disease experience significant hemorrhage, which represents a major challenge in clinical care, strains the laboratory and blood bank facilities, and is often the terminal event in these patients.[1,2] Alterations of hemostasis in patients with acute or chronic liver disease of any etiology are complex and notably multifaceted. Characteristically, it has been assumed that hemorrhage in chronic liver disease is simply because of defective hepatocyte synthesis of the vitamin K–dependent prothrombin complex factors, factors II, VII, IX, and X.[3] However, many other changes of hemostasis, including primary fibrinolysis, platelet dysfunction, and thrombocytopenia, must be appreciated to give effective therapy.[4,5] Disseminated intravascular coagulation may also play a role as chronic liver disease becomes terminal,[4,5] but this is more commonly a problem in acute hepatic failure and biliary stasis. The most common sequence of events in patients with chronic liver disease is the development of localized bleeding, usually from a ruptured esophageal varix, peptic ulcer disease, or hemorrhagic gastritis.[6] These bleeds then cascade into massive hemorrhage that is poorly responsive to the usual therapeutic modalities of Sengstaken-Blakemore tamponade, massive transfusions with whole blood, fresh frozen plasma, plasma expanders, and vasopressin infusion. The often ineffectual control of hemorrhage in patients with chronic liver disease is often because although many hemostasis defects are corrected, primarily defects in the prothrombin complex factors, many other defects are left essentially unattended, and effective hemostasis cannot be adequately achieved.

Alterations of hemostasis ocurring in acute and chronic liver disease are summarized in Table 8-1 in descending order of prevalence.

Coagulation Protein Changes

The hepatocyte is responsible for synthesizing factors I, II, V, VII, VIII:C, IX, X, XI, XII, and XIII, prekallikrein (Fletcher factor), high–molecular weight kininogen (Fitzgerald, Flaujeac, Williams, Reid, and Fujiwara factors), antithrombin III, protein C, protein S, alpha-2-macroglobulin, alpha-2-antiplasmin, and plasminogen.[2,7] Other sites of synthesis for factor VIII:C, plasminogen, and factor XIII may exist as well.[8,9] The patient with chronic liver disease commonly shows an early and significant decreased hepatic synthesis of the prothrombin complex factors (II, VII, IX, and X), factor V, fibrinogen, factors XI and XII, prekallikrein, high–molecular weight kininogen, AT III, proteins C and S, alpha-2-antiplasmin, and plasminogen.[1,7] However, the degree of decrease in each of these factors will be somewhat dependent on the degree of primary fibrinolysis present and the degree of elevation of those factors behaving as acute-phase reactants, including AT III, fibrinogen, factor V, factor VIII:C, and alpha-2-macroglobulin. The coagulation factor changes will be a clinical summation of many multifactorial events.[4,5] Patients with chronic liver disease show some degree of abnormal carboxylation leading to synthesis of abnormal factors II, VII, IX, and X or the synthesis of PIVKAs (proteins induced by vitamin K absence/antagonists).[10,11] The decrease in factor VII best correlates with the prothrombin time determination, whereas the decreases in factors IX and X best correlate with predisposition to clinical hemorrhage.

Patients with chronic liver disease may synthesize defective fibrinogen leading to a pseudodysfibrinogenemia. This process happens via many mechanisms, including not only the synthesis of an abnormal fibrinogen by the hepatocyte but by fibrinogen being mildly plasmin-degraded into a high-solubility, low–thrombin clottability type of abnormal fibrinogen. Fibrinogen may complex with FDPs and become

Table 8-1. Hemostasis Abnormalities in Liver Disease (Descending Order of Probability)

Acute liver disease
  Defective (PIVKA) synthesis (qualitative)
  Disseminated intravascular coagulation
  Thrombocytopenia
  Platelet dysfunction
  Decreased synthesis (quantitative)

Chronic liver disease
  Decreased synthesis (quantitative)
  Primary fibrinolysis
  Thrombocytopenia
  Platelet dysfunction
  Defective (PIVKA) synthesis (qualitative)
  Vascular defects
  Disseminated intravascular coagulation

Table 8-2. Impaired Synthesis in Chronic Liver Disease

Decreased synthesis of vitamin K–dependent factors
  Factor II
  Factor VII
  Factor IX
  Factor X
  Protein C
  Protein S

Abnormal (PIVKA) synthesis of vitamin K–dependent factors
  Factor II
  Factor VII
  Factor IX
  Factor X
  Protein C
  Protein S

Decreased (quantitative) synthesis of:
  Fibrinogen
  Factor V
  Factor VIII:C
  Factor XI
  Factor XII
  Prekallikrein
  Kininogens
  Antithrombin III
  Plasminogen
  Antiplasmin

dysfunctional.[12] Dysfibrinogenemia or pseudodysfibrinogenemia occurs by many multifaceted mechanisms in liver disease. If significant primary fibrinolysis is not present, however, hypofibrinogenemia is usually not of clinical significance with respect to clinical hemorrhage. Normal or increased fibrinogen levels may also be seen in patients with chronic liver disease, because fibrinogen may behave as an acute-phase reactant. Primary fibrinolysis and other defects are multifaceted determinants of the levels of all the clotting factors synthesized by the hepatocyte.

Many patients with chronic liver disease will have an acquired dysfibrinogenemia reflected by abnormal fibrin monomer polymerization and prolonged thrombin times and reptilase times, which may be caused by many multifaceted events, including abnormal carbohydrate content of fibrinogen.[13,14] As liver disease becomes end stage, decreased synthesis of factors V and VIII:C may occur. Alternatively, these factors may be markedly decreased simply resulting from significant activation of the fibrinolytic system and plasminemia. Early during chronic liver disease, however, these two factors may be elevated. The synthesis of prekallikrein and high–molecular weight kininogen is also decreased, but the clinical significance of this defect, if any, is unclear. Patients with chronic liver disease of any etiology usually show significantly decreased levels of AT III. The pathophysiology of this condition is unclear and may represent either a true decreased synthesis or the synthesis of a dysfunctional AT III molecule.[15,16] If DIC becomes a manifestation of end-stage chronic liver disease or if the patient has acute liver failure resulting from viral hepatitis, acute hepatitis of any infectious etiology, or liver failure because of acute drug-, chemical-, or toxin-induced hepatic failure, DIC may also develop, and then the typical findings of this fulminant syndrome may be operative (see chapter 7).[17-24] Some patients may have high or high-normal AT III levels if DIC is not present.[25] This alpha-2-globulin, like fibrinogen, also behaves as an acute-phase reactant.[26] The clinical significance of AT III findings in chronic liver disease is unclear with respect to clinical development of hypercoagulability or thrombosis.

Patients with acute hepatic failure of any etiology, especially that induced by viruses, drugs, toxins, or chemicals, may develop DIC with these findings present.[17-24] Patients developing long-term intrahepatic or extrahepatic cholestasis by biliary obstruction commonly develop decreased synthesis of the vitamin K–dependent factors resulting from inability of vitamin K to be utilized.[20,27-30] Vitamin K is lipid soluble and may be malabsorbed in these obstructive-type syndromes. These patients commonly show abnormal synthesis (PIVKA synthesis) of factors II, VII, IX, and X.[10,11,20,21] Patients may also, however, occasionally develop acute fulminant DIC (see chapter 7). Impaired synthesis-type defects in chronic liver disease are summarized in Table 8-2. Common defects of hemostasis in acute hepatic failure and cholestatic liver disease are summarized in Table 8-3.

Table 8-3. Hemostasis in Acute Hepatic Failure and Cholestasis

Acute hepatic failure
  Defective or decreased synthesis
  Thrombocytopenia
  Disseminated intravascular coagulation

Intrahepatic or extrahepatic cholestasis
  Defective (PIVKA) synthesis
  Disseminated intravascular coagulation

Table 8-4. Excessive Destruction in Chronic Liver Disease

Plasmin biodegradation
    Hypofibrinogenemia
    Dysfibrinogenemia
    Factor V
    Factor VIII:C
    Factor XI
    Factor XII
    Other plasmin proteins (ACTH, insulin, growth hormone, etc)

Fibrin(ogen) degradation products
    Dysfibrinogenemia
    Defective fibrin monomer polymerization
    Platelet function defects
    Hyperpyrexia

Plasmin-induced activation
    Factor XII activation
    Complement activation (C1 and C3)
    Prekallikrein activation
    Kinin generation

Table 8-5. Fibrinolytic Activation Pathways

Plasminogen elevation
Decreased fibrinolytic inhibitors
Increased fibrinolytic activators
Decreased activation inhibitors
Foreign surface activation of fibrinolysis
Drug-induced activation
Tumor material activation
Factor XII activation
Therapeutic thrombolytic activation

Excessive Destruction

The physiology of the fibrinolytic system was discussed in chapter 1; this section is concerned with pathologic fibrinolysis as it relates to liver disease. Excessive destruction-type defects in liver disease are summarized in Table 8-4. In most instances of pathologic activation of the fibrinolytic system, the precise mechanisms are unclear,[12] and many proposed mechanisms are only theoretic. Several potential pathologic activation mechanisms exist. (1) Elevated plasminogen levels may lead to pathologic activation of the fibrinolytic system, but usually in hyperplasminogenemia no such activation occurs. (2) Decreased inhibitors of the fibrinolytic system, primarily alpha-2-antiplasmin and alpha-2-macroglobulin, may lead to pathologic activation,[17] which may be, in part, responsible for primary activation processes in liver disease and liver failure. (3) Increased plasminogen activators, including tissue plasminogen activators (TPA), may cause pathologic activation. This mechanism, via poor hepatic clearance of activators, appears to be operative in hepatic cirrhosis. (4) Decreased activation inhibitors may be responsible for pathologic fibrinolytic system activation, but this is only hypothetic. (5) Exposure of blood and fibrinolytic system enzymes to foreign surfaces or abnormal vasculature may lead to activation: both may account for pathologic activation during cardiopulmonary bypass,[31,32] and the last may be operative in some instances of secondary activation in DIC.[18,19] (6) Drugs may activate the fibrinolytic system by unclear mechanisms. Certain antineoplastics, anabolic steroids, and nicotinic acid are known to have this property.[33,34] (7) Tumor-derived enzymes and extracts are capable of activating the plasminogen-plasmin system, which may clearly lead to primary fibrinolytic syndromes in selected malignancies.[35,36] (8) Pathologic activation of Hageman factor or pathologic activation of endothelial plasminogen activator may account for the secondary activation (release) of fibrinolysis in DIC.[18,19,37,38] (9) Streptokinase, urokinase, recombinant TPA and acyl-plasminogen-streptokinase activator complex (APSAC) are pharmacologic activators currently used clinically to induce a therapeutic thrombolytic state.[39] Thrombolytic therapy will be discussed in chapter 15. Potential activation mechanisms are summarized in Table 8-5. Pathologic activation pathways are summarized in Figure 8-1.

Fibrin(ogen) Degradation Products and Hemostasis

As plasmin begins to lyse fibrinogen and fibrin, the carboxy-terminal end of the A-alpha chain is destroyed (removed) first. This process then continues to destruction of the B-beta chain, and lastly the gamma chain is digested. This process of sequential digestion is responsible for the formation of the four major clinically recognized degradation products, the X, Y, D, and E fragments, called fibrin(ogen) degradation products or fibrin(ogen) split products (FDPs).[40,41] During any type of intravascular fibrino(geno)lysis, whether it be primary, secondary, or therapeutically induced, the titers of these four degradation products become significantly increased as the rate of formation exceeds the ability of the reticuloendothelial system to clear them from the circulation.[42] The titer can be used as an indirect approximation of fibrino(geno)lysis occurring. The scheme of fibrin(ogen) degradation by plasmin is depicted in Figure 8-2. These four degradation products exert significant biologic effects. Many of these effects have major deleterious consequences in hemostasis and may significantly enhance hemorrhage. Fragment X exerts a potent antithrombin action by still being clottable by thrombin, although more slowly than is intact fibrinogen. The Y fragment is derived from X fragment and appears to be a short-lived intermediate. The formation of this derivative involves cleavage of peptides from the amino-terminal part of the B-beta chains followed by asymmetric splitting of the three chains at one side of the partly degraded dimer. The Y derivative, like the X derivative, also prolongs the thrombin time when added to fibrinogen. Both fragments X and Y may form soluble fibrin monomer complexes (see chapter 7). Since one of the polymerization sites is found on the D area (others are found on the E area), it is understandable

Figure 8-1. Pathologic Activation of Fibrinolysis

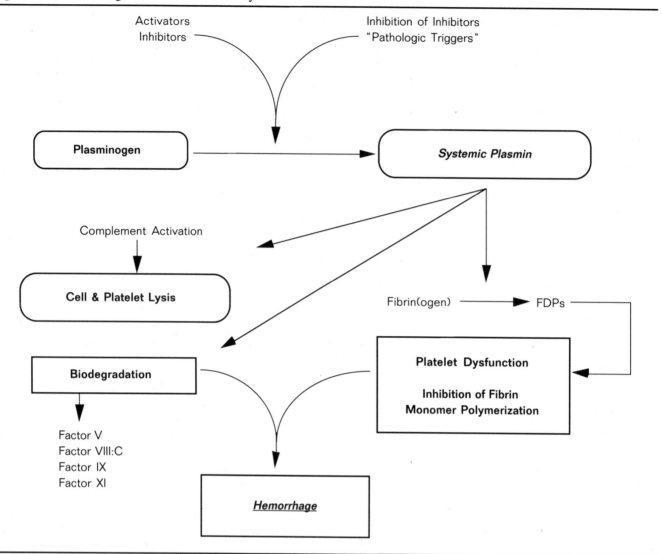

that in the presence of these fragments polymerization will be abnormal, since these fragments may complex with fibrin monomer and interfere with fibrin monomer polymerization. Further digestion of the Y fragment gives rise to a second D fragment and one final E fragment. Fragment D also interferes with normal polymerization. Anticoagulant activity of fragment E has not been determined with certainty.

As another insult to hemostasis, all four fragments show an affinity for platelet membranes and coat them, making platelets dysfunctional and causing a clinically significant platelet function defect.[12,43,44] Fragments D and E are the most pronounced in this action. Evidence suggests that FDPs may account for, at least in some instances, hyperpyrexia seen in hemorrhagic and thrombotic disorders. Another early activity of plasmin is to dissect B-beta 15-42 and related peptides from the B-beta chain. The noting of these peptides with the presence or absence of fibrinopeptide A is of benefit in the differential diagnosis between DIC-

type syndromes with secondary fibrinolysis and primary activation of the fibrinolytic system.[45,46]

As FDPs are formed from the plasmin-induced lysis of fibrinogen and fibrin, the biologic effects are the following: (1) inhibition of the hemostasis system by interference with fibrin monomer polymerization; (2) an antithrombin effect; and (3) interference with platelet function. These fragments may also induce hyperpyrexia. The biologic consequences of circulating FDPs are summarized in Table 8-6.

Clinical Consequences

The clinical and laboratory manifestations of pathologic fibrinolytic system activation are summarized in Figure 8-1. During pathologic fibrinolytic activation, plasmin-induced degradation of fibrinogen and fibrin rapidly creates FDPs, the X, Y, D, and E fragments. These fragments interfere with fibrin monomer polymerization, induce a platelet function defect, and are associated with hypofibrinogen-

Figure 8-2. Formation of Fibrin(ogen) Degradation Products

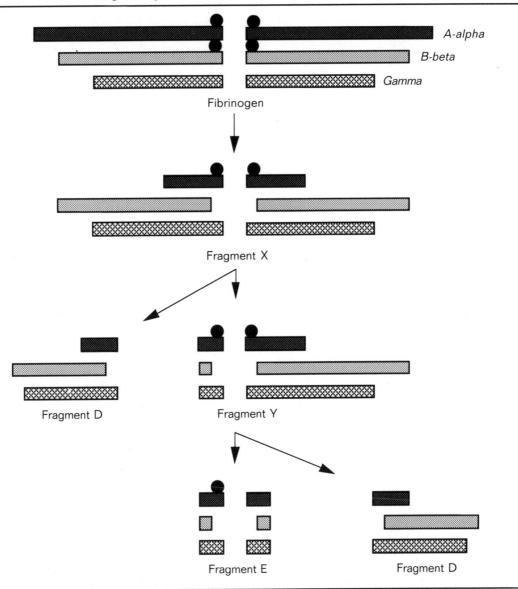

emia/dysfibrinogenemia. The net clinical result of these three events is hemorrhage.[12]

The hallmark laboratory findings of plasmin-induced lysis of fibrinogen or fibrin are an elevated titer of FDPs and elevated B-beta 15-42 and related peptide levels.[45] Laboratory manifestations of defective fibrin monomer polymerization are a prolonged thrombin time, a prolonged reptilase time, faulty clot formation and retraction, and occasional prolongation of the prothrombin time and activated partial thromboplastin time.[12,45] Hypoplasminogenemia and circulating plasmin may be found, and both proteins are readily assayed by synthetic substrate technique. Synthetic substrate-based assays are another potential aid for the assessment of pathologic fibrinolyis for tissue (endothelial) plasminogen activator activity.[45]

Fibrin(ogen) degradation product–induced platelet dysfunction is manifest in the laboratory as a prolonged template bleeding time and abnormal platelet aggregation and lumi-aggregation, although the patterns may not be consistent for the type of abnormalities seen.[45]

The laboratory findings of hypofibrinogenemia/dysfibrinogenemia induced by fibrinolysis and FDPs are prolongation of the thrombin time, prolongation of the reptilase time, and the noting of low fibrinogen levels by clotting assay, immunologic assay, or protein determination techniques.[12,18,19,45]

Since plasmin is a nonspecific proteolytic enzyme, it also degrades many coagulation factors. The primary factors degraded, besides fibrinogen (factor I), are factors V, VIII:C, IX, and XI.[12] This degradation may be pronounced with the clinical manifestation being hemorrhage.[12] The lab-

Table 8-6. Biologic Activity of Fibrin(ogen) Degradation Products

Hemostasis manifestations
    Interference with fibrin monomer polymerization
    Severe platelet dysfunction
    Thrombin inhibition
    Dysfibrinogenemia
    Hyperpyrexia

Laboratory manifestations
    Prothrombin time prolongation
    Activated partial thromboplastin time prolongation
    Thrombin time prolongation
    Reptilase time prolongation
    Hypofibrinogenemia
    Elevated fibrin(ogen) degradation products
    Template bleeding time prolongation
    Platelet aggregation abnormalities

Table 8-7. Activation of Fibrinolysis: Biologic Consequences

Lysis of coagulation proteins
    Hemorrhage

Activation of complement
    Platelet lysis
    Red blood cell lysis
    Hypotension
    Shock
    End-organ failure
    Hemorrhage

Activation of kinin system
    Hypotension
    Shock
    End-organ failure

oratory consequences of plasmin-induced coagulation factor degradation are prolongation of the prothrombin time, prolongation of the activated partial thromboplastin time, and abnormalities found on specific factor assays, including low levels of factor V, factor VIII:C, and others.[45] Another consequence of circulating plasmin is complement activation, a commonly neglected or ignored clinical aspect of primary activation of the fibrinolytic system.[9] The clinical manifestations of this activation pathway are increased vascular permeability, which leads to hypotension and shock, and cellular membrane changes, which lead to cell lysis, including red blood cell lysis and the lysis of platelets associated with release of procoagulant material.[18,19] This may be noted by abnormal complement assays, usually manifest as a decreased C3 level and decreased total hemolytic complement, and laboratory evidence of mild to moderate red blood cell hemolysis (low haptoglobin, elevated serum and urine iron levels, indirect hyperbilirubinemia, lactate dehydrogenase [LDH], and elevated reticulocyte count).[18,19]

A less common event after activation of the fibrinolytic system is kinin generation.[9] More commonly, the prekallikrein and then kinin systems are activated by mechanisms common to or before fibrinolytic system activation. The clinical consequences of kinin system activation are increased vascular permeability and vasodilatation leading to hypotension and shock.[18,19] Few clinical laboratory tools are yet available to document activation of the kinin system. The biologic consequences of pathologic activation of the fibrinolytic system are summarized in Table 8-7.

Until recently, primary activation of the fibrinolytic system was considered uncommon, and the only situations in which clinical fibrinolysis existed were assumed to be those secondary to DIC syndromes. These perceptions, however, were developed in an era when there were insufficient laboratory tools to analyze fibrinolytic activity in patients with disease. Early work in clinical fibrinolysis was limited to the use of the euglobulin lysis time, which is of no significance

in assessing clinical fibrinolytic activity.[47-49] With the advent of newer and more sophisticated techniques, such as determination of FDPs, plasminogen assays, plasmin assays, alpha-2-antiplasmin assays, and endothelial plasminogen activator assays, it is now known that primary activation of the fibrinolytic system is a common clinical event.[12] New assays for assessment of the fibrinolytic system are depicted in Table 8-8.

The conditions in which primary activation of the fibrinolytic system may happen are well defined and include chronic liver disease, cardiopulmonary bypass surgery, gastrointestinal bleeding, and malignancy.[12,36] Most patients with chronic liver disease experience a fibrino(geno)lytic syndrome resulting from increased circulating plasmin.[12,50] Primary fibrino(geno)lysis (circulating plasmin) causes many hemostatic defects. Hypofibrinogenemia and pseudodysfibrinogenemia are manifest in several forms, including the creation of high-solubility, low–thrombin clottability fibrinogen subspecies,[41] which represent fibrinogen that has undergone minimal cleavage by plasmin. Because of the fibrino(geno)lysis, patients with chronic liver disease show elevated levels of FDPs.[12] Early degradation products complex with fibrinogen and interfere with fibrin monomer polymerization, leading to a pseudodysfibrinogenemia. The fibrinogen degradation products cause severe platelet dysfunction. Circulating plasmin digests factor V, factor VIII:C, factor IX, and factor XI, further propagating hemorrhage.[4,5] These

Table 8-8. Fibrinolytic System Assays

Plasminogen
Plasmin
Alpha-2-antiplasmin
Alpha-2-macroglobulin
Fibrin(ogen) degradation products
Tissue plasminogen activator
Tissue plasminogen activator inhibitor

fibrino(geno)lytic insults to hemostasis must always be borne in mind when clinical care is being given to the patient with chronic liver disease.

Laboratory Manifestations

The consequences of circulating plasmin have been reported in detail.[12,45,46] The hallmark finding is elevated FDPs with associated severe platelet dysfunction, plasmin-induced degradation of clotting factors, and elevation of B-beta 15-42 and related peptides. D-Dimer titers usually remain normal.

Global tests of hemostasis, such as the prothrombin time and APTT, are often prolonged because of the presence of FDPs, the degradation of clotting factors V, VIII:C, IX, and XI, and FDP-induced defects in fibrin monomer polymerization. The thrombin time and reptilase time are usually prolonged as a result of interference of FDPs with fibrin monomer polymerization and plasmin-induced hypofibrinogenemia/dysfibrinogenemia. Specific factor assays usually show low levels of factors V, VIII:C, IX, and XI resulting from degradation, but these assays add little to a specific diagnosis. Assays for soluble fibrin monomer or D-dimer are usually negative since no significant fibrin monomer is formed without thrombin. Little or no AT III consumption is present; however, this test may not be of diagnostic significance since AT III levels are commonly low because of defective synthesis in patients with liver disease. Antithrombin III levels may be significantly decreased in patients with acute liver failure if a DIC-type syndrome is developing. Antithrombin III levels in liver disease are sometimes not of differential diagnostic significance.

Thrombocytopenia is highly variable depending on the underlying type of liver disease and often is not a reliable diagnostic test for distinguishing between primary fibrino(geno)lysis and DIC. Primary lysis itself will not induce thrombocytopenia, but many hepatic disorders are commonly associated with thrombocytopenia by independent mechanisms.

The keys to a laboratory diagnosis of primary fibrino(geno)lysis in liver disease are elevated FDPS, elevated levels of B-beta 15-42 and related peptides, normal fibrinopeptide A and D-dimer levels, usually negative results of the paracoagulation reaction, hypofibrinogenemia, and hypoplasminogenemia with elevated plasmin levels.[45,46] Decreased levels of alpha-2-antiplasmin will usually be found. Antithrombin III levels and platelet counts may or may not be of benefit, depending on the underlying disease process. In most instances of primary lysis, FDPs will be elevated, the B-beta 15-42 related peptides will be elevated, fibrinopeptide A levels will be normal, and results of the protamine sulfate or ethanol gelation test will usually be negative.[45,46,51] In most instances of DIC, FDPs will be elevated, the B-beta 15-42 peptides will be elevated, fibrinopeptides A or B and D-dimer levels will be elevated, the protamine sulfate or ethanol gelation test will be positive, plasminogen will be depressed, alpha-2-antiplasmin will be depressed,

Table 8-9. Molecular Markers for the Differential Diagnosis of Disseminated Intravascular Coagulation vs Primary Lysis

Marker	DIC	Primary lysis
Fibrinopeptide A	Elevated	Normal
Fibrinopeptide B	Elevated	Normal
B-beta 15-42 peptide	Elevated	Normal
B-beta 1-42 peptide	Elevated	Elevated
B-beta 1-118 peptide	Elevated	Elevated
Platelet factor 4	Elevated	Normal
Beta-thromboglobulin	Elevated	Normal
D-dimer	Elevated	Normal

circulating plasmin may be present, and AT III levels are markedly decreased.[18,19,45] Newer methods for the laboratory assessment of primary fibrino(geno)lysis are depicted in Table 8-8. Molecular marker profiling for rendering a differential diagnosis between DIC and primary fibrinolysis is depicted in Table 8-9.

Primary activation of the fibrinolytic system happens often in chronic liver disease, and this defect in hemostasis must, like other defects, be recalled in the patient with liver disease and hemorrhage, assessed from the laboratory standpoint, and treated appropriately if present. The usual therapy for primary fibrinolysis is the use of epsilon aminocaproic acid given as a 5- to 10-g slow intravenous push followed by 1 to 2 g/hour for 24 hours or tranexamic acid given as 500 mg every eight to 12 hours either orally or intravenously until fibrinolysis and subsequent hemorrhage stop.[4,5]

Platelet Defects

Thrombocytopenia

Thrombocytopenia is seen in up to 35% of patients with chronic liver disease (cirrhosis) of diverse causes.[52] The most common cause is portal hypertension with resultant congestive splenomegaly and hypersplenism.[53-55] Hypersplenism (increased splenic sequestration of platelets and other cellular elements) need not always be associated with significant splenomegaly. In most patients with chronic liver disease, however, thrombocytopenia correlates well with the degree of splenomegaly, and the degree of splenomegaly correlates well with the severity of hepatic damage.[56] This results in decreased platelet survival, and marrow megakaryocytes are usually normal to increased in number. Portacaval shunts will correct the thrombocytopenia of hypersplenism secondary to portal hypertension in about 30% of patients.[57]

Patients with cirrhosis may also have thrombocytopenia secondary to folate deficiency, which may arise from poor dietary intake, poor intestinal absorption, or enhanced requirements, such as patients with cirrhosis and hemolysis.

The archaic use of massive transfusions of banked whole blood to treat hemorrhage associated with liver disease may also significantly add to already existing thrombocytopenia or may independently induce thrombocytopenia.[20] This custom is to be condemned. Although whole blood supplies volume and oxygen-carrying capacity, its use in patients with acute or chronic liver disease is generally detrimental to the platelet count and to many other already impaired hemostasis systems and often leads to enhanced and uncontrollable hemorrhage.[4,5] The more modern approach to component therapy in patients with liver disease and hemorrhage, which has served to improve this problem, includes washed packed red blood cells, platelet concentrates, volume expanders, and occasional fresh frozen plasma. Thrombocytopenia may also arise because of DIC in patients with terminal chronic liver disease.[4,5] Disseminated intravascular coagulation is usually not associated with cirrhosis until cirrhosis reaches its terminal stage.[49] However, patients with chronic liver disease can develop DIC and associated severe thrombocytopenia if subjected to any of the usual triggers or disease entities, such as septicemia, shock, and the like, which may induce DIC (see chapter 7).

Significant thrombocytopenia may also be seen in acute liver failure of viral or drug- or chemical-induced etiology.[39] The thrombocytopenia of acute viral hepatitis, HIV, and hepatitis seen with mononucleosis or cytomegalovirus may be multifactorial. In these instances, an element of DIC may contribute to or account for thrombocytopenia via previously mentioned mechanisms (see chapter 7), megakaryopoiesis may be selectively suppressed, or the thrombocytopenia may be part of a pancytopenia associated with marrow aplasia that occasionally happens in patients with acute hepatic failure.[21,58,59] In acute hepatic failure of viral, drug, or chemical/toxin etiology, thrombocytopenia may result from the development of antiplatelet antibodies or the presence of circulating immune complexes.[60] In clinical practice, the thrombocytopenia of acute or chronic liver disease may be a compilation of several or all of these mechanisms.

If the patient with chronic liver disease is also an alcoholic, other mechanisms for the development of thrombocytopenia may be operative. Thrombocytopenia may be seen in up to 25% of ill patients who are actively drinking,[61,62] and 50% of these will have concomitant cirrhosis.[61-63] Ethanol appears to be directly toxic to megakaryocytes and may induce peripheral thrombocytopenia by causing ineffective megakaryopoiesis.[61,64-66] Additionally, ethanol induces a nonselective peripheral destruction of platelets, which does not necessarily result from splenic sequestration.[61,65,66] The reported findings of platelet size distribution profiles and platelet survival studies show ethanol to induce an increase in the percentage of small circulating platelets and a decrease in platelet survival. These findings are compatible with both ineffective megakaryopoiesis and enhanced peripheral destruction.[61,62,65] Folate deficiency associated with ethanol abuse, even without cirrhosis, may also contribute to or be responsible for thrombocytopenia.[61,64] Persis-

Table 8-10. Causes of Thrombocytopenia

Chronic liver disease
  Splenomegaly and hypersplenism
  Disseminated intravascular coagulation
  Massive transfusions with whole blood
  Folate deficiency
  Concurrent alcohol abuse

Acute liver disease
  Megakaryopoiesis suppression
  Aplastic anemia
  Disseminated intravascular coagulation
  Antiplatelet antibodies
  Circulating immune complexes
  Liver transplantation rejection

Ethanol abuse
  Splenomegaly and hypersplenism
  Ineffective megakaryopoiesis
  Nonselective peripheral destruction
  Folate deficiency
  Rebound thrombocytosis occurs in 30% with abstinence

tent thrombocytopenia is usually caused by portal hypertension, splenomegaly, and associated hypersplenism. If primarily caused by acute ethanol intoxication instead of splenic sequestration, the thrombocytopenia will usually abate within one to three weeks after abstinence.[61,62] In this regard, a rebound thrombocytosis may be seen in up to 30% of patients, which sometimes has been thought to be responsible for thrombotic episodes.[61,67] The template bleeding time may be two times prolonged with acute ethanol intoxication and up to five times prolonged with ethanol ingestion plus thrombocytopenia.[61] These findings should be viewed as multifactorial and are not only an ethanol- or cirrhosis-induced platelet function defect or thrombocytopenia but may also result from a vascular defect that may be present in alcoholic, cirrhotic patients.[5,7,68] The causes of thrombocytopenia associated with chronic liver disease, acute liver disease and acute hepatic failure, and alcohol are summarized in Table 8-10.

Many patients with chronic liver disease and ascites are subjected to LeVeen shunting, which may induce a DIC-type syndrome and associated severe thrombocytopenia (see chapters 7, 9, and 10).

It is unclear to what degree thrombocytopenia contributes to hemorrhage in patients with liver disease. Not only are the causes of thrombocytopenia itself multifaceted, but thrombocytopenia is only one of numerous alterations of hemostasis in patients with acute or chronic liver disease. Thrombocytopenia should be thought of as being part of a summation of multifactorial events when hemorrhage is present in these patients. Fortunately, however, thrombocytopenia is a defect that, if thought to be of clinical significance in the hemorrhaging patient with liver disease, can usually be readily corrected with the liberal use of platelet concentrates.

Platelet Dysfunction

Significant platelet dysfunction happens in patients with liver disease, although this hemostatic defect is less commonly appreciated and often goes unrecognized in patients with liver disease and hemorrhage.[12] As with thrombocytopenia, causes of platelet dysfunction in patients with liver disease are multifactorial in origin. Most patients with chronic liver disease have primary activation of the fibrinolytic system and resultant elevated circulating FDPs.[12] These circulating FDPs may severely compromise platelet function. Another reason for platelet dysfunction is an increase in older platelets, which are presumably less hemostatically active platelets, as noted by a decreased MPV in patients with liver disease.[65] Patients with both acute and chronic liver disease often show secondary aggregation defects or storage pool–type aggregation defects manifest as blunted aggregation to collagen, thrombin, and ristocetin and absent secondary aggregation waves after aggregation with ADP and epinephrine.[61,69] Platelet factor 3 release is commonly impaired.[70] Platelet dysfunction in liver disease may be a manifestation of altered platelet membrane palmate and sterate metabolism,[71] may result from coating of platelet membranes by FDPs,[12] or may be a combination of these defects. These defects may also be manifestations of many as yet undefined changes in platelet metabolic pathways.

If the patient with liver disease is an ethanol abuser, platelet function is further compromised. The ingestion of high doses of ethanol, even without significant liver disease, may induce a storage pool–type defect. Decreased storage pool ADP and ATP are induced by ethanol alone, and cyclic AMP levels are also reduced by ethanol-induced inhibition of adenylate cyclase.[61,69,72] As another insult, ethanol inhibits thromboxane A_2 synthesis.[61,69] Ethanol is known to inhibit monoamine oxidase but causes a 50% to 100% increase in intraplatelet serotonin, and the significance of this is unknown.[61,73-75] Ethanol induces significant changes in intraplatelet metabolism of adenine nucleotides, cyclic AMP, prostaglandins, and thromboxanes. Ethanol ingestion also impairs platelet factor 3 availability. Whether this results from previously mentioned changes or other undefined effects of ethanol, is unclear. Folate deficiency may accompany heavy ethanol ingestion without significant liver disease, and this also may induce a platelet function defect, independent of folate-associated thrombocytopenia.[20,61,76] Morphologic changes of platelets induced by ethanol, and presumably associated with defects in platelet function, have been described. These morphologic changes include vacuolization of both platelets and megakaryocytes, abnormal platelet granules, microtubular fragmentation, and the presence of giant platelets.[61,69] Platelet function defects, like thrombocytopenia, have also been seen in association with liver transplantation,[77] which is probably because of coating of platelets by FDPs resulting from a DIC-type syndrome. As with thrombocytopenia associated with transplantation rejection and resultant circulating immune complexes, these immune complexes will also compromise platelet function, since they are potent inducers of a platelet release reaction.

Table 8-11. Causes of Platelet Dysfunction

Chronic liver disease
  Elevated fibrin(ogen) degradation products
  Older circulating platelets
  Acquired storage pool defect
  Defective platelet factor 3 availability
  Defective platelet membrane receptors
  Folate deficiency

Acute liver disease
  Elevated fibrin(ogen) degradation products
  Acquired storage pool defect
  Abnormal platelet factor 3 availability

Alcohol abuse
  Acquired storage pool defect
  Deranged intraplatelet metabolism
  Folate deficiency

Hepatic transplantation rejection
  Elevated fibrin(ogen) degradation products
  Circulating immune complexes

Acute and chronic liver diseases are often associated with a severe and clinically significant platelet function defect. This defect is multifactorial and may result from altered intraplatelet metabolism of the compounds previously discussed and because of the presence of FDPs. If the patient is also an ethanol abuser, these defects are compounded. Ethanol itself, even without significant liver disease, may induce a significant platelet function defect. Most patients with acute and chronic liver disease do show significant platelet dysfunction. One cannot assume a false sense of security when examining a patient with liver disease, hemorrhage, and a normal or near normal platelet count, because the platelets circulating, although normal in number, may be significantly dysfunctional and contribute to hemorrhage that has remained unresponsive to infusions of fresh frozen plasma. When seeing patients with liver disease and hemorrhage, platelet dysfunction should be recalled, its presence or absence documented by aggregation or lumi-aggregtion, and if present, it should be treated with proper numbers of platelet concentrates despite the platelet count. Mechanisms of platelet function defects in chronic liver disease, acute liver disease, acute hepatic failure, and ethanol are summarized in Table 8-11.

Vascular Defects

The patient with chronic liver disease often harbors poorly defined vascular defects. This manifestation has often been ascribed to an estrogenlike effect on the vasculature, since these patients do have abnormal hepatic clearance and resultant hyperestrogenemia. This mechanism as a cause of the commonly seen vascular defect in patients is, however, poorly understood and undocumented. Despite the mechanism(s), the vascular defect may reach clinical significance, especially if the patient is subjected to surgery or trauma. This defect may also contribute to the prolonged template bleeding time seen in patients with chronic liver disease. Prolonged template bleeding times in patients with chronic liver disease may be the result of a combination of thrombocytopenia, platelet dysfunction, and a vascular defect.

Disseminated Intravascular Coagulation

Disseminated intravascular coagulation rarely, if ever, happens de novo as a hemostatic defect in patients with chronic liver disease,[12,18,19] but it may be operative in acute liver failure including hepatitis, acute liver failure of any origin, in patients subjected to LeVeen or Denver peritoneovenous shunting, and in patients with long-standing biliary obstruction and intrahepatic or extrahepatic cholestasis.[20,21,24,27,30] The patient with chronic liver disease is a candidate for DIC, as is any other patient, if one of the usual triggering events is involved, such as sepsis, massive transfusions with banked whole blood, transfusion reactions, shock, and other etiologic events known to trigger DIC.

Laboratory Findings

Most tests of hemostasis, including global screening tests, will be markedly abnormal in association with significant alterations of hemostasis associated with liver disease. The laboratory changes in patients with chronic liver disease will be a summation of not only the underlying type of defect (ie, acute liver disease, chronic liver disease, or cholestatic liver disease), but also a summary manifestation of all the defects that may be present and operative singularly or in any potential combination. Useful laboratory modalities for assessing hemostasis in patients with chronic liver disease are summarized in Table 8-12.[45] The mainstay of laboratory testing for assessing function of the prothrombin complex factors is the prothrombin time. In significantly decreased or dysfunctional synthesis of factors II, VII, IX, and X, the prothrombin time will be prolonged.[4,5] Whether the degree of prolongation is related to clinical hemorrhage is a subject of controversy. The decrease in factor VII closely correlates with prolongation of the prothrombin time; however, decreased/dysfunctional synthesis of factors IX and X more closely correlate with clinical hemorrhage. The prothrombin time may also be abnormal for other reasons. The presence of elevated FDPs or plasmin-induced biodegradation of factor V will also prolong the prothrombin time.[12] The APTT is also prolonged in patients with acute or chronic liver disease. This happens for reasons similar to those described for the prothrombin time, including plasmin-induced biodegradation of factor VIII:C and other factors susceptible to plasmin. Specific factor assays will usually show low levels, but values for some factors may be high or normal depending on the particular defect operative, amount of fibrinolysis, and the degree that several factors have increased as acute-phase reactants. High levels of factor VIII:C may be found unless significant plasmin is present, in which case low levels of factors VIII:C, V, and XI may be seen.[4,5] Lysis may contribute to the degree of decrease in factor XII, Fletcher factor, and high–molecular weight kininogen.

Table 8-12. Laboratory Evaluation of Hemostasis in Chronic Liver Disease

Coagulation protein defects
    Prothrombin time
    Activated partial thromboplastin time
    Fibrinogen level

Primary activation of fibrinolysis
    Plasminogen
    Plasmin
    Alpha-2-antiplasmin
    Alpha-2-macroglobulin
    Tissue plasminogen activator
    Tissue plasminogen activator inhibitor
    Fibrin(ogen) degradation products
    B-beta 15-42 and related peptides
    D-dimer

Platelet dysfunction
    Template bleeding time (not reliable)
    Platelet aggregation (lumi-aggregation)

Thrombocytopenia
    Peripheral smear evaluation
    Platelet count
    Computed tomographic scan of spleen

Tests for fibrinolysis will be abnormal in greater than 75% of patients with chronic liver disease and may be abnormal in patients with acute hepatic failure or cholestasis if DIC and secondary fibrinolysis are present.[12,50] Circulating plasmin and elevated FDP levels will be found in conjunction with decreased levels of plasminogen resulting from activation of the fibrinolytic system and plasminogen depletion. Good differential diagnostic tools in this respect for noting whether DIC is operative or whether low levels of clotting factors are present because of primary lysis are the B-beta 15-42 and related peptide determinations, in conjunction with fibrinopeptide A, D-dimer assay, the platelet release proteins, platelet factor 4 and beta-thromboglobulin, and a positive or negative paracoagulation reaction.[12]

Results of tests of platelet function will also be abnormal. Prolongation of the template bleeding time may result from a combination of platelet function defects, thrombocytopenia, or defects in the vasculature in patients with chronic liver disease or in patients with acute hepatic failure or cholestasis. However, no characteristic aggregation or lumi-aggregation patterns will be noted in these patients. In this regard, a template bleeding time should not be done in association with thrombocytopenia (platelet count less than 100 x 10^9/L [100,000/mm^3]), because this may be associated with unnecessary bleeding and will give results that are meaningless. Prolongation of the template bleeding time may be multifactorial, including induction by heavy ethanol ingestion. Whether the prolongation of the template bleeding time correlates with clinical propensity to hemorrhage, however, is a subject of controversy. The use of a thrombin time or reptilase time will offer an indication of the dysfibrinogenemia or hypofibrinogenemia present. Both laboratory modalities will also be prolonged with FDPs, rendering the results difficult to interpret with respect to precise reasons for the prolongation of these tests.

Clearly most tests of hemostasis will be markedly abnormal in patients with chronic or acute liver disease or cholestasis. Only with the use of a well-chosen hemostatic profile can each component of hemostasis be assessed with the type of liver disease defined, the precise defect or combination of defects therefore delineated, and a logical sequential approach to treatment of hemorrhage outlined.

Management

All clinicians are well aware of the catastrophic hemorrhage that happens in patients with chronic liver disease and the major challenge this disease presents for the laboratory, blood bank, pathologist, surgeon, hematologist, gastroenterologist, and internist. Unfortunately, the standard types of therapy in most patients are still limited to infusions of platelets, volume expanders, fresh frozen plasma, Sengstaken-Blakemore tamponade, gastric lavage, and vasopressin infusion.[78] However, many patients do not respond to these modalities of therapy. If the patient has significant fibrino-(geno)lysis, the concomitant or later use of antifibrinolytic agents, usually epsilon aminocaproic acid, may be indicated. Epsilon aminocaproic acid is used at a dosage of a 5- to 10-g slow intravenous push followed by 1 to 2 g/hour for 24 hours or until cessation of clinical hemorrhage is noted. Tranexamic acid is a newer and more potent antifibrinolytic agent and is not only effective in aborting systemic fibrinolysis but also in controlling diffuse hemorrhagic gastritis.[79-81] Tranexamic acid is given as 500 mg orally or intravenously every eight to 12 hours. If the patient is significantly thrombocytopenic, the liberal use of platelet concentrates should be considered. Platelet concentrates will correct the thrombocytopenia and will usually alleviate bleeding caused by the platelet function defect present. In patients failing to respond to these modalities of therapy, the use of prothrombin complex concentrates, with other components such as platelet concentrates and other indicated therapeutic modalities, may have to be employed.[82,83]

Another, although somewhat heroic approach, is to treat patients with exchange transfusions.[4,5] The use of exchange transfusion or the infusion of prothrombin complex concentrate to control hemorrhage is probably not indicated in patients with chronic liver disease and fulminant hemorrhage unless a surgically correctable bleeding point is proven, the patient is thought to be a surgical candidate, and the defect is thought to be correctable, because these modalities will only achieve hemostasis for a short time.[4,5] In reality many patients with fulminant hemorrhage survive if the treatment is approached in a logical and sequential manner that must include a precise delineation of the exact type of liver disease and hemostatic defect(s) present with each defect defined and treated individually. The patient with

Table 8-13. Therapy for Hemorrhage in Liver Disease

Coagulation protein defects
  Parenteral vitamin K
  Fresh or fresh frozen plasma (directed single donor for
    components if possible; discouraged)
  Prothrombin complex concentrates (hazards)
  Plasma exchange (investigational)

Primary fibrinolysis
  Tranexamic acid
  Aminocaproic acid

Platelet dysfunction or thrombocytopenia
  Platelet concentrates
  Portacaval shunting if indicated
  Immunosuppressive therapy if indicated

Disseminated intravascular coagulation
  Supportive therapy for shock
  Low-dose calcium heparin (generally not in chronic liver
    disease with disseminated intravascular coagulation)
  Platelet concentrates
  Antithrombin concentrates
  Immunosuppressive therapy if indicated

cholestasis and abnormal synthesis of the prothrombin complex factors will usually respond to the immediate parenteral administration of vitamin K with the usual dose of 30 mg intramuscularly or 1 mg/minute intravenously. If brisk bleeding is present, the use of fresh frozen plasma or prothrombin complex concentrates may stop hemorrhage. These patients may also develop a fulminant DIC-type syndrome, which must be treated appropriately if present.[49] Patients with acute liver disease or cholestasis who develop DIC rarely develop intravascular microthrombi, and the advisability of using heparin in patients with cholestasis or acute liver failure with DIC is debatable but must be individualized. This general approach to the patient with acute or chronic liver disease of varied etiologies allows successful blunting or arrest of hemorrhage to the point where the patient may become a reasonable candidate for surgical correction of the initiating event, which is most often peptic ulcer disease, a ruptured esophageal varix, or hemorrhagic gastritis. The patient with viral-, toxin-, or drug-induced acute liver failure is usually not a surgical candidate. The patient with cholestasis often is a surgical candidate, and the infusions of fresh frozen plasma, the recognition of the presence or absence of DIC, and the use of parenteral vitamin K may arrest hemorrhage. Therapeutic modalities available for the control of hemorrhage in liver disease are summarized in Table 8-13.

Liver Transplantation

Liver transplantation has now been successfully carried out in more than 2500 recipients during the last decade. However, liver transplantation is associated with severe coagulopathies of as yet uncertain origin and pathophysiology. Although the act of transplantation itself is associated with severe and rapid deterioration of the coagulation process, this is further complicated by the fact that most patients with chronic liver disease, usually cholangitis, primary biliary cirrhosis, or chronic active hepatitis, already have an associated severely compromised hemostasis system consisting of decreased or defective synthesis of coagulation factors, a primary fibrino(geno)lytic syndrome, platelet dysfunction, and thrombocytopenia.[4,84] Aside from an already compromised hemostasis system, the patient undergoing transplantation develops other derangements in hemostasis. The first transplantation-associated defect happens during the anhepatic phase and is generally associated with marked decreases in coagulation factors and platelets. The immediate posttransplantation phase is often associated with further deterioration in hemostasis by enhanced additional decreases in coagulation factors and platelets. Although all investigators note severe defects in hemostasis associated with hepatic transplantation, little agreement exists regarding the pathophysiology of deranged hemostasis in the anhepatic and posttransplantation phases. Disagreement also exists regarding whether the type of venovenous shunting has any positive or negative effect on hemostasis.

Owen, Rettke, and Bowie[85] have intensively studied hemostasis changes during the first 50 liver transplantation procedures done at the Mayo Clinic and concluded that DIC is the primary coagulopathy associated with the anhepatic and posttransplantation phases. They further concluded that although the venovenous shunt was not associated with heparin or other systemic anticoagulation therapy, this probably had little effect on the hemostasis changes, even though it was believed that some platelets might be trapped in the pump and certain coagulation factors could conceivably become activated on the walls of the pump.

Nakao, Kano, and Nonami[86] studied the application of an antithrombogenic Anthron bypass tube to coagulation and fibrinolysis in experimental liver transplantation using a method consisting of venous bypass from the inferior vena cava to the superior vena cava through one tube and from the portal vein to the superior vena cava by another tube. They noted no coagulation changes using this antithrombogenic Anthron bypass venovenous device. Tuman, Spiess, and McCarthy[87] reported that the use of an elaborate continuous arteriovenous hemofiltration bypass did not correct coagulation abnormalities, although it did have a positive impact on cardiac and renal complications. Regarding pathophysiology, Kang, Martin, and Marquez[88] studied 66 consecutive patients undergoing liver transplantation and noted that several defects occurred. These authors noted the following: (1) an exaggerated dilution effect resulting from the influx of organ preservation solution from the donor liver; (2) an active fibrinolytic syndrome in many of their patients thought to be caused by release of TPA from hepatic vascular endothelium; and (3) the loss of hepatic clearance function thought to contribute to the pathophysiology of deranged hemostasis. However, Sporn, Mauritz, and Schindler[89] studied 21 liver transplantation patients and noted that although they could not clearly define the pathophysiology of the defect, the use of preoperative plasmapheresis and preoperative platelet transfusions markedly reduced coagulopathy and total blood loss.

Grenvik and Gordon,[90] although again unable to define the type of coagulopathy, reported that the liberal use of packed red blood cells, fresh frozen plasma, platelet concentrates, cryoprecipitate, and epsilon aminocaproic acid resulted in only rare bleeding in the posttransplantation phase.

Bellani, Estrin, and Ascher[91] studied 66 hepatic transplantation patients and did not find primary fibrinolysis or DIC. Instead, they found that although most patients bled, the bleeding resulted from heparin, which they believed was caused by exogenous use but could also have been released endogenously during the procedure. Almost all patients stopped bleeding when protamine sulfate was delivered. Fibrinolysis was noted on rare occasion, but DIC was not documented in any of their 66 patients.

Dzik, Arkin, and Jenkins[92] carefully studied the hemostasis defects associated with hepatic transplantation in eight patients and noted extensive primary systemic fibrinolysis in five of the eight patients after recognizing a marked consumption of alpha-2-antiplasmin associated with fibrinogen degradation and concomitant appearance of FDPs. In association with these changes, they noted a significant increase in TPA activity and antigen levels. Fibrinolysis was most pronounced during the anhepatic phase of surgery and began to decrease after revascularization of the grafted liver. The operative course of patients developing TPA-associated primary fibrinolysis was characterized by transient shock, acidosis, generalized bleeding, and a need for greater blood product support during surgery. These authors lastly concluded that the primary systemic fibrinolytic defect is related to increased circulating plasma levels of TPA presumably resulting from a combination of increased intravascular release (presumably from vascular manipulation) and decreased hepatic clearance of already circulating TPA.

Although a serious and complex hemostatic compromise happens during allogeneic hepatic transplantation, authorities studying this problem do not agree on the pathophysiology of the defect. The primary theories are that this represents DIC, fibrinolysis, or a combination of both. A minority opinion appears to be that the defect primarily results from the use or release of heparin during the procedure. Indeed, since these patients already have severely compromised hemostasis because of the chronic liver disease necessitating transplantation, it would be extremely difficult to identify precisely the pathophysiologic mechanisms associated with the further deterioration of hemostasis during transplantation. A few case reports have been associated with massive thrombosis or thromboembolus during hepatic transplantation. Casella, Bontempo, and Markel[93] described a patient with homozygous protein C deficiency who underwent successful hepatic transplantation. This patient had an extraordinary thrombotic history before transplantation and developed hepatic artery and portal vein thrombosis during the transplantation operative procedure. Apparently the child did not have serious bleeding during the transplantation procedure. Navalgund, Kang, and Sarner[94] reported a case of fatal massive pulmonary embolus during the transplantation procedure. This patient, like the other, did not appear to undergo massive bleeding or significant hemostasis defects during the transplant itself. The cause of pulmonary embolism in this patient was uncertain, as in patients with end-stage liver disease, and decreased levels of coagulation factors and platelets would suggest that thrombus formation would be unlikely. Pulmonary embolism after hepatic transplantation has also been reported.[94] Although there are conflicting reports concerning whether DIC or a primary fibrino(geno)lytic syndrome is generally responsible for the severe deterioration of hemostasis during the anhepatic and posttransplantation phases, many investigators believe DIC to be the pathophysiologic defect and many incriminate primary fibrinolysis as the primary hemostatic defect.[95]

Hemorrhage in the patient with chronic liver disease can no longer be attributed to a simple decrease in the synthesis of factors II, VII, IX, and X. Many defects may happen, and when significant or life-threatening hemorrhage develops, this may be because of any one or a combination of these defects. When treating the patient with hemorrhage in association with chronic liver disease it is a major clinical and laboratory challenge to define precisely those defects most probably at fault in causing hemorrhage and then to deliver specific, logical, and effective therapy. If primary fibrino(geno)lysis is the major cause of hemorrhage, as it often is, the proper therapy is antifibrinolytic. Fresh frozen plasma may be used to correct hemorrhage associated with decreased or dysfunctional synthesis of factors II, VII, IX, and X. Vitamin K is used to reverse dysfunctional synthesis. If significant thrombocytopenia or platelet dysfunction is present, infusion of platelet concentrates is indicated. When the patient does not respond to specific therapy directed at clearly defined defects, the use of prothrombin complex concentrates in combination with other components may have to be used. This is an investigational method, however, and those choosing to use these therapeutic modalities should be aware of the potential for disseminated thromboses and hepatitis. All blood products are associated with blood-borne infection, including HIV, and must be used wisely, always weighing the benefits vs the risks. The same arguments apply for the patient with acute liver failure or cholestasis: multifactorial defects may be present, including a fulminant DIC-type syndrome. One must recall all of these defects and document the presence or absence of DIC when designing effective and logical therapy for these patients.

Renal Disease

Dialysis

Renal hemodialysis is the mainstay of therapy for acute and chronic renal failure and for the alleviation of selected acute toxicity or poisoning. However, the formation of fibrin-platelet thrombi on the dialysis membrane reduces its efficiency and provides a focus for embolization, with later potential complications.[96,97] Renal hemodialysis is commonly associated with neutrophil adherence and complement activation on the dialysis membrane.[98] The complement activation may further add to clinical problems by the release of the anaphylatoxins C3a and C5a with subsequent leukoembolization as well. Since thrombosis and thromboembolism are major clinical problems associated with renal hemodialysis, systemic or regional heparinization is used.[96,97] Regional heparinization consists of adding heparin to the arterial line as blood leaves the patient and neutralizing heparin with protamine in the venous line as blood returns to the patient. Some have considered heparin rebound to be a clinical problem with regional heparinization.[99] Platelet-suppressive therapy has decreased platelet adhesion to dialysis membranes. Antiplatelet agents must be used cautiously in uremic patients with already compromised platelet function (see chapter 5).[96,97,100,101]

Many hemostatic defects are associated with underlying renal disease, but these defects may be difficult to distinguish from defects induced by dialysis. The role of the hemostasis system as a mediator of renal vascular and glomerular damage is unclear. Evidence suggesting participation of the hemostasis system in renal disease is based on morphologic, histochemical, serologic, and radioisotope studies and the noting of abnormal test results of hemostasis.[96,97] Renal diseases associated with a microangiopathic hemolytic anemia as a prominent feature are accompanied by activation of the hemostasis system with later fibrin deposition, which is responsible for progressive renal damage. However, the role of the hemostasis system and the pathogenesis of other glomerular diseases is less clear, and it is often impossible to know if activation of the hemostasis system leads to renal damage or disease, or, alternatively, if renal disease leads to activation of the hemostasis system with subsequent renal microvascular fibrin deposition. The mechanisms responsible for accelerating fibrin deposition in renal disease are also unclear.[96,97] However, fibrin deposition in glomeruli assumes an important pathogenetic role in crescent formation and eventual glomerular degeneration.[102] Fibrin is not only deposited within capillaries but also in Bowman's space where it probably stimulates epithelial cell proliferation with later crescent formation. Fibrin leakage through capillary walls is thought to result from focal membrane disruption. Crescent formation progresses through three well-defined stages: cellular, fibrocellular, and fibrotic. Crescent formation is a prominent feature of idiopathic extracapillary glomerulonephritis. In other glomerular diseases, however, including acute poststreptococcal nephritis, lupus nephritis, and anaphylactoid purpura, crescent formation is less pronounced.[96,97]

Immunofluorescent microscopy appears to be the best single technique for consistently detecting fibrinogen, fibrin, or FDPs in the kidney.[96,97] These deposits have been consistently shown by immunofluorescence, even when histologic stains for fibrin or electron microscopy studies have been negative.[103] Fibrinogen, fibrin, and FDP deposits have been detected by immunochemical techniques either along the basement membrane within the mesangium or in the vascular walls in a variety of renal diseases, including hemolytic-uremic syndrome, scleroderma, malignant hypertension, acute homograft rejection, postpartum renal failure, and rapidly progressive glomerulonephritis.[104-106] Additionally, in hemolytic-uremic syndrome, postpartum renal failure, acute homograft rejection, scleroderma, and malignant hypertension, factor VIII is present in the same areas as fibrinogen.[107] This finding suggests an active participation of the hemostasis system that leads to later fibrin deposition in these disorders. Factor VIII has not been found in epithelial cell crescents in proliferative nephritis or in the mesangium of patients with anaphylactoid purpura, all of which are areas of intense fibrinogen, fibrin, and FDP deposition. This finding suggests that differing mechanisms of fibrin deposition and hemostasis activation may exist in differing renal diseases.[108] Factor VIII:C levels may be of prognostic significance in patients with glomerulonephritis: high levels are associated with a poor prognosis and a low probability of renal function returning to normal.[109] Furthermore, this increase is attributed to progressive vascular endothelial damage.

The clearance of deposited fibrin in the kidney may happen because of endothelial cell or mesangial cell phagocytosis or because of fibrino(geno)lysis by plasminogen activators in the associated vascular endothelium. Human kidney endothelial cells produce a potent plasminogen activator: urokinase. In the normal kidney, plasminogen activator activity may be demonstrated in glomeruli, arteries, arterioles, and veins.[110] An unclear relationship exists between glomerular fibrin deposition and glomerular fibrinolysis in kidneys from patients with a wide variety of renal diseases. Plasminogen activator activity is absent in the cortex of patients with acute renal homograft rejection, although the mechanisms responsible for loss of fibrinolytic activator activity are unknown.[111]

Generally, serum FDPs are elevated in most of these renal diseases and vary with the activity and severity of the disease process.[96,97,112] Extrarenal sites of fibrino(geno)lysis, however, will also lead to elevated serum FDP levels, which are found in several renal diseases, including lupus nephritis, poststreptococcal progressive glomerulonephritis, anaphylactic purpura, hemolytic-uremic syndrome, nephrotic syndrome, focal sclerosis with hypertension, renal failure, and membranous nephropathy.[96,97] Urinary FDPs correlate much better with disease activity and fibrin deposition than do serum FDP levels.[113-115] Urinary FDP excretion may not correlate with disease activity, since variability may be noted with the degree of protein selectivity.[116] Others, however, have found that urinary FDPs are indicative of renal fibrin deposition and not of protein excretion selectivity.[117]

The role of platelets as mediators of renal disease is unclear and confusing. However, abnormal platelet turnover, manifest by decreased platelet survival, increased platelet consumption, and abnormal platelet aggregation patterns, has been noted in hemolytic-uremic syndrome, acute homograft rejection, membranoproliferative nephritis, glomerulosclerosis, diffuse proliferative nephritis, and diabetic nephropathy.[96,97,114] Bilateral nephrectomy results in normalization of platelet survival in a variety of renal diseases, which suggests the presence of intrarenal platelet deposition.[114] Despite these findings, it is unclear whether improvement in renal function will happen in patients treated with anticoagulant or platelet-suppressive therapy, although such therapy tends to lead to normal platelet survival. Increased platelet aggregability has been documented in patients with Alport's syndrome, nephrotic syndrome, active glomerulonephritis, and in patients with diabetic nephropathy.[118] Immune complex–induced endothelial injury and changes of the renal basement membrane and other subendothelial surfaces may certainly lead to primary platelet activation. This event may provide procoagulant material for later activation of the blood proteins and subsequent fibrin deposition in similar morphologic areas.[96,97]

The precise role of the hemostasis system as a modulator of renal disease is unclear.[96,97] The presence of decreased platelet survival, FDPs, and factor VIII by immunofluorescent studies and the noting of elevated urine and serum FDPs in most renal diseases present highly suggestive evidence of active participation of hemostasis in immune-mediated glomerular disease. Unfortunately, what is unclear is whether activation of the hemostasis system may lead to renal microvascular fibrin deposition with later renal disease or, alternatively, whether exposure of the hemostasis system to subendothelial collagen or other materials in the renal microenvironment will later activate the hemostasis system.[96,97]

In patients with various renal disorders, the determination of serum and urinary FDPs is useful for aiding in a diagnosis, assessing severity of disease, and monitoring disease activity and potential efficacy of therapy. Generally, the urinary FDP titer appears better correlated with severity and activity of disease. Urinary FDP titers of up to 50 µg/dL have been noted in active renal disorders, including hydronephrosis, lupus nephritis, and proliferative glomerular nephritis, and these levels are generally noted to correlate well with disease activity.[96,97,119] In contrast, patients with minimal renal disease or membranous lesions have FDP levels rarely exceeding 2 µg/dL, which provides an important laboratory diagnostic tool.[96,97] In both types of lesions, including those associated with minimal nephrotic syndrome, serum FDP levels may be abnormally elevated. Studies have shown that urinary FDP levels decrease when therapy for glomerular lesions is effective.[119,120]

In pediatric renal disease, including chronic glomerular nephritis, Henoch-Schönlein glomerulonephritis, and hemolytic-uremic syndrome, high serum FDP levels are often noted.[96,97] In the presence of disease progression, urinary FDP levels may begin to rise, and when monitored in association with blood pressure, they may provide evidence

Figure 8-3. Platelet Function in Uremia (Lumi-Aggregation)

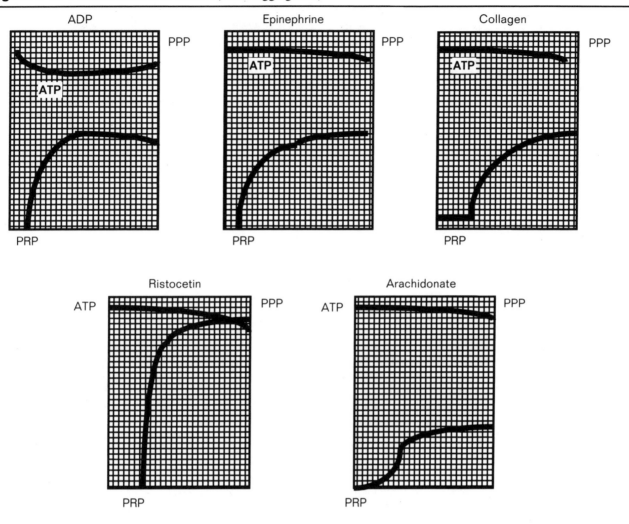

PRP = Platelet-Rich Plasma
PPP = Platelet-Poor Plasma
ATP = ATP Release

of effective therapy when decreases in titer and blood pressure are noted.[120]

Patients with upper urinary tract infections usually have elevated urinary FDP titers. The urinary FDP titer appears to help in distinguishing the site of urinary tract infections.[121]

Patients with recent renal homograft transplants often show elevated levels of FDPs in serum and urine as the donor kidney begins to function. Although several investigators have reported that the determination of urinary FDPs appears to be of little value in the diagnosis of early acute rejection but may be helpful in chronic rejection,[96,97,122,123] other investigators have shown that the assay of FDPs in urine and serum does indeed provide a sensitive laboratory index of impending rejection.[96,97,124] The failure to note rising urinary FDPs to decrease after enhancing immunosuppressive therapy seems to correlate with rejection and may

indicate the need for still more intensive therapy in trying to salvage the graft.[96,97,123] Sustained increased FDP titers appear to correlate with early graft rejection and herald the need for more aggressive therapy.[96,97,124]

Current evidence would suggest that serum and urine FDP titers may be a useful guide in the diagnosis, determination of severity and disease activity, and efficacy of therapy in many renal diseases. The determination of urinary FDPs may aid in the differential diagnosis between membranous and glomerular lesions and in site of urinary tract infection. Current, although incomplete, evidence suggests that the determination of serum and urinary FDPs may be useful in assessing the efficacy of successful steroid, immunosuppressive, anticoagulant, and platelet suppressive therapy in a wide variety of renal diseases. Some evidence suggests that decreased platelet survival and increased platelet turnover may be of diagnostic aid in assessing severity of renal disease and, more importantly, may be an effective way of monitoring efficacy of anticoagulant therapy or platelet suppressive therapy in a variety of renal diseases, including lupus nephritis and diabetic nephropathy. It appears that the pathophysiology of renal transplant rejection represents a DIC-type syndrome, probably induced by circulating immune complexes.[46,96,97]

Platelet Dysfunction in Uremia

Platelet function defects are an almost universal finding in patients with uremia.[125-127] In uremic patients, it is thought that circulating quanidinosuccinic and hydroxyphenolic acids interfere with platelet function by eliminating platelet factor 3 activity.[128-130] Both compounds are dialyzable, and dialysis often corrects or improves platelet function. Other mechanisms of altered platelet function in uremia, including altered prostaglandin metabolism or intraplatelet nucleotides, have also been suggested.[131-137] Studies have demonstrated an abnormality in the interaction between von Willebrand factor and the platelet membrane glycoprotein IIb/IIIa complex in uremic patients. Platelet membrane glycoproteins Ib, IIb, and IIIa are quantitatively normal in uremia.[138,139] These findings suggest a functional defect in the von Willebrand factor–IIb/IIIa adhesive interaction. Like the other acquired platelet function defects, aggregation pattern abnormalities are not uniform or characteristic, and any combination of defects may be seen (Figure 8-3). Platelet concentrates are indicated for most instances of severe or life-threatening bleeding in uremia. Other modes of therapy that have been noted to correct the prolonged bleeding time in a variety of disorders will also not only correct the bleeding time but often control significant hemorrhage in uremic patients. These modalities are cryoprecipitate, DDAVP (intravenous, intramuscular, or intranasal), and estrogen compounds.[140-146] Dialysis tends to correct the platelet function defect, and the degree of correction toward normal appears to correlate with frequency of dialysis.[147-150]

Summary

This chapter has outlined the complex hemostasis changes associated with both liver and renal diseases. Altered coagulation noted with both liver and renal transplantation are also presented. The keys to successful diagnosis and therapy in these complex disorders are familiarity and understanding of all the defects that may potentially be present, delineation of those defects present by appropriate clinical and laboratory evaluation, and then delivery of specific therapy.

References

1. Lechner K, H Niesser, E Thaler: Coagulation abnormalities in liver disease. Semin Thromb Hemost 4:40, 1977.

2. Aledort LM: Clotting abnormalities in liver disease. Prog Liver Dis 5:350, 1976.

3. Donaldson GWK, SR Davies, S Darg, J Richmond: Coagulation factors in chronic liver disease. J Clin Pathol 22:109, 1969.

4. Bick RL: Liver disease, ch 7. In: Disorders of Hemostasis and Thrombosis: Principles of Clinical Practice. Thieme, Inc., New York, 1985, p 205.

5. Bick RL: Syndromes associated with hyperfibrino(geno)lysis, ch 3. In: Disseminated Intravascular Coagulation and Related Syndromes. CRC Press, Boca Raton, FL, 1983, p 105.

6. Amir-Ahmadi N, RS McGray, F Marton, W Mitch, P Kantrowitz, N Zamcheck: Reassessment of massive upper gastrointestinal hemorrhage on the wards of the Boston city hospital. Surg Clin North Am 49:715, 1980.

7. Workman EF, RL Lundblad: The role of the liver in biosynthesis of the non–vitamin K–dependent clotting factors. Semin Thromb Hemost 4:15, 1977.

8. Barnhart MI, JM Riddle: Cellular localization of profibrinolysin (plasminogen). Blood 21:306, 1963.

9. Murano G: Plasma protein function in hemostasis, ch 4. In: G Murano, RL Bick (Eds): Basic Concepts of Hemostasis and Thrombosis. CRC Press, Boca Raton, FL, 1980, p 43.

10. Denson KWR: The levels of Factor II, VII, IX, and X by antibody neutralization techniques in the plasma of patients receiving phenindione therapy. Br J Haematol 20:643, 1971.

11. Stenflo J: Vitamin K, prothrombin, and gamma-carboxyglutamic acid. N Engl J Med 296:624, 1977.

12. Bick RL: The clinical significance of fibrinogen degradation products. Semin Thromb Hemost 8:302, 1982.

13. Green G, JM Thompson, L Poller, IW Dymock: Abnormal fibrin monomer polymerization in liver disease. Gut 16:827, 1975.

14. Lane PA, MF Scully, DP Thomas, VV Kakkar, R Williams: Acquired dysfibrinogenemia in acute and chronic liver disease. Br J Haematol 35:301, 1977.

15. Abildgaard U, MK Fagerhol, O Egeberg: Comparison of progressive antithrombin activity and the concentrations of three thrombin inhibitors in human plasma. Scand J Clin Lab Invest 26:349, 1970.

16. Braunstein KM, K Evrenius: Minimal heparin cofactor activity in disseminated intravascular coagulation and cirrhosis. Am J Clin Pathol 66:48, 1976.

17. Stump DC, FB Taylo, ME Nesheim: Pathologic fibrinolysis as a cause of clinical bleeding. Semin Hemost Thromb 16: 260, 1990.

18. Bick RL: Disseminated intravascular coagulation (DIC) and related syndromes, ch 6. In: Disorders of Hemostasis and Thrombosis: Principles of Clinical Practice. Thieme, Inc., New York, 1985, p 157.

19. Bick RL: Disseminated intravascular coagulation, ch 2. In: Disseminated Intravascular Coagulation and Related Syndromes. CRC Press, Boca Raton, FL, 1983, p 31.

20. Ratnoff OD: Hemostatic defects in liver and biliary tract disease and disorders of vitamin K metabolism, ch 15. In: OD Ratnoff, CD Forbes (Eds): Disorders of Hemostasis. WB Saunders, Philadelphia, 1991, p 459.

21. Rake MO, PT Flute, G Panell, R Williams: Intravascular coagulation in acute hepatic necrosis. Lancet 1:533, 1970.

22. Wardle EN: Fibrinogen in liver disease. Arch Surg 109:741, 1974.

23. Coccheri S, G Palareti, PR Dalmonte, M Poggi, O Boggian: Investigations on intravascular coagulation in liver disease: soluble fibrin monomer complexes in liver cirrhosis. Haemostasis 8:8, 1979.

24. Straub PW: Diffuse intravascular coagulation in liver disease. Semin Thromb Hemost 4:29, 1977.

25. Bick RL: Clinical relevance of antithrombin III. Semin Thromb Hemost 8:276, 1982.

26. Bick RL: Alterations of hemostasis associated with malignancy, ch 11. In: G Murano, RL Bick (Eds): Basic Concepts of Hemostasis and Thrombosis. CRC Press, Boca Raton, FL, 1980, p 213.

27. Cederblad G, K Korstan-Bengsten, R Olsen: Observation of increased levels of blood coagulation factors and other plasma proteins in cholestatic liver disease. Scand J Gastroenterol 11:391, 1976.

28. Quick AJ, M Stanley-Brown, FW Bancroft: A study of the coagulation defect in hemophilia and in jaundice. Am J Med Sci 190:501, 1935.

29. Brinkhous KM, HP Smith, ED Warner: Prothrombin deficiency and the bleeding tendency of obstructive jaundice and in biliary fistula. Effect of feeding bile and alfalfa (vitamin K). Am J Med Sci 196:50, 1938.

30. Lord JW, W Andrus: Differentiation of intrahepatic and extrahepatic jaundice. Response of the plasma prothrombin to intramuscular injection of menadione (2-methyl-1, 4-naphthoquinone) as a diagnostic aid. Arch Intern Med 68:199, 1941.

31. Bick RL: Alterations of hemostasis associated with cardiopulmonary bypass: etiology, pathophysiology, diagnosis and management. Semin Thromb Hemost 3:59, 1976.

32. Bick RL, WR Schmalhorst, NR Arbegast: Alterations of hemostasis associated with cardiopulmonary bypass. Thromb Res 8:285, 1976.

33. Kumada T, Y Abiko: Enhancement of fibrinolytic and thrombolytic potential in the rat by treatment with an anabolic steroid, Furazabol. Thromb Haemost 36:451, 1976.

34. Walker ID, JF Davidson, P Young, JA Conkie: Plasma fibrinolytic activity following oral anabolic steroid therapy. Thromb Diath Haemorrh 34:236, 1975.

35. Bick RL: Alterations of hemostasis in malignancy, ch 10. In: Disorders of Hemostasis and Thrombosis: Principles of Clinical Practice. Thieme, Inc., New York, 1985, p 262.

36. Bick RL: Alterations of hemostasis associated with malignancy: etiology, pathophysiology, diagnosis and management. Semin Thromb Hemost 5:1, 1978.

37. Bick RL: Disseminated intravascular coagulation and related syndromes: etiology, pathophysiology, diagnosis and management. Am J Hematol 5:265, 1978.

38. Bick RL: Disseminated intravascular coagulation and related syndromes. In: J Fareed, H Messmore, J Fenton, KM Brinkhous (Eds): Perspectives in Hemostasis. Pergamon Press, New York, 1981, p 122.

39. Dymock IW, JS Tucker, EL Woolf, L Poller, JM Thompson: Coagulation studies as a prognostic index in acute liver failure. Br J Haematol 29:385, 1975.

40. Marder VJ, AZ Budzynski: The structure of fibrinogen degradation products. Prog Hemost Thromb 2:141, 1974.

41. Mossesson M: Fibrinogen catabolic pathways. Semin Thromb Hemost 1:63, 1974.

42. Reeve EB, JJ Franks: Fibrinogen synthesis, distribution, and degradation. Semin Thromb Hemost 1:129, 1974.

43. Kopec M, Z Wegrzynowicz, AZ Budynski, ZS Latallo, B Lipinski, E Kowalski: Interaction of fibrinogen degradation products (FDP) with platelets. Exp Biol Med 3:73, 1968.

44. Kowalski E: Fibrinogen derivatives and their biological activities. Semin Hematol 5:45, 1968.

45. Bick RL: Clinical hemostasis practice: the major impact of laboratory automation. Semin Thromb Hemost 9:139, 1983.

46. Bick RL: Clinical implications of molecular markers in hemostasis and thrombosis. Semin Thromb Hemost 10:290, 1984.

47. Kowalski E, M Kopec, S Niewiarowski: An evaluation of the euglobulin method for the determination of fibrinolysis. J Clin Pathol 12:215, 1959.

48. Menon IS: A study of the possible correlation of euglobulin lysis time and dilute blood clot lysis time in the determination of fibrinolytic activity. Lab Pract 17:334, 1968.

49. Bick RL: Disseminated intravascular coagulation: a clinical review. Semin Thromb Hemost 14:299, 1988.

50. Pises P, RL Bick, B Siegal: Hyperfibrinolysis in cirrhosis. Am J Gastroenterol 60:280, 1973.

51. Bick RL, J Fareed, G Squillaci: Molecular markers of hemostatic processes. Implications in diagnostic and therapeutic management of thrombotic and hemorrhagic disorders. Fed Proc 42:4, 1983.

52. Penny R, FC Rosenberg, BG Firkin: The splenic platelet pool. Blood 17:1, 1966.

53. Tocantins LM: The hemorrhagic tendency in congestive splenomegaly (Banti's syndrome): its mechanism and management. JAMA 136:616, 1948.

54. Aster RH: Pooling of platelet in the spleen. Role in the pathogenesis of "hypersplenic" thrombocytopenia. J Clin Invest 45:654, 1966.

55. Bick RL: Platelet defects, ch 4. In: Disorders of Hemostasis and Thrombosis: Principles of Clinical Practice. Thieme, Inc., New York, 1985, p 65.

56. Frick W: Thrombocytopenie und lebercirrhose. Schweiz Med Wochenschr 97:407, 1967.

57. Bick RL: Pathophysiology of hemostasis and thrombosis. In: WA Sodeman, TM Sodeman (Eds): Pathologic Physiology: Mechanisms of Disease. WB Saunders, Philadelphia, 1985, p 705.

58. Straub PW: Intravascular coagulation in acute hepatic necrosis. Lancet 1:1339, 1970.

59. Hillenbrand P, SP Parbhoo, A Jedrychowski, S Sherlock: Significance of intravascular coagulation and fibrinolysis in acute hepatic failure. Gut 15:83, 1974.

60. Karpatkin S, N Strick, MB Karpatkin, GW Siskind: Cumulative experience in the detection of antiplatelet antibody in 234 patients with idiopathic thrombocytopenic purpura, systemic lupus erythematosus, and other clinical disorders. Am J Med 52:776, 1972.

61. Cowan DH: Effect of alcoholism on hemostasis. Semin Hematol 17:137, 1980.

62. Cowan DH, JD Hines: Thrombocytopenia of severe alcoholism. Ann Intern Med 74:37, 1971.

63. Eichner ER, RS Hillman: The evolution of anemia in alcoholic patients. Am J Med 50:218, 1971.

64. Cowan DH: Thrombokinetic studies in alcohol-related thrombocytopenia. J Lab Clin Med 81:64, 1973.

65. Ashud MA: Platelet size and number in alcoholic thrombocytopenia. N Engl J Med 286:355, 1972.

66. Sullivan LW, V Herbert: Suppression of hematopoiesis by ethanol. J Clin Invest 43:2048, 1964.

67. Haselager EM, J Vreeken: Rebound thrombocytosis after alcohol abuse: a possible factor in the pathogenesis of thromboembolic disease. Lancet 1:774, 1977.

68. Bick RL: Vascular disorders associated with thrombohemorrhagic phenomena. Semin Thromb Hemost 5:167, 1979.

69. Cowan DH, RC Graham Jr: Studies on the platelet defect in alcoholism. Thromb Diath Haemorrh 33:310, 1975.

70. Haut MJ, DH Cowan: The effect of ethanol on hemostatic properties of human blood platelets. Am J Med 56:22, 1974.

71. Thomas DP, VJ Ream, RK Stuart: Platelet aggregation patients with cirrhosis of the liver. N Engl J Med 276:1344, 1967.

72. Cowan DH, M Kikta, D Baunach: Alteration of platelet cyclic AMP (cAMP) by ethanol. Thromb Haemost 38:270, 1977.

73. Brown JB: Platelet MAO and alcoholism. Am J Psychiatry 134:206, 1977.

74. Major LF, DL Murphy: Platelet and plasma amine oxidase activity in alcoholic individuals. Br J Psychiatry 132:548, 1978.

75. Cowan DH, P Shook: Effects of ethanol on platelet serotonin metabolism. Thromb Haemost 38:33, 1977.

76. Jandl JH, AA Lear: The metabolism of folic acid in cirrhosis. Ann Intern Med 45:1027, 1956.

77. Bohmig HJ: The coagulation disorders of orthoptic hepatic transplantation. Semin Thromb Hemost 4:57, 1977.

78. Gilberg DA, FE Silverstein, DC Auth, CE Rubin: Nonsurgical management of acute nonvariceal upper gastrointestinal bleeding. Prog Hemost Thromb 4:349, 1978.

79. Biggs JC, TB Hugh, AJ Dodds: Tranexamic acid and upper gastrointestinal hemorrhage: a double-blind study. Gut 17:729, 1976.

80. Cormack F, RR Chakrabarti, AJ Jouhar: Tranexamic acid in upper gastrointestinal hemorrhage. Lancet 1:1207, 1973.

81. Engqvist A, O Brostrom, F von Feilitzen: Tranexamic acid in massive hemorrhage from the upper gastrointestinal tract: a double-blind study. Scand J Gastroenterol 14:839, 1979.

82. Bick RL, WR Schmalhorst, E Shanbrom: Prothrombin complex concentrate: use in controlling the hemorrhagic diathesis of chronic liver disease. Am J Dig Dis 20:1, 1975.

83. Sandler SG, CE Rath, A Ruder: Prothrombin complex concentrate in acquired hypoprothrombinemia. Ann Intern Med 79:485, 1973.

84. Bick RL, S Scates: Qualitative platelet defects. Lab Med. 23:95, 1992.

85. Owen CA, SR Rettke, EJW Bowie: Hemostatic evaluation of patients undergoing liver transplantation. Mayo Clin Proc 62:761, 1987.

86. Nakao A, T Kano, T Nonami: Application of an antithrombogenic Anthron bypass tube to experimental orthotopic liver transplantation. Trans Am Soc Artif Organs 32:503, 1986.

87. Tuman KJ, BD Spiess, RJ McCarthy: Effects of continuous hemofiltration on cardiopulmonary abnormalities during anesthesia for orthoptic liver transplantation. Anesth Analg 67:363, 1988.

88. Kang YG, DJ Martin, J Marquez: Intraoperative changes in blood coagulation and thromboelastographic monitoring in liver transplantation. Anesth Analg 64:888, 1985.

89. Sporn P, W Mauritz, I Schindler: Zur problematik des blutersatzes bei libertransplantationen. Insfusionstherapie 12:187, 1985.

90. Grenvik A, R Gordon: Postoperative care and problems in liver transplantation. Transpl Proc 19:26, 1987.

91. Bellani KG, JA Estrin, NL Ascher: Reperfusion coagulopathy during human liver transplantation. Transpl Proc 19:71, 1987.

92. Dzik WH, CF Arkin, RL Jenkins: Fibrinolysis during liver transplantation in humans: role of tissue-type plasminogen activator. Blood 71:1090, 1988.

93. Casella JF, FA Bontempo, H Markel: Successful treatment of homozygous protein C deficiency by hepatic transplantation. Lancet 1:435, 1988.

94. Navalgund AA, Y Kang, JB Sarner: Massive pulmonary thromboembolism during liver transplantation. Anesth Analg 67:400, 1988.

95. Bick RL, N Tse: Hemostasis in cardiac surgery and organ transplantation. Lab Med. In press.

96. Bick RL: Alterations of hemostasis associated with surgery, cardiovascular surgery, prosthetic devices and transplantation, ch 13. In: OD Ratnoff, CD Forbes (Eds): Disorders of Hemostasis. WB Saunders, Philadelphia, 1991, p 382.

97. Bick RL: Hemostasis defects in general surgery, cardiac surgery, transplantation and the use of prosthetic devices, ch 8. In: Disorders of Hemostasis and Thrombosis: Principles of Clinical Practice. Thieme, Inc., New York, 1985, p 223.

98. Kapplow LS, JA Goffinet: Profound neutropenia during early phase of haemodialysis. JAMA 203:133, 1968.

99. Hampers CL, MD Blanfox, JP Merrill: Anticoagulation rebound after hemodialysis. N Engl J Med 275:776, 1966.

100. Lindsay RM, CRM Prentice, JF Davidson: Hemostatic changes during dialysis, associated with thrombus formation on dialysis membranes. Br Med J 4:454, 1972.

101. Woods JF, G Ash, MJ Weston: Sulfinpyrazone reduced deposition of fibrinon dialyser membranes. Thromb Haemost 42:401, 1979.

102. Morita T, Y Susuki, J Churg: Structure and development of glomerular crescent. Am J Pathol 72:349, 1973.

103. Davidson AM, D Thomson, MK MacDonald: Identification of intrarenal fibrin deposition. J Clin Pathol 26:102, 1973.

104. Koffler N, F Paronetto: Immunofluorescent localization of immunoglobulins, complement and fibrinogen in human disease. J Clin Invest 44:1665, 1965.

105. MacDonald MK, AR Clarkson, AM Davidson: The role of coagulation in renal disease. In: P Kincaid-Smith, TH Mathew, EL Becker (Eds): Glomerulonephritis. John Wiley & Sons, New York, 1973, p 923.

106. McCluskey RT, R Vassalli, G Gallo: An immunofluorescent study of pathogenic mechanism in glomerular disease. N Engl J Med 274:695, 1966.

107. Hoyer JR, AF Michael, LW Hower: Immunofluorescent localization of antihemophilic factor and fibrinogen in human renal diseases. J Clin Invest 53:1375, 1974.

108. Sixma JJ, L Kater, BN Bouma: Immunofluorescent localization of Factor VIII–related antigen, fibrinogen, and several other plasma proteins in hemostatic plugs in humans. J Lab Clin Med 87:112, 1976.

109. Ekgerg M, IM Nilsson: Factor VIII and glomerulonephritis. Lancet 2:1111, 1975.

110. Isacson S, IM Nilsson: The kidneys and the fibrinolytic activity of the blood. Thromb Diath Haemorrh 22:211, 1969.

111. Bergstein JM, AF Michael: Glomerular plasminogen activation activity in renal homograft rejection. Transplantation 17:443, 1974.

112. Steihm ER, CW Trygstad: Split products of fibrin in human renal disease. Am J Med 46:774, 1969.

113. Hedner U, IM Nilsson: Renal diseases and fibrinogen degradation products. In: J Hamburger, J Crosnier, MH Maxwell (Eds): Advances in Nephrology. Year Book Medical Publishers, Chicago, 1974, p 241.

114. Hedner U: Urinary fibrin/fibrinogen derivatives. Thromb Diath Haemorrh 34:693, 1975.

115. Portemont G, J Vermylen, MB Donati: Urinary excretion of fibrinogen/fibrin related antigen in glomerulonephritis. In: P Kincaid-Smith, TH Mathew, EL Becker (Eds): Glomerulonephritis. John Wiley & Sons, New York, 1973, p 829.

116. Ekert H, TM Barratt, C Chantler, MW Turner: Immunologically reactive equivalents of fibrinogen in sera and urine of children with renal disease. N Y State J Med 74:1396, 1974.

117. McNicol GP, CRM Prentice, JD Briggs: Fibrinogen degradation products or FDP in renal disease: estimation and significance of FDP in urine. Scand J Haematol (suppl) 13:329, 1971.

118. Bang NU, CW Trystad, JE Schroeder: Enhanced platelet function in glomerular renal disease. J Lab Clin Med 81:651, 1973.

119. Pitcher FM: Fibrinogen degradation products. Lab Equip Dig 11:109, 1973.

120. Ambrus JL, TR Baliah, CM Ambrus: Fibrin-fibrinogen degradation products in children with renal disease. N Y State J Med 74:1396, 1974.

121. Whitworth JA, KF Fairley, MA McIvor: Urinary fibrin degradation products and the site of urinary infection. Lancet 1:234, 1973.

122. Case JD, AR Clarkson: Serum and urinary fibrin/fibrinogen degradation products in renal disease. Scand J Haematol (suppl) 13:331, 1971.

123. Clarkson AR, JB Morton, JD Cash: Urinary fibrin/fibrinogen degradation products after renal homotransplantation. Lancet 2:1220, 1970.

124. Naish P, DK Peters, R Shackman: Increased urinary fibrinogen derivatives after renal allotransplantation. Lancet 1:1280, 1973.

125. Rabiner SF: Uremic bleeding. Prog Hemost Thromb 1:233, 1972.

126. Lewis JH, MB Zucker, JH Ferguson: Bleeding tendency in uremia. Blood 11:1073, 1956.

127. Castaldi PA: Hemostasis and renal disease, ch 15. In: OD Ratnoff, CD Forbes (Eds): Disorders of Hemostasis. Grune and Stratton, New York, 1991, p 473.

128. Horowitz HI, DB Cohen, P Martinez, M Papayoanov: Defective ADP-induced platelet factor 3 activation in uremia. Blood 30:331, 1967.

129. Horowitz HI, IM Stein, DB Cohen, JG White: Further studies on the platelet-inhibiting effect of guanidine succinic acid and its role in uremic bleeding. Am J Med 49:339, 1970.

130. Rabiner SF, F Molinas: The role of phenol and phenolic acids on the thrombocytopathy and defective platelet aggregation of patients with renal failure. Am J Med 49:346, 1970.

131. Evans EP, GR Jones, AL Bloom: Abnormal breakdown of adenosine diphosphate in uraemic plasma and its possible relationship to defective platelet aggregation. Thromb Res 1:323, 1972.

132. Schondorf TH, D Hey: Platelet function tests in uraemia and under acetylsalicylic acid administration. Haemostasis 3:129, 1974.

133. Remuzzi G, M Livio, AE Cavenaghi, D Marchesi, G Mecca, MB Donati, G de Gaetano: Unbalanced prostaglandin synthesis and plasma factors in uraemic bleeding: a hypothesis. Thromb Res 13:531, 1978.

134. Kamoun P, D Kleinknecht, H Duerot, H Jerome: Platelet-serotonin in uraemia. Lancet 1:782, 1970.

135. Remuzzi G, AE Cavenaghi, G Mecca, MB Donati, G de Gaetano: Prostacyclin (PGI2) and bleeding time in uremic patients. Thromb Res 11:919, 1977.

136. Albertazzi A, C Spisni, PF Palmieri: Nucleotide deficit and functional platelet alterations in patients on regular dialysis treatment. Life Support Systems 3:77, 1985.

137. Ware JA, BA Clark, M Smith: Abnormalities of cytoplasmic Ca++ in platelets from patients with uremia. Blood 73:172, 1989.

138. Escolar G, A Casa, E Bestidi: Uremic platelets have a functional defect affecting the interaction of von Willebrand factor with glycoprotein IIb-IIIa. Blood 76:1336, 1990.

139. Komarnicki M, T Twardowski: Platelet glycoprotein concentrations in patients with chronic uraemia. Folia Haematol 114:642, 1987.

140. Jubelirer SJ: Hemostatic abnormalities in renal disease. Am J Kidney Dis 5:219, 1985.

141. Rydzewski A, M Rowinski, M Mysiwiec: Shortening of bleeding time after intranasal administration of 1-deamino-8-arginine vasopressin to patients with chronic uremia. Folia Haematol 113:823, 1986.

142. Manucci PM: Desmopressin (DDAVP) for treatment of disorders of hemostasis. Prog Hemost Thromb 8:19, 1986.

143. Gotti E, G Mecca, C Valentino, E Cortinovis, T Bertanit, G Remuzzi: Renal biopsy in patients with acute renal failure and prolonged bleeding time: a preliminary report. Am J Kidney Dis 6:397, 1985.

144. Livio M, P Mannucci, G Vigano, G Mignardi, R Lombardi, G Mecca, G Remuzzi: Conjugated estrogens for the management of bleeding associated with renal failure. N Engl J Med 315:731, 1986.

145. Vigano GL, PM Mannucci, A Lattuada: Subcutaneous desmopressin (DDAVP) shortens the bleeding time in uremia. Am J Hematol 31:32, 1989.

146. Vigano G, F Gaspari, M Locatelli: Dose-effect and pharmacokinetics of estrogens given to correct bleeding time in uremia. Kidney Int 34:853, 1988.

147. Harker LA: Acquired disorders of platelet function. Ann N Y Acad Sci 509:188, 1987.

148. Carvalho AC: Acquired platelet dysfunction in patients with uremia. Hematol Oncol Clin North Am 4:129, 1990.

149. Gordge MP, RW Faint, PB Rylance: Platelet function and the bleeding time in progressive renal failure. Thromb Haemost 60:83, 1988.

150. Lindsay RM, AV Moorthy, F Koens: Platelet function in dialyzed and non-dialyzed patients with chronic renal failure. Clin Nephrol 4:52, 1975.

CHAPTER
9

Hemostasis Defects With Cardiac Surgery, General Surgery, and Prosthetic Devices

The use of prosthetic devices and diverse types of extracorporeal circuits, especially cardiopulmonary bypass (CPB), has become conventional in clinical medicine. A preeminent challenge with devices and extracorporeal circuits is that most induce mild or severe defects in hemostasis that may dramatically compromise morbidity or mortality of patients. In addition, many, if not most, patients undergoing extracorporeal bypass or implantation of a prosthetic device are often candidates for other defects in the hemostasis system secondary to their underlying disease process being treated by any of these special modalities. It is not only compelling to be acquainted with all aberrations in hemostasis that may materialize with extracorporeal circuits and prosthetic devices but also to be familiar with those rudimentary defects of hemostasis apt to be established in patients who are candidates for these devices and procedures. Furthermore, many patients who are candidates for a prosthetic device or shunt must experience a general surgical procedure for device placement, and this also requires that those dealing with these patients must be acquainted with the underlying disease conditions requiring devices and the affiliated defects in hemostasis that may be present and may be compounded or exaggerated by the implantation of a prosthetic device with its own particular associated anomalies of hemostasis.[1]

Prevention of Surgical Bleeding

General surgery is mandatory for placement of most devices, and common hemorrhagic problems are associated with the underlying disease states that make patients candidates for prosthetic devices and extracorporeal circuits. Hemorrhage associated with surgery may be devastating and life threatening. Overcautiousness regarding prevention, differential diagnosis, and rapid effective therapy is essential. Exceptional awareness must be given to preventing surgical hemorrhage by uncovering hereditary, acquired, or drug-induced bleeding tendencies before subjecting a patient to general surgery, prosthetic devices, cardiopulmonary bypass, or other extracorporeal circuits. A preexisting bleeding diathesis, although mild, when coupled with surgery or the changes of hemostasis induced by cardiac surgery or an implanted device, may lead to calamitous results.[2]

History Taking

Many cases of surgical or cardiac surgical hemorrhage could be thwarted by simply obtaining a competent hemostasis history. Ideally, this should be elicited before hospital admission to allocate time for proper assessment if a potential problem with hemostasis is exposed. Most historical data essential for detecting obvious or obscure bleeding tendencies are well known.[2,3] Crucial questions often suggesting a bleeding diathesis are the following: Does the patient suffer significant gingival bleeding with toothbrushing? Is there easy or spontaneous bruising? Has the patient experienced excessive bleeding following dental extraction or prior surgical procedures? Is there a childhood history of epistaxis? Is menstrual flow normal or profuse? These simple questions surely do not constitute a comprehensive historical scrutiny for disorders of hemostasis, but a positive reply is a good indication of the possibility of an underlying bleeding tendency. Obviously, all patients considered for prosthetic devices, extracorporeal circulation, or cardiac surgery should also be asked regarding epistaxis, hemoptysis, hematemesis, melena, hematochezia, and hematuria.

The family history should always include inquiries about bleeding tendencies in relatives (especially aunts, uncles, parents, siblings, and children), which may uncover a hereditary bleeding tendency that has remained silent in the patient because the hemostasis system has never been stressed by surgery or trauma. Of paramount importance, and typically neglected, is a detailed drug history. Many instances of cardiac surgical hemorrhage or hemorrhage with devices can be explained in retrospect by noting the ingestion of drugs known to interfere with hemostasis, usually platelet or, less commonly, vascular function.[3] Many drugs interfere with hemostasis, and frequently the bleeding is mild and only considered bothersome. When drug-induced defects are combined with general surgery, prosthetic devices, or cardiac surgery, however, hemorrhage may reach alarming dimensions. Drugs may interfere with hemostasis by many mechanisms, most commonly by interfering with platelet function.[4] If the drug history is positive and cardiac surgery is elective instead of emergent, surgery should be cancelled for a full 14 days. Most drugs interfering with platelet function are ordinarily effective for as long as 10 to 14 days, and this period may be needed for platelet function to return to normal and the planned procedure to be done safely. If the drug history is positive for antiplatelet agents, the drug has been ingested within 14 days, and a procedure is emergent instead of elective, the patient should be given an appropriate quantity of platelet concentrates (6 to 8 units for an adult) before surgery.[5] In addition, for cardiac surgery, the patient should receive a similar dose of platelet concentrates before leaving the operating room and then each morning for two postoperative days. This approach is somewhat vigorous but is important if life-threatening CPB hemorrhage is to be avoided. For general surgical procedures necessary for device placement or transplantation, platelets are given preoperatively if the template bleeding time is greater than 15 minutes.[1,5] Platelets are then kept on hold for two days postoperatively and given only if bleeding happens.[1,5] If the template bleeding time is less than 15 minutes, platelets are not infused preoperatively but are kept immediately available and used if bleeding occurs.[1,5] Obviously, presurgical patients should be asked about the prior use of warfarin or heparin anticoagulants. Patients previously taking warfarin, although the prothrombin time has returned to normal, have an increased bleeding risk with surgery.[1,5,6]

Physical Findings

The patient's general appearance often provides hints of a bleeding tendency. All the hereditary and acquired connective tissue disorders are often associated with a significant vascular defect and the potential for surgical or cardiac surgical hemorrhage. Most of the hereditary collagen vascular disorders are accompanied by inadequately defined platelet function defects. Clinical clues heralding the presence of a collagen vascular disorder are well known to most clinicians and include the body habitus of Marfan's syndrome, blue sclerae, skeletal deformities, hyperextensible joints and skin, and nodular, spiderlike, or pinpoint telangiectasia (see chapter 3). These suggestive signs should promote a more comprehensive investigation for a collagen vascular disorder before surgery is undertaken. The hereditary and acquired collagen vascular disorders most likely to be associated with general surgical bleeding will be discussed. Other disorders that may be associated with a vascular defect and surgical bleeding include Cushing's syndrome, malignant paraprotein disorders, the allergic purpuras, and hereditary hemorrhagic telangiectasia.[2]

Other subtle hints of an occult bleeding tendency are found by rigorous surveillance of the integument and mucous membranes. Mucosal petechiae, purpura, or significant telangiectasia should be searched for and explained if present (see chapters 3, 4, and 5). Likewise, petechiae, significant ecchymoses (bruises greater than 2 cm in diameter), or telangiectasia of the skin, nailbeds, or sublingual areas must be sought. These findings are often suggestive of a vascular defect, platelet function defect, or significant thrombocytopenia. If any of these findings are present, they should be explored and thoroughly explained. The usual physical findings of the more common clinical disorders associated with a significant bleeding tendency, such as chronic liver disease, hypersplenism, chronic renal disease, rheumatoid arthritis, and systemic lupus erythematosus, are well known (see chapters 3 and 8). In addition, prior laboratory screening will usually suggest the presence of any of these disorders if characteristic physical findings are absent. If the personal, family, or drug history or physical examination suggests a potential or real bleeding tendency, surgery for device placement or cardiac surgery should be postponed until the defect is ruled out or until it is fully delineated and a therapeutic plan for hemostasis has been painstakingly designed. A bleeding disorder of any type is rarely, if ever, a contraindication to doing general surgical procedures or cardiac surgery if the defect is elucidated and a sound approach to correcting hemostasis during surgery and the postoperative period is designed.[5,7]

Laboratory Screening

Any preoperative laboratory and hemostasis screening should generally be simple and incur a minimum of expense to the patient while providing adequate information. Repeatedly, however, presurgical or precardiac bypass hemostasis screenings are insufficient.[3,5,8] As with an adequate history and physical examination, one must be knowledgeable in screening for defects in hemostasis when a surgical procedure or device placement is planned. When preexisting hemostatic defects are combined with general surgical procedures to place prosthetic devices (disruption of the vasculature) or the defects in hemostasis created by cardiopulmonary bypass or the prosthetic device itself, the resultant hemorrhage is often catastrophic but frequently can be averted by wise screening of patients. The SMA 12/60 biochemical screening survey, electrolyte level, and complete blood cell and platelet counts, which are usually ordered, will detect the common acquired disorders often associated with a bleeding tendency, such as chronic liver disease, renal disease, and instances of hypersplenism or bone marrow failure. Most commonly, a presurgical screen consists only of a prothrombin time, APTT, and a platelet count. Although these simple tests will detect most coagulation protein problems and thrombocytopenia, they provide absolutely no information about vascular or platelet function and disregard the possibility of pathologic fibrinolysis.

Most nontechnical hemorrhage associated with general surgical procedures or cardiac surgery hemorrhage is caused

Table 9-1. Presurgical Hemostasis Screen (Minimal Requirements)

Complete blood cell and platelet count
Prothrombin time
Partial thromboplastin time
Template bleeding time (duplicate)
Thrombin time (CPB surgery; observe clot for five minutes)
Cryoglobulins and cold agglutinins (hypothermic CPB)

Table 9-2. Vascular Disorders Commonly Found in Surgical Candidates

Hereditary hemorrhagic telangiectasia (Osler-Weber-Rendu)
Cushing's syndrome
Collagen vascular disease
Multiple myeloma
Aspirin induced

by platelet function defects and, less commonly, coagulation protein or vascular defects. Platelet defects are a more common cause of surgical bleeding than are coagulation protein problems. Therefore, one simple procedure is added to the routine preoperative surgical screening: the standardized template bleeding time. As described by Mielke and coworkers,[9] this test is done on all patients before a general surgical procedure, providing a reasonable screen for adequate vascular and platelet function.[10] The template bleeding time should not be done until adequate platelet numbers (greater than 100 x 10⁹/L [100,000/mm³]) are documented by count or smear evaluation. For cardiac bypass surgery patients, in addition to the template bleeding time, a thrombin time is added to the preoperative cardiac surgery screen.[11,12] The resultant clot is observed for five minutes after the test is done. A normal thrombin time assures the absence of significant hypofibrinogenemia, dysfibrinogenemia, fibrinolysis, or FDP elevation. The use of one or both tests in the routine presurgical screen adds only minimal cost and laboratory time while providing valuable information not given by a simple prothrombin time, APTT, or platelet count. For cardiac surgery, if hypothermic perfusion is to be done, cryoglobulins and cold agglutinins should also be assessed before bypass.[13-18] The preoperative surgical and bypass hemostasis screening tests are summarized in Table 9-1.[9,19-22]

Hemostasis in General Surgery

Vascular Defects

Most prosthetic devices and transplantation procedures call for a local or general surgical procedure. Although most vascular defects are not strictly hematologic diseases, many are characterized or accompanied by a significant hemorrhagic diathesis and often present in this manner.[23] In addition, most, if not all, of these disorders can be accompanied by significant surgical hemorrhage. The surgeon should be aware of the more common vascular disorders, especially those that may lead to vascular hemorrhage with surgery and placement of a prosthetic device. Vascular disorders are characteristically manifest by petechiae, purpura, ecchymoses, or telangiectasia.[23,24] Although these are the most common manifestations, mucosal membrane bleeding (including epistaxis, genitourinary, pulmonary, and gastrointestinal bleeding) also commonly occurs. Other characteris-

tics often found in vascular disorders are a history of gingival bleeding with toothbrushing, bleeding after dental extraction, and a history of easy and spontaneous bruising.[14-16] Most vascular disorders and their propensity to surgical hemorrhage will be detected by noting an abnormal template bleeding time and usually a normal platelet function test. The vascular disorders that most commonly lead to hemorrhage in surgical patients are listed in Table 9-2 and include hereditary hemorrhagic telangiectasia (HHT), collagen vascular disorders with a microvascular component, Cushing's syndrome, malignant paraprotein disorders, amyloidosis, allergic purpuras, and aspirin ingestion (see chapter 3).[25] With a known vascular disorder, little can be done to prevent hemorrhage other than the use of meticulous surgical technique. However, if the patient with a vascular disorder and a propensity to surgical hemorrhage has not taken antiplatelet agents before surgery, and careful surgical hemostasis is strictly controlled, significant intraoperative or postoperative hemorrhage rarely happens. The surgeon, however, should know if one of these disorders and the possibility of surgical hemorrhage exist before subjecting a patient to a surgical procedure, especially if it is elective. The template bleeding time is commonly normal in HHT and the allergic purpuras, so an adequate history and physical examination are compulsory.

Thrombocytopenia

Thrombocytopenia is not uncommonly encountered in general surgical practice and especially in candidates for prosthetic devices or transplantation. The causes of thrombocytopenia most commonly seen by the surgeon are depicted in Table 9-3. These are almost always, if not always, detected by the presurgical platelet count or careful evaluation of the peripheral blood smear. In the busy laboratory, however, severe thrombocytopenia may be missed on a smear evaluation, and presurgical patients should always have a quantitative platelet count. When thrombocytopenia is noted, the etiology should be delineated before surgery is undertaken. The most common etiologic mechanisms are listed in Table 9-3. The common drugs causing thrombocytopenia in surgical patients are listed in Table 9-4, and the patient should be asked about any drug use when encountering presurgical thrombocytopenia. Surgical bleeding commonly does not occur with a platelet count greater than 100 x 10⁹/L (100,000/mm³). If a patient has a platelet count below 100 x 10⁹/L (100,000/mm³) and does not have immune thrombocy-

Table 9-3. Common Causes of Thrombocytopenia in Surgical Patient Populations

Aplastic anemia
Drug induced
Hemolytic-uremic syndrome
Immune thrombocytopenia purpura (ITP)
Infection
Liver disease
Low-grade disseminated intravascular coagulation
Metastatic malignancy
Multiple blood transfusions
Myeloproliferative disorders
Severe iron deficiency
Splenomegaly/hypersplenism

Table 9-5. Common Platelet Function Defects Seen in Surgical Patient Populations

Acquired storage pool disease
Circulating FDPs
Drug induced
Hereditary storage pool disease
Liver disease
Low-grade DIC
Multiple myeloma
Myeloproliferative disorders
Uremia

topenia, proper numbers of platelet concentrates are usually given before surgery and 6 to 8 units are kept on hold for the possibility of postsurgical hemorrhage. If the platelet count is greater than 100 x 10⁹/L (100,000/mm³), but below normal, the patient is subjected to the surgical procedure with platelets on hold and given only if significant bleeding occurs intraoperatively or postoperatively. In my experience the most common causes of presurgical thrombocytopenia are malignancy and attendant chemotherapy, radiation therapy, marrow metastases, unrecognized DIC, liver disease, or drug-induced thrombocytopenia.[3,7,10,26] Quantitative platelet defects were discussed in chapter 5.

Platelet Function Defects

Platelet function defects clearly account for more than 50% of nontechnical surgical hemorrhage.[3,8,10] Most of the hereditary platelet function defects are clinical oddities and extremely rare. The one most commonly seen that leads to surgical hemorrhage is a hereditary storage pool defect, typically manifest by absent second-wave aggregation to adenosine diphosphate (ADP) and epinephrine and totally absent aggregation to collagen with normal ristocetin-induced platelet agglutination. In addition, the possibility of a storage pool defect should be considered when noting normal

platelet counts and a prolonged template bleeding time. More commonly, however, the surgeon will be challenged with acquired or drug-induced platelet function defects. Those common clinical disorders associated with abnormal platelet function are depicted in Table 9-5, and the common drugs that interfere with platelet function and lead to surgical hemorrhage are depicted in Table 9-6. These are only the common drugs inducing postsurgical hemorrhage, and several excellent reviews provide more extensive lists.[27-30] Drug-induced platelet dysfuction was thoroughly discussed in chapter 4. If presurgical template bleeding times are not done, these disorders will not be detected by the routine presurgical screen consisting only of a prothrombin time, APTT, and platelet count. When surgical bleeding is thought to be potentially because of a platelet function defect, a template bleeding time should be performed immediately, and if prolonged, platelet aggregation should be measured and a diligent drug and bleeding history taken from the patient.

Platelet function defects are treated in the same manner as thrombocytopenia. If a patient has a platelet function defect that has been uncovered preoperatively and a template bleed-

Table 9-4. Common Drugs Causing Thrombocytopenia in Surgical Patient Populations

Acetaminophen
Aspirin
Cephalosporins
Chlorpropamide
Digitalis preparations
Meprobamate
Penicillin compounds
Phenobarbital
Phenytoin
Quinidine
Streptomycin
Thiazide diuretics

Table 9-6. Common Drugs Interfering With Platelet Function in Surgical Patient Populations

Ampicillin
Aspirin
Benadryl
Carbenicillin
Clofibrate
Dipyridamole
Furosemide
Gentamicin
Glycerol guaiacolate
Indocin
Motrin
Nitrofurantoin
Papaverine
Penicillin
Phenothiazines
Propanolol
Sulfinpyrazone
Tricyclic amines

ing time of more than 15 minutes, the patient is infused with 6 to 8 units of platelet concentrates before the surgical procedure.[1,7,8] If, however, the template bleeding time is less than 15 minutes (normal, four to nine minutes), then platelets are kept on hold and infused only if significant intraoperative or postoperative hemorrhage happens.[1,7,8] Alternatively, if the defect is not uncovered before surgery and postsurgical bleeding occurs or if the template bleeding time is prolonged and platelet aggregation abnormalities are noted, appropriate numbers of platelet concentrates are given immediately to abort hemorrhage, usually 6 to 8 units in the adult, given twice a day or every morning, depending on the site and severity of hemorrhage.[1,7,8] My practice and recommendation is to infuse platelets until significant hemorrhage stops.

Isolated Coagulation Factor Deficiencies

Isolated coagulation factor deficiencies are rarely encountered in surgical practice, except in centers specializing in hemophilia and other congenital coagulation protein problems. Far more commonly, however, the general and subspecialty surgeon will be faced with acquired multiple compartment defects. The most common of these defects are DIC and the hypoprothrombinemic problems seen with chronic liver disease, biliary obstruction, renal disease, or disseminated malignancy. The defect of chronic liver disease consists not only of coagulation factor problems, including deficiencies of the vitamin K–dependent clotting factors, but also of vascular and platelet defects. The platelet defect(s) present in patients with liver disease may be quantitative or qualitative. Hypoprothrombinemic bleeding may be seen in warfarin-treated patients, in patients with acute liver insults, including hepatitis, and in patients with hepatic cirrhosis. Most of these defects are detected by a careful history and adequate presurgical laboratory screening. Although a patient taking warfarin before surgery may have a prothrombin time that has returned to normal, the patient still has an increased bleeding risk with a surgical procedure.[1,5,6,8] When vitamin K–dependent, clotting factor deficiency–type bleeding occurs, whether because of liver disease or resulting from presurgical use of warfarin, it is best managed by phytonadione, 20 mg intravenously (1 mg/min) or 30 mg intramuscularly, and occasionally the use of fresh frozen plasma, 2 to 4 units as necessary, as the site and severity of bleeding dictate.[1,7,8] If bleeding is truly emergent and life threatening, the use of prothrombin complex concentrates to correct the hemostatic defect quickly may be considered.[31] The use of these concentrates is not without hazard, and they should be infused only by individuals highly experienced in management of serious thrombohemorrhagic phenomena. Congenital coagulation factor defects were discussed in chapter 6, and acquired coagulation protein defects are discussed in appropriate chapters.

Disseminated Intravascular Coagulation

Disseminated intravascular coagulation–type syndromes not uncommonly lead to significant surgical hemorrhage.

Table 9-7. Common Settings for Disseminated Intravascular Coagulation Syndromes in Surgical Patient Populations

Acidosis/shock
Biliary obstruction/cholestasis
Collagen vascular disorders
Crush injuries
Extensive burns
Hemolysis
Infection/sepsis
Metastatic malignancy
Obstetric accidents
Prosthetic devices
Transfusion reactions
Ulcerative colitis

Typically, a patient with a disorder associated with low-grade underlying DIC is subjected to a surgical procedure, which then precipitates an acute, fulminant DIC syndrome. Those conditions most commonly associated with low-grade or subacute underlying DIC processes in patients who are candidates for prosthetic devices or general surgical procedures are depicted in Table 9-7 and include septicemia (often unrecognized), disseminated solid malignancy, crush injuries, tissue necrosis, burns, selected liver and biliary diseases, and obstetric accidents including amniotic fluid embolism, placental abruption, toxemia, and the retained fetus syndrome.[32-35] The surgeon should be aware of the disorders that may be associated with a low-grade DIC process and that may not be detected using routine presurgical screening. Primary fibrino(geno)lysis has been commonly blamed for many instances of posttransurethral prostatectomy (TURP) hemorrhage. In my experience, however, although primary fibrino(geno)lysis is occasionally seen and may account for massive post-TURP hematuria, far more common causes of post-TURP bleeding are drug-induced platelet function defects and a low-grade underlying DIC syndrome.[36] It has been suggested that a minimum DIC evaluation be performed on all patients undergoing TURP, because this may identify patients who are predisposed to post-TURP hemorrhage.[37]

The general or subspecialty surgeon who is responsible for implanting a prosthetic device or extracorporeal circuit should not only be familiar with the particular hemostasis changes associated with the device or particular procedure but also the hemostasis defects commonly present in a general surgical population, particularly those defects found in patients whose underlying disease renders them candidates for prosthetic devices.

Hemostasis in Cardiac Surgery

Cardiac surgery using cardiopulmonary bypass (CPB) is now a common procedure and, with popularization of coronary artery bypass grafting (CABG), is no longer limited to large centers but is now done in many community hospitals. Widespread use of CPB has rejuvenated awareness of the catastrophic intraoperative or postoperative hemorrhage sometimes associated with this procedure. Hemorrhage during or after bypass is of more than fleeting significance because it may lead to substantial morbidity and mortality from an elective procedure, places formidable demands on blood bank facilities, and can lead to prolonged, expensive hospitalizations.[1,7,12,38,39] The actual incidence of life-threatening hemorrhage associated with CPB varies from 5% to 25%.[1,6,12,39-42]

Formerly, the pathophysiology of altered hemostasis created by CPB was inadequately understood. Previous failures to explain the pathophysiology of altered hemostasis during CPB have, quite understandably, prevented the development of uniform concepts of successful prevention, adequate and rapid diagnosis, and effective control of CPB hemorrhage and also have led to expensive, often inappropriate, and unsuccessful approaches to management. Lack of understanding of CPB hemorrhagic syndromes has derived from several factors. Many past studies of hemostasis during CPB examined only isolated aspects of blood coagulation and ignored the complexities and interrelationships of the hemostasis system. Many previous studies did not use coagulationists or hematologists, which sometimes led to the inappropriate choice of test systems and unclear or inappropriate interpretation of results. Despite available and sophisticated advances in modalities to assess the hemostatic system, many previous studies used insensitive, inaccurate, or inappropriate test systems. For example, the euglobulin lysis time has been a commonly used modality for studying CPB fibrinolysis, although this test system is unquestionably obsolete, inaccurate, and provides no information about clinically significant fibrinolysis.[1,43-46]

Various investigators have attributed the hemorrhagic syndrome of CPB to an assorted spectrum of defects. Moreover, each investigator has prioritized diverse degrees of importance on each defect, depending on which particular hemostatic parameters were monitored. In the past, the abnormalities most frequently evoked to account for CPB hemorrhage have included inadequate heparin neutralization, protamine excess, heparin rebound, thrombocytopenia, hypofibrinogenemia, primary fibrino(geno)lysis, DIC, isolated coagulation factor deficiencies, transfusion reactions, and hypocalcemia. The suggestion that all of these defects may contribute to CPB hemorrhage clearly shows that despite the finding of multiple defects in hemostasis, the basic pathophysiology of altered hemostasis during CPB is bewildering to many. These basic mechanisms of altered hemostasis associated with CPB must be completely understood and appreciated before an appropriate approach to rapid diagnosis and effective therapy can be rationally designed.

Thrombocytopenia

Early studies of hemostasis during CPB noted significant thrombocytopenia, with a platelet count of about 50 x 10⁹/L

(50,000/mm³) in patients undergoing bypass surgery, which many authors thought to be responsible for bypass hemorrhage. In addition, Kevy and associates[47] noted that thrombocytopenia was related to time on bypass and was more pronounced with perfusions lasting greater than 60 minutes. A relationship between thrombocytopenia and time on bypass was also reported by Signori, Penner, and Kahn.[48] Later studies noted similar findings.[49,50] Porter and Silver[49] observed that in most patients undergoing CPB, the platelet count fell to one third of the preoperative level. In addition, they found that thrombocytopenia did not abate until several days after CPB.[49] Earlier studies by Wright, Darte, and Mustard[51] and von Kaulla and Swan[52] also recognized thrombocytopenia in association with CPB, but these investigators concluded that thrombocytopenia bore little, if any, relationship to actual bypass hemorrhage. Some studies finding thrombocytopenia during CPB concluded that this represented thrombocytopenia of DIC.[53-56] Bick[7,8,12,57-60] and others[61-63] have failed to find significant thrombocytopenia during CPB. This wide variability in experience probably represents different surgical and pumping techniques, such as flow rates, normothermic or hypothermic perfusion, the oxygenation system used, time on bypass, and the priming solution.

Figure 9-1 shows changes in platelet number during CPB. The dotted line represents the mean platelet counts after membrane oxygenation pumping, and the solid line represents platelet counts after bubble oxygenation pumping.[7,8,64] The results of 300 consecutive patients are depicted. In our experience, the type of oxygenation mechanism used appears to play little role, if any, in causing clinically significant thrombocytopenia.[7,8,64] Thrombocytopenia with bubble oxygenators is slightly greater than that seen with membrane oxygenators, but this does not often reach clinical significance. The most commonly cited mechanisms for the development of CPB thrombocytopenia are hemodilution, formation of intravascular platelet thrombi, platelet utilization in the pump or oxygenation system, and peripheral utilization because of DIC. We have failed to find a correlation between CPB hematocrit and platelet count, which suggests that hemodilution is not a major factor.[5,60,65] Indeed, the role, if any, of these mechanisms in producing CPB thrombocytopenia is totally unclear.

Platelet Function Defects

In contrast to the prolific investigations regarding platelet number during CPB, a surprising lack of interest exists in assessing platelet function during this procedure. Early investigators suspected that abnormalities of platelet function might occur, since faulty clot retraction was noted.[48] These results were of unclear significance, however, since other changes known to affect clot retraction, such as hypofibrinogenemia and thrombocytopenia, were also present. Another early study assessed platelet function before performing CPB but did not evaluate platelet function during or after bypass.[66] In this study, abnormal preoperative platelet adhesion in glass bead columns was associated with

Figure 9-1. Platelet Counts During CPB

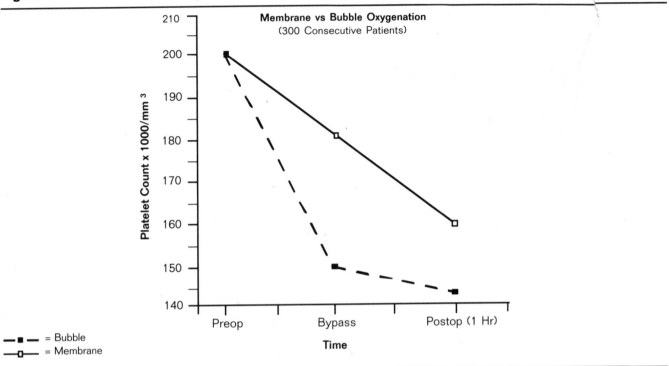

increased postoperative bleeding. Salzman[67] studied platelet adhesion before, during, and after bypass and noted decreased adhesion to glass bead columns in patients during bypass. The significance of this defect was difficult to evaluate, however, since all patients had marked thrombocytopenia, which is definitely known to alter adhesion studies,[68-70] and in addition, adhesion studies are now generally thought to be without any particular clinical significance.[10,71,72] Further information from this study was that heparin, in doses used during CPB, did not alter platelet adhesion. This study concluded that a circulating anticoagulant might be responsible for the platelet function defect noted, because plasma from patients undergoing CPB altered adhesion when added to normal platelets. This circulating anticoagulant probably represented fibrin(ogen) degradation products.[12,46] Salzman's study also noted that perfusion temperature and the type of priming solution did not correlate with the development of abnormal platelet function.

More recently, platelet adhesion studies have been performed in patients undergoing CPB without significant thrombocytopenia.[57,59,60,65] In these studies platelet function, as measured by adhesion, decreased profoundly in all patients at the initiation of bypass. Most patients showed adhesion that decreased to 17% of the preoperative levels. Bick and associates[59] noted little correlation between hematocrit, fibrinogen level, or FDP titer and abnormal adhesion. In addition, poor correlation was noted between chest tube blood loss and abnormal platelet function, as assessed by adhesion. Figure 9-2 depicts platelet adhesion changes during CPB. Recent studies have questioned the clinical significance of platelet adhesion by the glass bead column technique.[10,71,72] However, this degree of abnormal platelet function would surely be expected to compromise hemostasis severely. Membrane oxygenation procedures are depicted by a dashed line, and bubble oxygenation procedures are depicted by a solid line.[64] The platelet function defect is slightly more severe and tends to correct more slowly when a membrane oxygenator is used as compared to a bubble oxygenator. Platelet function as assessed by template bleeding times, platelet aggregation, or lumi-aggregation is abnormal in patients with platelet function defects,[10,70] von Willebrand's syndrome (ristocetin aggregation only),[69] and myeloproliferative disorders.[73] Many factors, some possibly altered by CPB, may affect platelet function, including pH, absolute platelet count, hematocrit, drugs, the presence of FDPs, the type of pump prime, and the type of oxygenation system used.[12,28,46,74-78] Although most studies do not clearly define the reasons for abnormal platelet function during CPB, they do suggest that several of these mechanisms are probably not involved. The finding of platelet counts greater than 100 x 10^9/L (100,000/mm³) and hematocrits greater than .30 (30%) in most patients with marked platelet dysfunction one hour after CPB suggests that the absolute platelet count and the hematocrit do not account for altered platelet function. In addition, most patients have a normal or near normal pH one hour after bypass surgery, so a change in pH is unlikely to account for abnormal platelet function during bypass surgery. Heparin, at levels higher than those attained in patients undergoing CPB, has been shown to not alter platelet function.[1,67,70] Circulating FDPs are known to

Figure 9-2. Platelet Adhesion During CPB

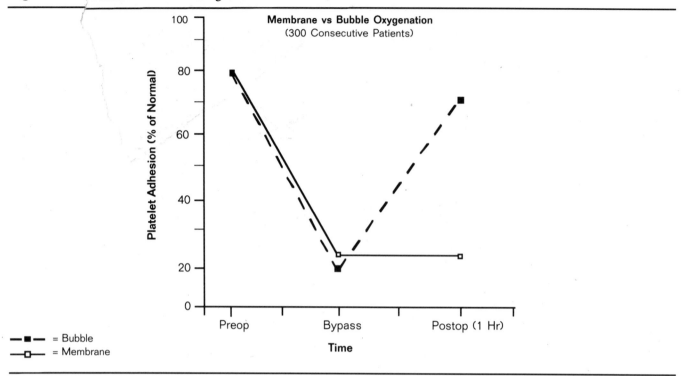

interfere with platelet function, and these are present in about 85% of patients undergoing CPB.[12,46,77] However, poor correlation exists between levels of circulating FDPs and abnormal platelet function during bypass surgery.[59,65] In addition, defective platelet function occurs in all patients undergoing CPB, and thus, circulating FDPs cannot account for altered platelet function in many instances.[5,7,12,59,65]

Other possible mechanisms of altered platelet function during CPB include platelet membrane damage by shearing force or contact with foreign material, resulting in a partial release of platelet contents, platelet membrane coating with nonspecific proteins or protein degradation products, or incomplete release reaction or nonspecific platelet damage induced by flow rates. Recent studies by Harker and associates[79] have shown selective platelet degranulation to happen during bypass surgery. However, no studies reported yet allow conclusions to be drawn regarding the contribution of any of these mechanisms to altered platelet function during CPB. One preliminary study has reported platelet aggregation studies during CPB. In this series of 29 patients, only 20% developed aggregation abnormalities during CPB. After heparin reversal with protamine sulfate, 90% of patients developed aggregation abnormalities. These authors attributed this finding to a protamine/platelet interaction and not because of bypass itself.[80] We have recently evaluated platelets by lumi-aggregation in patients undergoing CPB, and in all patients platelet aggregation and platelet release was markedly altered.[1,7,81] Typical midbypass and postbypass lumi-aggregation patterns seen in cardiac surgery patients are depicted in Figures 9-3 and 9-4. In addition, in all patients assessed, the aggregation and release reaction defect happened within 10 to 15 minutes of starting the bypass procedure. We have also noted that in all patients platelet factor 4 levels rise rapidly with the initiation of bypass. The aggregation defects appear to be similar with both membrane- and bubble-type oxygenators. The type of priming solution, albumin vs hydroxyethyl starch, does seem to change the type of defects seen.[81]

Despite the mechanism(s) involved, studies to date clearly disclose a significant platelet function defect that is induced in all patients undergoing CPB. The magnitude of this defect would certainly be expected to have potential serious consequences for hemostasis during and after bypass. In addition, patients who have ingested drugs known to interfere with platelet function would be expected to have more blood loss than those not ingesting such agents. In such patients, drug ingestion would be expected to compound the defects already induced by CPB and potentiate the chance for hemorrhage. One small study has provided evidence for this conclusion.[76] This platelet function defect is of major significance in post-CPB hemorrhage. The use of platelet concentrates in association with a normal platelet count will usually promptly correct or significantly reduce most episodes of CPB or post-CPB hemorrhage. DDAVP (desmopressin acetate) was initially thought to decrease bleeding after open-heart surgery. Because of this finding, many surgeons began the empiric, and sometimes irrational, use of DDAVP during and after open-heart surgery. More recent masked randomized trials have failed to show any significant differences in post-CPB blood loss between DDAVP and placebo.[82-84] DDAVP releases tissue (endothelial) plasminogen activator, potential-

Figure 9-3. Cardiopulmonary Bypass Surgery (Midbypass)

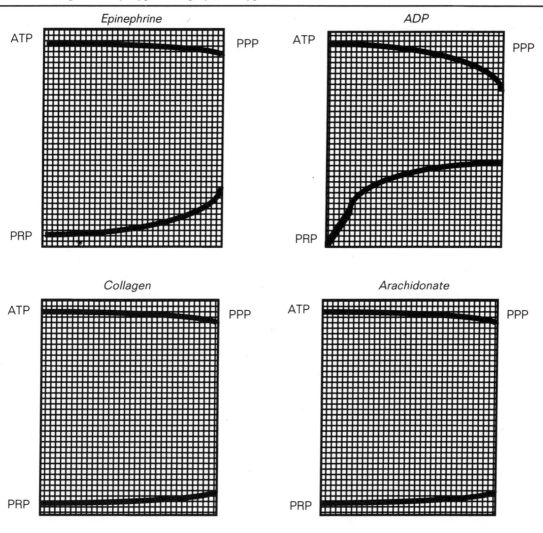

PRP = Platelet-Rich Plasma
PPP = Platelet-Poor Plasma
ATP = ATP Release

ly activating the fibrinolytic system and enhancing or inducing hemorrhage. Therefore, many physicians using this agent recommend the concomitant use of aminocaproic acid to abort any possible hemorrhage.[85-88] Based on current evidence, little, if any, rationale exists for the empiric use of DDAVP during CPB. Those using this agent should be aware of the potential for enhancing hemorrhage and for increased risk of coronary artery and cerebrovascular thrombosis.

Vascular Defects

Few studies of vascular defects during CPB have been reported. A syndrome of mild to moderate thrombocytopenic purpura accompanied by splenomegaly and atypical lymphocytosis following CPB has been reported by Behrendt and coworkers.[89] In this series the purpura was benign, self-limited, and frequently manifest only after discharge from the hospital. Only one patient of seven had a complication following the development of this syndrome, which was glomerulonephritis of the type often seen in Henoch-Schönlein purpura. A case of fatal purpura fulminans was reported following extracorporeal circulation for coronary artery bypass grafting.[90] These two reports suggest that an inflammatory vasculitis may be associated with CPB, and the most benign forms, purpura simplex and rarely purpura fulminans (without DIC), may happen. Cardiac surgeons should be aware of this potential complication of bypass surgery. Except for these two reports, no mention has been made in the literature of vascular defects associated with CPB.

Isolated Coagulation Factor Defects

Many studies have examined and reported coagulation factor deficiencies during CPB. A wide variety of findings

Figure 9-4. Cardiopulmonary Bypass Surgery (Postbypass)

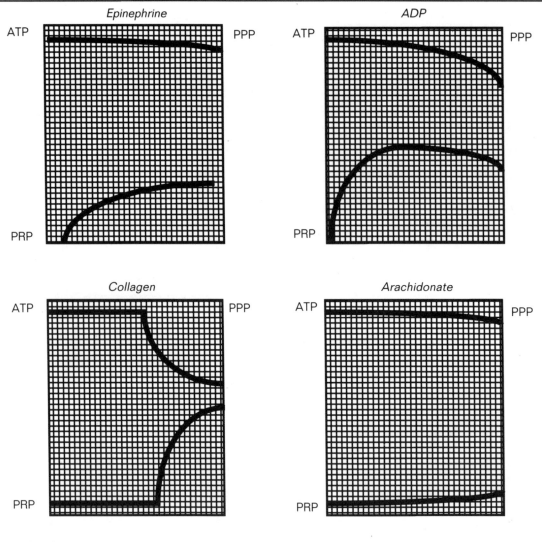

PRP = Platelet-Rich Plasma
PPP = Platelet-Poor Plasma
ATP = ATP Release

have been observed and, like the finding of thrombocytopenia, may only reflect differences in surgical or pumping techniques, such as flow rate, priming solution, and the like. Most studies have noted significant hypofibrinogenemia, which does not seem to be correlated with perfusion time.[40,49-51,59,60] We [46,59,60] and others [40,50] have found fibrinogen levels to be correlated closely with CPB fibrinolysis. However, other investigators report little correlation between hypofibrinogenemia and degree of CPB fibrino-(geno)lysis.[47,91] Figure 9-5 depicts correlations noted between fibrinogen, plasminogen, circulating plasmin, and FDP during CPB. The dashed lines represent membrane pumping procedures, and the solid lines represent bubble oxygenator pumping procedures.[5,7,64] Some studies have concluded that hypofibrinogenemia happens primarily because of DIC during pump surgery.[53,55,56] Others have

failed to find hypofibrinogenemia during CPB.[92,93] It seems reasonable to conclude from the studies reported that hypofibrinogenemia secondary to hyperfibrinolysis may be a frequent occurrence during CPB. This appears to be a consistent finding in these carefully studied series and is probably a major cause of hypofibrinogenemia associated with CPB. Fibrino(geno)lysis occurs in about 85% of patients undergoing bypass surgery. Most studies have also noted other coagulation deficiencies in association with CPB, and those most commonly decreased and reported to play a role in CPB hemorrhage are factor II, factor V, and factor VIII:C.[40,47,50,51,53,56] Some patients undergoing CPB for valvular heart disease have low–factor VIII:vWF, high–molecular weight monomers, which may increase during the CPB procedure.[83] Some conclude that these changes are secondary to DIC,[53,63] whereas others describe these decreases to a primary fibri-

Figure 9-5. Fibrinolytic Activity During Cardiopulmonary Bypass

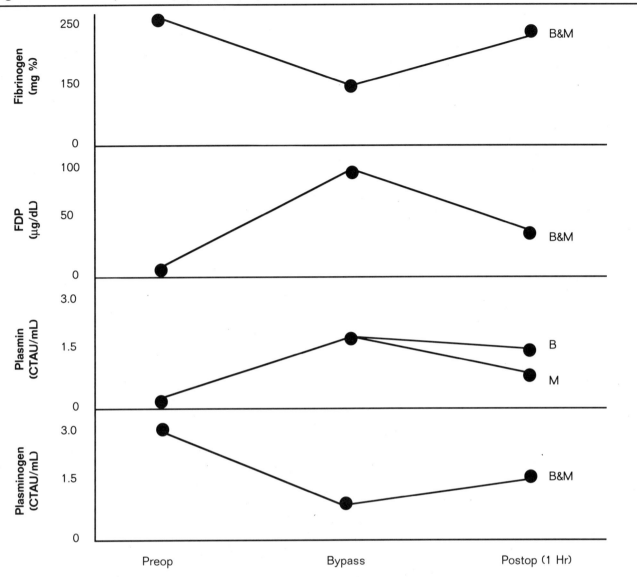

no(geno)lytic syndrome and plasmin-induced degradation of coagulation proteins.[5,12,40,46,59,60] Still others have failed to find a significant decrease in most coagulation factors during bypass surgery,[47,92,93] and two authors have reported increased factor VIII:C levels during perfusion.[92,94]

Disseminated Intravascular Coagulation

The question of DIC developing during bypass surgery has caused much confusion regarding altered hemostasis both during and after bypass. Many early studies of hemostasis during CPB concluded that DIC occurred.[53,55,56,95,96] However, many such studies monitored only isolated coagulation factors, and the measured decreases were empirically ascribed to presumed DIC, since no other obvious explanation was evident. Specifically, the findings of isolated fibrinogen, factor VIII:C,[51,55] or prothrombin complex factor deficiencies[62] were often assumed, usually erroneously, to be secondary to DIC,

without proper confirmatory laboratory testing. In addition, two more recent reports have concluded that DIC accounts for altered hemostasis during CPB.[63,97] In these reports of nine patients, the authors concluded that DIC was present after noting that several parameters of hemostasis worsened following heparin reversal with protamine. Specifically, FDP elevation, hypofibrinogenemia, and hypoplasminogenemia appeared to become accentuated following the infusion of protamine. However, my experience[1,5,8,12,59,60] and that of others[40,48,49,52,93,98] have been the opposite: hypofibrinogenemia, hypoplasminogenemia, and FDP elevation are usually noted to correct rapidly and uniformly after the administration of protamine sulfate.

These findings would suggest that DIC is not generally associated with CPB. Disseminated intravascular coagulation during cardiac surgery also seems unlikely in view of massive heparinization and the absence of significant or uni-

Figure 9-6. Pathologic Activation of the Fibrinolytic System

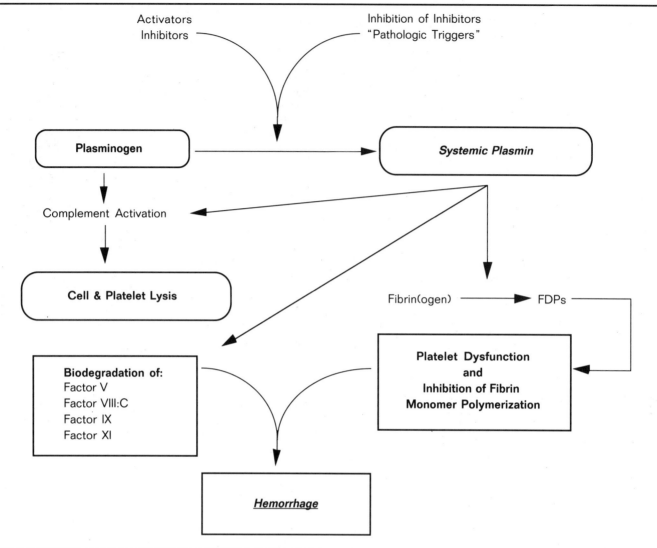

form thrombocytopenia reported in many studies in which hemostasis appears to be markedly abnormal. Another finding that would surely suggest that DIC is not present during CPB is the presence of normal or near normal AT III levels during CPB.[1,5,40,65] Prevailing evidence suggests that decreased AT III levels are a good indicator of the development of acute or chronic DIC.[33,34,45,99] Only one study has shown decreased AT III during CPB[63]; however, in the nine patients described, all had low levels of AT III before bypass was started. In addition, the method used was old and possibly influenced by the presence of FDP or heparin, making interpretation of these results ambiguous. Another consideration negating the probability that DIC happens during CPB is the following: if DIC were present in patients undergoing CPB, the infusion of intravenous protamine sulfate would be expected to cause a massive precipitation of soluble fibrin monomer, with resultant extensive microvascular or macrovascular occlusion. In my experience, only two out of several thousand patients have had DIC in association

with CPB.[5,7,12] Both patients developed DIC before CPB: one from cardiac arrest and the other from septicemia. In these two instances, bypass surgery was accomplished without incidence. When protamine sulfate was infused, however, massive vascular occlusion, including carotid and renal artery thrombosis, suddenly occurred.

Although most early and several recent studies have detected primary fibrino(geno)lysis in association with CPB, a few authors have concluded that DIC might occur. These conclusions probably emanate from the marked superficial similarities between primary fibrino(geno)lysis, DIC, and the usual secondary fibrinolytic response and from the difficulty in making a clear-cut differential diagnosis between these two states without sophisticated and complete coagulation studies.

Primary Fibrino(geno)lysis

Fibrinolytic activity is generally decreased or inhibited during and after most general surgical procedures.[100-103] However, most studies using a variety of laboratory modalities have found increased fibrinolysis during and after CPB.[5,7,12,40,46-49,59-61,81,91,93,98,104] Many earlier studies of hemostasis during CPB assessed fibrinolysis with the euglobulin lysis time, and the finding of fibrinolysis was of unclear significance for a long time.[43,44] More recent studies of CPB hemostasis,[1,5,7,49,59,60,65] which have used more specific methods for assessing fibrinolysis, primarily synthetic substrate assays,[45,105-109] have confirmed earlier reports of a primary fibrino(geno)lytic syndrome in most patients undergoing CPB. Because of early reports detecting primary fibrino(geno)lysis during CPB, the empiric use of antifibrinolytics, usually epsilon aminocaproic acid (EACA), has become commonplace. Despite the attendant hazards of this agent, which include hypokalemia, hypotension, ventricular arrhythmias, local or disseminated thromboses, and DIC syndromes,[110,111] many cardiovascular surgeons have frequently used this drug. Controlled studies with and without antifibrinolytics have failed to show any clear-cut differences in CPB hemorrhage.[6,40,50,91,112] Gomes and McGoon[98] and Tsuji and associates[93] have shown a definite increase in post-CPB hemorrhage with the empiric use of antifibrinolytics. The need to use EACA to control CPB hemorrhage is extremely rare.[5,7,8,12] This agent should only be used when concrete laboratory evidence of primary fibrino(geno)lysis is noted in the severely hemorrhaging CPB patient who has failed to respond to adequate platelet transfusions.

Several investigators finding primary fibrino(geno)lysis during CPB have concluded this to be inconsequential as a cause of postperfusion hemorrhage,[48,50] whereas others have thought that this syndrome is triggered only by specific events such as pyrogenicity of equipment, the use of Rheomacrodex, or induction of anesthesia.[52,113,114] Since primary fibrino(geno)lysis occurs in most patients subjected to CPB, it seems likelier that activation of the fibrinolytic system may be happening in the oxygenation mechanism or, alternatively, that pump-induced accelerated flow rates may activate the plasminogen-plasmin system or may alter endothelial plasminogen activator or inhibitor activity. Factor XII is markedly activated in patients undergoing CPB with about 70% of factor XII being converted to factor XIIa.[115] This is another potential activation pathway for the initiation of a primary fibrino(geno)lytic syndrome. However, the pathogenesis of fibrinolytic activation during CPB is unclear. Although many investigators have noted enhanced fibrinolysis during CPB, a few studies have found only elevated fibrinolytic activator activity, with no systemically circulating plasmin.[47,91,95] A few studies have failed to find any evidence of primary fibrino(geno)lysis in association with cardiopulmonary bypass.[6,50,51,95]

The pathophysiology of primary fibrino(geno)lysis is familiar (Figure 9-6). Hemostasis is significantly altered when plasmin circulates systemically; the attendant systemic hypofibrinogenemia and plasmin-induced biodegradation of factors V, VIII, and IX may severely compromise the hemostasis system.[12,46,116-118] In addition, the resultant FDPs further derange hemostasis by interfering with thrombin activ-

Table 9-8. Molecular Marker Profiling in the Differential Diagnosis of Disseminated Intravascular Coagulation vs Primary Fibrino(geno)lysis

Marker	DIC	Primary Lysis
Fibrinopeptide A	Elevated	Normal
Fibrinopeptide B	Elevated	Normal
B-beta 15-42 peptide	Elevated	Normal
B-beta 1-42 peptide	Elevated	Elevated
B-beta 1-118 peptide	Elevated	Elevated
Platelet factor 4	Elevated	Normal
Beta thromboglobulin	Elevated	Normal
Fibrin(ogen) degradation products	Elevated	Elevated
D-dimer	Elevated	Normal

ity, interfering with fibrin monomer polymerization, and radically altering platelet function.[12,34,46,77,78,119-121] These changes in hemostasis would certainly be expected to be associated with a significant hemorrhagic potential. In addition, it is easy to see how these changes in hemostasis could be superficially confused with DIC and secondary fibrinolysis. A molecular marker profile can be used to diagnose differentially between primary fibrinolysis and DIC (Table 9-8).[121]

Other Defects in Cardiac Surgery

Heparin rebound has received significant attention as a potential cause of CPB hemorrhage,[114,122-125] although this was observed more often in earlier studies. With today's generally accepted doses of both heparin and protamine, both heparin rebound and inadequate heparinization are rarely, if ever, seen.[5,7,12,59,60,63,65] Neither heparin rebound nor inadequate heparin neutralization have ever been documented as actual causes of CPB hemorrhage.[5,7,8,54,56] Similarly, protamine excess has occasionally been incriminated as a source of CPB hemorrhage, although several series have failed to note this phenomena in a single patient undergoing CPB.[12,42,59-61,123,126] In addition, although protamine sulfate is a well-known in vitro anticoagulant, it is unlikely that this agent is the cause of in vivo altered hemostasis or clinical hemorrhage.[127]

Several authors have reported that both coagulation defects and significant CPB hemorrhage may be associated with hypothermic perfusion.[6,50,52,114] Our experience in comparing normothermic to hypothermic perfusions have led to the same conclusion.[104] Gomes and McGoon[98] and Porter and Silver[49] have found no increased incidence of CPB hemorrhage resulting from hypothermic perfusion. Many patients undergoing coronary artery bypass grafting for coronary occlusive disease have been taking warfarin-type drugs. Verska, Lonser, and Brewer[6] have noted that although the prothrombin time returns to normal before CPB, patients previously receiving warfarin therapy show more hemorrhage than those not taking these agents. This observation applies to general surgery patients as well. Quick, Stanley-Brown, and Bancroft[22] noted that increased hemorrhage was associated with a repeat bypass procedure. Others, however, have noted no increased hemorrhage in association with a second procedure.[56,98] In addition, patients undergoing CPB for correction of cyanotic heart disease appear to have more severe derangements in hemostasis during perfusion and a propensity to hemorrhage than those operated on for noncyanotic heart disease.[48,98] Increased hemorrhagic risk during and after CPB is associated with the prior use of warfarin drugs, hypothermic perfusion, surgery for correction of cyanotic heart disease, repeat bypass procedure, long perfusion times, and preoperative ingestion of drugs interfering with platelet function.[1,5,7,8] Advancing age does not appear to be associated with increased risk of hemorrhage with CPB.[128,129]

Pathophysiology

Many conclusions regarding altered hemostasis and resultant hemorrhage during CPB are of questionable significance. For example, it appears that overheparinization, heparin rebound, inadequate protamine neutralization, and protamine excess, although receiving at least theoretic attention as potential sources of CPB hemorrhage, have not been documented as being responsible for bleeding associated with bypass surgery. Similarly, thrombocytopenia, almost surely a potential source of hemorrhage, is an inconsistent finding during cardiac bypass surgery. The finding of isolated coagulation defects during CPB has added little, except confusion, to an understanding of altered hemostasis during bypass surgery. Probably, these isolated findings simply represent isolated measurements of the results of fibrino-(geno)lysis and systemically circulating plasmin.

Although DIC has been thought by some to occur during CPB, most carefully done studies did not document this. The significant doses of heparin used during CPB, the absence of consistent thrombocytopenia, and the general correction of hypofibrinogenemia, hypoplasminogenemia, and elevated FDP levels after heparin neutralization all suggest that the presence of DIC during cardiac surgery is a very rare event. Disseminated intravascular coagulation may be associated with cardiac surgery when another triggering event is provided, such as sepsis, shock, massive transfusions, or a frank hemolytic transfusion reaction.

Predisposing factors associated with enhanced cardiac surgery hemorrhage are long perfusion times, prior ingestion of warfarin-type drugs, cyanotic heart disease, hypothermic perfusions, the preoperative ingestion of drugs known to interfere with platelet function, and prolonged perfusion times. These predisposing risk factors are summarized in Table 9-9. Prevailing evidence suggests that most patients undergoing CPB develop a primary fibrino(geno)lytic syndrome, although the exact triggering mechanisms are unclear, which may be the result of factor XII activation. The resultant secondary derangements in hemostasis will certainly create a potential for CPB hemorrhage. In addition, most patients undergoing CPB develop severe platelet dysfunction. It is unclear if this defect is the result of coating of platelet surfaces by FDPs, membrane damage from the oxy-

Table 9-9. Factors Predisposing to Hemorrhage During Cardiopulmonary Bypass

Long perfusion times
Prior use of warfarins
Cyanotic heart disease
Hypothermic perfusion
Preoperative ingestion of antiplatelet drugs
Repeat bypass procedure

genation mechanism, platelet damage from fast flow rates, or other unrecognized mechanisms. Whatever the triggering mechanism(s), the most significant alterations in hemostasis associated with CPB are defective platelet function and primary fibrino(geno)lysis. These two defects alone or in combination certainly account for most nonsurgical and nontechnical hemorrhage in patients undergoing CPB. Platelet function defects account for far more hemorrhagic episodes than primary fibrino(geno)lysis.

Diagnosis

When bleeding happens during or after bypass it is obviously extremely important to define the defect as quickly as possible, so specific and effective therapy can be delivered.[7,8,12,42,130] Many instances of CPB hemorrhage are clearly caused by inadequate surgical technique, but alterations of hemostasis may also be responsible for accentuating CPB hemorrhage. This discussion will be limited to nontechnical causes of cardiopulmonary bypass hemorrhage. The types of hemorrhage that occur during CPB are somewhat limited and are depicted in Table 9-10 in descending order of probability.

The primary distinction to be made is between strictly surgical bleeding, defects in hemostasis, or a combination of the two. This distinction becomes more difficult and more important after the patient has left the operating room. During this period, a decision must be made regarding reexploration and the adequacy of hemostasis for reexploration. In distinguishing between surgical and nonsurgical bleeding, many physical findings are helpful, such as whether the bleeding is localized or systemic. If the patient is already in the recovery room, the recognition of hematuria in association with petechiae and purpura, oozing from intravenous

Table 9-10. Hemorrhagic Syndromes Seen With Cardiopulmonary Bypass Surgery (Descending Order of Probability)

Severe platelet dysfunction
    Cardiopulmonary bypass induced
    Drug induced

Primary fibrinolytic syndrome

Thrombocytopenia

Hyperheparinemia or rebound ?

Disseminated intravascular coagulation (exceedingly rare)

Table 9-11. Clinical Evaluation of Hemorrhage in the CPB Patient

Chest tube blood loss only, or associated with:
Petechiae, purpura, or ecchymoses
Hematuria
Oozing from intra-arterial line sites
Oozing from intravenous sites
Oozing from venipunctures
Oozing from sternotomy wound
Oozing from saphenous vein graft site
Other systemic bleeding sites
Clots forming in chest tube

Table 9-12. Laboratory Evaluation of Bypass Hemorrhage (Ordered Stat)

Platelet count and complete blood cell count
Peripheral blood smear evaluation
Prothrombin time
Partial thromboplastin time
FDP titer
D-dimer assay
Heparin assay*
Thrombin time**
Plasminogen assay*
Plasmin assay*

* Synthetic substrate assay
** Observe for clot lysis at five minutes

sites in conjunction with increased chest tube blood loss, and oozing from surgical sites, including the sternotomy wound and saphenous vein harvest site, suggest a defect in hemostasis. Increased chest tube blood loss alone, however, often signifies a technical bleeding problem. When the patient is in the operating room, these same findings hold true, and the surgeon will usually note bleeding or oozing throughout the surgical field in nontechnical bleeding. It is important, therefore, that communication between the surgeon and the hematologist or internist occur. Clinical suggestions of a systemic instead of a local cause of CPB hemorrhage are depicted in Table 9-11.

When CPB hemorrhage is seen or suspected the following laboratory tests are ordered: prothrombin time, activated partial thromboplastin time, complete blood cell and platelet counts, examination of a peripheral smear, FDP level, heparin assay by synthetic substrate, thrombin or reptilase time, and plasminogen/plasmin levels by synthetic substrate methods.[1,7,8,42] Evaluation of the heparin level will provide rapid information regarding the status of heparin and its potential effects on other tests of hemostasis. The resultant clot from the thrombin or reptilase time is always observed for five minutes for evidence of lysis, supplying rapid additional information regarding the presence or absence of a clinically significant primary fibrino(geno)lytic syndrome. More evidence for or against primary lysis is obtained by noting the FDP and D-dimer levels.[34,131-133] A peripheral blood smear and platelet count are invaluable to rapid evaluation of the potential for thrombocytopenic bleeding. Plasminogen and plasmin levels obtained by synthetic substrate technique are not time consuming but are not used for an immediate diagnosis; however, they are invaluable in making decisions regarding antifibrinolytic therapy later.[1,7,8,42] If significant primary fibrino(geno)lysis is present, FDPs will be significantly elevated, and the D-dimer level will be normal or near normal, and hypoplasminogenemia and circulating plasmin will be detected. If available, fibrinopeptide A levels will not be elevated, but B-beta 15-42–related peptides will be elevated. If, conversely, excess heparin is a potential problem, this is noted by the heparin assay, and the thrombin time will be markedly prolonged. If no significant clot lysis is observed, the clot formed during measurement of the

thrombin time, and significant FDP elevation is not present, primary fibrino(geno)lysis should not be suspected.

All patients undergoing CPB display a platelet function defect. When bleeding occurs, I assume this defect is always present, and although it might not be the primary reason for hemorrhage, platelet dysfunction can be assumed to be additive to any other defect whether surgical or resulting from altered hemostasis. Therefore, no tests of platelet function are routinely done, but platelet concentrates are immediately ordered for any patient who demonstrates intrabypass or postbypass hemorrhage.[5,7,8] The time period when hemorrhage occurs (ie, intraoperatively, after heparin neutralization, or in the recovery room) appears to have little relationship to the etiology of the primary hemostatic defect responsible for hemorrhage. Exceptions to this are thrombocytopenic bleeding, which usually happens after the patient is in the recovery room, and a significant drug-induced platelet function defect, which is usually manifest as significant oozing immediately after the operative procedure is started. Tests ordered for the differential diagnosis of the etiology of hemorrhage during CPB are listed in Table 9-12.

Management

When first encountering a patient with CPB hemorrhage, whether intraoperative or postoperative, it is important to note the type of bleeding (systemic vs local), to order a stat laboratory screen as outlined earlier, and to administer 6 to 8 units of platelet concentrates as quickly as possible. Although the use of platelet concentrates is somewhat empiric at this point, it is done for several sound reasons: all patients have a significant platelet function defect, which may be the primary reason for hemorrhage and usually is if it is a nontechnical bleed; or this defect is likely to be accentuating bleeding from other causes, whether it be a surgical defect or defective hemostasis. The quick administration of platelet concentrates while awaiting the laboratory evaluation will often stop or significantly reduce most instances of nontechnical CPB hemorrhage.[5,7,8] Recently, a fibrin glue in paste or spray form has been applied with reasonable success to bleeding sites in patients undergoing CPB hemorrhage. The source for this fibrin glue may be autologous or allogeneic.[134-137]

When bleeding begins immediately after initiation of surgery, a platelet function defect, usually drug induced, can be assumed to be present until further laboratory investigation can be done. In this instance, the patient should be given 6 to 8 units of platelet concentrates as quickly as possible, and the surgical wound should be closed if feasible. If a platelet function defect is responsible for the hemorrhage (no laboratory evidence of significant fibrinolysis or hyperheparinemia), 6 to 8 units of platelet concentrates should be repeated the evening after surgery and for two postoperative mornings. Thrombocytopenic CPB hemorrhage should be controlled in the same manner, although greater numbers of platelet concentrates may be needed as dictated by the initial platelet count, the site and severity of hemorrhage, and the response to platelet transfusions. Hyperheparinemia and heparin rebound, if thought to be a real clinical problem as documented by synthetic substrate assays, are managed by delivering 25% of the original calculated protamine sulfate dose, repeated every 30 to 60 minutes until bleeding stops. Hyperheparinemia and heparin rebound are unlikely to be responsible for bleeding and should not be suspected unless concrete laboratory proof of hyperheparinemia is present and evidence of primary fibrino(geno)lysis is clearly absent. I have seen many instances of excessive heparinization resulting from mistakes in calculations and solution preparation, although none of these instances were associated with significant cardiac surgical hemorrhage. Similarly, protamine excess is rarely, if ever, a clinical problem. This situation should never call for therapy and should not be suspected at the risk of ignoring other potential defects in hemostasis.

Primary fibrino(geno)lysis is commonly present, may or may not be responsible for hemorrhage, and should not be treated empirically. Antifibrinolytic therapy should be considered if the patient has failed to respond to platelet concentrates and laboratory evidence for this syndrome has been documented, as noted by the presence of hypoplasminogenemia, circulating plasmin, and elevated FDP levels. In addition, for physicians who have appropriate testing systems available, the absence of elevated fibrinopeptide A levels, the absence of elevated D-dimer levels, and the presence of elevated B-beta 15-42–related peptides offer further evidence for primary lysis. Primary fibrino(geno)lytic bleeding is generally treated with epsilon aminocaproic acid given as an initial dose of a 5- to 10-g slow intravenous push followed by 1 to 2 g per hour until bleeding stops or slows to a non–life-threatening level. It should be recalled that the use of EACA may be associated with ventricular arrhythmias (tachycardia or fibrillation), hypotension, hypokalemia, localized or diffuse thrombosis, and frank DIC. This agent should be injected slowly, and cardiac status, renal output, blood pressure, and electrolytes should be monitored carefully. A newer and more potent antifibrinolytic agent now available is tranexamic acid, which is usually delivered at a dosage of about 2 to 4 g intravenously every 24 hours.[138]

Hemostasis With Prosthetic Devices and Extracorporeal Circuits

Exposure of the blood to foreign surfaces is often linked with thrombosis, which provides a major clinical obstacle to the use of prosthetic devices. The use of prosthetic devices and extracorporeal circuits has become commonplace for the treatment of patients with cardiovascular disease and renal disease, for chemotherapy, for long-term parenteral hyperalimentation, and for common angiographic studies or therapeutic angioplasty.[1,7,139] The hemostatic complications following the insertion of prosthetic devices include consumption of coagulation factors, other plasma proteins, or platelets, the generation of microthrombi of little clinical consequences, and thrombosis or thromboembolism that may give rise to serious, life-threatening, or terminal vaso-occlusion. Under normal circumstances, the blood stays fluid because of many obvious factors, including a nonthrombogenic endothelial surface, endogenous fibrinolytic activity, natural protease inhibitors such as AT III, protein C, and protein S, and the dilution and dispersion of procoagulant components of the blood.[140-143] These protective mechanisms are lost, to some degree, with the use of prosthetic devices.[1,7,8]

Generally, slow flow rates are associated with local thrombotic events; however, fast flow rates are more commonly associated with a high shear force and embolization.[132] In addition, smooth prosthetic surfaces tend to favor little adhesiveness of a formed thrombus, and embolization is more likely to occur than with a rough surface, which tends to favor firm fibrin clot formation and eventual neovascularization.[144] When blood is exposed to prosthetic devices or any foreign surface, including extracorporeal circuits, plasma proteins are immediately absorbed, primarily fibrinogen, albumin, alpha and beta globulins, gamma globulin, factor VIII:C, factor XII, factor XI, and thrombin.[145,146] Factors XII and XI may simply be absorbed or, alternatively, may become activated. Fibrinogen appears to be the major plasma protein absorbed and promotes later platelet adhesion, with platelets adhering as a monolayer and then aggregating. Platelet adhesion will be enhanced or induced not only by fibrinogen but also by gamma globulin, thrombin, and subsequent factor XII and factor XI activation.[147] In addition, the activation of factors XII or XI may induce intrinsic coagulation, with further fibrin formation generating a platelet-fibrin thrombus. As thrombotic surfaces form and embolize in this manner, they may eventually overwhelm the ability of the reticuloendothelial system to clear them, and subsequent thromboembolization with vascular occlusion and later end-organ infarction may occur.[148]

The most common defects that may generally happen with prosthetic devices are as follows: frank coagulation factor and platelet consumption with subsequent thrombocytopenia and resultant hemorrhage; devices may cause partial platelet degranulation, with later defective platelet function and resultant hemorrhage; in cases of oxygenation/dialysis membranes, fibrin-platelet deposition will make the exchange ineffective and provide a focus for thromboembolus; and microthromboemboli or macrothromboemboli of platelets and/or fibrin may give rise to serious clinical vaso-occlusive problems.[1,8] Anticoagulants, including warfarin-type drugs, heparin, and platelet suppressive agents, tend to normalize thrombotic and thromboembolic complications with prosthetic devices.[1,8] The problem, however, is clinically significant, especially during CPB, hemodialysis, angiographic studies, prosthetic heart valve placement, long-term intravenous catheterization, the use of LeVeen or Denver shunts, and implantation of total artificial hearts (TAHs).[1,8]

Arterial and Venous Catheters

Intra-arterial or intravenous catheters become coated with fibrin and platelet aggregates when used for angiographic studies, therapeutic angioplasty, long-term chemotherapy, infusions of fluids, and long-term parenteral hyperalimentation.[1,7,8,149] Thromboembolism happens in about 2% of individuals catheterized for angiographic studies.[1,7,8,150] Another complication is that an existing atherosclerotic plaque may be disrupted and embolize. The thromboembolic complications of short-term or long-term catheterization are usually minimized by low-dose intravenous heparin. In addition to the intra-arterial catheters, intravenous catheters can also be associated with thrombotic events but are most usually associated with localized phlebitis around the introduction site. This complication can happen in up to 20% to 30% of patients, and only 10% of these conditions are diagnosed before the intravenous catheter is removed.[151] The diagnosis of phlebitis may be made between 60 and 80 hours after starting the IV and appears to occur later in patients with diabetes and earlier in patients with intravenous catheters for peripheral hyperalimentation.[1,7,151] In addition, an inordinately increased incidence of local phlebitis is noted in those patients who are undergoing intravenous therapy and have an associated infectious process.[152]

Intra-Aortic Balloon Pumping

Intra-aortic balloon pumping (IABP) has been in clinical use since 1968 and is commonly used for the control of cardiogenic shock or low-output failure following CPB.[153-155] Common current indications also include the following: acute myocardial infarction with cardiogenic shock remaining unresponsive to immediate medical management; unstable cardiac status following cardiac catheterization, coronary angiography, or coronary angioplasty; impaired left ventricular function; refractory low cardiac output following CPB procedures; and arrhythmias occasionally.[153-156]

These devices are usually constructed of polyurethane and are inserted surgically or percutaneously into the left common femoral artery.[153] The most common complications of intra-aortic balloon pumping are leg ischemia from diverse causes, local or distal arterial injury/thrombosis, aortic dissection, destruction or activation of many blood elements including red blood cells, platelets, and coagulation proteins, and infections that are, of course, more common

when the percutaneous insertion route is used.[1,157,158] Despite the high frequency of thrombus and thromboembolus formation, no uniform anticoagulation regimen is used with these devices. Some clinicians advocate the routine use of heparin to be delivered before, during, and until removal of these balloons.[159] Others, however, use heparin only in medical patients and use aspirin and/or low–molecular weight dextrans in surgical patients.[1,7,156] Even other clinicians use no anticoagulants unless another underlying indication besides balloon assistance is present.[160] Another approach has been to use dextran plus heparin.[155] Although it has been suggested that the routine use of anticoagulants may decrease the chance of thrombus or thromboembolus,[157,160] no randomized studies confirm this opinion.

Several operative mechanisms induce thrombus, thromboembolus, and resultant end-organ infarction in patients undergoing intra-aortic balloon pumping. Patients often develop thrombi adherent to the aortic intima along the path of the balloon, and emboli may easily develop.[158] These mural thrombi may detach fragments of existing thrombus, denuded endothelium, and/or platelet macroaggregates, which may embolize downstream (during systole) or upstream (during diastole) and may infarct essentially any end organ or any other site, including the upper or lower extremities, depending on the direction of embolization and the size of the embolus.[158,161] After three days of balloon assist, marked denuding of aortic endothelium next to the balloon has been noted. Following this, the usual expected platelet hyperactivity with subsequent platelet activation and release of procoagulant and vasoactive materials occur, leading to more platelet activation, activation of the coagulation system, more thrombi, emboli, thromboembolic showers, and vasoconstriction.[5] Embolization can frequently be to the upper extremities, lower extremities, central nervous system, kidneys, spleen, superior mesenteric artery, or small bowel.[157,158,161,162] Embolization is noted to happen most frequently in debilitated patients or in patients with severe cardiac failure.

Leg ischemia can develop from local thrombus formation in the aortic or iliofemoral vessels or from emboli.[156-158] Local thrombosis is especially common if the insertion is inadvertently made into the superficial femoral artery.[157] Leg ischemia resulting from thrombus or thromboembolus is the most frequent early complication of intra-aortic balloon assist devices.[157] The use of heparin has been suggested to decrease the chance of this serious complication.[1,7,39,157] Leg ischemia resulting from local thrombosis or thromboembolus may be severe enough to give rise to an anterior compartment syndrome necessitating fasciotomy or even amputation in severe cases.[156] The incidence of leg ischemia secondary to thrombosis or thromboembolus is thought to be related to the time undergoing balloon assistance.[157] In addition, the presence of atherosclerosis in the iliofemoral system is another important predisposing factor for vaso-occlusion and the development of leg ischemia, and the use of heparin will obviously not be preventive with this mechanism.[157] The type of balloon may also influence the incidence of thrombus or thromboembolus.[156] Even bilateral renal artery thrombi have been noted in association with IABP.[162] Limb ischemia because of thrombosis or thromboembolus associated with intra-aortic balloon pump is common, occurring in up to 36% of patients.[1,7,155,156] Since this complication can lead to obviously serious morbidity or even mortality, attentive monitoring and the use of anticoagulants, preferably heparin in nonsurgical patients, is mandatory. Evaluation of the dorsalis pedis and posterior tibial pulses coupled with Doppler ultrasonography of the thigh vessels should be performed every four hours in these patients.[156,157] The capillaries of the dorsum of the feet are inspected to assess capillary filling every four hours.[157] The development of leg ischemia dictates immediate removal of the balloon if medically possible.

Hemorrhage is another potentially serious complication of IABP. Wound hemorrhage is the most common bleeding seen, but retroperitoneal hemorrhage, gastrointestinal bleeding, genitourinary bleeding, central nervous system bleeding, and frank DIC may also occur.[1,7,8,155,157] The most common etiologic mechanism for hemorrhage associated with IABP is thrombocytopenia.[8,155,157] Thrombocytopenia is clearly related to the time the device is used and may be of multiple etiologies including consumption in an aortic mural thrombus or consumption secondary to DIC. The development of DIC also appears to be related to the time the device is used. I have only noted DIC to develop in patients undergoing at least five days of IABP, although DIC has also been noted to occur at only one day of balloon assistance.[161] Disseminated intravascular coagulation may develop in patients undergoing IABP by multiple mechanisms, including activation of the hemostasis system by massive platelet release and consumption resulting from massive aortic intramural thrombus formation. Intravascular hemolysis may commonly develop, especially if the device is used for more than two days,[157] which may also trigger DIC.[34] In this regard, balloon-induced hemolytic anemia and thrombocytopenia may be so severe that support with washed packed red blood cells and platelet concentrates is required.[157] Another triggering event for DIC is the high incidence of bacteremia, which is most commonly seen in patients receiving the balloon by percutaneous insertion.[157]

Intra-aortic balloon pumping has now become a common therapeutic modality for patients with selected indications, including cardiogenic shock and weaning from CPB in association with unstable hemodynamics or left ventricular dysfunction. These devices can be associated with extremely severe thrombotic, thromboembolic, and hemorrhagic problems of multifaceted origins. Generally, the careful monitoring of patients in association with the judicious use of anticoagulants and a familiarity with the types of thrombotic or hemorrhagic disorders that may develop are important to ward off these serious complications.

Vascular Shunts

Access shunts in the form of surgically created arteriovenous (A-V) shunts or prosthetic A-V shunts are necessary for patients undergoing hemodialysis, frequent transfusion, long-term parenteral hyperalimentation, long-term chemotherapy, and long-term commitment to apheresis programs.[5,16] Surgically created A-V shunts tend to have fewer thrombotic complications than prosthetic shunts.[163] Although thrombosis of the shunt is the major significant problem with these devices, infection is also of concern. Prosthetic shunts and surgically created shunts are usually declotted by surgery, streptokinase, or urokinase with good success.[8,164,165] Anticoagulant therapy has not become commonplace for patients with A-V shunts; however, dipyridamole has been shown to correct decreased platelet survival and increased platelet consumption in patients with these devices.[166] Aspirin alone will not decrease the chance of shunt thrombosis. Prosthetic vascular grafts are primarily constructed of Dacron with enough porosity to allow for neovascularization, thrombus organization, and nutrient blood flow. Thrombotic occlusion of prosthetic grafts is not well controlled with heparin or warfarin-type drugs and is now most commonly treated with platelet suppressive therapy.[1,7,8]

Peritoneovenous shunting using a LeVeen or Denver valve has become a palliative procedure for the treatment of intractable ascites associated with severe liver disease and malignant ascites.[167,168] A generalized hemorrhagic diathesis is frequently seen with the use of LeVeen shunts and appears to represent a straightforward DIC-type syndrome associated with accelerated fibrinogen and platelet destruction.[7,8,34,35,169-172] The removal of ascitic fluid at the time of valve implantation and the use of anticoagulants have been advocated to abort DIC in patients receiving LeVeen shunts.[8,34] Placing the patient in an upright position will often totally abort or significantly blunt the DIC process and should be used as a short-term palliative measure in patients with LeVeen shunts who are developing DIC.[34]

Apheresis Procedures

Apheresis (plasmapheresis, plasma exchange, leukopheresis, plateletpheresis, and peripheral stem cell harvest for bone marrow transplantation) has become a common procedure for the treatment of patients with a wide variety of hematologic and immunologic diseases, including thrombotic thrombocytopenic purpura, hemolytic-uremic syndrome, collagen vascular disorders, myasthenia gravis, hyperviscosity syndromes, and some instances of immune hemolytic anemias.[1,7,8] Hemorrhage and/or thrombosis may occur with any of these apheresis procedures. Thrombosis and thromboembolism may occur in vivo and frequently occur ex vivo in the apheresis equipment and tubing.[173] Thrombocytopenia occurs in most patients undergoing apheresis procedures, and commonly the platelet count will drop to between 15% and 50% of the initial platelet count. The platelet loss is less with discontinuous flow systems than with continuous flow systems. Another problem that happens during apheresis procedures is defective platelet function, which has been documented by the Borchgrevink technique and has also been studied by use of the glass bead column adhesion method. By the Borchgrevink technique about 80% of patients undergoing apheresis procedures have decreases in platelet adhesion.[174] The glass bead column technique, however, did not show this abnormality, which is in harmony with recent suggestions that the glass bead column test is not of clinical significance.[8,10,72,73]

Other severe derangements in hemostasis also happen during apheresis procedures. The most pronounced changes in coagulation appear to be decreases in fibrinogen and factor XI.[175] The fibrinogen level may drop to 50% of prepheresis levels and may remain depressed chronically for up to 72 hours. However, in most studies the fibrinogen level has not dropped below .5 g/L (50 mg/dL) and thrombin times are only rarely prolonged.[173-176] If greater than a 3.5-L exchange occurs, the prothrombin time, APTT, and thrombin time commonly become prolonged.[177] If a 2- to 5-L exchange occurs, fibrinogen levels will fall from 50% to 25% of normal and may not return to normal levels until about three days' postpheresis.[173,177] However, this change in fibrinogen is commonly not associated with bleeding unless large amounts of heparin are also used during the apheresis procedure. Factor IX levels will decrease from 60% to 70% of normal if greater than a 4-L exchange occurs. Other changes in coagulation are the noting of a 60% to 70% decrease in factors II, V, VII, X, XI, and XII.[173] In addition, factor V and factor VII levels will usually be normalized within 24 hours; however, factor II, factor X, factor XI, and factor XII levels will usually not normalize until about 48 hours postpheresis.[173,175]

Another complication of apheresis is a significant decrease in AT III, which may lead to thrombosis in up to 25% of patients.[173,178] The thrombotic events and AT III depletion associated with apheresis can be markedly blunted or eradicated using heparin in the replacement fluid or by the infusion of fresh frozen plasma as a source of AT III. This practice has, again, been noted to reduce or blunt the in vivo and ex vivo thrombotic and thromboembolic problems associated with apheresis.[178] Complement activation with the release of C3a and C5a and later potential leukoembolization and endothelial damage may also occur with apheresis procedures.[179] In addition, if activation of the complement system proceeds to C8,9 this may potentially also lead to or contribute to platelet and red blood cell release of procoagulant materials and subsequent thrombus formation.[32-34]

Apheresis is associated with significant changes in the hemostasis system, including thrombocytopenia, platelet dysfunction, and decreasing coagulation factor levels, with the most profound decreases being those of fibrinogen and factor XI. Most of these parameters return to normal in 24 to 48 hours postpheresis. Antithrombin III levels tend to decrease significantly during apheresis procedures, and unless heparin is used or AT III is replaced by fresh frozen plasma, thrombosis and thromboembolus can be a problem in up to 25% of patients undergoing apheresis procedures.

Prosthetic Heart Valves

The use of prosthetic heart valves has become common and has greatly reduced morbidity and mortality in patients with valvular heart disease. Complications of these devices, which include thromboembolism, infection, hemolysis, and detachment, may also significantly alter morbidity and mortality.[180] Of these complications, thromboembolism is the most common and can be the most serious. The likeliest sites of embolism are the central nervous system, coronary arteries, retinal vessels, and extremities.[181] Early in the history of cardiac valve placement, it was found that warfarin could decrease but not alleviate the thromboembolic events occurring with mitral and aortic valves.[182] Thromboembolism is more common with mitral valves than aortic valves, especially if atrial fibrillation or left atrial enlargement is present.[180,182-184] Early valves that had metal exposed to blood were associated with a 50% chance of thromboembolism, which could be reduced to 13% with the use of warfarin.[185] Original aortic valves were associated with a 35% chance of thromboembolism, which was reduced to 8% with the use of warfarin.[186] Valvular thromboemboli arise from platelets: after valve replacement, platelets adhere to the foreign surface by adhesion and aggregation.[1,7,8,139,180,187,188] Another impetus for platelet aggregation may come from ADP, liberated during red blood cell hemolysis.[139] Because of platelet consumption on valvular surfaces, many patients with prosthetic valves demonstrate decreased platelet survival and increased platelet turnover. The decreased survival appears to correlate well with the incidence of thromboemboli.[189-191] However, patients with rheumatic valve disease without prosthetic valves also show decreased platelet survival, increased platelet consumption, and an increased chance of thromboembolism.[192] Valvular platelet consumption has decreased progressively with new valve design but still has not been totally alleviated. Platelet deposits and thromboemboli were most pronounced with the early metal valves, and decreased in incidence with second-generation cloth-bound valves, which would induce neoendothelialization of the valve surface and an inert valve. New xenograft (porcine) valves are associated with an even greater reduction in thromboembolic complications. Despite this improvement, however, a significant chance of serious thromboembolism in patients with prosthetic aortic or mitral valves still exists, and most patients with valves are committed to long-term or life-long anticoagulation of some type.

Both dipyridamole and sulfinpyrazone will normalize decreased platelet survival in patients with prosthetic valves, but aspirin alone does not demonstrate this effect.[189,193] Aspirin will potentiate the effect of dipyridamole in normalizing platelet survival in patients.[189] The mechanisms for this are unclear, because the doses of dipyridamole and sulfinpyrazone that will normalize platelet survival are lower than doses needed to alter platelet aggregation in vitro. Sulfinpyrazone will normalize decreased platelet survival in patients with rheumatic mitral valvular disease who do not have prosthetic valves.[192] These observations led to interest in anti-platelet drugs for the control of thromboembolism associated with prosthetic heart valves, and many clinical trials have proven the efficacy of several agents, including aspirin and dipyridamole.[194-198] One early trial showed a reduction from a 14% to a 1.3% incidence of thromboemboli by adding dipyridamole to a warfarin regimen.[194] Another early trial showed that the addition of aspirin to the warfarin regimen decreased the chance of thromboembolism by 80%.[195] The efficacy of antiplatelet agents alone is unclear: one trial has found aspirin plus dipyridamole alone (no warfarin) to be effective,[199] but another trial found this regimen to be ineffective.[200]

Although the role of antiplatelet agents alone is unclear, an antiplatelet agent should be used with warfarin in patients with prosthetic valves. At the present time, no uniformity in anticoagulant regimens for patients with prosthetic cardiac valves exists. One suggestion has been that the chance of thromboembolism decreases with time, and after a given period of time an anticoagulant is no longer needed in selected patients.[74,201,202] Another recommendation is to use adequate doses of warfarin (2.5 times the control time) plus aspirin or dipyridamole.[188] Yet another recommended regimen is to use warfarin in patients with mitral or double valve replacement but antiplatelet agents alone in patients with aortic valves.[184] Another author suggests combination antiplatelet agents alone in patients with prosthetic valves; the aspirin dosage suggested is 330 mg, three times daily, and the dipyridamole dosage recommended is 75 mg, three times daily.[190] Probably the safest recommendation is that of Frankl[180] who recommends that patients with aortic valves receive adequate doses of aspirin plus dipyridamole, and patients with mitral valve replacement or double valve replacement should be treated with aspirin plus dipyridamole plus warfarin.

Recently, specific anticoagulant recommendations for patients with mechanical or bioprosthetic heart valves have been offered by a national panel conference of the National Heart, Lung, and Blood Institute and the American College of Chest Physicians.[203] This conference resulted in the following recommendations for mechanical prosthetic heart valves: (1) All patients with mechanical prosthetic heart valves should be given anticoagulants of long-term warfarin at a dose appropriate to prolong the prothrombin time to 1.5 to 2.0 times the control (using rabbit brain thromboplastin), and it was recommended that the addition of dipyridamole to this regimen may be considered an additional acceptable option. (2) If patients with a mechanical prosthetic heart valve have systemic embolization, then dipyridamole, at a dosage of 400 mg per day, should be added to the warfarin dose. (3) Antiplatelet agents alone were not considered adequate protection in patients with mechanical prosthetic heart valves. (4) When a major bleeding episode happens in a patient with a mechanical prosthetic heart valve being treated with long-term warfarin, lower doses of warfarin appropriate to give a prothrombin time ratio of 1.3 to 1.5 times the control should be started.

The specific recommendations for patients with bioprosthetic heart valves are the following: (1) All patients with bioprosthetic heart valves in the mitral position should be treated for the first three months with appropriate warfarin to render a prothrombin time ratio of 1.3 to 1.5 times the control, and, similarly, if patients have been implanted with bioprosthetic valves in the aortic position and remain in normal sinus rhythm, warfarin therapy may be considered optional. (2) Patients with bioprosthetic heart valves who have a history of systemic embolization, who demonstrated a left atrial thrombus at surgery, or who have atrial fibrillation should be treated with long-term warfarin therapy, although ideal doses are unclear. (3) Patients with bioprosthetic heart valves in regular sinus rhythm may, optionally, be treated with long-term aspirin at 500 mg per day.

Total Artificial Heart Transplantation

Cardiac transplantation has become a routine medical procedure. Unfortunately, many patients awaiting transplantation die before a human transplant becomes available or develop cardiogenic shock that cannot be controlled by medication. Because of the number of patients awaiting transplantation, the use of a total artificial heart (TAH) has come into use, usually as a temporizing measure while a human allogeneic transplant is awaited. The use of the total artificial heart has been associated with many complications, the most important of which is thrombus formation followed by cerebral thromboembolization. This complication, thus far, occurs in greater than 50% of patients implanted with the TAH while awaiting human allogeneic heart transplant.[1,204] Most studies regarding both the hemodynamics and the thrombotic and thromboembolic problems with the total artificial heart have primarily come from animal studies, the majority being done in calves. Calves, however, do not have as high an incidence of cerebrovascular thrombosis as do humans, probably because of anatomic species differences. About 30% to 40% of calves do show cerebral thromboemboli, but a higher percentage develop renal emboli.[205]

The mechanisms of thrombus and subsequent thromboembolic formation have primarily been studied in the bovine species. Hartmannova and associates[206] implanted TAHs in eight calves, and four died of thromboembolic disease or hemorrhage. The total artificial heart was made out of polymethylacrylate with valves made of polyurethane. Of those with thromboemboli, the majority were to the brain stem, although mesenteric thromboembolic events were also noted. These investigators noticed that a fibrous capsule with a pseudointima formed in the total artificial heart, which was later followed by surface thrombi, primarily platelet thrombi. Noted as another complication of the TAH was venostasis leading to a "nutmeg liver" or congestive hepatomegaly from less than ideal pump efficiency.

Vasku,[207] in studying transplanted bovine species, noted that thromboemboli arose from calcification of indigenous thrombi formed on the artificial surfaces. The first event appears to be a platelet or fibrin thrombus, most commonly platelet thrombi, which later become calcified, and the thromboemboli may be calcific, thrombotic, or a combination thereof. Vasku also noted calcification and thromboembolic events to the arteries and veins of the gastrointestinal tract and cerebrovascular tissue. Thromboembolic events did not occur in the first two to three months of implantation of the TAH, and it was concluded that temporary transplantation of the total artificial heart could be free from serious thromboembolic events if allogeneic transplant were carried out early on. The development of a nidus of thrombus and subsequently the potential for thromboembolization depended on the biochemistry and physics of the TAH and was thought to be primarily related to the carbohydrate content of the coating of the biomaterial and its subsequent stretching and porosity characteristics. Vasku also noted that calcium deposits not only led to microthrombi and macrothrombi but also decreased driving ability of the TAH and mechanical damage to the driving diaphragms.

Tolpekin and coworkers[208] implanted the TAH into 25 calves, 16 of which developed thrombi of the valves within four to six days, despite anticoagulation with heparin at 50 units per kg and aspirin. After three days of this anticoagulant regimen, the therapy was changed to warfarin and pentoxifylline (Trental). During the warfarin and pentoxifylline phase, the valves tended to thrombose. These investigators also noted transient thrombocytopenia to occur during the first 24 to 48 hours in calves receiving a total artificial heart.

Shumakov and associates[209] implanted TAHs in five calves with a non–Jarvik-type device that was specifically designed with an elliptic shape. Vigorous anticoagulation with warfarin, aspirin, and dipyridamole (doses not specified) were instituted to keep the prothrombin time and partial thromboplastin time significantly prolonged. None of these five calves had thrombotic or thromboembolic disease. They concluded that this was because of vigorous anticoagulation and "better hemodynamic conditions" created with an elliptically shaped total artificial heart.

Hughes and associates[210] studied two groups of calves receiving a total artificial heart of the Jarvik type. Group I consisted of 11 calves implanted with the Jarvik total artificial heart, no warfarin was used, but 36% of the calves were given combination platelet suppressive therapy with aspirin and dipyridamole. Group II consisted of 11 calves also implanted with a Jarvik-type total artificial heart, and warfarin was used. In those animals who were taking warfarin (Group II), the dose was adjusted to give a prothrombin ratio of 1.5 to 3.0 (15 to 20 seconds). In the calves not receiving warfarin (but 36% received a combination of aspirin/dipyridamole), calcified thrombi developed in 9 of the 11. In Group II animals, however, of the seven that were given warfarin, all seven developed calcific thrombi of the diaphragm/valvular area. The authors concluded that endogenous biomaterial surface defects led to thrombi that then usually became calcified, providing a source for thromboemboli, but that this could be moderately reduced with adequate warfarin.

Iwaya and associates[211] studied 27 calves with a TAH made of polyurethane material and noted that 19% of these animals died of thrombi primarily of the inflow or outflow of valvular tracts. The mechanism of death in these particular animals was that thrombi of the inflow and outflow tracts led to mechanical failure, and this was more commonly noted as a cause of death than thromboembolic disease.

Dostal and associates[212] studied seven calves with a polymethylacrylate TAH supplied with polyurethane valves, and all animals implanted survived for longer than 100 days. Vigorous anticoagulation with warfarin, aspirin, dipyridamole, and alpha tocopherol was given to the animals. In this group of animals, only two of seven died of thromboembolic events both to the central nervous system. Therefore, these authors concluded that the warfarin plus combined platelet suppressive therapy does offer adequate long-term anticoagulation for the implanted TAH.

Human studies with the TAH have been far fewer than the animal studies yet published. Of the original seven Jarvik-VII TAHs implanted, over 50% of patients developed serious thromboembolic events to the brain.[1,205] This continues to be a problem with the Jarvik-VII device. However, Griffith and coinvestigators[213] have implanted six temporary Jarvik-VII hearts for a total of 52 patient-days and noted no clinical thrombotic or thromboembolic events in any patient. When removing the device for allogeneic human heart transplantation, however, all TAHs had microscopic deposits of platelet and fibrin thrombi. During the time of Jarvik heart implantation, these patients were postoperatively treated with heparin to keep the PTT at 2.0 to 2.5 times the control and were also treated with dipyridamole at 75 mg every eight hours. As in calf studies, these authors also noted transient thrombocytopenia during the postoperative period, which then abated. Of the six explanted TAHs, two showed large macrothrombi that were fibrin-rich but did not interfere with function of the device and did not embolize. The thrombi were primarily found on the valves and valve housings. The authors concluded that all six patients failed to show clinical evidence of thrombotic or thromboembolic events, and this was owed to good fortune, short-term use of the total artificial heart, and vigorous anticoagulation therapy. The first seven patients implanted with a Jarvik TAH had thrombi, emboli, or hemorrhage most often to the central nervous system.

Kolff[205] pointed out that the decreased incidence of cerebral thromboemboli seen in calves vs humans with the same Jarvik-VII–type device is probably because of central nervous system vascular anatomic differences, because the calves do demonstrate a high incidence of renal thromboembolic events. This same investigator has noted that TAHs with a rough Dacron fibril intima, the absence of quick disconnect devices, and the use of tissue valves instead of mechanical valves may be the safest options yet available.

Trubel and coworkers[214] described three patients implanted with a TAH while awaiting allogeneic heart transplants. Only one of the three died of a cerebrovascular thromboembolic event. All three patients were given intravenous heparin to keep the thrombin time at 20 to 30 seconds and intravenous aspirin. All three patients had excessive postoperative bleeding, commonly seen in most patients receiving TAHs with vigorous postoperative anticoagulation. These investigators believed that their vigorous anticoagulation prevented thromboembolic complications in two of the three patients.

Green and associates[215] described a patient implanted with a Jarvik-VII heart who developed DIC postoperatively. The DIC was manifest by an increased D-dimer and fibrinopeptide A level, with a twofold to threefold elevated level of thromboxane A_2, which happened while the patient was being treated with heparin, warfarin, and enteric-coated aspirin. Elevating the levels of enteric-coated aspirin was believed to be associated with alleviation of the DIC. As the aspirin was tapered, however, the patient had a serious cerebrovascular thrombotic event followed by intracranial hemorrhage resulting from anticoagulant therapy.

Coleman and coworkers[216] described a patient who sustained a transplant of a Jarvik-VII TAH for 112 days followed by death. At autopsy, a careful examination noted no evidence of calcification, vegetation, or thrombus formation in the implanted device. Small platelet thrombi were noted along the suture line in the right atrium but did not obstruct blood flow or valve function. Microscopic thrombi, however, were noted in the pumping diaphragm, which were only found by scanning electron microscopy. Levinson and coworkers[204] implanted a Jarvik-VII TAH in a patient who was then given a vigorous anticoagulant mechanism with heparin. Despite this, the patient developed a cerebrovascular thrombotic event on the seventh postoperative day. The patient recovered and subsequently has received an allogeneic human heart transplant.

The use of a total artificial heart appears extremely desirable for use in suitable human candidates who are awaiting an allogeneic human transplantation. The indications are particularly for those individuals who develop cardiogenic shock unresponsive to medication. However, vigorous anticoagulation often consisting of warfarin, heparin, and platelet suppressive therapy in various forms has failed to alleviate an extremely high incidence of thrombotic and thromboembolic cerebral disease. The use of vigorous anticoagulation has also been associated with significant postoperative hemorrhage, which often, however, is not fatal. It is hoped that the future will be associated with major advances in biomaterials so that the serious problem of thrombogenicity, which in the total artificial heart is the rate-limiting factor, can be alleviated.

Summary

This discussion has provided a review of the available literature regarding alterations of hemostasis associated with cardiopulmonary bypass, the use of prosthetic devices, and apheresis. The key to prevention of CPB hemorrhage is to obtain an adequate preoperative work-up. Of extreme importance is an adequate history for bleeding tendencies and thrombotic tendencies in both the patient and the family; of equal importance is a careful history regarding the use of drugs affecting hemostasis, especially drugs known to interfere with platelet function. A careful physical examination, searching for clues of a real or potential bleeding diathesis, may also prevent catastrophic cases of hemorrhage. Adequate presurgical screening must be done in surgical and transplantation patients. In addition to the usual prothrombin time, partial thromboplastin time, and platelet count, a standardized template bleeding time (and thrombin time in patients subjected to CPB) should be done. The use of these simple testing modalities will guard against significant defects in vascular and platelet function. Most instances of nontechnical surgical and cardiovascular surgical hemorrhage are caused by several well-defined defects in hemostasis, which should be readily controlled if approached in a logical manner as a team effort among all surgeons, cardiac surgeons, pathologists, and hematologists.

References

1. Bick RL: Alterations of hemostasis associated with surgery, cardiopulmonary bypass surgery, and prosthetic devices. In: OD Ratnoff, CD Forbes (Eds): Disorders of Hemostasis, ed 2. WB Saunders, Philadelphia, 1991, p 379.

2. Bick RL: Clinical approach to the patient with hemorrhage, ch 2. In: Disorders of Hemostasis and Thrombosis: Principles of Clinical Practice. Thieme, Inc., New York, 1985, p 36.

3. Bick RL: A systemic approach to the diagnosis of bleeding disorders, ch 4. In: G Murano, RL Bick (Eds): Basic Concepts of Hemostasis and Thrombosis. CRC Press, Boca Raton, FL, 1980, p 81.

4. Coller BS: Platelets and their disorders. In: OD Ratnoff, CD Forbes (Eds): Disorders of Hemostasis, ed 2. WB Saunders, Philadelphia, 1991, p 73.

5. Bick RL: Alterations of hemostasis associated with cardiopulmonary bypass: pathophysiology, prevention, diagnosis, and management. Semin Thromb Hemost 3:59, 1976.

6. Verska JJ, ER Lonser, LA Brewer: Predisposing factors and management of hemorrhage following open-heart surgery. J Cardiovasc Surg 13:361, 1972.

7. Bick RL: Hemostasis defects associated with cardiac surgery, prosthetic devices, and other extracorporeal circuits. Semin Thromb Hemost 11:249, 1985.

8. Bick RL: Hemostasis defects in general surgery, cardiac surgery, transplantation, and the use of prosthetic devices, ch 8. In: Disorders of Hemostasis and Thrombosis: Principles of Clinical Practice. Thieme, Inc., New York, 1985, p 223.

9. Mielke CH, MM Kaneshiro, LA Maher, J Weiner, SI Rapaport: The standardized normal Ivy bleeding time and its prolongation by aspirin. Blood 34:204, 1969.

10. Bick RL: Platelet defects, ch 4. In: Disorders of Hemostasis and Thrombosis: Principles of Clinical Practice. Thieme, Inc., New York, 1985, p 65.

11. Bick RL, G Murano: Primary hyperfibrino(geno)lytic syndromes, ch 9. In: G Murano, RL Bick (Eds): Basic Concepts

of Hemostasis and Thrombosis. CRC Press, Boca Raton, FL, 1980, p 181.

12. Bick RL: Syndromes associated with hyperfibrino(geno)lysis, ch 3. In: Disseminated Intravascular Coagulation. CRC Press, Boca Raton, FL, 1983, p 105.

13. Shahian DM, SR Wallach, MM Bern: Open heart surgery in patients with cold-reactive proteins. Surg Clin North Am 65:315, 1985.

14. Landymore R, W Isom, B Barlam: Management of patients with cold agglutinins who require open-heart surgery. Can J Surg 26:79, 1983.

15. Guena L, KA Kwabena, A Addei: Intraoperative hypothermia in a patient with cold agglutinin disease. JAMA 74:691, 1982.

16. Klein HG, LL Faltz, CL McIntosh, FR Appelbaum, AB Deisseroth, PV Holland: Surgical hypothermia in a patient with a cold agglutinin. Transfusion 20:354, 1980.

17. Leach AB, GL Van Hasselt, JC Edwards: Cold agglutinins and deep hypothermia. Anaesthesia 38:140, 1983.

18. Moore RA, EA Geller, ES Mathews, SB Botros, AB Jose, DL Clark: The effect of hypothermic cardiopulmonary bypass on patients with low-titer, non-specific cold agglutinins. Ann Thorac Surg 37:233, 1984.

19. Brecker G, EP Cronkite: Morphology and enumeration of human blood platelets. J Appl Physiol 3:365, 1950.

20. Hougie C: Fundamentals of Blood Coagulation in Clinical Medicine. McGraw-Hill, New York, 1963, p 241.

21. Proctor RR, SI Rapaport: The partial thromboplastin time with kaolin. A simple screening test for first-stage plasma clotting factor deficiencies. Am J Clin Pathol 36:212, 1961.

22. Quick AJ, M Stanley-Brown, FW Bancroft: A study of the coagulation defect in hemophilia and in jaundice. Am J Med Sci 190:501, 1935.

23. Bick RL: Vascular disorders associated with thrombohemorrhagic phenomenon. Semin Thromb Hemost 5:167, 1979.

24. Bick RL: Vascular disorders associated with thrombohemorrhagic phenomenon, ch 3. In: Disorders of Hemostasis and Thrombosis: Principles of Clinical Practice. Thieme, Inc., New York, 1985, p 44.

25. Bick RL: Vascular disorders. In: G Murano, RL Bick (Eds): Basic Concepts of Hemostasis and Thrombosis. CRC Press, Boca Raton, FL, 1980, p 89.

26. Bick RL: Alterations of hemostasis associated with malignancy: etiology, pathophysiology, diagnosis, and management. Semin Thromb Hemost 5:1, 1978.

27. Cohen LS: Clinical pharmacology of acetylsalicylic acid. Semin Thromb Hemost 2:146, 1976.

28. Mustard JF, MA Packham: Factors influencing platelet function: adhesion, release, and aggregation. Pharmacol Rev 23:97, 1970.

29. Triplett DA: Quantitative or functional disorders of platelets. In: DA Triplett (Ed): Platelet Function. ASCP Press, Chicago, 1978, p 123.

30. Triplett DA: Platelet disorders. In: G Murano, RL Bick (Eds): Basic Concepts of Hemostasis and Thrombosis. CRC Press, Boca Raton, FL, 1980, p 95.

31. Bick RL, WR Schmalhorst, E Shanbrom: Prothrombin complex concentrates: use in controlling the hemorrhagic diathesis of chronic liver disease. Am J Dig Dis 20:741, 1975.

32. Bick RL: Disseminated intravascular coagulation and related syndromes: etiology, pathophysiology, diagnosis and management. Am J Hematol 5:265, 1978.

33. Bick RL: Disseminated intravascular coagulation and related syndromes, ch 6. In: Disorders of Hemostasis and Thrombosis: Principles of Clinical Practice. Thieme, Inc., New York, 1985, p 157.

34. Bick RL: Disseminated intravascular coagulation and related syndromes: a clinical review. Semin Thromb Hemost 14:299, 1988.

35. Bick RL: Disseminated intravascular coagulation, ch 2. In: Disseminated Intravascular Coagulation. CRC Press, Boca Raton, FL, 1983, p 31.

36. Bick RL: Disseminated intravascular coagulation and related syndromes. In: J Fareed, J Messmore, J Fenton, et al (Eds): Perspectives in Hemostasis. Pergamon Press, New York, 1981, p 122.

37. Mertens BF, LF Greene, EJW Bowie, LR Elveback, CA Owen: Fibrinolytic split products and ethanol gelation test in preoperative evaluation of patients with prostatic disease. Mayo Clin Proc 49:642, 1974.

38. Beall C, EM Yow, RD Blodwell, G Hallman, D Cooley: Open heart surgery without blood transfusion. Arch Surg 94:567, 1967.

39. Cordell AR: Hematological complications of extracorporeal circulation. In: AR Cordell, RG Ellison (Eds): Complications of Intrathoracic Surgery. Little, Brown, and Company, Boston, 1979, p 27.

40. Mammen EF: Natural proteinase inhibitors in extracorporeal circulation. Ann N Y Acad Sci 146:754, 1968.

41. Koets MH, BC Washington, LW Wolk, et al: Hemostasis changes during cardiovascular bypass surgery. Semin Thromb Hemost 11:281, 1985.

42. Bick RL: Pathophysiology of Hemostasis and Thrombosis, ch 24. In: WA Sodeman, TA Sodeman: Pathologic Physiology, Mechanisms of Disease, ed 7. WB Saunders, Philadelphia, 1985, p 705.

43. Graeff H, FK Beller: Fibrinolytic activity in whole blood, dilute blood, and euglobulin lysis time tests. In: N Bang, FK Beller, E Deutsch (Eds): Thrombosis and Bleeding Disorders, Theory and Methods. Academic Press, New York, 1970, p 328.

44. Menon IS: A study of the possible correlation of euglobulin lysis time and dilute blood clot lysis time in the determination of fibrinolytic activity. Lab Pract 17:334, 1968.

45. Bick RL: Clinical hemostasis practice: the major impact of laboratory automation. Semin Thromb Hemost 9:139, 1983.

46. Bick RL: The clinical significance of fibrinogen degradation products. Semin Thromb Hemost 8:302, 1982.

47. Kevy SV, RM Glickman, WF Bernhard, L Diamond, R Gross: The pathogenesis and control of the hemorrhagic defect in open-heart surgery. Surg Gynecol Obstet 123:313, 1966.

48. Signori EE, JA Penner, DR Kahn: Coagulation defects and bleeding in open heart surgery. Ann Thorac Surg 8:521, 1969.

49. Porter JM, D Silver: Alterations in fibrinolysis and coagulation associated with cardiopulmonary bypass. J Thorac Cardiovasc Surg 56:869, 1968.

50. Tice DA, MH Worth: Recognition and treatment of postoperative bleeding associated with open heart surgery. Ann N Y Acad Sci 146:745, 1968.

51. Wright TA, J Darte, WT Mustard: Postoperative bleeding after extracorporeal circulation. Can J Surg 2:142, 1959.

52. von Kaulla KN, H Swan: Clotting deviations in man during cardiac bypass: fibrinolysis and circulating anticoagulants. J Thorac Surg 36:519, 1958.

53. Blomback M, I Noren, A Senning: Coagulation disturbances during extracorporeal circulation and the postoperative period. Acta Chir Scand 127:433, 1964.

54. Deiter RA, WE Neville, R Piffare, M Jasuja: Preoperative coagulation profiles and posthemodilution cardiopulmonary bypass hemorrhage. Am J Surg 121:689, 1971.

55. Penick GD, HE Averette, RM Peters, KM Brinkhous: The hemorrhagic syndrome complicating extracorporeal shunting of blood: an experimental study of its pathogenesis. Thromb Diath Haemorrh 2:218, 1958.

56. Trimble AS, R Herst, M Grady, J Crookston: Blood loss in open heart surgery. Arch Surg 93:323, 1966.

57. Bick RL, NR Arbegast, N Holtermann, L Crawford, WR Schmalhorst: Platelet function abnormalities in cardiopulmonary bypass. Circulation (suppl) 50:301, 1974.

58. Bick RL, WR Schmalhorst, L Crawford, M Holtermann, NR Arbegast: The hemorrhagic diathesis created by cardiopulmonary bypass. Am J Clin Pathol 63:588, 1975.

59. Bick RL, NR Arbegast, L Crawford, L Holtermann, T Adams, WR Schmalhorst: Hemostatic defects induced by cardiopulmonary bypass. Vasc Surg 9:228, 1975.

60. Bick RL, WR Schmalhorst, NR Arbegast: Alterations of hemostasis associated with cardiopulmonary bypass. Am J Clin Pathol 63:588, 1975.

61. Casteneda AR: Must heparin be neutralized following open heart operations? J Thorac Cardiovasc Surg 52:716, 1966.

62. deVries SI, S von Creveld, P Green, E Muller, M Wettermark: Studies on the coagulation of the blood in patients treated with extracorporeal circulation. Thromb Diath Haemorrh 5:426, 1961.

63. Muller N, S Popov-Cenic, W Buttner, RG Kladetsky, H Egli: Studies of fibrinolytic and coagulation factors during open-heart surgery, II: postoperative bleeding tendencies and changes in the coagulation system. Thromb Res 7:589, 1975.

64. Bick RL: Alterations of hemostasis during cardiopulmonary bypass: a comparison between membrane and bubble oxygenators. Am J Clin Pathol 73:300, 1980.

65. Bick RL, WR Schmalhorst, NR Arbegast: Alterations of hemostasis associated with cardiopulmonary bypass. Thromb Res 8:285, 1976.

66. Holswade GR, RL Nachman, T Killip: Thrombocytopathies in patients with open-heart surgery. Preoperative treatment with corticosteroids. Arch Surg 94:365, 1967.

67. Salzman WE: Blood platelets and extracorporeal circulation. Transfusion 3:274, 1963.

68. Bick RL, T Adams, WR Schmalhorst: Bleeding times, platelet adhesion, and aspirin. Am J Clin Pathol 65:69, 1976.

69. Bowie EJW, CA Owen, JH Thompson: Platelet adhesiveness in von Willebrand's disease. Am J Clin Pathol 52:69, 1969.

70. Bowie EJW, CA Owen: The value of measuring platelet adhesiveness in the diagnosis of bleeding diseases. Am J Clin Pathol 60:302, 1973.

71. Hirsh J: Laboratory diagnosis of thrombosis, ch 58. In: RW Coleman, J Hirsh, VJ Marder, EW Salzman (Eds): Hemostasis and Thrombosis: Basic Principles and Clinical Practice. JB Lippincott, Philadelphia, 1982, p 789.

72. Zimmerman TS, D Meyer: Factor VIII–von Willebrand factor and the molecular basis of von Willebrand's disease, ch 5. In: RW Coleman, J Hirsh, VJ Marder, EW Salzman (Eds): Hemostasis and Thrombosis: Basic Principles and Clinical Practice. JB Lippincott, Philadelphia, 1982, p 54.

73. Adams T, L Schutz, L Goldberg: Platelet function abnormalities in the myeloproliferative disorders. Scand J Haematol 13:215, 1975.

74. Sarin CL, E Yalav, AJ Clement, MV Braimbridge: Thromboembolism after Starr valve replacement. Br Heart J 33:111, 1971.

75. Hellem AJ: The advances of human blood platelets in vitro. Scand J Clin Lab Invest (suppl) 51:1, 1960.

76. Bick RL, LF Fekete: Cardiopulmonary bypass hemorrhage: aggrevation by pre-op ingestion of antiplatelet agents. Vasc Surg 13:277, 1979.

77. Kowalski E, M Kopec, Z Wegrzynowicz: Influence of fibrinogen degradation products (FDP) on platelet aggregation, adhesiveness, and viscous metamorphosis. Thromb Diath Haemorrh 10:406, 1963.

78. Kowalski E: Fibrinogen derivatives and their biologic activities. Semin Hematol 5:45, 1968.

79. Harker LA, TW Malpass, HE Branson, EA Hessel, SJ Slichter: Mechanisms of abnormal bleeding in patients undergoing cardiopulmonary bypass: acquired transient platelet dysfunction associated with selective alpha-granule release. Blood 56:824, 1980.

80. Stass S, C Bishop, R Fosberg, M Hartley, M Cramer: Platelets as affected by cardiopulmonary bypass. Am J Clin Pathol 66:459, 1976.

81. Saunders CR, L Carlisle, RL Bick: Hydroxyethyl starch versus albumin in cardiopulmonary bypass prime solutions. Ann Thorac Surg 35:532, 1983.

82. Salzman EW, MJ Weinstein, RM Weintraub, JA Ware, RL Thurer, L Robertson, A Donovan, T Gaffney, V Bertele, J Troll, M Smith, LE Chute: Treatment with desmopressin acetate to reduce blood loss after cardiac surgery. N Engl J Med 314:1402, 1986.

83. Weinstein M, JA Ware, J Troll, EW Salzman: Changes in von Willebrand factor during cardiac surgery: effect of desmopressin acetate. Blood 71:1648, 1988.

84. Rocha E, R Llorens, JA Paramo, R Arcas, B Cuesta, AM Trenor: Does desmopressin acetate reduce blood loss after surgery in patients on cardiopulmonary bypass? Circulation 77:1319, 1988.

85. Mannucci PM: Desmopressin (DDAVP) for treatment of disorders of hemostasis. Prog Hemost Thromb 8:19, 1986.

86. Warrier I, JM Lusher: DDAVP: a useful alternative to blood components in moderate hemophilia A and von Willebrand's disease. J Pediatr 102:228, 1983.

87. Mariani G, N Ciavarella, MG Mazzucconi: Evaluation of the effectiveness of DDAVP in surgery and in bleeding episodes in hemophilia and von Willebrand's disease: a study of 43 patients. Clin Lab Haematol 6:229, 1984.

88. De La Fuente B, CK Kasper, FR Rickles: Response of patients with mild hemophilia A and von Willebrand's disease to treatment with desmopressin. Ann Intern Med 103:6, 1985.

89. Behrendt DM, SE Epstein, AG Morrow: Postperfusion nonthrombocytopenic purpura: an uncommon sequel of open heart surgery. Am J Cardiol 22:631, 1968.

90. Bick RL, TP Comer, NR Arbegast: Fatal purpura fulminans following total cardiopulmonary bypass. J Cardiovasc Surg 14:569, 1973.

91. Derman UM, PW Rand, N Barker: Fibrinolysis after cardiopulmonary bypass and its relationship to fibrinogen. J Thorac Cardiovasc Surg 51:223, 1966.

92. Bachmann F, R McKenna, ER Cole, HJ Maiafi: The hemostatic mechanisms after open-heart surgery. I. Studies on plasma coagulation factors and fibrinolysis in 512 patients after extracorporeal circulation. J Thorac Cardiovasc Surg 70:76, 1975.

93. Tsuji HK, JV Redington, JH Kay, RK Goesswald: The study of fibrinolytic and coagulation factors during open heart surgery. Ann N Y Acad Sci 146:763, 1968.

94. Woods JE, JW Kirklin, CA Owen, JH Thompson, HF Taswell: The effect of bypass surgery on coagulation sensitive clotting factors. Mayo Clin Proc 42:724, 1967.

95. Gans H, V Subramanian, S John, AR Casteneda, CW Lillehei: Theoretical and practical (clinical) considerations concerning proteolytic enzymes and their inhibitors with particular reference to changes in the plasminogen-plasmin system during assisted circulation in man. Ann N Y Acad Sci 146:721, 1968.

96. Palester-Chlebowzyk M, E Strzyzewska, W Sitowski, K Olender: Detection of the intravascular coagulation of blood clotting. II. Results of the paracoagulation test in patients undergoing open-heart surgery, with extracorporeal circulation. Pol Med J 11:59, 1972.

97. Kladetsky RG, S Popov-Cenic, W Buttner, N Muller, H Egli: Studies of fibrinolytic and coagulation factors during open-heart surgery with ECC. Thromb Res 7:579, 1975.

98. Gomes MM, D McGoon: Bleeding patterns after open heart surgery. J Thorac Cardiovasc Surg 60:87, 1970.

99. Bick RL, I Kovacs, LF Fekete: A new two-stage functional assay for antithrombin III (heparin cofactor): clinical and laboratory evaluation. Thromb Res 8:745, 1976.

100. Lackner H, JP Javid: The clinical significance of the plasminogen level. Am J Clin Pathol 60:175, 1973.

101. Tsitouris G, S Bellet, R Eilberg, L Feinberg, H Sandberg: Effects of major surgery on plasmin-plasminogen systems. Arch Intern Med 108:98, 1961.

102. Wuelfing D, KP Brandau: Fibrinolytic activity after surgery. Minn Med 51:1503, 1968.

103. Ygge J: Changes in blood coagulation and fibrinolysis during the postoperative period. Am J Surg 119:225, 1970.

104. Bick RL, RC Bishop, M Warren, E Stemmer: Changes in fibrinolysis and fibrinolytic enzymes during extracorporeal circulation. Trans Am Soc Hematol 38:109, 1971.

105. Bick RL, RC Bishop, ES Shanbrom: Fibrinolytic activity in acute myocardial infarction. Am J Clin Pathol 57:359, 1972.

106. Bishop RC, H Ekert, G Gilchrist, E Shanbrom, LF Fekete: The preparation and evaluation of a standardized fibrin plate for the assessment of fibrinolytic activity. Thromb Diath Haemorrh 23:202, 1970.

107. Fareed J: New methods in hemostatic testing. In: J Fareed, H Messmore, J Fenton (Eds): Perspectives in Hemostasis. Pergamon Press, New York, 1981, p 310.

108. Fareed J, HL Messmore, EW Bermes: New perspectives in coagulation testing. Clin Chem 26:1380, 1980.

109. Huseby RM, RE Smith: Synthetic oligopeptide substrates: their diagnostic application in blood coagulation, fibrinolysis, and other pathologic states. Semin Thromb Hemost 6:173, 1980.

110. Naeye RL: Thrombotic state after a hemorrhagic diathesis: a possible complication of therapy with epsilon amino-caproic acid. Blood 19:694, 1962.

111. Ratnoff OD: Epsilon aminocaproic acid: a dangerous weapon. N Engl J Med 280:1124, 1969.

112. Verska J: Letter to the editor. Ann Thorac Surg 13:87, 1972.

113. Brooks DH, HT Bahnson: An outbreak of hemorrhage following cardiopulmonary bypass. J Thorac Cardiovasc Surg 63:449, 1972.

114. O'Neill JA, N Ende, IS Collins, HA Collins: A quantitative determination of perfusion fibrinolysis. Surgery 60:809, 1966.

115. Bick RL, BL Frazier, CL Saunders, NR Arbegast: Alterations of hemostasis during cardiopulmonary bypass: the potential role of Factor XII activation in inducing primary fibrino(geno)lysis. Blood 64:(5)926, 1984.

116. Pechet L: Fibrinolysis. N Engl J Med 273:966, 1965.

117. Sharp AA: The significance of fibrinolysis. Proc R Soc Lond (Biol) 173:311, 1969.

118. Sherry S, AP Fletcher, N Alkjaersig: Fibrinolysis and fibrinolytic activity in man. Physiol Rev 39:343, 1959.

119. Larrieu MJ, L Dray, N Ardaillou: Biological effects of fibrinogen-fibrin degradation products. Thromb Diath Haemorrh 34:686, 1975.

120. Alkjaersig N, AP Fletcher, S Sherry: Pathogenesis of the coagulation defect developing during pathological plasma proteolytic ("fibrinolytic") states. II. The significance, mechanism, and consequences of defective fibrin polymerization. J Clin Invest 41:917, 1962.

121. Bick RL: Clinical implications of molecular markers in hemostasis and thrombosis. Semin Thromb Hemost 10:290, 1984.

122. Akkerman JW, WC Runne, JJ Sixma, AE Zimmerman: Improved survival rates in dogs after extracorporeal circulation by improved control of heparin levels. J Thorac Cardiovasc Surg 68:59, 1974.

123. Ellison N, CP Betty, DR Blake, H Wurzel, H MacVaugh: Heparin rebound: studies in patients and volunteers. J Thorac Cardiovasc Surg 67:723, 1974.

124. Gollub S: Heparin rebound in open-heart surgery. Surg Gynecol Obstet 124:337, 1967.

125. Jaberi M, WR Bell, DW Benson: Control of heparin therapy in open-heart surgery. J Thorac Cardiovasc Surg 67:133, 1974.

126. Ellison N, AJ Ominsky, H Wollman: Is protamine a clinically important anticoagulant? A negative answer. Anesthesiology 35:621, 1971.

127. Ollendorff P: The nature of the anticoagulant effect of heparin, protamine, Polybrene, and toluidine blue. Scand J Clin Lab Invest 14:267, 1962.

128. Tsai TP, JM Matloff, RJ Gray, A Chaux, RM Kass, ME Lee, LS Czer: Cardiac surgery in the octagenerian. J Thorac Surg 91:924, 1986.

129. Horneffer PJ, TJ Gardner, TA Manolio, SJ Hoff, MF Rykiel, TA Pearson, VL Gott, WA Baumgartner: The effects of age on outcome after coronary bypass surgery. Circulation 76:v-6, 1987.

130. Soloway HB, BM Cornett, JV Donahoo, SP Cox: Differentiation of bleeding diathesis which occurs following protamine correction of heparin anticoagulation. Am J Clin Pathol 60:188, 1973.

131. Lewis JH, HJ Wilson, JM Brandon: Counterelectrophoresis test for molecules immunologically similar to fibrinogen. Am J Clin Pathol 58:400, 1972.

132. Salzman EW: The events that lead to thrombosis. Bull N Y Acad Med 48:225, 1972.

133. Bick RL, WF Baker: Diagnostic efficacy of the D-Dimer assay in DIC and related disorders. Blood 68:329, 1986.

134. Rousou JA, RM Engelman, RH Breyer: Fibrin glue: an efective hemostatic agent for nonsuturable intraoperative bleeding. Ann Thorac Surg 38:409, 1984.

135. Rousou J: Randomized clinical trial of fibrin glue sealant in patients undergoing resternotomy or reoperation after cardiac operations: a multicenter study. J Thorac Surg 97:194, 1989.

136. Garcia-Rinaldi R, P Simmons, V Salcedo, C Howland: A technique for spot application of fibrin glue during open heart operations. Ann Thorac Surg 47:59, 1989.

137. Dresdale A, FO Bowman, JR Malm, K Reemtsma, CR Smith, HM Spotnitz, EA Rose: Hemostatic effectiveness of fibrin glue derived from single-donor fresh frozen plasma. Ann Thorac Surg 40:385, 1985.

138. Verstraete M: Clinical application of inhibitors of fibrinolysis. Drugs 29:236, 1985.

139. Forbes CD: Thrombosis and artificial surfaces. In: CRM Prentice (Ed): Thrombosis. Clin Haematol 10:653, 1981.

140. Bick RL: Basic mechanisms of hemostasis pertaining to DIC, ch 1. In: Disseminated Intravascular Coagulation. CRC Press, Boca Raton, FL, 1983, p 1.

141. Bick RL: Clinical relevance of antithrombin III. Semin Thromb Hemost 8:276, 1982.

142. Seegers WH: Basic principles of blood coagulation. Semin Thromb Hemost 7:180, 1981.

143. Esmon CT: Protein C: biochemistry, physiology, and clinical implications. Blood 62:1155, 1983.

144. Braunwald NS, L Bonchek: Prevention of thrombus formation on rigid prosthetic heart valves by the ingrowth of autogenous tissue. J Thorac Cardiovasc Surg 54:630, 1967.

145. Bagnall RD: Absorption of plasma proteins on hydrophobic surfaces. II. Fibrinogen and fibrinogen-containing protein mixtures. Biomed Biomater Res 12:203, 1978.

146. Hubbard D, GL Lucas: Ionic charges of glass surfaces and other materials and their possible role in the coagulation of blood. J Appl Physiol 15:265, 1960.

147. Mason RG: The interaction of blood hemostatic elements with artificial surfaces. In: TH Spaet (Ed): Progress in Hemostasis and Thrombosis. Grune & Stratton, New York, 1972, p 141.

148. Knieriem HJ, AB Chandler: The effect of warfarin sodium on the duration of platelet aggregation. Thromb Diath Haemorrh 18:766, 1967.

149. Lessin LS, WH Jensen, GA Kelser: Scanning electron microscopy of thrombogenesis on vascular catheter surfaces. N Engl J Med 286:139, 1972.

150. Moore CH, FJ Wolma, RW Brown, JR Derrick: Complications of cardiovascular radiology. A review of 1204 cases. Am J Surg 120:591, 1970.

151. Hershey CO, JW Tomford, CE McLaren, DK Porter, DI Cohen: The natural history of intravenous catheter-associated phlebitis. Arch Intern Med 144:1373, 1984.

152. Tomford JW, CO Hershey: The effect of an intravenous therapy team on peripheral venous catheter associated phlebitis. Clin Res 30:770A, 1982.

153. Bolooki H: Indications for use of IABP. In: Clinical Application of Intra-Aortic Balloon Pump. Futura Publications, Mt. Kisco, New York, 1984, p 293.

154. Okada M, T Shiozawa, M Iizuka, KO Kuno, CC Chen, S Matsuda, K Yoneda, A Yano, M Kawai, S Asada: Experimental and clinical studies on the effect of intra-aortic balloon pumping for cardiogenic shock following acute myocardial infarction. Artif Organs 3:271, 1979.

155. McEnany MT, HR Kay, MJ Buckley, WM Daggett, AJ Erdmann, ED Mundth, RS Rao, J DeTouef, WG Austen: Clinical experience with intra-aortic balloon pump support in 728 patients. Circulation 58:124, 1978.

156. Alpert J, EK Bhaktan, I Gielchinsky, L Gilbert, BJ Brener, DK Brief, V Parsonnet: Vascular complications of intra-aortic balloon pumping. Arch Surg 111:1190, 1976.

157. Balooki H: Complications of balloon pumping: diagnosis, prevention, and treatment. In: Clinical Application of Intra-Aortic Balloon Pump. Futura Publications, Mt. Kisco, New York, 1984, p 133.

158. Isner JM, SR Cohen, R Virmani, W Lawrinson, WC Roberts: Complications of the intra-aortic ballon counter-pulsation device: clinical and morphologic observations in 45 necropsy patients. Am J Cardiol 45:260, 1980.

159. Karlson K: Discussion. In: Vascular complications of intra-aortic balloon pumping. Arch Surg 111:1190, 1976.

160. Curtis JJ, DA Barnhorst, JR Pluth, GK Danielson, CE Harrison, RB Wallace: Intra-aortic balloon assist: initial Mayo Clinic experience and current concepts. Mayo Clin Proc 52:723, 1977.

161. Schneider MD, MP Kaye, SJ Blatt, HG Tobin, FAO Eckner: Safety of intra-aortic balloon pumping: II. Physical injury to aortic endothelium due to mechanical pump action. Thromb Res 4:399, 1974.

162. Baciewicz FA, BM Kaplan, TE Murphy, HL Neiman: Bilateral renal artery thrombotic occlusion: a unique complication following removal of a transthoracic intra-aortic balloon. Ann Thorac Surg 33:631, 1982.

163. Kuruvila KC, EG Beven: Arteriovenous shunts and fistulas for hemodialysis. Surg Clin North Am 51:1219, 1971.

164. Murano G, RL Bick: Thrombolytic therapy. In: G Murano, RL Bick (Eds): Basic Concepts of Hemostasis and Thrombosis. CRC Press, Boca Raton, FL, 1980, p 259.

165. Bick RL: Thrombolytic therapy, ch 14. In: Disorders of Hemostasis and Thrombosis: Principles of Clinical Practice. Thieme, Inc., New York, 1985, p 352.

166. Harker LA, SJ Slichter: Platelet and fibrinogen survival in man. N Engl J Med 287:999, 1972.

167. LeVeen HH, G Christoudias, M Ip, R Luft, G Falk, S Grosberg: Peritoneovenous shunting for ascites. Ann Surg 180:580, 1974.

168. Reinhardt GF, MM Stanley: Peritoneovenous shunting for ascites. Surg Gynecol Obstet 145:419, 1977.

169. Lerner RG, JC Nelson, P Corines, LRM del Guercio: Disseminated intravascular coagulation: complication of LeVeen peritoneovenous shunts. JAMA 240:2064, 1978.

170. Harmon DC, Z Demirjian, L Ellman, J Fischer: Disseminated intravascular coagulation with the peritoneovenous shunt. Ann Intern Med 90:774, 1979.

171. Strin SF, JT Fulenwider, JD Ansley, BL Evatt, B Nordlinger, P Melemore, L Schwotzer, CS Wideman: Accelerated fibrinogen and platelet destruction after peritoneovenous shunting. Arch Intern Med 141:1149, 1981.

172. Baker WF: Clinical aspects of disseminated intravascular coagulation. Semin Thromb Hemost 15:1, 1989.

173. Urbaniac SJ, CV Prowse: Hemostatic changes during plasma exchange. Plasma Ther Transf Technol 4:21, 1983.

174. Smith DA, WP Monaghan, WD Hann, H Schumacher: Evaluation of in vivo platelet adhesiveness during discontinuous-flow centrifugal thrombocytapheresis. Plasma Ther Transf Technol 4:37, 1983.

175. Simon TL: Coagulation disorders with plasma exchange. Plasma Ther Transf Technol 3:147, 1983.

176. Domen RE, MS Kennedy, LL Jones, DA Senhauser: Hemostatic imbalances produced by plasma exchange. Transfusion 24:336, 1984.

177. Orlin JB, EM Berkman: Partial plasma exchange using albumin replacement. Removal and recovery of normal plasma constituents. Blood 56:1055, 1981.

178. Spiva DA, CS Robinson, JW Langley: Acute changes in antithrombin III levels during apheresis procedures. Plasma Ther Transf Technol 3:137, 1982.

179. Wegmuller E, MD Kazatchkine, UE Nydegger: Complement activation during extracorporeal blood bypass. Plasma Ther Transf Technol 4:361, 1983.

180. Frankl WS: Indications for anticoagulants in cardiovascular disease. In: JH Jepson, WS Frankl (Eds): Hematological Complications in Cardiac Practice. WB Saunders, Philadelphia, 1975, p 182.

181. Kaltman AJ: Late complications of heart valve replacement. Ann Rev Med 2:343, 1971.

182. Fraser RS, J Waddell: Systemic embolization after aortic valve replacement. J Thorac Cardiovasc Surg 54:81, 1967.

183. Effler DB, R Favaloro, LK Groves: Heart valve replacement: clinical experience. Ann Thorac Surg 1:4, 1965.

184. Mason RG, HYK Chuang, SF Mohammad, HI Saba: Thrombosis and artificial surfaces. In: J van de Loo, CRM Prentice, FK Beller (Eds): The Thromboembolic Disorders. Schattauer Verlag, Stuttgart, 1983, p 533.

185. Akbarian M, WG Austen, PM Yurchak, JG Scannel: Thromboembolic complications of prosthetic cardiac valves. Circulation 37:826, 1968.

186. Duvoisin GE, RO Brandenburg, DC McGoon: Factors affecting thromboembolism associated with prosthetic heart valves. Circulation 35:70, 1967.

187. Berger S, EW Salzman: Thromboembolic complications of prosthetic devices. Prog Hemost Thromb 2:273, 1974.

188. Weiss HJ: Antiplatelet drugs in clinical medicine. In: Platelets: Pathophysiology and Antiplatelet Drug Therapy. Alan R. Liss, Inc., New York, 1982, p 75.

189. Harker LA, SJ Slichter: Studies of platelet and fibrinogen kinetics in patients with prosthetic heart valves. N Engl J Med 283:1302, 1970.

190. Harker LA, J Hirsh, M Gent, E Genton: Critical evaluation of platelet-inhibiting drugs in thrombotic disease. Prog Hematol 9:229, 1975.

191. Weily HS, PP Steele, H Davies, G Pappas, E Genton: Platelet survival in patients with substitute heart valves. N Engl J Med 290:534, 1974.

192. Steele PP, HS Weily, H Davies, E Genton: Platelet survival in patients with rheumatic heart disease. N Engl J Med 290:537, 1974.

193. Weily HW, E Genton: Altered platelet function in patients with prosthetic mitral valves. Effects of sulfinpyrazone therapy. Circulation 42:967, 1970.

194. Sullivan JM, DE Harken, R Gorlin: Pharmacologic control of thromboembolic complications of cardiac-valve replacement. N Engl J Med 284:1391, 1971.

195. Dale J, E Myhre, A Storstein, H Stormorken, L Efskind: Prevention of arterial thromboembolism with acetylsalicylic acid. Am Heart J 94:101, 1977.

196. Dale J, E Myhre, D Lowe: Bleeding during acetylsalicylic acid and anticoagulant therapy in patients with reduced platelet reactivity after aortic valve replacement. Am Heart J 99:746, 1980.

197. Altman R, F Boullon, J Rouvier, P Raca, L de la Fuente, R Favaloro: Aspirin and prophylaxis of thromboembolic complications in patients with substitute heart valves. J Thorac Cardiovasc Surg 72:127, 1976.

198. Arrants JE, E Hairston: Use of persantine in preventing thromboembolism following valve replacement. Ann Surg 38:432, 1972.

199. Taguchi K, H Matsumura, T Washizu, M Kirao, K Kato, E Kato, T Mochizuki: Effect of athrombogenic therapy, especially high-dose therapy of dipyridamole, after prosthetic valve replacement. J Cardiovasc Surg 16:8, 1975.

200. Bjork VO, A Henz: Management of thromboembolism after aortic valve replacement with the Bjork-Shiley tilting disc valve. Scand J Thorac Cardiovasc Surg 9:183, 1975.

201. Gadboys HL, RS Litwak, J Niemetz, N Wisch: Role of anticoagulants in preventing embolization from prosthetic heart valves. JAMA 202:282, 1967.

202. Friedli B, N Aerichide, P Grondin, L Campeau: Thromboembolic complications of heart valve prostheses. Am Heart J 81:702, 1971.

203. Dalen JE, Hirsh J: American College of Chest Physician and the National Heart Lung Blood Institute National Conference on Antithrombotic Therapy. Chest 95:107, 1989.

204. Levinson MM, RG Smith, RC Cork, et al: Thromboembolic complications of the Jarvik-7 total artificial heart: case report. Artif Organs 10:236, 1986.

205. Kolff WJ: Experiences and practical considerations for the future of artificial hearts and of mankind. Artif Organs 12:89, 1988.

206. Hartmannova B, J Vasku, S Dolezi, et al: Mechanisms causing the death of 8 calves surviving with implanted artificial heart from 31 to 173 days. Exp Pathol 26:221, 1984.

207. Vasku J: Calcification of the driving diaphragm in a total artificial heart. Czech Med 10:16, 1987.

208. Tolpekin VE, GD Ioseliani, VA Dobyshev, et al: Development of methods of assisted circulation with artificial heart ventricles. Artif Organs 7:112, 1983.

209. Shumakov VI, NK Zimin, AA Drobyshev, et al: Use of an ellipsoid artificial heart. Artif Organs 11:16, 1987.

210. Hughes SD, DL Coleman, PA Dew, et al: Proc Trans Am Soc Artif Intern Organs 30:75, 1984.

211. Iwaya F, S Hoshino, T Igari, et al: Experimental studies in total artificial heart replacement. Jap Circ J 48:312, 1984.

212. Dostal M, J Vasku, J Cerny, et al: Hematological and biochemical studies in calves living over 1090 days with the polymethylmethacrylate total artificial heart TNS Brno II. Int J Artif Organs 9:39, 1986.

213. Griffith BP, RL Hardesty, RL Kormos, et al: Temporary use of the Jarvik-7 total artificial heart before transplantation. N Engl J Med 316:130, 1987.

214. Trubel W, U Losert, H Schima, et al: Total artificial heart bridging: a temporary support for deteriorating heart transplantation candidates: methods and results. Thorac Cardiovasc Surg 35:277, 1987.

215. Green K, J Liska, N Egberg, et al: Hemostatic disturbances associated with implantation of an artificial heart. Thromb Res 48:349, 1987.

216. Coleman DL, HLC Meuzelaar, TR Kessler, et al: Retrieval and analysis of a clinical total artificial heart. J Biomed Mater Res 20:417, 1986.

Acquired Circulating Anticoagulants

cquired circulating anticoagulants (inhibitors) direct-ed against single factors or several factors are ex-tremely rare causes of clinical hemorrhage. Acquired circulating anticoagulants are often associated with well-defined disease entities, drugs, or other clinical situa-tions and may happen in otherwise normal individuals. Any coagulation factor may be affected. This chapter is con-cerned with acquired circulating anticoagulants in otherwise hemostatically healthy individuals. For further discussion of anticoagulants in congenital coagulation factor defects, see chapter 6.

Clearly the most common circulating anticoagulants of clinical significance are fibrin(ogen) degradation products. The mechanisms of action of FDPs in interfering with hemostasis include impairment of fibrin monomer polymer-ization and interference with platelet function (see chapters 7 and 8).[1,2] The next most common circulating anticoagulant of clinical relevance is malignant paraprotein, and the mecha-nism(s) of action for paraprotein hinderance of hemostasis and thrombosis will be discussed in chapter 12.[3,4,5] When suspecting circulating anticoagulants, Munchausen's syn-drome, the deliberate self-administration of warfarin-type drugs,[6,7] and the potentially unrecorded yet very real covert use of heparin in hospitalized patients (eg, to keep intra-venous lines open) must be considered. Several early excel-lent reviews have recognized the importance of circulating anticoagulants and have paved the way for a more thorough understanding of them and the clinical situations in which they arise. The first early large review of circulating antico-agulants was presented by Margolius, Jackson, and Ratnoff[8] followed by excellent reviews by Duetsch and Lechner,[9] Feinstein and Rapaport,[10] and Shapiro and Siegel.[11]

Acquired inhibitors in noncongenitally deficient patients may generally be divided into two types. The first type includes inhibitors that inactivate individual coagulation fac-tors, commonly in a progressive, usually irreversible, time-dependent manner.[3,8,10-12] Most are immunoglobulins (specif-ic antifactor antibodies). Subtyping of these inhibitors show most to be IgG, and the most common subtype is IgG4.

Kappa light chains are more common than lambda light chains in circulating IgG anticoagulants.[3,11,12] The second type of circulating inhibitor is characterized by being reversible (or partly reversible), immediate in action, and usually representing a protein-protein interaction (complex formation) with either a specific coagulation factor or group of factors.[3,4,11] These types of anticoagulants often do not destroy the coagulation factor attacked, and the biologic activity of the coagulation factor may be recovered if the complex can be dissociated. These types of anticoagulants are most commonly seen in malignant or benign paraprotein disorders with the interaction being between paraprotein and a specific clotting factor or group of clotting factors. Circu-lating anticoagulants should be strongly suspected when an otherwise healthy individual begins to develop unexplained bleeding, when the prothrombin time, activated partial thromboplastin time, or thrombin time are unexplainably prolonged, or when coagulation testing gives contradictory or confusing results.[3,11,12]

Acquired Inhibitors to Specific Coagulation Factors

Fibrinogen Inhibitors

Very few instances of acquired inhibitors to fibrinogen have been reported, and of these, two have occurred in trans-fused afibrinogenemic patients.[13,14] In noncongenitally defi-cient patients, the anticoagulant has been associated with autoimmune disorders (two cases of systemic lupus erythe-matosus), chronic inflammatory disorders (chronic active hepatitis),[15,16] and Down's syndrome.[17] One instance was noted in a multiple transfused patient who, retrospectively, probably had disseminated intravascular coagulation.[18] In these cases, the antibody was identified as an IgG. The anti-body has been found to interfere with the release of fi-brinopeptide A or with fibrin monomer polymerization.[19] In some patients a mild hemorrhagic tendency has been present, but in others no clinically significant hemostasis defects were encountered.

Prothrombin Inhibitors

Antiprothrombin (factor II) antibodies in cases of non-congenital factor II deficiency are extremely rare and have usually been seen in patients with systemic lupus erythematosus.[20-22] A clear-cut distinction between a specific anti–factor II antibody and a lupus anticoagulant has been unclear.[20-22] Some patients have had no bleeding with antiprothrombin anticoagulants.[21,23]

Factor V Inhibitors

Acquired antibody to factor V has occurred in many patients, and the common denominator in many is a surgical procedure. In about 70% of patients developing an anti–factor V antibody, the development of the antibody was preceded by a surgical procedure. To further complicate etiologic factors, 50% of the surgical patients described had ingested streptomycin or other antibiotics during their operative course.[10,24-43] An anti–factor V antibody has also been associated with the use of streptomycin in several nonsurgical patients, in association with coeliac disease and Crohn's disease,[44] and have occurred spontaneously, without apparent associated diseases.[45] Most patients have had a mild bleeding problem, but bleeding has been severe or fatal in a few isolated cases.[34-37] Both IgG and IgM immunoglobulins have been incriminated. Therapy, when necessary, is generally limited to fresh frozen plasma. One patient, however, was treated successfully with platelet concentrates.[34]

Factor VII Inhibitors

Anti–factor VII antibodies have only been reported once, in association with a case of probable carcinoma of the lung.[46] The antibody was determined to be an IgG. Surgery was not done because of a bleeding risk. The diagnosis was not confirmed, and the cell type was unknown.

Factor VIII:C Inhibitors

Anti–factor VIII antibodies happen in 8% to 10% of patients with hemophilia A. Anti–factor VIII antibodies commonly occur as circulating anticoagulants in otherwise healthy individuals and in selected clinical situations and should be suspected in healthy individuals who suddenly develop an unexplained hemorrhagic diathesis.[3,8-12,47,48] An anti–factor VIII antibody is the likeliest circulating anticoagulant to be present in the patient without lupus who develops a circulating anticoagulant in the absence of malignant paraprotein or elevated FDP levels.[3,12,47,48]

Green and Lechner[49] surveyed 215 nonhemophilic patients with inhibitors to factor VIII, which provided significant understanding of the clinical manifestations of anti–factor VIII antibodies in these patients. More than 46% of patients had no discernible underlying disease condition; 8% developed an anti–factor VIII antibody in association with rheumatoid arthritis; more than 7% developed an anti–factor VIII antibody during a normal postpartum course; almost 7% had an associated disseminated malignancy; slightly more than 5% had associated drug ingestion; approximately 5% had associated systemic lupus; more than 4% had associated less common autoimmune disorders; 4.5% had associated dermatologic disorders; and about 10% had other rare clinical disorders associated. The peak incidence occurred between 50 and 80 years of age, and this group comprised greater than 65% of all patients developing an anti–factor VIII antibody. The clinical result in postpartum patients was good; 85% of patients survived the development of an anti–factor VIII antibody, which eventually disappeared. Of the survivors, 36% were not treated, and the remainder received some type of immunosuppressive therapy. This survey also showed that patients developing a circulating anticoagulant in association with an autoimmune disorder did poorly, and persistence of the antibody and/or death occurred in 36% of patients. The remainder survived with the use of immunosuppressive therapy. When evaluating the total number of cases in this large survey, 56% of patients survived the development of an anti–factor VIII antibody, and 44% died from a hemorrhagic complication of the circulating anti–factor VIII antibody. Of those surviving, the majority received some type of immunosuppressive therapy, while of those not surviving, the majority (62%) received no immunosuppressive therapy. This finding confirms suggestions that the use of immunosuppressive therapy in nonhemophilic patients who develop an anti–factor VIII antibody is clearly warranted.[50] Factor VIII:C antibodies are seen in almost all autoimmune disorders, including rheumatoid arthritis and polymyositis.[51,52] Anti–factor VIII:C antibody has been found in T-immunoblastic lymphoma,[53] breast cancer, other malignancies, and other varied medical disorders.[54-60] Interestingly, nonhemophilic patients who develop an acquired anti–factor VIII antibody only uncommonly have the types of bleeding usually associated with hemophilia A, including intra-articular bleeding, deep intramuscular bleeding, or intracranial bleeding, but more commonly have large subcutaneous ecchymoses.

Acquired von Willebrand's Disease

Acquired von Willebrand's disease, or the development of an acquired anticoagulant to the von Willebrand part of the factor VIII macromolecular complex, has been described in many individuals.[8-10,12,47-85] Most patients had an autoimmune disorder, lymphoma, or a malignant paraprotein disorder. The interaction between malignant or benign paraprotein and coagulation factors will be discussed in chapter 12. Anti–von Willebrand antibody has also been noted in hypothyroidism and in almost all the myeloproliferative syndromes.[86-93] One individual developed an anti–von Willebrand factor antibody after pesticide exposure,[94] and one patient developed this antibody in association with Wilm's tumor,[72] which improved with surgical resection. Usually, the bleeding has not been severe and has been compatible with a mild acquired von Willebrand's syndrome. Therapy has included immunosuppression, cryoprecipitate, DDAVP, and other proper measures to control the underlying disease process whether it be a myeloproliferative disease, myeloma, other paraprotein disorders, or autoimmunity.

Factor IX Inhibitors

Anti–factor IX antibodies most commonly occur in patients with hemophilia B[95] and only rarely happen in postpartum females, patients with systemic lupus, and rarely in patients with rheumatic fever.[8-10,12,47,96-99] Like anti–factor VIII antibody in the nonhemophilic patient, the anti–factor IX antibody often abates with the use of immunosuppressive therapy, such as prednisone, azathioprine, or cyclophosphamide.

Factor X Inhibitors

Only two cases of an anti–factor X antibody have been reported, both in patients with leprosy.[100] One patient was ingesting dapsone; however, the patient was untreated when developing the antibody, and leprosy, instead of drug ingestion, appeared to be the common denominator. Neither patient had a clinically significant bleeding diathesis. Of more clinical interest is the association of a selective factor X deficiency and systemic amyloidosis. Although an anti–factor X antibody has not clearly been found in the circulation, amyloid fibrils may selectively bind with factor X and remove it from the circulation.[101-104] Although a circulating anticoagulant cannot be shown, amyloid may represent an extracirculatory factor X inhibitor via the interaction of factor X and amyloid fibrils. In vivo recovery studies support this mechanism.[103,104]

Factor XI Inhibitors

Anti–factor XI antibodies in noncongenitally deficient patients have occurred in less than 20 patients. Most patients had an autoimmune disorder,[8,11,12,47,105-113] and one individual had pneumonia resulting from an adenovirus.[114]

Factor XII Inhibitors

Acquired factor XII antibody has been noted in systemic lupus, Waldenström's macroglobulinemia, and glomerulonephritis.[95,115,116] Severe deficiency of factor XII has been associated with angioimmunoblastic lymphadenopathy, but a circulating anticoagulant could not conclusively be proved.[117]

Factor XIII Inhibitors

Acquired factor XIII antibody has happened in at least eight otherwise hemostatically normal individuals.[8-10,12,47,118-128] Many patients received isoniazid therapy, and one patient developed an anti–factor XIII antibody in association with a drug-induced systemic lupus syndrome.[129] The inhibitor is believed either to react with the thrombin activation site on the alpha chain of factor XIII or, alternatively, to prevent fibrin cross-linking by reacting with sites on fibrinogen.[10,12,47] Some individuals developing an anti–factor XIII antibody have had profuse bleeding.

Thrombin Inhibitors

An inhibitor to thrombin has been reported in patients taking suramin for metastatic adrenal cell carcinoma. The inhibitor was thought to be directed against enzymes responsible for degrading endogenous heparan sulfate and dermatan sulfate, leading to exacerbated antithrombin activity of these two vascular glycosaminoglycans.[130] Another inhibitor to thrombin activity has been noted in association with posthepatic cirrhosis.[131]

Lupus Anticoagulants

The lupus anticoagulant has long been described and many excellent reviews have begun to shed light on this elusive anticoagulant.[8-12,20,132-137] Lupus anticoagulants are immunoglobulins interfering with phospholipid-dependent coagulation tests.[11,12,20,136] Unlike the other inhibitors, lupus anticoagulants do not inhibit the activity of specific coagulation factors. Lupus anticoagulants may occur in about 10% of patients with systemic lupus erythematosus.[137,138] Lupus anticoagulants are commonly associated with HIV infection, being reported in up to 50% of patients,[139-144] scleroderma,[145,146] and gastric Castleman's disease.[147] Lupus anticoagulant in children can follow a viral-type syndrome but is usually unassociated with thrombosis.[148] The frequency of bleeding resulting from the lupus anticoagulant is clearly less than 1% of patients developing this anticoagulant.[12,20,135-137] Almost 25% of patients with systemic lupus and the lupus anticoagulant will have a concomitant prothrombin deficiency, and over 40% of patients with systemic lupus and the lupus anticoagulant have thrombocytopenia.[11,12,20] Patients who bleed with the lupus anticoagulant almost always have associated hypoprothrombinemia or thrombocytopenia. No increase in surgical hemorrhage occurs in patients with the lupus anticoagulant alone.[20] Isolated prothrombin deficiency may happen in patients with systemic lupus who do not have the lupus anticoagulant, but the mechanisms are unknown.[10,12,20,48] Infusions of plasma have failed to correct isolated factor II deficiency adequately in patients with lupus, which suggests the presence of an anti–factor II antibody.[149,150] Biologic false-positive test results for syphilis are seen in about 40% of patients with systemic lupus,[20,151] but these results are seen in greater than 50% and up to 90% of patients with systemic lupus plus the lupus anticoagulant.[11,20,48,134] Almost 40% of patients with biologic false-positive test results for syphilis will have a lupus anticoagulant, which should be searched for in this clinical situation. Thromboembolism happens in about 10% of patients with systemic lupus. However, if a patient with systemic lupus also has the lupus anticoagulant, thromboembolism is a complication in 25% to 50% of cases.[11,12,20,152-155] Lupus anticoagulants may happen in normal individuals and in other disease states besides lupus and may occur in association with drug

Figure 10-1. Laboratory Evaluation of Circulating Anticoagulant

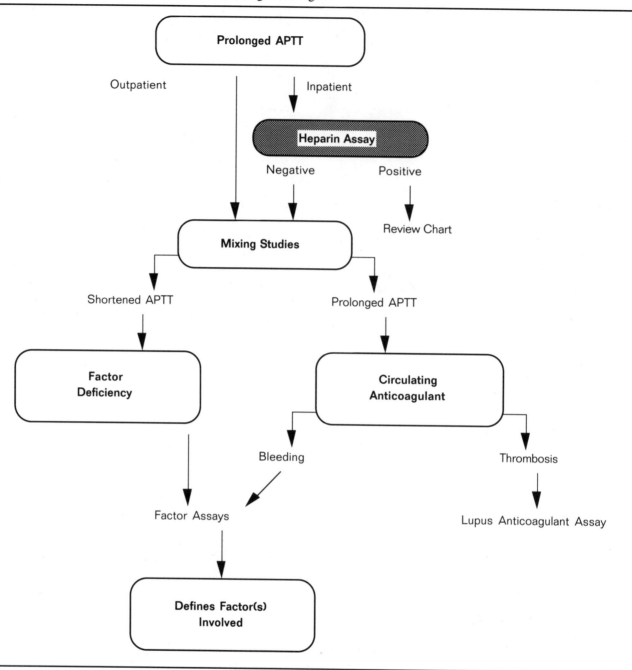

ingestion, with the most commonly cited drugs being chlor-promazine, pronestyl, Fansidar, and phenothiazine.[156-162]

Lupus inhibitors can be associated with the development of renal microvascular disease (microvascular thrombosis) and thrombosis of the dermal vessels.[163,164] However, they are most commonly associated with deep vein thrombosis, pulmonary emboli, and thrombosis of other vessels.[12] Lupus anticoagulants and detection methods will be discussed in chapter 13.

Diagnosis

The screening tests of coagulation protein function, the prothrombin time, activated partial thromboplastin time, and the thrombin time, are also the principle screening tests for circulating anticoagulants.[12] Of these, most circulating anti-coagulants will be detected by prolongation of the APTT. Only anti–factor VII antibodies are associated with a long prothrombin time and a normal APTT, and these are extremely rare. The APTT will be prolonged in most cases of acquired circulating anticoagulants, and the thrombin time will detect most paraproteins acting as circulating anticoagulants by interference with fibrin monomer polymerization.[3,12,165] In this instance, the APTT may not be prolonged, so the thrombin time should be considered in patients with paraprotein disease suspected of harboring a circulating anticoagulant. If the APTT is prolonged in an outpatient, mixing studies to assess the possibility of an acquired circulating anticoagulant are then done. For inpatients with an unexplained prolonged APTT, however, a heparin assay or attentive chart review for occult delivery of heparin should be done before embarking on laborious mixing studies. After heparin has been ruled out, mixing studies to determine if a deficiency or a circulating anticoagulant exists are then done. The most reliable method is that of Lossing and coworkers.[166] Using this technique, the APTT is repeated on a 50:50 mix of patient plasma and normal control plasma. If correction is noted, a deficiency is assumed; if no correction is noted, a circulating anticoagulant is assumed, as it will also inactivate the factor(s) in the added normal control plasma. Once this has been shown, specific factor assays are then done in logical sequential order to find out which factor is inhibited by the circulating anticoagulant. To demonstrate factor VIII:C inhibitors, the APTT and normal plasma mixture often must be incubated for 30, 60, 90, or 120 minutes to demonstrate the anti–factor VIII:C antibody. Prolonged incubation is not needed to demonstrate antibodies to other factors. If a lupus anticoagulant is suspected, one of the lupus anticoagulant assays, as outlined in chapter 13, is done. A flow diagram for evaluating plasma suspected of harboring a circulating anticoagulant is provided in Figure 10-1.

Management

The mainstay of therapy for circulating anticoagulants in patients with acquired circulating anticoagulants is treatment of the underlying disease process or withdrawal from suspected drugs. Treatment of the underlying disease process thought associated with the acquired circulating anticoagulant is particularly important in autoimmune diseases, malignancy, neoplastic paraprotein disorders, or the myeloproliferative syndromes. In instances where severe bleeding is present or impending, specific treatment modalities have included immunosuppression with corticosteroids, intravenous immunoglobulin, azathioprine, cyclophosphamide, and other agents.[167-174] Other more specific modalities used, with varying degrees of success, have included plasma exchange and plasmapheresis, immunoadsorption with staphylococcal A columns, and the additional use of DDAVP with vWF or factor VIII:C inhibition.[49,175-184] Treatment modalities for acquired circulating anticoagulants are summarized in Table 10-1.

Table 10-1. Treatment Methods for Acquired Circulating Anticoagulants

Intravenous immunoglobulin
Azathioprine
Cyclophosphamide
Plasmapheresis
Plasma exchange
Protein A immunoadsorption columns
DDAVP (VIII:C, vWF)
Factor concentrates (uncommonly warranted)

Summary

This chapter has summarized the clinical aspects of those rare clinical instances of acquired circulating anticoagulants in noncongenitally deficient patients. Although these circulating anticoagulants are extremely interesting and may sometimes give rise to significant or fatal hemorrhage, these anticoagulants are exceedingly rare. Circulating FDPs and malignant paraprotein acting as "circulating anticoagulant" are more common causes of significant hemorrhage than are the specific antifactor antibodies discussed in this chapter. When suspecting circulating anticoagulants in the absence of circulating FDPs or paraprotein, the likeliest to be found in clinical practice are an anti–factor VIII:C antibody or the lupus anticoagulant.

References

1. Bick RL: The clinical significance of fibrinogen degradation products. Semin Thromb Hemost 8:302, 1982.

2. Bick RL: Disseminated intravascular coagulation, ch 2. In: Disseminated Intravascular Coagulation and Related Syndromes. CRC Press, Boca Raton, FL, 1983, p 31.

3. Bick RL: Acquired circulating anticoagulants and defective hemostasis in malignant paraprotein disorders, ch 10. In: G Murano, RL Bick (Eds): Basic Concepts of Hemostasis and Thrombosis. CRC Press, Boca Raton, FL, 1980, p 205.

4. Lackner H: Hemostatic abnormalities associated with dysproteinemias. Semin Hematol 10:125, 1973.

5. Patterson WP, CW Caldwell, DC Doll: Hyperviscosity syndromes and coagulopathies. Semin Oncol 17:210, 1990.

6. Agle DP, OD Ratnoff, GK Spring: The anticoagulant malingerer. Psychiatric studies in three patients. Ann Intern Med 73:67, 1970.

7. O'Reilly RA, PM Aggeler: Covert anticoagulant ingestion: study of 25 patients and review of world literature. Medicine 55:389, 1976.

8. Margolius A, DP Jackson, OD Ratnoff: Circulating anticoagulants: a study of 40 cases and a review of the literature. Medicine 40:145, 1961.

9. Deutsch E, K Lechner: Circulating anticoagulants. In: NU Bang, FK Beller, E Deutsch, EF Mammen (Eds): Thrombosis

and Bleeding Disorders. Georg Thieme Verlag, Stuttgart, 1971, p 286.

10. Feinstein DI, SI Rapaport: Acquired inhibitors of blood coagulation. Prog Hemost Thromb 1:39, 1972.

11. Shapiro SS, JE Siegel: Hemorrhagic disorders associated with circulating inhibitors, ch 7. In: OD Ratnoff, CD Forbes (Eds): Disorders of Hemostasis. WB Saunders, Philadelphia, 1991, p 245.

12. Bick RL: Circulating anticoagulants, ch 9. In: Disorders of Hemostasis and Thrombosis. Thieme, Inc., New York, 1985, p 254.

13. DeVries A, T Rosenberg, S Kochwa, JH Boss: Precipitating antifibrinogen antibody appearing after fibrinogen infusions in a patient with congenital afibrinogenemia. Am J Med 30:486, 1961.

14. Menache D: Abnormal fibrinogens. Thromb Diath Haemorrh 29:525, 1973.

15. Galankis DK, EM Ginzler, SM Fikrig: Monoclonal IgG anticoagulants delaying fibrin aggregation in two patients with systemic lupus erythematosus (SLE). Blood 52:1037, 1978.

16. Hoots WK, NA Carrell, RH Wagner: A naturally occurring antibody that inhibits fibrin polymerization. N Engl J Med 304:857, 1981.

17. Marceniak E, MF Greenwood: Acquired coagulation inhibitor delaying fibrinopeptide release. Blood 53:81, 1979.

18. Mammen EF, KP Schmidt, MI Barnhart: Thrombophlebitis migrans associated with circulating antibodies against fibrinogen. Thromb Diath Haemorrh 18:605, 1967.

19. Ghosh S, P McEvoy, BA McVerry: Idiopathic autoantibody that inhibits fibrin monomer polymerization. Br J Haematol 53:65, 1983.

20. Shapiro SS, P Thagarajan: Lupus anticoagulants. Prog Hemost Thromb 6:263, 1982.

21. Scully MF, V Ellis, VV Kakkar: An acquired coagulation inhibitor to Factor II. Br J Haematol 50:655, 1986.

22. Struzik T, Z Haricki, R Hawiger: Cryo-coagulopathy with presence of immuno antithrombin in the course of lupus erythematosus disseminatus. Acta Med Pol 5:61, 1964.

23. Bajaj SP, SI Rapaport, S Barclay: Acquired hypoprothrombinemia due to nonneutralizing antibodies to prothrombin: mechanism and management. Blood 65:1538, 1985.

24. Lopez VA, R Pfugshaupt, R Butler: A specific inhibitor of human clotting factor V. Acta Haematol 40:275, 1968.

25. Feinstein DI, SI Rapaport, WG McGehee: Factor V anticoagulants: clinical, biochemical, and immunologic observations. J Clin Invest 49:1578, 1970.

26. Ferguson JH, CL Johnston, DA Howell: A circulating inhibitor (anti-AcG) specific for the labile factor V of the blood-clotting mechanism. Blood 13:382, 1958.

27. Handley DA, BM Duncan: A circulating anticoagulant specific for Factor V. Pathology 1:265, 1969.

28. Crowell EB: A spontaneous Factor V inhibitor in an elderly man. Clin Res 19:664, 1971.

29. Blecker SM, AC Williams: Postextraction bleeding in a patient with an acquired circulating anticoagulant against Factor V. Oral Surg 32:533, 1971.

30. Feinstein DI, SI Rapaport, MMY Chong: Factor V inhibitor: report of a case, with comments on a possible effect of streptomycin. Ann Intern Med 78:385, 1973.

31. Nilsson IM, U Hedner, M Ekberg: A circulating anticoagulant against Factor V. Acta Med Scand 195:73, 1974.

32. Feinstein DI: Acquired inhibitors of Factor V. Thromb Haemost 39:663, 1978.

33. Lust A, A Bellon: A circulating anticoagulant against Factor V. Acta Clin Belg 33:62, 1978.

34. Chediak J, JB Ashenhurst, I Garlick: Successful management of bleeding in a patient with Factor V inhibitor by platelet transfusions. Blood 56:835, 1980.

35. Stirling ML, AC Parker, AJ Keller: Factor V inhibitor and bullous pemphigoid. Br Med J 2:677, 1977.

36. Coots MC, AF Muhleman, HI Glueck: Hemorrhagic death associated with a high titer Factor V inhibitor. Am J Hematol 4:193, 1978.

37. Wajima T, DA Schenk, TR Maloney: Severe bleeding associated with circulating anticoagulant to Factor V. Blood 54:308, 1979.

38. Massignon D, S Roullit, D Espinosa: Apparition d'un anticoagulant circulant antifacteur V apres intervention chirurgicale. Ann Fr Anesth Reanim 8:70, 1989.

39. Mazzuccon MG, S Solinas, A Christolini: Inhibitor of factor V in severe factor V congenital deficiency. Nouv Rev Fr Hematol 27:303, 1985.

40. Chong LL, YC Yong: A case of factor V inhibitor. Am J Hematol 19:395, 1985.

41. Chiu HC, AK Rao, C Beckett: Immune complexes containing factor V in a patient with an acquired neutralizing antibody. Blood 65:810, 1985.

42. Vickars LM, RW Coupland, SC Nainman: The response of an acquired factor V inhibitor to activated factor IX concentrate. Transfusion 25:51, 1985.

43. Lazerchick J, CM Wolff, SH Pepkowitz: Factor V inhibitor associated with immune complex formation. Arch Pathol Lab Med 110:448, 1986.

44. Taillan B, JG Fuzibet, H Vinti, A Pesce: Anticoagulant circulant specifique du facteur V et enteropathy deux observations. Presse Med 19:211, 1990.

45. Brandt JT, A Britton, E Kraut: A spontaneous Factor V inhibitor with unexpected laboratory features. Arch Pathol Lab Med 110:224, 1986.

46. Campbell E, S Sanal, J Mattson, L Walker, S Estry, L Mueller, M Schwarz, S Hampton: Factor VII inhibitor. Am J Med 68:962, 1980.

47. Shapiro SS, M Hultin: Acquired inhibitors to the blood coagulation factors. Semin Thromb Hemost 1:336, 1975.

48. Lechner K: Acquired inhibitors in nonhemophilic patients. Haemostasis 3:65, 1974.

49. Green D, K Lechner: A survey of 215 non-hemophilic patients with inhibitors to Factor VIII. Thromb Haemost 45:200, 1981.

50. Penner JA, PA Kelly: Management of patients with Factor VIII or IX inhibitors. Semin Thromb Hemost 1:386, 1975.

51. Soriano RM, JM Matthews, E Guerado-Parra: Acquired hemophilia and rheumatoid arthritis. Br J Rheumatol 26:381, 1987.

52. Corbett AJ, WR Bell, MC Hochberg: A circulating anticoagulant to Factor VIII in a patient with polymyositis: successful treatment with azathioprine. J Rheumatol 12:1026, 1985.

53. Casas E, J Garcia-Puig, A Villar: Sindrome hemorrhagico asociado a un inhibidor del factor VIII:C en un paciente con linfoma. Med Clin 93:23, 1989.

54. Bick RL: Anti-VIII:C antibody in a case of breast cancer. Personal observation.

55. Waddell CC, DE Lehane, MA Zubler: Acquired factor VIII inhibitor in a patient with mycosis fungoides. Cancer 47:2901, 1981.

56. Lottenberg R, TB Kentro, CS Kitchens: Acquired hemophilia: a natural history study of 16 patients with factor VIII inhibitors receiving little or no therapy. Arch Intern Med 147:1077, 1987.

57. Legrand JC, P van der Auwera, A Bailly: Circulating inhibitor of factor VIII during treatment with teicoplanin and rifampicin. J Antimicrob Chemother 19:850, 1987.

58. Ganly PS, JD Isaacs, MA Laffan: Acquired factor VIII inhibitor associated with lung abcess. Br Med J 295:811, 1987.

59. Singal U, EF Mammen: Concomitant occurrence of disseminated intravascular coagulation and factor VIII inhibitor in a patient with prostatic cancer. Am J Hematol 25:237, 1987.

60. Hoyle C, CA Lundlam: Acquired factor VIII inhibitor associated with multiple sclerosis, successfully treated with porcine factor VIII. Thromb Haemost 57:233, 1987.

61. Simone JV, JA Cornet, CF Abildgaard: Acquired von Willebrand's syndrome in systemic lupus erythematosus. Blood 31:806, 1968.

62. Ingram GI, PG Kingston, J Leslie: Four cases of acquired von Willebrand's syndrome. Br J Haematol 21:189, 1979.

63. Pool-Wilson PA: Acquired von Willebrand's syndrome and systemic lupus erythematosus. Proc R Soc Med 65:561, 1972.

64. Ingram GI, CR Prentice, CD Forbes: Low Factor VIII–like antigen in acquired von Willebrand's syndrome and response to treatment. Br J Haematol 25:137, 1973.

65. Mant MJ, J Hirst, J Gauldie: von Willebrand's syndrome presenting as an acquired bleeding disorder in association with a monoclonal gammopathy. Blood 42:429, 1973.

66. Handin RI, V Martin, WL Moloney: Antibody-induced von Willebrand's disease: a newly defined inhibitor syndrome. Blood 48:393, 1976.

67. Stabelforth P, GC Tamagnini, KM Dormandy: Acquired von Willebrand syndrome with inhibitors both to Factor VIII clotting activity and ristocetin-induced platelet aggregation. Br J Haematol 33:565, 1976.

68. Joist HH, JF Cowan, TS Zimmerman: Acquired von Willebrand's disease: evidence for a quantitative and qualitative Factor VIII disorder. N Engl J Med 298:988, 1978.

69. Zettervall O, IM Nilsson: Acquired von Willebrand's disease caused by a monoclonal antibody. Acta Med Scand 204:521, 1978.

70. Govault-Heilmann M, MD Dumond, L Intrator: Acquired von Willebrand syndrome with IgM inhibitor against von Willebrand's factor. J Clin Path 32:1030, 1979.

71. McGrath KM, CA Johnson, JJ Stuart: Acquired von Willebrand disease associated with an inhibitor to factor VIII antigen and gastrointestinal telangiectasia. Am J Med 67:693, 1979.

72. Noronha PA, HA Hruby, HS Maurer: Acquired von Willebrand disease in a patient with Wilms tumor. J Pediatr 95:997, 1979.

73. Gan TE, RJ Sawers, J Koutts: Pathogenesis of antibody-induced acquired von Willebrand syndrome. Am J Hematol 9:363, 1980.

74. Wautier JL, S Levy-Toledano, JP Caen: Acquired von Willebrand's syndrome and thrombopathy in a patient with chronic lymphocytic leukemia. Scand J Haematol 16:128, 1976.

75. Brody J, M Haider, RE Rossman: A haemorrhagic syndrome in Waldenström's macroglobulinemia, secondary to immune absorption to Factor VIII. N Engl J Med 300:408, 1979.

76. Leone G, P Pola, G Guerrera: Sindrome di von Willebrand acquisitita in corso di malattia disreattiva. Haematologica 59:212, 1974.

77. Matsuda S, I Acki, M Kikuchi: A case of acquired von Willebrand's syndrome associated with IgG myeloma. Rinsho Ketsueki 18:1007, 1977.

78. Fricke WA, KM Brinkhous, JB Garris: Comparison of inhibitory and binding characteristics of an antibody causing acquired von Willebrand's syndrome: an assay for von Willebrand factor binding by antibody. Blood 66:562, 1985.

79. Brinkhous KM, WA Fricke, MS Read: Determinants of von Willebrand factor activity elicited by ristocetin and botrocetin: studies on a human von Willebrand factor–binding antibody. Semin Thromb Hemost 11:337, 1985.

80. Richard C, MC Sedano, MA Cuadrado: Acquired von Willebrand's syndrome associated with hydatid disease of the spleen: disappearance after splenectomy. Thromb Haemost 52:90, 1984.

81. Mohri H, T Noguchi, F Kodama: Acquired von Willebrand disease due to inhibitor of human myeloma protein specific for von Willebrand factor. Am J Clin Pathol 87:663, 1987.

82. Bovill EG, WB Ershler, EA Golden: A human myeloma-produced monoclonal protein directed against the active subpopulation of von Willebrand factor. Am J Clin Pathol 85:115, 1986.

83. Takahashi H, R Nagayama, Y Tanabe: DDAVP in acquired von Willebrand syndrome associated with multiple myeloma. Am J Hematol 22:21, 1986.

84. Mannucci PM, R Lomnardi, R Bader: Studies of the pathophysiology of acquired von Willebrand's disease in seven patients with lymphoproliferative disorders or benign monoclonal gammopathies. Blood 64:614, 1984.

85. Tran-thang C, PM Mannucci, PH Schneider: Profound alterations of the multimeric structure of von Willebrand factor in a patient with malignant lymphoma. Br J Haematol 61:307, 1985.

86. Takahashi H, M Yamada, A Shibata: Acquired von Willebrand's disease in hypothyroidism. Thromb Haemost 58:1095, 1987.

87. Dalton RG, MS Dewar, GF Savidge: Hypothyroidism as a cause of acquired von Willebrand's disease. Lancet 1:1007, 1987.

88. Mohri H: Acquired von Willebrand disease in patients with polycythemia rubra vera. Am J Hematol 26:135, 1987.

89. Budde U, JA Dent, SD Berkowitz: Subunit composition of plasma von Willebrand factor in patients with the myeloproliferative syndrome. Blood 68:1213, 1986.

90. Fabris F, A Casonato, M Grazia Del Ben: Abnormalities of von Willebrand factor in myeloproliferative disease: a relationship with bleeding diathesis. Br J Haematol 63:75, 1986.

91. Budde U, G Schaefer, N Mueller: Acquired von Willebrand's disease in the myeloproliferative syndrome. Blood 64:981, 1984.

92. Mohri H: Acquired von Willebrand disease and storage pool disease in chronic myelocytic leukemia. Am J Hematol 22:391, 1986.

93. Casonato A, A Girolami: Acquired type I von Willebrand's disease in a patient with essential thrombocytosis. Acta Haematol (Basel) 75:188, 1986.

94. Veltkamp JJ, P Stevens, MV Plas: Production site of bleeding factor (acquired morbus von Willebrand). Thromb Diath Haemorrh 23:412, 1970.

95. Bateman D, R Gokal, R Prescott: Minimal-change glomerulonephritis associated with circulating anticoagulant to Factor XII. Br Med J 281:358, 1980.

96. Miller K, JE Neeley, W Krivit: Spontaneously acquired Factor IX inhibitor in a nonhemophilic child. J Pediatr 93:232, 1978.

97. Torres A, JF Lucia, A Oliveros: Anti-Factor IX circulating anticoagulant and immune thrombocytopenia in a case of Takayasu's arteritis. Acta Haematol 64:338, 1980.

98. Largo R, P Sigg, A von Felton: Acquired Factor IX inhibitor in a nonhemophilic patient with autoimmune disease. Br J Haematol 26:129, 1974.

99. Collins HW, MF Gonzalez: Acquired factor IX inhibitor in a patient with adenocarcinoma of the colon. Acta Haematol (Basel) 64:338, 1980.

100. Nes PM, PG Hymas, D Gesme: An unusual Factor-X inhibitor in leprosy. Am J Hematol 8:397, 1980.

101. Spero JA, JH Lewis, U Hasiba, LD Ellis: Treatment of amyloidosis associated with Factor X deficiency. Thromb Haemost 35:377, 1976.

102. Greipp PR, RA Kyle, EJW Bowie: Factor-X deficiency in amyloidosis: a critical review. Am J Hematol 11:443, 1981.

103. Furie B, E Greene, BC Furie: Syndrome of acquired Factor X deficiency and systemic amyloidosis. In vivo studies of the metabolic fate of Factor X. N Engl J Med 297:81, 1975.

104. Furie B, L Voo, PWG McAdam: Mechanism of Factor X deficiency in systemic amyloidosis. N Engl J Med 304:827, 1981.

105. DiSabatino CA, LP Clyne, SE Malawista: A circulating anticoagulant directed against Factor XIa in systemic lupus erythematosus. Arthritis Rheum 22:1135, 1979.

106. Fischer DS, LP Clyne: Circulating Factor XI and disseminated intravascular coagulation. Arch Intern Med 141:515, 1981.

107. Vercellotti GM, DF Mosher: Acquired Factor XI deficiency in systemic lupus erythematosus. Thromb Haemost 48:250, 1982.

108. Krieger H, RT Breckenridge: Circulating anticoagulant interfering with the action of Factor XIa in lupus. Blood 42:1002, 1974.

109. Castro O, LR Farber, LP Clyne: Circulating anticoagulants against Factors IX and XI in systemic lupus erythematosus. Ann Intern Med 77:543, 1972.

110. Aberg H, IM Nilsson: Recurrent thrombosis in a young woman with a circulating anticoagulant directed against Factors XI and XII. Acta Med Scand 192:419, 1972.

111. Cronberg S, IM Nilsson: Circulating anticoagulant against Factors XI and XII together with massive spontaneous platelet aggregation. Scand J Haematol 10:309, 1973.

112. Rustgi RN, FM La Duca, KD Tourbaf: Circulating inhibitor against factor XI in psoriasis. J Med 13:289, 1982.

113. Reece EA, LP Clyne, R Romero: Spontaneous factor XI inhibitors: seven additional cases and a review of the literature. Arch Intern Med 144:525, 1984.

114. Beck DW, RGH Strauss, CT Kisker: An intrinsic coagulation pathway inhibitor in a 3-year-old child. Am J Clin Pathol 71:470, 1979.

115. Gandolfo GM, A Afeltra, A Amoroso: Circulating anticoagulant against Factor XII and platelet antibodies in systemic lupus erythematosus. Acta Haematol 57:135, 1977.

116. Raz I, A Ramon, M Lahav: Inhibition of blood coagulation Factor XI-XII by monoclonal IgM. Isr J Med Sci 11:1392, 1975.

117. Londino AV, FJ Luparello: Factor XII deficiency in a man with gout and angioimmunoblastic lymphadenopathy. Arch Intern Med 144:1497, 1984.

118. Lorand L, N Maldonado, J Fradera: Haemorrhagic syndrome of autoimmune origin with a specific inhibitor against fibrin stabilizing factor (Factor XIII). Br J Haematol 23:17, 1972.

119. Rosenberg RD, RW Colman, L Lorand: A new haemorrhagic disorder with defective fibrin stabilization and cryo-fibrinogenaemia. Br J Haematol 26:269, 1974.

120. McDevitt NB, J McDonagh, HL Taylor: An acquired inhibitor to Factor XIII. Arch Intern Med 130:772, 1972.

121. Flore PA, LD Ellis, HL Dameshek: XIII inhibitor and antituberculous therapy. Clin Res 19:418, 1971.

122. McGehee WG, DI Feinstein, G Carpenter: Factor XIII inhibitor in a patient receiving INH. Arch Intern Med 130:772, 1972.

123. Godal HC: An inhibitor to fibrin stabilizing factor (FSF, Factor XIII). Scand J Haematol 7:43, 1970.

124. Lewis JH, ILF Szeto, LD Ellis: An acquired inhibitor to coagulation Factor XIII. Johns Hopkins Med J 120:401, 1967.

125. Lopaciuk S, K Bykowska, JM McDonagh: Differences between Type I autoimmune inhibitors of fibrin stabilization in two patients with severe hemorrhagic disorder. J Clin Invest 61:1196, 1978.

126. Fear JD, KJ Miloszewski, MS Losawsky: An acquired inhibitor of factor XIII with a qualitative abnormality of fibrin cross-linking. Acta Haematol (Basel) 71:304, 1984.

127. Lorand L, PT Valesco, JR Rinne: Autoimmune antibody (IgG Kansas) against the fibrin stabilizing (factor XIII) system. Proc Natl Acad Sci 85:232, 1988.

128. Nakamura S, A Kato, Y Sakata: Bleeding tendency caused by IgG inhibitor to factor XIII treated successfully by cyclophosphamide. Br J Haematol 68:313, 1988.

129. Wilner GR, PJL Holt, J Bottomley: Practolol therapy associated with a systemic lupus erythematosus-like syndrome and inhibitor to Factor XIII. J Clin Pathol 30:770, 1977.

130. Horne MK, CA Stein, RV LaRocca: Circulating glycosaminoglycan anticoagulants associated with suramin treatment. Blood 71:273, 1988.

131. Shojania AM, G Meilleur, AW Alvi: An autoantibody with potent antithrombin activity whose action could be inhibited by toluidine blue or methylene blue. Am J Hematol 24:207, 1987.

132. Gonyea L, R Herdman, RA Bridges: The coagulation abnormalities in systemic lupus erythematosus. Thromb Diath Haemorrh 20:457, 1968.

133. Breckenridge RT, OD Ratnoff: Studies on the site of action of a circulating anticoagulant in disseminated lupus erythematosus. Am J Med 35:813, 1963.

134. Schleinder MA, RL Nachman, EAS Jaffe: A clinical study of the lupus anticoagulant. Blood 48:499, 1976.

135. Coots MC, MA Miller, HI Glucck: The lupus inhibitor: a study of its heterogeneity. Thromb Haemost 46:734, 1981.

136. Veltkamp JJ, P Kerkhoven, EA Loeliger: Circulating anticoagulant in disseminated lupus erythematosus. Haemostasis 2:253, 1974.

137. Lee SL, AB Miotti: Disorders of hemostatic function in patients with systemic lupus erythematosus. Semin Arthritis Rheum 4:241, 1975.

138. Frick PG: Acquired circulating anticoagulants in systemic "collagen disease." Autoimmune thromboplastin deficiency. Blood 10:691, 1955.

139. Taillan B, C Roul, JG Fuzibet: Les anticoagulants circulants au cours de l'infection par le virus de l'immunodeficience humaine: resultats d'une etude prospective effectuee chez 157 patients seropositifs. Ann Med Interne (Paris) 140:405, 1989.

140. Taillan B, C Roul, JG Fuzibet: Circulating anticoagulant in patients seropositive for human immunodeficiency virus. Am J Med 87:238, 1989.

141. Burns, ER, BZ Frieger, L Bernstein, A Rubenstein: Acquired circulating anticoagulants in children with acquired immunodeficiency syndrome. Pediatrics 82:763, 1988.

142. LeFrere JJ, D Gozin, J Lerable: Circulating anticoagulant in asymptomatic persones seropositive for human immunodeficiency virus. Ann Intern Med 108:771, 1988.

143. LeFrere JJ, D Gozin, J Modai: Circulating anticoagulant in the acquired immunodeficiency syndrome. Ann Intern Med 107:429, 1987.

144. Cohen AJ, TM Phillips, CM Kessler: Circulating coagulation inhibitors in the acquired immunodeficiency syndrome. Ann Intern Med 104:175, 1986.

145. Saveuse H, E Rouveix, J Roussi: Sclerodermie et anticoagulant circulant de type antiprothrombinase. Ann Med Interne (Paris) 139:230, 1988.

146. Freeman WE, JL Lesher, JG Smith: Connective tissue disease associated with sclerodermoid features, early abortion, and circulating anticoagulant. J Am Acad Dermatol 19:932, 1988.

147. Yebra M, JA Vargas, MJ Menendez, JR Cabrera: Gastric Castleman's disease with a lupus-like circulating anticoagulant. Am J Gastroenterol 84:566, 1989.

148. Munzer M, C Behar, C Droulle: Les anticoagulants acquis de l'enfant: a propos d'une serie pediatrique de 35 cas. Arch Fr Pediatr 45:629, 1988.

149. Rapaport SI, SB Ames, BJ Duvall: A plasma coagulation defect in systemic lupus erythematosus arising from hypoprothrombinemia combined with antiprothrombinase activity. Blood 15:212, 1960.

150. Corrigan JJ, JH Patterson, NE May: Incoagulability of the blood in systemic lupus erythematosus. A case due to hypoprothrombinemia and a circulating anticoagulant. Am J Dis Child 119:365, 1970.

151. Harvey AM, LE Shulman, PA Tumulty: Systemic lupus erythematosus. Review of the literature and clinical analysis of 138 cases. Medicine 33:291, 1954.

152. Peck B, GS Hoffman, WA Franck: Thrombophlebitis in systemic lupus erythematosus. JAMA 240:1728, 1978.

153. Gladman DD, MB Urowitz: Venous syndromes and pulmonary embolism in systemic lupus erythematosus. Ann Rheum Dis 39:340, 1980.

154. Mueh JR, KD Herbst, SI Rapaport: Thrombosis in patients with the lupus anticoagulant. Ann Intern Med 92:156, 1980.

155. Harvey AM, LE Shulman: Systemic lupus erythematosus and biologic false-positive test for syphilis. In: EL Dubois (Ed): Lupus Erythematosus. University of Southern California Press, Los Angeles, CA, 1974, p 196.

156. Canoso RT, RA Hutton, D Deykin: A chlorpromazine-induced inhibitor of blood coagulation. Am J Hematol 2:183, 1977.

157. Zarrabi MH, S Zucker, F Miller: Immunologic and coagulation disorders in chlorpromazine-treated patients. Ann Intern Med 91:194, 1979.

158. Zucker S, MH Zarrabi, GS Romano: IgM inhibitors of the contact ativation phase of coagulation in chlorpromazine-treated patients. Br J Haematol 40:447, 1978.

159. Bell WR, GR Boss, JS Wolfson: Circulating anticoagulant in the procainamide-induced lupus syndrome. Arch Intern Med 137:1471, 1977.

160. Davis S, BC Furie, JH Griffin: Circulating inhibitors of blood coagulation associated with procainamide-induced lupus erythematosus. Am J Hematol 4:401, 1978.

161. Jeffrey, RF: Transient lupus anticoagulant with Fansidar therapy. Postgrad Med J 62:893, 1986.

162. Steen VD, R Ramsey-Goldman: Phenothiazine-induced systemic lupus erythematosus with superior vena cava syndrome: case report and review of the literature. Arthritis Rheum 31:923, 1988.

163. Kleinknecht D, G Bobrie, O Meyer: Recurrent thrombosis and renal vascular disease in patients with a lupus anticoagulant. Nephrol Dial Transplant 4:854, 1989.

164. Francis C, B Tribout, S Boisnic: Cutaneous necrosis associated with the lupus anticoagulant. Dermatologica 178:194, 1989.

165. Bick RL: Alterations of hemostasis in malignancy, ch 10. In: Disorders of Hemostasis and Thrombosis: Principles of Clinical Practice. Thieme, Inc., New York, 1985, p 262.

166. Lossing TS, CK Kasper, DI Feinstein: Detection of Factor VIII inhibitors with the partial thromboplastin time. Blood 49:793, 1977.

167. Hultin MB, SS Shapiro, HS Bowman: Immunosuppressive therapy of factor VIII inhibitors. Blood 48:95, 1976.

168. Nilsson IM, SB Sundqvist, RL Jung: Suppression of secondary antibody response by intravenous immunoglobulin in a patient with hemophilia B and antibodies. Scand J Haematol 30:458, 1983.

169. Nilsson IM, E Berntorp, O Zettervall: Induction of immune tolerance in patients with hemophilia and antibodies to factor VIII by combined treatment with intravenous IgG, cyclophosphamide and factor VIII. N Engl J Med 318:947, 1988.

170. Seifried E, G Gaedicke, G Pindur: The treatment of hemophilia A inhibitor with high-dose intravenous immunoglobulin. Blut 48:397, 1984.

171. Greene D, PT Schuette, WH Wallace: Factor VIII antibodies in rheumatoid arthritis: effect of cyclophosphamide. Arch Intern Med 140:1232, 1980.

172. Spero JA, JH Lewis, U Hasiba: Corticosteroid therapy for acquired factor VIII:C inhibitors. Br J Haematol 48:635, 1981.

173. Lian EC, AF Larcada, AY Chiu: Combination immunosuppressive therapy after factor VIII infusion for acquired factor VIII inhibitor. Ann Intern Med 110:774, 1989.

174. Macik BG, DA Gabriel, CG White: The use of high-dose intravenous gamma globulin in acquired von Willebrand syndrome. Arch Pathol Lab Med 112:143, 1988.

175. Francesconi M, C Korninger, E Thaler: Plasmapheresis: its value in the management of patients with antibodies to factor VIII. Haemostasis 11:79, 1982.

176. Wensley RT, RE Stevens, AM Bevin: Plasma exchange and human factor VIII concentrate in managing hemophilia A with factor VIII inhibitors. Br Med J 281:1388, 1980.

177. Bona RD, DN Pasquale, RI Kalish: Porcine factor VIII and plasmapheresis in the management of hemophiliac patients with inhibitors. Am J Hematol 21:201, 1986.

178. Uehlinger J, R Watt, L Aledort: Extracorporeal immunoadsorption: an alternative treatment for hemophiliacs with high-responding inhibitors. Blood 70:334, 1987.

179. Nilsson IM, SB Sundqvist, C Freiburghaus: Extracorporeal protein A-Sepharose and specific affinity chromatography for removal of antibodies. Prog Clin Biol Res 150:225, 1984.

180. De La Fuente B, S Panek, LW Hoyer: The effect of 1-deamino-8-D-arginine vasopressin (DDAVP) in a nonhemophilic patient with an acquired type II factor VIII inhibitor. Br J Haematol 59:127, 1985.

181. Vincente V, I Alberca, G Gonzalez: DDAVP in a non-hemophilic patient with an acquired factor VIII inhibitor. Br J Haematol 60:585, 1985.

182. Takahashi H, R Nagayama, Y Tanabe: DDAVP in acquired von Willebrand syndrome associated with multiple myeloma. Am J Hematol 22:421, 1986.

183. Silberstein LE, J Abraham, SJ Shattil: The efficacy of intense plasma exchange in acquired von Willebrand's disease. Transfusion 27:234, 1987.

184. Neva FA, EL Murphy, A Gam: Successful treatment of an acquired von Willebrand antibody by extracorporeal immunoadsorption. N Engl J Med 320:252, 1989.

C H A P T E R
11

Assessment of Patients
With Thrombosis, Thromboembolus,
and Pulmonary Embolus

Thrombosis, thromboembolus, and pulmonary embolus are substantial clinical problems seen in a broad spectrum of clinical practices. Pulmonary embolus is a leading cause of death in the United States. Therefore, it is critical to diagnose this condition promptly in those individuals who are predisposed to thrombosis and thromboembolus and to treat immediately those individuals who already harbor thrombosis. As in all domains of medicine a comprehensive clinical assessment of the patient is the mainstay of diagnosis, and only after a rigorous clinical evaluation should adjunct studies, including laboratory assessment, radiographic examination, nuclear imaging studies, and invasive procedures, such as angiography, be performed. Only in the appropriate clinical circumstance can the results of these ancillary investigations be appropriately interpreted and a reliable diagnosis made, resulting in precise, effective, and expeditious therapy. The clinical circumstances associated with arterial thrombosis are summarized in Table 11-1, the situations affiliated with venous thrombosis are summarized in Table 11-2, and the disorders related to either arterial or venous thrombosis are denoted in Table 11-3.

Obtaining the History

When examining patients with a predisposition to thrombus formation or a suspected thrombotic event, it is customary to secure a chief complaint, including the symptoms and how long they have been present. Next, one must painstakingly question the patient about affiliated disease conditions with emphasis on those conditions and situations known to be associated with a predisposition to venous or arterial thrombotic events. Of particular priority regarding increased risk of venous thrombotic events, one must ask the patient about oral contraceptive use, obesity, a history of malignancy, a history of abdominal, thoracic, obstetric, or orthopedic surgery, pregnancy, the presence or absence of heart disease, a history of venous thrombosis, a history of chronic venous

insufficiency or varicosities, and suggestions of other rarer predisposing disorders, such as Behçet's syndrome and cystathionine beta synthetase deficiency. If a predisposition to arterial thrombotic events is suspected, the patient should be questioned about the presence or absence of ischemic heart disease, hypertension, hypercholesterolemia, hyperlipidemia, tobacco use, hyperglycemia, peripheral vascular disease, prior myocardial infarction, angina, a history of high dietary fat intake, and a lack of exercise. The sex of the patient may be relevant.

Following this, the physician should inquire about diseases known to be associated with an enhanced predisposition to venous or arterial thrombotic events. The patient must be carefully asked about any regular drug intake with particular attention to the use of contraceptive agents, estrogens, or progestational agents. A history regarding the use of aspirin, aspirin-containing compounds, antihypertensives, cough medications, digitalis, hormones, cortisone, insulin, diabetic medications, thyroid medications, analgesics, weight-reducing pills, anticoagulants, dilantin, diuretics, antibiotics, barbiturates, tranquilizers, or antidepressants must be elicited.

A medical history of angina, coronary artery disease, heart disease, diabetes, emphysema, recurrent bronchitis, recurrent pneumonia, asthma, tuberculosis, herpes zoster, measles, mumps, chickenpox, rheumatic fever, scarlet fever, hepatitis, peptic ulcer disease, liver disease, jaundice, renal disease, hives, venereal disease, anemia, seizures, mental disease, chronic venous insufficiency, any type of arterial or venous thrombotic event, or varicosities should be prompted and recorded. A complete surgical history should be obtained, particularly for abdominal, thoracic, gynecologic, or orthopedic surgery. The patient must be questioned about any recent injuries or accidents, especially those involving the extremities or chest. The patient should be asked about any known allergy to medications or any other agents.

Next, a meticulous review of systems should be executed, including a personal history of generalized weakness, pruri-

Table 11-1. Positive Risk Factors for Arterial Thrombosis and Thromboembolus

Atherosclerosis
Male sex
Cigarettes
Hypertension
Diabetes mellitus
LDL cholesterol
Hypertriglyceridemia
Family history
High hematocrit
Left ventricular hypertrophy
Oral contraceptives
Lipoprotein A

Table 11-2. Positive Risk Factors for Venous Thrombosis and Thromboembolus

Obesity
Oral contraceptives
Varicose veins
Infection
Trauma
Surgery
General anesthesia
Pregnancy
Malignancy
Immobility
Congestive heart failure
Nephrotic syndrome
Blood protein defects

tus, fevers, chills, skin rashes, poorly healing sores, enlarging moles, drenching night sweats, weight loss, loss of appetite, recurrent localized headaches, dizzy spells, or any unexplored loss of consciousness. A careful history must be acquired regarding blurred vision, double vision, persistent scotomata, tinnitus, hearing loss, lateralization of hearing, or sore tongue. The patient must be asked about gingival bleeding with toothbrushing, the presence of dentures, frequent upper respiratory tract infections, difficulty in swallowing, unexplained hoarseness, cervical pain, or the noting of supraclavicular, cervical, submental, axillary, epitrochlear, inguinal, or deep iliac adenopathy. The patient should be questioned about productive cough, hemoptysis, blood-tinged sputum, coughing episodes, dyspnea at rest or exertion, angina or other types of chest pain, a history of heart disease, hypertension, tachycardia, palpitations, or ankle edema. The patient should also be asked about frequent preprandial or postprandial epigastric distress, epigastric pain, nausea, emesis, hematemesis, melena, hematochezia or deviations in bowel habits within the last six months. A genitourinary history should include a history of burning or stinging on urination, nocturia, hematuria, port wine– or root beer–colored urine, and a history of renal stones or renal disease. A history of joint pain, back pain, or bone pain should also be prompted.

In the female patient, the age of onset of menses and the age of first pregnancy should be recorded. The presence or absence of continued menses should be noted, including the date of the last menstrual period, the year menses stopped, and whether it stopped naturally or by surgical means. The patient must be asked about ingesting any type of oral contraceptives, the exact nature of these contraceptives, and exactly when and why they were stopped. The female patient should be asked about excessive vaginal discharge, recurrent vaginal infections, intramenstrual bleeding, or the noting of lumps, discharge, or irritation of her breasts. The date of the last Pap smear and pelvic examination should be obtained. Following this, a pregnancy history should be taken including numbers of pregnancies, miscarriages, premature births, children born alive, cesarean sections, stillborn births, abortions, and any potential complications of pregnancy, including any suspi-

cion of pre-eclampsia or eclampsia, the blood pressure during these episodes, and any thrombotic problems. Male patients should be asked about difficulty in starting the urinary stream, a history and type of prostatic disease if present, and whether the patient has been circumcised.

Then, a personal history is done, including a detailed smoking history incorporating the amount smoked per day and whether the patient smokes cigarettes, pipe, cigars, or uses snuff or chewing tobacco. An ethanol history, including the amount ingested per day and the specific type of ethanol consumed, should be specified. After that, a dietary history should be obtained including any special diets, food faddism, and an indication of type of meals apropos to cholesterol/lipid intake. Thereafter, a careful occupational history should be obtained, including inquiry into the potential exposure to radiation, carbon tetrachloride, benzene, industrial toxins, lead, asbestos, and pesticides. Any potential injuries, especially to the extremities and chest, should be recorded.

A family history must incorporate the presence or absence of any venous or arterial thrombotic events, pulmonary emboli, hypertension, cerebral vascular thrombotic events, renal disease, myocardial infarction, or any other situations known to be associated with increased family risk. The patient should be asked about the general health of the spouse and children. A comprehensive family history must be obtained for cerebral vascular thrombosis, hypertension, tuberculosis, diabetes mellitus, thyroid disease, gout, arthritis, any type of bleeding or thrombotic trends, coronary

Table 11-3. Positive Risk Factors for Arterial and Venous Thrombosis

Age
Obesity
Blood group A
Oral contraceptives
Homocystinuria
Behçet's syndrome
Thromboangiitis obliterans?

artery disease, pulmonary disease, pulmonary emboli, gastrointestinal disease, gastric or duodenal ulcer, ulcerative colitis, renal disease, anemia, or other hematologic disease.

Physical Examination

The physical examination should begin with an evaluation of body habitus and general health, the noting of the presence or absence of obesity, muscle wasting, skin complexion, skin turgor, and the presence or absence of acceptable hygiene. Following this, the vital signs are recorded, including the height, weight, body surface area, temperature, sitting, standing, and supine blood pressure, and the recording, character, and regularity of the pulse. Next, the head is examined carefully for any subcutaneous nodules in the scalp followed by an evaluation of occipital, periauricular, cervical, submental, or supraclavicular lymphadenopathy. The pupils must be appraised for reactivity to light and accommodation, and the conjunctivae, both palpebral and bulbar, must be evaluated. The equality of the pupils should be recorded. A careful ophthalmoscopic examination must be done. If a pulmonary embolus is suspected, the detection of retinal venous dilation is indicative of a pulmonary artery pressure greater than 30 mm Hg. Hearing should be carefully appraised by both Weber and Rinne testing; Weber testing may lateralize in the presence of transient ischemic attacks, small stroke syndromes, or a frank cerebral vascular thrombotic event. The oral mucosa and the sublingual area must be explored for vascular anomalies. The carotid pulses should be evaluated, and auscultation should be performed for detecting bruits. The noting of jugular venous distension suggests a pulmonary artery pressure of greater than 30 to 35 mm Hg, which indicates a sizable pulmonary embolus in the appropriate clinical setting. Next, the patient should be examined for tenderness of the sternum, ribs, cervix, chest, lumbosacral spine, and costovertebral angle. The chest should be carefully auscultated and percussed, and diaphragmatic excursion should be documented.

The physical findings of a patient with a pulmonary embolus may be unremarkable, may be compatible with pleural effusion, or may include tachypnea, localized inspiratory wheezing, rhonchi, or rales. A pleural friction rub, findings of consolidation, or findings harmonious with pleural effusion, increased tactile fremitus, dullness to percussion, or tubular breath sounds may be noted. An evaluation of the heart must next be accomplished with recording of the heart sounds, murmurs, and findings suggestive of acute cor pulmonale, including a right ventricular heave, a right-sided gallop, accentuated second heart sound, or a murmur of tricuspid insufficiency. Again, the presence or absence of distended jugular veins and a positive hepatojugular reflex should be recorded when a pulmonary embolus is suspected. These findings are suggestive of increased pulmonary artery pressure. Following evaluation of the heart and heart sounds, the peripheral pulses should be evaluated, including the

brachial, radial, ulnar, femoral, popliteal, dorsalis pedis, and posterior tibial pulses. The femoral arteries and the aorta should be auscultated for murmurs. The popliteal, posterior tibial, and dorsalis pedis pulses are usually evaluated simultaneously with assessment of the extremities.

Following the cardiorespiratory evaluation, the abdomen should be examined for tenderness, normal bowel sounds, hepatomegaly, hepatic tenderness, splenomegaly, splenic tenderness, costovertebral angle tenderness or bruits, and abdominal masses. A rectal examination is done unless a contraindication is present. Prostatic enlargement and localized tenderness should be recorded, and the stool specimen should be analyzed for occult blood. The genitalia are examined for testicular swelling or tenderness in males, and a pelvic examination is performed in females. Assessment of the extremities is crucial in a patient with suspected venous thrombosis, since the physical findings are inconclusive. The reliability of these findings, however, is amplified by rigorous examination. A search for findings of chronic venous insufficiency should be done, including varicosities, ankle edema, and chronic hemosiderin deposits. The popliteal, dorsalis pedis, and posterior tibial pulses must be appraised not only for presence or absence but also for intensity. The toes and toenails should be examined for evidence of pallor, cyanosis, chronic ulcerative changes, or chronic atrophic changes suggestive of chronic vascular insufficiency. The inguinal areas, anterior medial thighs, popliteal fossae, and calfs should be carefully evaluated for evidence of erythema, tenderness, swelling, hyperpyrexia, or the demonstration of a frank venous cord. In this regard the palpation of a distinct cord is the most dependable physical finding of a venous thrombus. Detection of demonstrable increases in diameter of the calf, popliteal area, or thigh and associated edema are also reliable findings. Homan's sign is less reliable. In the presence of substantial venous thrombosis, a compartmental compression syndrome may occur, either anterior tibial, posterior tibial, or of the thigh (extensor or flexor compartment). Arterial and neurologic (neurovascular bundle impairment) compromise may occur as well with not only extreme pain, cyanosis, redness, swelling, and tenderness in the area of a cord noted in association with venous disease but also interference with arterial vascular flow leading to more cyanosis, pallor, intensified swelling, and a dull persistent ache with decreased or absent pulses by palpation. The pulses, however, are usually demonstrable by Doppler.

After a careful evaluation of the extremities for the physical findings of venous thrombosis or arterial disease, the integument should be inspected for petechiae, purpura, ecchymoses, or any unexplained cyanosis, edema, clubbing, discoloration, or rash. Following this, a careful neurologic examination is done. The cerebrum, cerebellum, cranial nerves, biceps, triceps, ulnar reflexes, and the patellar and Achilles reflexes should be assessed. Pinpoint sensation, two-point sensation, and vibratory sensation should be appraised.

Figure 11-1. Positive Thromboscintogram

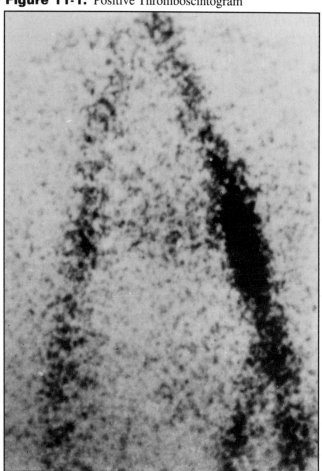

Figure 11-2. Perfusion Scan

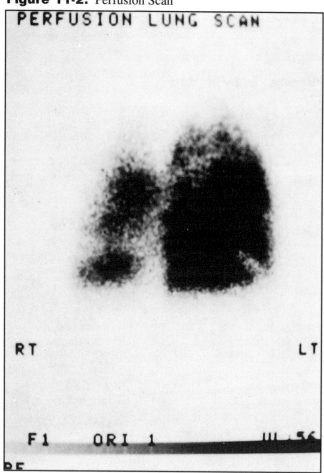

Ancillary Studies

Ancillary studies are usually called for when assessing patients who are hypercoagulable or are suspected of having venous or arterial thrombotic or thromboembolic events or pulmonary embolus. For pulmonary embolus, ancillary diagnostic aids are readily available; however, they must be interpreted in the appropriate clinical setting. Usually, elevated enzyme levels will be noted, including lactate dehydrogenase (LDH), serum glutamic-oxaloacetic transaminase (SGOT), and creatine phosphokinase (CPK). However, these are nonspecific findings. Close to 90% of patients with a pulmonary embolus will have a partial oxygen pressure (pO$_2$) of less than 80 mm Hg. Further laboratory tests that often yield positive results include elevated FDP and D-dimer levels, circulating soluble fibrin monomer, depressed antithrombin III, and depressed protein C and protein S. Moreover, elevated fibrinopeptide A and B, platelet factor 4, and beta-thromboglobulin levels are frequently observed in patients with pulmonary embolus or extensive deep venous thrombosis. A baseline electrocardiogram (EKG) should always be done in a patient with venous thrombosis or suspected pulmonary embolus. The results of the EKG may be normal but more typically will exhibit findings of acute cor pulmonale and right ventricular failure. Almost always a sinus tachycardia will be present, and transient atrial premature systoles, atrial flutter, or atrial fibrillation may also be present in association with a large pulmonary embolus. The extremity leads commonly show an S-1, Q-3 pattern consisting of a deep S wave in lead 1, a prominent Q wave and an inverted T wave in lead 3, and depression of ST segments in leads 2 and 1. The precordial leads will often show T-wave inversions in right precordial leads, a complete or incomplete right bundle branch block, and a QR pattern in leads V-3, V-1, and V-2 in association with negative T waves. Because of widespread myocardial ischemia, the precordial leads may show ST segment depressions or T-wave inversions. The following patterns are strongly suggestive of an acute pulmonary embolus and acute right heart failure: S-1, Q-3, T-3 pattern associated with T-wave inversion in the right precordial leads; S-1, T-3 pattern or T-wave inversion in lead 3 and the right precordial leads; and an S-1, Q-3, T-3 pattern in association with a complete or incomplete right bundle branch block.

Similarly, a baseline chest roentgenogram must always be obtained in patients with suspected thrombus or pulmonary embolus. Most individuals with a pulmonary embolus will have abnormal results of a chest roentgenogram, although

Figure 11-3. Positive Venogram

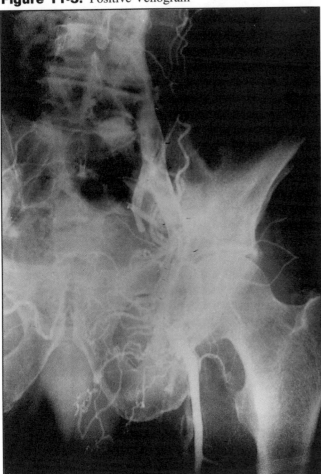

Figure 11-4. Pulmonary Angiogram

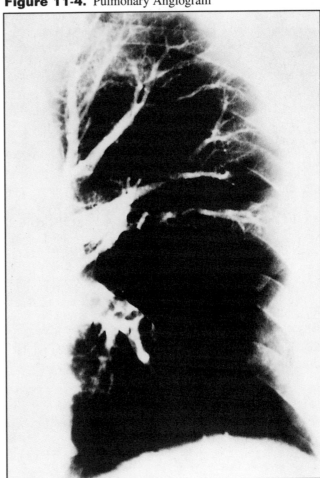

many findings are not usually diagnostic. The most common defect found is a patchy infiltrate, but characteristic hump-shaped infarcts at the lung base or in other areas of the pulmonary parenchyma may also be found. Less commonly, a pleural effusion, local constriction of pulmonary vessels, fullness of pulmonary arteries at the hilus, and an area of oligemia (Westermark's sign) may be noted. These findings must be correlated with ventilation perfusion lung scans using technetium-99–labeled macroaggregated albumin. Usually, perfusion defects will be noted in the same areas as pulmonary infiltrates. If the pulmonary infiltrate is smaller than the perfusion defect, a pulmonary embolus is probable. Alternatively, if the infiltrative anomaly on the chest roentgenogram is larger than the perfusion defect, the probability of pulmonary embolus is doubtful. Ventilation scans of low probability for a pulmonary embolus are those showing single or multiple defects less than 3 to 4 cm in diameter or a perfusion defect that is smaller than a radiographic infiltrate. However, the presence of a perfusion defect that is larger than a radiographic infiltrate or a perfusion defect that is larger than a segment in size may be considered positive. Perfusion defects equal to or smaller than chest roentgenogram infiltrates fall into an intermediate probability category. In this instance, the patient should be treated for a pulmonary

embolus or should be subjected to pulmonary angiography if the findings will change the proposed therapy. The noting of normal results of a ventilation perfusion lung scan is strong evidence that the patient has not sustained a pulmonary embolus. However, the finding of normal results of a chest roentgenogram is not compelling verification for the absence of a pulmonary embolus. When appropriate clinical suspicion is aroused, a ventilation perfusion scan must always be done. Absolute confirmation may require pulmonary angiography.

About 95% of pulmonary emboli arise from deep venous thrombi of the lower extremities, and about 25% are from calf veins. These venous thrombi are most commonly proximal to the popliteal vein and are less commonly noted to be present in the calf veins. When a patient has a documented pulmonary embolus, a search for venous thrombi should be done. Pulmonary emboli may sporadically emanate from thrombi in the subclavian, basilic, or ovarian veins and the inferior vena cava. Alternatively, in the patient without a pulmonary embolus but with only clinically suspected deep venous thrombosis, confirmatory procedures must be done.

Lively dispute exists regarding the comparative proficiency and safety of ascending contrast venography vs radioactive (I^{125}) fibrinogen scans vs ascending thromboscintography and whole blood pool venograms, using technetium-

99–labeled macroaggregated albumin for the former and technetium-99–labeled red blood cells for the latter. I prefer ascending thromboscintography or pooled blood venograms, since a ventilation/perfusion scan can be done simultaneously. Difficulties are associated with other invasive procedures. The radioactive fibrinogen scan is associated with a high chance of false-negative and false-positive results and is insensitive to thrombi above the lower thigh because of increased radioactive background activity in the pelvic vessels and bladder. Moreover, positive results will emanate from perivascular hemorrhage or inflammation. Furthermore, radioactive fibrinogen scanning cannot discriminate between old and new thrombi. Doppler ultrasonography is of high reliability except for lesions below the knee; however, the results may be influenced by collateral circulation and venous recanalization. New techniques using color Doppler flow imaging are very reliable. Contrast venography is the customary technique to prove venous thrombi of the lower extremities. This method, however, is exceedingly painful, time consuming, and associated with allergic reactions. I seldom use this procedure because of the associated 10% chance of postvenogram venous thrombosis. Thromboscintography is exceptionally dependable. Experienced radiologists can distinguish between an old and new thrombus, a simultaneous pulmonary perfusion/ventilation scan for pulmonary embolus can be performed, and the procedure is generally unassociated with side effects, procedure-related thrombosis, or allergic reactions. Figure 11-1 demonstrates a positive thromboscintogram, and Figure 11-2 is a perfusion scan from the same patient. Figures 11-3 and 11-4 show a positive venogram and pulmonary angiogram in another patient. Radiographic techniques for diagnosis of deep vein thrombosis will be discussed in more detail in chapter 13.

Summary

Because thrombotic or thromboembolic events are common irreversible events potentially leading to significant morbidity and mortality in patients, adequate assessment of these patients from the clinical standpoint is extremely important, including the use of ancillary testing procedures. This principle applies to patients who are hypercoagulable and who have recently sustained a thrombotic event. Only in this manner can prophylactic therapy or therapy to treat the underlying event be started before the patient has sustained an unalterable and often catastrophic insult that will lead to prolonged morbidity or to mortality.

CHAPTER
12

Hemostasis in Malignancy

lterations of hemostasis in malignancy have long
been appreciated. Trousseau[1] was the first to acknowl-
edge this association in 1865, and Morrison[2] began a
considerable study of altered hemostasis in patients
with malignancy in 1932. Aberrations of hemostasis in
patients with malignancy are unusually complex and present
major clinical challenges and problems. Many instances of
bleeding or thrombosis in patients with malignancy are
caused by unexplained mechanisms[3]; however, frequently
the mechanisms are understood and will be discussed.
Changes of hemostasis secondary to malignancy are decid-
edly multifaceted, and the development of clinically significant hemorrhage or thrombosis in these patients often represents a total clinical expression of many changes in the
hemostatic system.[4,5] This chapter describes the major
changes of hemostasis developing in patients with malignancy, emphasizing those believed to be most clinically significant for morbidity and mortality.

Hypercoagulability and Thrombosis

Pathophysiology

The first described abnormality of hemostasis in malignancy was hypercoagulability and thrombosis, and the first
large study of blood changes in patients with cancer showed
accelerated bleeding times in more than 60% of patients
studied.[1,2] After these classic descriptions, many authors
have reported hypercoagulability and thrombosis in association with most kinds of malignancy.[5-14] Many have found
elevated clotting factors in patients with malignancy, with
the factors most commonly implicated being factors I, V,
VIII:C, IX, and XI.[6,7,12,16] Many patients with malignancy
have shortened activated or nonactivated partial thromboplastin times, accelerated prothrombin times, and accelerated clotting times.[5,12,16] Although these parameters have usually been assumed to be indicative of hypercoagulability, no
proof of this association has been documented.[3,5] None of

these laboratory parameters correlate with the development
of a clinical thrombotic episode in an individual patient.[3,4]

Increased fibrinogen and platelet catabolism (increased
turnover and decreased survival) happens in many patients
with disseminated malignancy.[17] Increased titers of FDPs,
D-dimer, fibrinopeptides A and B, cryofibrinogens, fibrin
monomer, B-beta 15-42 and related peptides, platelet factor
4, beta-thromboglobulin, and altered fibronectin and
antithrombin levels are seen in many individuals with disseminated malignancy.[7,17-27] These laboratory findings imply
vividly that many patients with cancer have a low-grade disseminated intravascular clotting process.[28,29] The shortened
survival of fibrinogen, platelets, and other coagulation proteins is often followed by an overcompensatory increase in
coagulation factors and fibrinolytic enzymes, although these
latter proteins may be decreased in selected myeloproliferative disorders.[30] These changes are frequently accompanied
by significant decreases in major coagulation inhibitors
including AT III, protein C, and protein S, although the
exact mechanisms of decreases in AT III and protein C are a
source of controversy and may be because of consumption
or the result of defective hepatic synthesis.[10,12,30,31] This
sequence of changes, however, alters the balance between
coagulation, fibrinolysis, and inhibition of the clotting and
fibrinolytic system and may make patients highly susceptible to a significant clinical event secondary only to minor
changes in the hemostatic system. This may then predispose
the patient to localized intravascular coagulation (thrombosis or thromboembolism) or a classic DIC-type syndrome
associated with hemorrhage or thrombosis.[28,29,32] Thrombus
formation is the more common of the two expressions of
intravascular coagulation in patients with solid tumors and
may approach 40% to 50% in some populations of patients
with cancer.[5,33] Sometimes, changes in coagulation factors
have been correlated with the bulk of tumor present and
overall patient survival. Some coagulation abnormalities
tend to normalize following initiation of therapy for the particular malignancy. This phenomenon may be noted following surgery, radiation therapy, chemotherapy, biotherapeutic

or hormonal manipulation.[5-7,17] Hormonal therapy has been noted to lead to decreases in AT III and make the patient more susceptible to thrombotic events.[34]

The mechanisms by which malignant tissues may initiate localized or disseminated intravascular coagulation are highly complex. Many malignant tissues can release procoagulant materials and sometimes fibrinolytic materials into the systemic circulation. Despite the mechanisms, when compared to normal tissue, most malignant tissue can begin the clotting process via many multifaceted processes, and many pathologic tumor specimens are commonly noted to be associated with encircling fibrin formation. Many malignant tissues can initiate fibrin formation without apparent later activation of the fibrinolytic system.[35,36] Many malignant tissues are also capable of releasing a thromboplastinlike activity and may provide this activity either systemically or locally to start a clotting process. The amount released will most probably dictate whether a localized intravascular coagulation event (thrombus) or a systemic DIC-type syndrome happens. Low levels of AT III, despite its cause, will allow this process to start more readily and to proceed without normal inhibition once it has begun[5,12] (eg, in the patient with significant liver metastases and later decreased or defective AT III synthesis[31]).

Mucinous adenocarcinomas are tumors commonly associated with thrombus formation. In these malignancies the sialic acid moiety of secreted mucin can initiate coagulation by the nonenzymatic activation of factor X to factor Xa.[5,8,16,37] In pancreatic carcinoma, the release of systemic trypsin triggers intravascular coagulation events.[5,38] Trypsin release has been shown to correlate with the magnitude of disseminated thrombi. Patients with carcinoma of the body or tail of the pancreas have minimal ductal obstruction, large amounts of trypsin release, and far more thrombotic and thromboembolic episodes than patients with carcinoma of the head of the pancreas, who have maximal ductal obstruction and minimal trypsin release.[5,32]

Disseminated intravascular coagulation represents the coagulopathy of adenocarcinoma of the prostate.[39,40] Malignant prostatic tissue not only activates the procoagulant system but also independently activates the fibrinolytic system. In this instance, both DIC and secondary fibrinolysis occur in association with inordinantly excessive fibrino(geno)lysis from both primary activation and activation secondary to DIC. This coagulopathy is more often manifest as hemorrhage instead of thrombosis, showing the wide variability of clinical expression in DIC depending on the balance between activation of the procoagulant system vs activation of the fibrino(geno)lytic system. Therapy for prostatic carcinoma is often followed by an alleviation of general hemostasis abnormalities, including changes of the procoagulant and fibrinolytic systems. This is noted particularly with administration of estrogens, whereas testosterone has been noted to enhance coagulation abnormalities in many patients.[19,41,42]

Hypercoagulability in patients with cancer may also arise from platelet abnormalities. The role of platelets in contributing to thrombosis in malignancy was suspected many years ago, and the first large study of this phenomenon was initiated by Moolten et al in 1949.[43] These studies showed abnormal increases in platelet numbers and abnormal morphology, platelet lysis, and defective adhesion to glass wool. A correlation was noted between platelet adhesiveness and the development of thrombosis; increased platelet adhesion was better correlated with thrombosis in malignancy than was thrombocytosis. Increased platelet adhesion, as measured by shortened bleeding times, accelerated thromboplastin generation, shortened prothrombin consumption, and increased adhesion to glass, has been studied in many populations of patients with cancer and appears to be a uniform abnormality in a variety of solid tumors.[2,6,7,12,44] However, it is unclear whether these changes are primary disturbances caused by the malignancy or whether these platelet abnormalities are caused by initial earlier changes in the coagulation system that activate platelets and make them hyperaggregable.[5] Thrombocytosis is a well-recognized accompaniment of malignancy and most commonly is associated with carcinoma of the pancreas, lung, gastrointestinal tract, ovary, breast, and myeloproliferative syndromes. Patients undergoing bone marrow suppressive chemotherapy have less thrombocytosis than patients not being so treated.[2,5,7,12,44] The most pronounced instances of thrombocytosis are usually noted in the myeloproliferative disorders.[5,45] As with coagulation protein abnormalities and hypercoagulability, thrombocytosis and increased platelet aggregability generally correlate poorly with the actual development of a clinical thrombotic event in an individual patient, and, therefore, the significance of these in vitro laboratory findings is unclear.

Various mechanisms enable malignant tissue to induce changes in coagulation factors and platelets to create a hypercoagulable state (ie, an increased predisposition to thrombosis) as an expression of an underlying intravascular clotting process that may be systemic or may stay localized.[5,29] Intravascular coagulation may be mild and manifest only by abnormal results of laboratory tests of hemostasis, such as elevated levels of FDPs, D-dimer, B-beta 15-42 and related peptides, fibrinopeptide A or B, circulating fibrin monomer, and other tests generally interpreted as representing hypercoagulability.[46] However, intravascular coagulation may proceed to more than a laboratory phenomenon and become expressed clinically as localized thrombosis or thromboembolus or, in more extreme cases, may manifest as a systemic (or disseminated) intravascular coagulation event associated with hemorrhage and thrombosis. The malignancies most commonly associated with thrombosis are depicted in Table 12-1. The general incidence of thrombosis in malignancy is about 15%, but this may be higher in specific tumors, such as pancreatic carcinoma, being seen in more than 50% of patients.[3-5,10,14] Patients with malignancy are more likely to develop postoperative deep venous thrombosis than are patients without cancer. For cancer of the gastrointestinal tract, the chance of postoperative thrombosis and thromboembolus approaches 40%.[3,4,8,16,37,47]

Table 12-1. Malignancies Commonly Associated With Thrombosis

Colon
Gallbladder
Gastric
Lung (any cell type)
Myeloproliferative syndromes
Ovary
Pancreas
Paraprotein disorders

Table 12-2. Antithrombin Changes in Liver Metastases

Malignancy	Antithrombin (%)	Liver
Breast	33	Involved
Hodgkin's	75	Involved
Breast	80	Involved
Breast	58	Involved
Ovary	76	Involved
Colon	83	Involved
Breast	71	Involved
Colon	92	Involved
Carcinoid	160	Involved
Colon	160	Involved
Hodgkin's	120	Clear
Breast	92	Clear
Lung	121	Clear
Lung	117	Clear
Breast	112	Clear
Ovary	92	Clear
Pancreas	104	Clear
Breast	140	Clear
Breast	104	Clear
Breast	150	Clear

Management

Antineoplastic therapy is associated with some correction of abnormal hemostasis, which is especially appreciated in prostatic carcinoma. Because of this, treated patients are less susceptible to thrombosis and thromboembolus. When thrombotic episodes develop in untreated patients, consideration should be given to antineoplastic therapy. The use of both warfarin and heparin anticoagulants or antiplatelet agents, usually as aspirin plus dipyridamole, is associated with some correction of altered coagulation factors and normalization of both fibrinogen and platelet consumption (increased turnover and decreased survival).[3,4,7,17,41] Despite these findings, however, patients with cancer are notoriously resistant to anticoagulant therapy, and thrombotic events commonly continue after initiation of antithrombotic therapy.[3-5,48]

Warfarin and less commonly intravenous heparin are not only often ineffective but may be associated with significant bleeding problems in patients with malignancy, probably resulting from large areas of necrotic tumor surface.[3-5,48] This problem has also been experienced by others who have noted a high chance of fatal hemorrhage associated with the use of intravenous heparin in patients with malignancy.[17] Many patients with malignancy have decreased AT III levels,[5,31] and responses to heparin may be less than optimal. This problem is especially frequent in patients with liver metastases, as shown in Table 12-2. Experience with antiplatelet agents in patients with malignancy has been acceptable.[5] I commonly use enteric-coated aspirin, 300 to 600 mg twice daily with 30 mL of liquid antacid in combination with dipyridamole, 50 to 75 mg four times daily in patients with cancer and thrombosis.[3-5,29,48] This regimen is often effective for the immediate prophylaxis of extension of thrombi and for long-term prophylactic therapy in patients with cancer with recurrent thrombosis. Warfarin and heparin are generally contraindicated in patients with malignancy and thrombosis or thromboembolus if central nervous system metastases, abscesses, or infection are present.[3,4,48] The use of aspirin and dipyridamole preoperatively or immediately postoperatively seems effective for prophylaxis in those patients with tumors known to be associated with a high rate of postoperative thrombosis. Usually, bleeding complications are not noted in association with antiplatelet therapy even in patients with recent gastrointestinal surgery. The importance of using concomitant liquid antacids and enteric-coated aspirin cannot be overstressed. Alternatively, low-dose subcutaneous heparin can safely be used in most preoperative patients with malignancy as prophylaxis for postoperative thrombosis or pulmonary embolus, but intravenous or high-dose heparin therapy should not be used in this instance.[5,29] The antiplatelet effect may last for four to 10 days after the last dose, and this should be considered in the event of bleeding, planned nonemergent surgery, or other invasive procedures. However, bleeding from antiplatelet therapy can easily be controlled with proper numbers of platelet concentrates, as was outlined in chapters 4 and 5. When the patient with malignancy has life-threatening thrombosis and has adequate levels of AT III, low-dose heparin is most useful, appears to be equally effective as large doses of heparin, and is not often associated with bleeding from tumor surfaces as frequently as with intravenous heparin.

Leukemias

Hemorrhage

Hemorrhage may precede the overt clinical diagnosis of leukemia by several months and is most frequently noted in

Table 12-3. Clinical Hemorrhage in Acute Leukemia

Hemorrhage may precede diagnosis by months; petechiae, purpura, and ecchymoses most common

Up to 70% of patients have petechiae and purpura at diagnosis

Retinal hemorrhage in 15% of patients at diagnosis and in 50% of patients during course of disease

Most patients will have hemorrhage of skin and/or mucosal membranes during course of disease

Hemorrhage is the cause of death in 40% of patients

Table 12-4. Propensity to Hemorrhage in Leukemia (Descending Order of Probability)

Acute promyelocytic leukemia
Acute myelomonocytic leukemia
Acute myeloblastic leukemia
Chronic myelogenous leukemia
Chronic lymphocytic leukemia
Monocytic leukemia

acute leukemias.[49-52] Petechiae, purpura, and ecchymoses are the most common prediagnostic manifestations, and these or other less commonly noted sites of hemorrhage are present at the time of diagnosis in about 40% to 70% of patients with acute leukemia.[5,53-55] The most prevalent sites of hemorrhage in patients with acute leukemia are the skin, eye, and mucosal membranes including epistaxis, gingival bleeding, and gastrointestinal tract bleeding.[5,50,51] Retinal bleeding can be found in about 15% of patients at presentation and in 50% of patients with acute leukemia as the disease progresses.[5,52,53,56] In acute leukemia, hemorrhage is a commmon cause of death and accounts for the mechanism of death in about 40% of patients.[52,53,57] During the past two decades, infection has surpassed hemorrhage as the most common cause of death in patients with acute leukemia, probably resulting from more intensive chemotherapy and attendent immunosuppression and the major impact of the development of platelet concentrate therapy to help control thrombocytopenia, the most common cause of fatal hemorrhage in acute leukemia.[5,50-52,58] Clinical bleeding manifestations in acute leukemias are summarized in Table 12-3.

Hemorrhage is less commonly a problem in the chronic myeloid or lymphoid leukemias.[3-5,50-52,59] In both chronic myelogenous leukemia or chronic lymphocytic leukemia, however, local or diffuse thromboses or thromboembolism frequently happen.[3,4,48,60] Many patients with chronic leukemia have bothersome bleeding, usually manifest as petechiae, purpura, ecchymoses, or oozing from mucosal membranes, including the gastrointestinal and genitourinary tracts.[5] Only rarely do these patients have retinal bleeding or other serious life-threatening bleeding unless severe thrombocytopenia (usually drug induced) or thrombocytosis and thrombocythemia develop.[5] Alterations of hemostasis associated with malignant thrombocytosis and thrombocythemia were discussed in chapter 5. As with chronic myelogenous leukemias, chronic lymphocytic leukemia is also more commonly associated with thrombosis or thromboembolus in the early course of the disease.[3,4,60] Hemorrhage, however, becomes a problem later during the disease when thrombocytopenia from chemotherapy or marrow infiltration, liver infiltration, or other hemostasis defects, including DIC secondary to the leukemia itself, sepsis, transfusions, or other causes, may become manifest.[3-5,28,29,32,48,61]

Hemorrhage may happen in any of the leukemias but is most common in acute promyelocytic (FAB M3) leukemia, acute myelomonocytic (FAB M4) leukemia, and acute granulocytic (FAB M1 and M2) leukemia. Life-threatening or severe hemorrhage is less commonly seen in chronic myelogenous leukemia and chronic lymphocytic leukemia and is less commonly seen in pure monocytic leukemia.[3,4,50-52,62-64] Propensity to hemorrhage in leukemias is depicted in Table 12-4.

The development of significant or life-threatening hemorrhage in all leukemias occurs by many mechanisms, and these will be discussed as categories of defects, including platelets, the coagulation proteins, mechanisms for the development of DIC, abnormalities of the vasculature, and the leukemia cell as a source of various clot-promoting materials, fibrino(geno)lytic materials, and other products that may modify or disrupt the hemostasis system.[5,52]

Platelets

The most common single cause of serious or life-threatening hemorrhage in acute or chronic leukemias is thrombocytopenia.[3,4,50,51] Thrombocytopenia is most commonly caused by chemotherapy or marrow infiltration. The grades of thrombocytopenia and the chemotherapeutic agents likeliest to cause thrombocytopenia were outlined in chapter 5. Less common causes of thrombocytopenia in patients with leukemia include the development of DIC with consumption of platelets, infection-induced immune or nonimmune thrombocytopenia, or the development of splenomegaly and associated hypersplenism with increased platelet sequestration. In clinical practice when noting severe thrombocytopenia in patients with leukemia, these mechanisms must be recalled even though the most common causes of thrombocytopenia are drugs or marrow infiltration. Any combination of several or many of these mechanisms may be operative and must be corrected if life-threatening hemorrhage is to be treated successfully. Mechanisms of thrombocytopenia in leukemia are summarized in Table 12-5.

In patients with acute myelogenous leukemia the platelet count commonly decreases to below 10×10^9/L (10,000/mm³) during remission induction therapy.[5,52,65,66] Bleeding is uncommon with a platelet count of greater than 10×10^9/L (10,000/mm³) in patients undergoing remission induction. When the platelet count drops to below 5×10^9/L (5,000/mm³), however, severe hemorrhage is frequent. During remission induction, a daily urine test for red blood cells and a daily

Table 12-5. Mechanisms of Thrombocytopenia in Leukemia

Bone marrow infiltration (myelophthisis)
Chemotherapy
Radiation therapy
Bacteremia
Disseminated intravascular coagulation
Infection induced (immune and nonimmune)
Splenomegaly and hypersplenism
Immune thrombocytopenia purpura
Myelofibrosis
Richter's syndrome (CLL)

---

stool guaiac test should be obtained when the platelet count drops to below 50 x 10⁹/L (50,000/mm³). If either of these tests becomes positive, serious hemorrhage may be impending.[5] If the urine and stool samples are negative, prophylactic platelet concentrate therapy should not be empirically given unless the platelet count is less than 5 x 10⁹/L (5,000/mm³).[5] If the urine or stool samples are positive or if the platelet count is less than 5 x 10⁹/L (5,000/mm³), the daily infusion of 6 to 8 units of platelet concentrates each day is appropriate to circumvent irreversible or life-threatening hemorrhage and should be continued until the platelet count is consistently greater than 10 x 10⁹/L (10,000/mm³) and no significant bleeding or early signs of bleeding, as manifest by guaiac tests or blood in the urine, are noted.[5] If possible, directed single-donor platelets are used.

Chronic myelogenous leukemia is only rarely associated with platelet counts of less than 10 x 10⁹/L (10,000/mm³).[3-5,50-52] As in acute leukemias, however, when the platelet count is less than 50 x 10⁹/L (50,000/mm³) these same principles of management also apply.[5] More commonly, chronic myeloid leukemias are associated with hemorrhage and/or thrombosis secondary to a profound thrombocytosis/thrombocythemia. The general characteristics of this complication, including the diagnostic problems and therapeutic approach to essential thrombocythemia or secondary thrombocythemia in patients with leukemias, were discussed in chapter 5.

Like chronic myelogenous leukemia (CML), chronic lymphocytic leukemia (CLL) is rarely, at least in the early course of the disease, associated with platelet counts of less than 50 x 10⁹/L (50,000/mm³).[5] As CLL begins to enter a terminal phase, thrombocytopenia may become a significant problem, resulting from the institution of more vigorous chemotherapy, severe marrow replacement, infections, or the development of various immune-mediated thrombocytopenic problems including Richter's syndrome or an ITP-type syndrome. Severe thrombocytopenia may also happen following the development of significant hypersplenism or a frank DIC syndrome. The same management principles, as outlined earlier, should be instituted, specifically depending on the mechanism or combination of mechanisms involved.[5]

Platelet Dysfunction

Significant platelet dysfunction, even in the face of normal or elevated platelet counts, is almost uniformly noted in chronic myelogenous leukemia, essential thrombocythemia, and other myeloproliferative syndromes.[3-5,45,50,52] The characteristics of platelet dysfunction in essential thrombocythemia were discussed in chapter 5. Generally, characteristic platelet function defects are noted in CML, and these often lead to or contribute to significant hemorrhage. Although many types of defects are seen, the most common are impaired aggregation to ADP and epinephrine and defective platelet factor 3 release.[67-69] A deficiency or absence of alpha granules occurs in patients with myeloproliferative syndromes and platelet function defects.[70] The platelet function defect associated with chronic myelogenous leukemia or essential thrombocythemia commonly leads to or contributes to significant clinical hemorrhage, especially if coupled with other defects in the hemostasis system.[3,4,62,71,72] If the platelet count is decreased or normal, the defect can be overcome using proper numbers of platelet concentrates. Platelet dysfunction associated with hemorrhage and an elevated platelet count (greater than 700 x 10⁹/L [700,000/mm³]) is rapidly corrected by plateletcytapheresis. Clinically significant platelet dysfunction happens in about 70% of patients with polycythemia vera, about 50% of patients with myelofibrosis, and about 30% of patients with chronic myelogenous leukemia.[73] Platelet dysfunction is less commonly a problem in acute leukemias. Some authors have reported normal platelet function to most usual aggregating agents,[74] while others have noted impaired platelet function as assessed by platelet aggregation to thrombin, ADP, epinephrine, and collagen in patients with acute leukemias.[75] Abnormal release of platelet factor 3 is noted in patients with acute leukemia.[50,52] Although platelet function defects in chronic myelogenous leukemia and other myeloproliferative disorders are known to contribute to significant hemorrhage, the role of abnormal platelet function as a dominant cause of hemorrhage in acute leukemias is less clearly defined. Platelet dysfunction is much less commonly seen in chronic lymphocytic leukemia and in monocytic leukemia than in the myelogenous leukemias or other myeloproliferative syndromes.[5,50,52]

Coagulation Protein Abnormalities

Liver infiltration with ensuing defective or decreased synthesis of the vitamin K–dependent factors is commonly a problem in acute leukemias, and impaired synthesis of other factors may also evolve.[50,52,76] Therefore, if a patient with acute leukemia develops significant liver infiltration, defective or decreased synthesis may occur of any combination of factors II, VII, IX, X, V, VIII:C, XI, XII, and XIII, fibrinogen, prekallikrein, high–molecular weight kininogen, plasminogen, AT III, protein S, and protein C.[3-5,30,50-52] Fibronectin levels are typically decreased in acute leukemia, probably because of decreased synthesis or possibly consumption from the development of a DIC syndrome. This phenomenon correlates appropriately with infectious episodes, and DIC instead of defective synthesis appears to be incriminated as the mechanism for decreased levels of fibronectin in patients with acute leukemia.[30] Cholestasis occurs in a noteworthy number of patients with acute leukemia, may lead to defective synthesis of the vitamin K–dependent clotting factors, and sometimes may also lead to frank DIC.[50,51,77]

Chronic lymphocytic leukemia may also be associated with substantial liver infiltration, especially as the disease progresses and approaches terminal stages.[5,50,52,76,78] As in the acute leukemias, this condition may lead to impaired or decreased synthesis of the vitamin K–dependent factors, any other combination of factors, and proteins synthesized by the liver. Many patients with chronic lymphocytic leukemia exhibit prolonged prothrombin times, which may correct with more intensive appropriate chemotherapeutic agents. Factors V and VIII:C and fibrinogen may behave as acute-phase reactants, and these levels may be high, low, or normal in patients with chronic lymphocytic leukemia.[5] Accordingly, the APTT may be remarkably inconsistent because of the variable levels of factors V and VIII:C and fibrinogen. Defective hepatic synthesis of coagulation factors resulting from hepatic infiltration in chronic lymphocytic leukemia is an uncommon cause of life-threatening hemorrhage. Chronic myelogenous leukemias may also be associated with significant hepatic infiltration, but this is much less commonly a problem than in acute leukemias or chronic lymphocytic leukemia.[50,62] Patients with chronic myelogenous leukemia who do not have DIC will usually manifest normal or near normal global tests of hemostasis, and defective hepatic synthesis resulting from leukemic infiltrates is infrequently a singular problem accounting for hemorrhage in patients with chronic myelogenous leukemia.[5]

Acquired von Willebrand's syndrome has been noted in association with many hematologic malignancies, including chronic lymphocytic leukemia, hairy cell leukemia, myelodysplastic syndromes, multiple myeloma, chronic myelogenous leukemia, polycythemia vera, essential thrombocythemia, and myelofibrosis.[79-86] In these cases, the variant has been classified as type II. The two mechanisms yet defined have been the development of a circulating inhibitor to von Willebrand factor or proteolysis of von Willebrand factor. Sometimes, treatment of the underlying malignant disorder has been accompanied by partial or complete correction of the bleeding diathesis. The use of DDAVP has alleviated bleeding in some patients with malignancies associated with von Willebrand's syndrome (Table 12-6).

Fibrinolysis

Many changes in the fibrinolytic system of patients with acute leukemia have been reported; however, these findings have been inconsistent, with increased fibrinolytic activity reported by some[74] and decreased fibrinolytic activity noted by others.[87] One study noted a correlation between leukocytosis, subsequent leukostasis, and enhanced fibrinolytic

Table 12-6. Malignancies Associated With Acquired von Willebrand's Disease

Wilm's tumor
Renal cell carcinoma
Malignant lymphoma
Waldenström's disease
Multiple myeloma
Chronic lymphocytic leukemia
Hairy cell leukemia
Chronic myelogenous leukemia
Polycythemia vera
Essential (primary) thrombocythemia
Myelodysplastic syndromes

activity; however, this is an isolated report that remains unconfirmed.[88] Generally, noteworthy changes in the fibrinolytic system components have not been noted in patients with chronic myelogenous leukemia or chronic lymphocytic leukemia.[50,62,78] High plasminogen activator activity has been noted in association with chronic myeloid leukemias[89,90] but not lymphocytic leukemias.[5,50,52,78] One study has shown that 30% of patients with acute leukemia have excessive fibrinolytic activity; these patients also exhibited low antiplasmin levels and the presence of circulating plasmin-antiplasmin complexes. These findings did not correlate with findings suggestive of procoagulant activity or findings of DIC, and these fibrinolytic changes appear to be independent of intravascular procoagulant activity.[91]

Disseminated Intravascular Coagulation

Myeloblasts, promyelocytes, monocytes, and lymphoblasts all contain and can release procoagulant materials or enzymes in patients with acute leukemia.[3-5,50-52,64,92-97] As expected, DIC may complicate the course of acute leukemia in about 50% of patients.[98,99] Blast cells may have fibrinolytic activity or fibrinolytic system activator activity.[3-5,50,51,88,94,101-103] Granulocytes of chronic granulocytic leukemia are capable of releasing procoagulant enzymes, procoagulant activity, and antithrombin-type materials.[50,62] Granulocytes of chronic myelogenous leukemia release an antiheparinlike substance that is derived from myeloperoxidase.[50,104] Mature lymphocytes of chronic lymphocytic leukemia also release procoagulant materials that are phospholipoproteinlike or thromboplastinlike in composition.[5,50,52,60,78] Because of this ability to release procoagulant materials into the systemic circulation and potentially activate the coagulation system, essentially any leukemia may be associated with low-grade or fulminant DIC.[3,4,28,29,105-107] The most common leukemia associated with DIC is acute promyelocytic leukemia (FAB M3), followed by acute myelomonocytic leukemia (FAB M4), acute myeloblastic leukemia (FAB M1 and M2), and acute lymphoblastic leukemia (FAB L1-3), in descending order of probability.[5,28,29,105,106] Acute DIC is seen much less frequently in chronic leukemias than in acute leukemias and is more likely to

Table 12-7. Defective Hemostasis in Leukemia (Descending Order of Probability)

Thrombocytopenia

Platelet dysfunction

Disseminated intravascular coagulation
    Leukemia cell procoagulant activity
    Bacteremia
    Massive transfusions
    Shock

Coagulation protein defects
    Liver infiltration
    Cholestasis
    Drug induced

Primary fibrinolysis
    Leukemia cell proteolytic activity
    Drug induced

Vascular defects
    Infiltration
    Hyperviscosity/leukostasis
    Extramedullary hematopoiesis

Table 12-8. Malignancies Associated With Disseminated Intravascular Coagulation

Acute promyelocytic leukemia
Acute myelomonocytic leukemia
Acute myeloblastic leukemia
Lymphomas (immunoblastic)
Hodgkin's disease
Biliary cancer
Breast cancer
Colon cancer
Gastric cancer
Lung cancer
Malignant melanoma
Ovarian cancer
Prostate cancer

Disseminated Intravascular Coagulation

Hemorrhage and Solid Tumors

Although thrombosis is more commonly manifest with solid tumors and hemorrhage is more commonly associated with acute leukemias, hemorrhage may be a significant clinical problem in patients with solid tumors as well.[3,4] Intravascular coagulation is present in many patients with malignancy and manifests various clinical expressions, the most extreme form being acute fulminant DIC and catastrophic hemorrhage and thrombosis. Disseminated intravascular coagulation in patients with cancer may be low grade or fulminant.[5,28,32,48,105-107] The low-grade form is slightly more common and is manifest clinically by mild to moderate bleeding, usually of the integument or mucous membranes.[5,29,32,105] Easy and spontaneous bruising, petechiae and purpura, ecchymoses, gingival bleeding, and minor gastrointestinal bleeding coupled with thrombosis are the usual manifestations. In contrast, fulminant DIC is characterized by an explosive catastrophic hemorrhage, with bleeding usually being from at least three unrelated sites simultaneously.[29,32] The most commonly noted abnormalities are petechiae, purpura, and ecchymoses seen with significant gastrointestinal, pulmonary, or genitourinary hemorrhage. Most patients with acute DIC will manifest oozing from intravenous sites or sites of other invasive procedures, such as intra-arterial lines, subclavian catheters, and hepatic artery catheters.[3,4,28,29,32,105-107] Although these are the most common bleeding manifestations, more life-threatening bleeding, such as intracranial and intrapulmonary hemorrhage with massive hemoptysis, may also happen. This form of DIC has been noted in association with almost all types of solid tumors and is most commonly seen in carcinoma of the lung, gallbladder, stomach, colon, breast, ovary, malignant melanoma,[5,12,16,37,113-115] and prostate.[19,39,40,117] Table 12-8 lists the malignancies most commonly associated with DIC. In these latter disorders, initiation of chemotherapy has occasionally been associated

evolve with chronic myelogenous leukemia than with chronic lymphocytic leukemia. The development of DIC is of profound gravity for survival in acute leukemias and is a frequent complication in acute promyelocytic leukemia (FAB M3). The survival of patients with acute promyelocytic leukemia can be dramatically improved by suppressing development of DIC or by attenuating an existing DIC with the early application of low-dose (subcutaneous) heparin.[5,28,29,105,106,108,109]

Vascular Defects

Noteworthy vascular defects, which are repeatedly neglected or forgotten, may evolve in patients with acute leukemia. Vascular defects in leukemia may be responsible for or contribute to significant hemorrhage.[5,50,51] Although vascular defects are of clinical significance in acute leukemias, they are unlikely to be a clinical problem in chronic leukemias. Patients with acute leukemias commonly display increased vascular permeability because of infiltration of the vasculature by leukemic cells, hyperviscosity or leukostasis of the vasa vasorum, or foci of extramedullary hematopoiesis in the vessel wall.[5,110-112]

Many defects of hemostasis may be associated with acute and chronic leukemias, and when significant hemorrhage happens, the defects may be multifactorial and are a combination of any one, several, or all the earlier described defects. Only by carefully examining the patient from both the clinical and laboratory standpoint and carefully delineating the presence or absence of each of these defects can rational and effective therapy be delivered. Hemostasis syndromes associated with leukemia are summarized in Table 12-7.

with triggering or acceleration of DIC.[7,92,105,115,118] The initiation or enhancement of DIC in association with starting antineoplastic therapy is presumably caused by release of thromboplastinlike or other clot-promoting materials or enzymes from necrotic tumor cells. In acute promyelocytic leukemia, low-dose heparin therapy, given before starting cytotoxic drugs, may protect against this development.[105,108,109,119] Most patients with disseminated solid malignancy have some laboratory or clinical evidence of DIC, whereas many patients with malignancy never develop clinical manifestations of DIC, but laboratory findings of DIC are usually present. The patient with disseminated malignancy represents a special problem since DIC may be manifest as a fulminant, subacute, or low-grade form and, therefore, may be manifest as local thrombosis, diffuse thrombosis, thromboembolism, minor hemorrhage, diffuse hemorrhage, or any combination of these.[3,4,105-107]

There are many potential mechanisms by which malignancy provides triggers for DIC. The hemorrhagic syndrome associated with prostatic carcinoma was poorly understood for a long time. Many authors considered this to represent DIC with secondary fibrinolysis, while others thought the hemorrhage associated with prostatic carcinoma was a primary hyperfibrinolytic syndrome.[40,120] Both processes are clearly recognized to happen in malignant prostatic disease and may happen to a lesser extent in benign prostatic disease as well. Malignant prostatic tissue contains procoagulant materials that may be released into the circulation, triggering a disseminated intravascular clotting process with the usual secondary fibrinolytic response.[5] Malignant prostatic tissue may independently activate the fibrinolytic system either directly or indirectly, leading to a primary fibrino(geno)lytic syndrome.[5] Prostatic carcinoma is commonly associated with DIC and the usual secondary fibrinolytic response plus a primary fibrino(geno)lytic syndrome. This explains why, from the clinical and laboratory standpoint, prostatic carcinoma more often presents as an overwhelming fibrino(geno)lytic syndrome, a minimal procoagulant problem, and the clinical manifestation of this is, as expected, hemorrhage instead of diffuse thrombosis.[5] One study noted evidence for DIC, as defined by elevated FDPs and the presence of soluble fibrin monomer, in many patients before surgery for malignant prostatic disease.[121] Post–transurethral prostatic resection (TURP) blood loss appears to be correlated with preoperative evidence of DIC. These findings suggest that it is indicated to look for laboratory manifestations of DIC before undertaking TURP in patients with prostatic disease, since these parameters may predict postoperative bleeding, blood loss, and necessity of blood component replacement.[105,121]

Disseminated intravascular coagulation is commonly associated with pancreatic carcinoma. In this circumstance, DIC is more commonly manifest as diffuse thrombosis instead of diffuse hemorrhage, because the procoagulant activity dominates and secondary fibrinolysis is minimal. Disseminated intravascular coagulation, manifest as acute disseminated thrombosis, is more commonly seen in carci-

Table 12-9. Coagulation Abnormalities in Metastatic Malignancy

Elevated fibrinogen (with decreased survival)
Elevated fibrin(ogen) degradation products
Circulating soluble fibrin monomer
Elevated fibrinopeptide A
Elevated fibrinopeptide B
Cryofibrinogenemia
Decreased plasminogen
Elevated plasmin
Elevated B-beta 15-42–related peptides
Decreased fibronectin
Decreased antithrombin III
Decreased protein C
Elevated factor VIII:C
Thrombocytosis (with decreased survival)
Thrombocytopenia (with decreased survival)
Elevated platelet factor 4
Elevated beta-thromboglobulin

noma of the body and tail of the pancreas, because little ductal obstruction occurs and large amounts of trypsin are released, which have thrombinlike activity. In carcinoma of the head of the pancreas, more ductal obstruction occurs, less trypsin is released into the systemic circulation, and a DIC-type syndrome is less commonly associated.[5,38]

In patients with adenocarcinoma of many primary sites, the mechanism for DIC may be multifaceted. The sialic acid moiety of secreted mucin from adenocarcinomatous tissue can invoke the nonenzymatic activation of factor X to factor Xa.[16,37] This sequence can easily provide a trigger for systemic thrombin generation and a later course of fulminant or subacute DIC[105,122] or thrombosis alone.[5,105-107] It is probable that other less clearly defined mechanisms exist for initiating DIC in malignancy. The systemic release of necrotic tumor tissue and/or enzymes with procoagulant or phospholipoproteinlike activity may activate the early phases of coagulation and/or platelet release. Many tumors undergo neovascularization, which could potentially produce abnormal endothelial cell lining that may either cause a platelet release or cause generation of factors XIIa and XIa with subsequent procoagulant activation and the development of a fulminant, subacute, or low-grade DIC process.[105-107,123,124] Table 12-9 lists the usual laboratory features found in most patients with disseminated malignancy and disrupted hemostasis. These findings are often associated with and are interpreted as a hypercoagulable state or a propensity to thrombus formation, but they usually represent complicated changes of a subacute or low-grade disseminated intravascular clotting process that may or may not become clinically manifest.[5,28,29,46]

Another not uncommon trigger for DIC in the patient with malignancy is the use of LeVeen or Denver shunts for malignant ascites. Patients with malignant ascites must be carefully chosen for this procedure. If ascitic fluid is positive for malignant cells, the placement of a LeVeen shunt is usually not successful,[125] does not lead to significant prolongation of good-quality life, and is commonly associated with the development of a DIC process.[28,29,32,127-129] Disseminated intravascular coagulation may be blunted or aborted by removal of ascitic fluid at the time of shunt placement.[130] A less common although significant complication of LeVeen shunting in the patient with malignant ascites is thromboembolism.[125]

A significant amount of discussion has concerned the association of malignancy and DIC, which is one of the most common clinical settings where clinicians must contend with fulminant, subacute, or low-grade DIC. Disseminated intravascular coagulation may display highly varied clinical manifestations especially in malignancy. For example, the patient with malignancy may show accelerated procoagulant activity with minimal fibrinolytic response and diffuse thrombosis or may have a moderate procoagulant drive with overwhelming secondary fibrinolytic activation and subsequent purely hemorrhagic manifestations.[3,4,28,29,105-107] Any combination between these two extremes may be seen in patients with metastatic solid tumor.[3,4] The patient with malignancy and associated DIC presents a major problem in treatment, and a clear understanding and definition of possible triggering events is desirable and often necessary for efficacious control of the intravascular clotting process.[5,28,29,32]

Clinical Diagnosis

The clinical diagnosis of DIC need not be difficult to determine. The key to a high index of suspicion is simply to note the appropriate type of bleeding in the patient with malignancy.[3,4,105] The type of bleeding manifest by most patients with fulminant or subacute DIC suggests multiple hemostatic compartment defects. For example, most patients with fulminant DIC will bleed from at least three unrelated sites simultaneously.[3,4,28,29,105] This may be expressed in a wide variety of ways and commonly is seen as melena and hematochezia, epistaxis, or hemoptysis, in association with oozing from intra-arterial or intravenous invasion sites, hematuria, and associated findings of petechiae and purpura.[105-107] This type of bleeding or these combinations of bleeding should immediately suggest that multiple hemostatic compartments are involved. When noting this type of bleeding in patients with cancer, one can be almost assured of a diagnosis of DIC. Most patients with cancer and fulminant DIC also display shock and associated end-organ hypoxia and ischemic changes.[5,105] This may be manifest in a wide variety of ways, depending on end-organ involvement and degree of occlusive changes. Renal failure, resulting from fibrin thrombi deposited in the renal microvasculature, is a frequent manifestation as is pulmonary failure or central nervous system symptomatology. The interplay between coagulation proteins and other protein systems also must be recalled. Specifically, kinin generation and complement activation in these patients often account for many attendant signs and symptoms in these bleeding or thrombosing individuals, including pain and shock. Many patients with malignancy and subacute or low-grade DIC will not display

Table 12-10. Common Laboratory Manifestations of Fulminant DIC in Metastatic Malignancy

Microangiopathic hemolytic anemia
Shistocytosis
Reticulocytosis
Leukocytosis
Elevated fibrin(ogen) degradation products
Circulating soluble fibrin monomer
Decreased antithrombin III
Decreased protein C
Elevated fibrinopeptide A
Elevated B-beta 15-42–related peptides
Decreased fibronectin
Clotting factors: normal, up, or down
Hypoplasminogenemia
Circulating plasmin
Decreased antiplasmin
Thrombocytopenia
Decreased platelet survival
Large "young" platelets
Elevated platelet factor 4
Elevated beta-thromboglobulin

fulminant and multiple site bleeding, as is more typically seen in those with fulminant DIC. Patients with low-grade DIC more commonly have minor mucosal membrane bleeding often manifest as excessive gingival bleeding with toothbrushing, minor hemoptysis, bothersome epistaxis, and sometimes hematuria.[5,29,48,105-107] Patients with malignancy often have easy and spontaneous bruising and petechiae and purpura, which may not be noticed by the patient and may only represent minimal findings found by the clinician after attentive examination. When the patient with malignancy presents with diffuse thrombosis, this may only be a manifestation of the opposite clinical spectrum of DIC. In this setting, DIC should be strongly considered, and the patient appropriately examined for confirmatory proof. Proper therapy should be started if the diagnosis is confirmed.[48,105-107,131]

Laboratory Diagnosis

The laboratory diagnosis of DIC was discussed in detail in chapter 7; however, for those readers who are primarily interested in oncology the salient features will be discussed here. Although noting the appropriate type of bleeding in the appropriate clinical setting can essentially assure a diagnosis of DIC, laboratory confirmation is desirable, if not mandatory, before instituting a regimen of heparin, low-dose heparin, or other antiprocoagulant therapy in the patient with cancer. Understanding the pathophysiology of DIC makes it clear that these patients have innumerous abnormal laboratory test results of hemostasis. Most laboratory tests that are abnormal in DIC are only abnormal in the fulminant form of DIC. In subacute or low-grade DIC associated with malignancy, many laboratory parameters of hemostasis may be difficult to interpret or are within normal limits.[5,105-107,131] Table 12-10 lists the laboratory tests typically abnormal in

Table 12-11. Common Laboratory Manifestations of Low-Grade DIC in Metastatic Malignancy

Microangiopathic hemolytic anemia
Shistocytosis
Reticulocytosis
Leukocytosis
Fibrinogen borderline or normal
Clotting factors borderline or normal
Antithrombin III normal or decreased
Protein C normal or decreased
Circulating soluble fibrin monomer
Elevated fibrin(ogen) degradation products
Elevated fibrinopeptide A
Circulating plasmin
Plasminogen normal or decreased
Elevated B-beta 15-42 peptides
Platelets normal or borderline low
Large "young" platelets
Decreased platelet survival
Elevated platelet factor 4
Elevated beta-thromboglobulin

Table 12-12. Sequential Treatment of Disseminated Intravascular Coagulation in Malignancy

Treat the malignancy
    Surgery as indicated
    Radiation as indicated
    Chemotherapy and hormonal therapy as indicated

Stop intravascular clotting process
    Antiplatelet drug therapy
    Subcutaneous heparin, intravenous heparin (contraindicated
        with central nervous system metastases)

Component therapy as indicated
    Platelet concentrates
    Packed red blood cells (washed)
    Fresh frozen plasma
    Antithrombin III concentrates

Inhibit residual fibrino(geno)lysis
    Rarely, if ever, indicated
    Tranexamic acid, aminocaproic acid

Individualize therapy
    Type of malignancy
    Site(s) of bleeding and thrombosis
    Age
    Hemodynamic and medical status

fulminant DIC in patients with malignancy. Table 12-11 lists typical laboratory findings in patients with subacute or low-grade DIC. In addition to malignancy itself, other common complications of cancer may act as triggers for DIC, including sepsis, initiation of radiation therapy, microangiopathic hemolytic anemia, hemolysis of any etiology, hemolytic transfusion reactions, and transfusions of large amounts of banked whole blood.[28,29,32,105,106]

Therapy

Therapy for DIC in the patient with cancer represents a major clinical challenge. My approach is outlined in Table 12-12. Effective therapy is multiphasic and must be approached in a sequential and logical manner.[28,29,32,105,132] The first and essential modality is to treat the malignancy, since this supplies the trigger of procoagulant material for intravascular coagulation to evolve. Treatment may include surgery, radiotherapy, chemotherapy, or endocrine manipulation as the clinical situation warrants. Treatment of the trigger (tumor) is often associated with cessation or significant improvement of DIC. Until attempts at antineoplastic therapy are introduced, later therapy of bleeding or thrombosis is often unsuccessful. This is especially true if the manifestation of DIC and malignancy is thrombosis. Unless the malignancy is well controlled, patients with cancer are notoriously resistent to anticoagulant therapy.[3-5,48,105] Therapy must be highly individualized, depending on the overall medical condition of the patient, sites and severity of hemorrhage and thrombosis, sites of metastases, hemodynamic status, and age of the patient. If significant bleeding continues after reasonable attempts to control the malignancy, anticoagulant therapy must be considered. For the patient with malignancy and fulminant DIC, low-dose heparin therapy at 80 to 100 units/kg is given subcutaneously three to four times per day as the site and severity of hemorrhage or thrombosis dictate.[5,29,105] Patients with low-grade DIC and bothersome but not life-threatening hemorrhage may be given antiplatelet agents, such as aspirin and dipyridamole,[5] which are usually successful at stopping a low-grade intravascular clotting process. Antiplatelet agents in chronic DIC will usually require 24 to 36 hours to stop the intravascular clotting process, but low-dose heparin will usually stop the process within four to eight hours.[5,29]

Other Defects

Patients with cancer may also develop bleeding from other coagulation factor abnormalities, which are less common and are usually associated with less serious hemorrhage than that in DIC. Patients with malignancy, especially those with liver metastases, may acquire deficiencies of the vitamin K–dependent factors.[12,117] When this results in significant or life-threatening bleeding, vitamin K is usually ineffective, and the hemorrhage must be controlled with fresh frozen plasma or prothrombin complex concentrates.[133] Before using these modalities as primary approaches to therapy, however, DIC must be excluded. If the patient with malignancy develops extrahepatic or intrahepatic biliary obstruction and cholestasis, because of tumor at any site in the biliary tree, malabsorption of vitamin K and defective synthesis of the vitamin K–dependent factors are often associated.[5] In this setting, DIC may also happen, although this is less commonly a complication than simple defective synthesis of the vitamin K–dependent proteins.

Factor XIII deficiency or dysfunction is common in malignancy and is most pronounced in patients with liver metastases.[116,134] This deficiency may be the result of decreased factor XIII activators or impaired removal of factor XIII inhibitors by the invaded liver.[5] Factor XIII is associated with albumin, and patients with cancer and hypoalbuminemia may be factor XIII–deficient, although usually not to a clinically significant degree. In patients with cancer, acquired factor XIII deficiency may or may not cause hemorrhage. More commonly, impaired clot formation and poor wound healing are noted. Factor XIII deficiency thought to cause or contribute to hemorrhage in patients with cancer is managed by transfusions with fresh frozen plasma given at a dose of 5 mL/kg every seven to 10 days.[135]

Patients with liver metastases often have low levels of other clotting factors synthesized in the liver including fibrinogen, factor V, factor VIII:C, factor XI, factor XII, prekallikrein, high–molecular weight kininogen, plasminogen, AT III, protein C, protein S, and fibronectin.[5] The decreased synthesis of these are of unclear clinical significance. The development of a dysfibrinogenemia with either primary hepatoma or liver metastases is of particular concern in malignancy. Abnormalities in fibrin monomer polymerization are manifestations of this dysfibrinogenemia and may lead to hemorrhage in patients with disseminated malignancy and liver metastases or primary hepatoma.[3-5]

Acquired circulating anticoagulants may materialize in a wide variety of tumors, but these have been isolated findings in patients with cancer and often have an unclear relationship to actual hemorrhage. Many are heparinoid in nature and are found in association with carcinoma of the lung and myeloma.[3-5,48,136-140] Some appear to inhibit the activation phase of coagulation or act as antithrombins, and these have been most commonly noted in association with carcinoma of the breast.[134] Of more clinical significance, circulating anticoagulants in the form of FDPs may assume paramount clinical importance in patients with cancer with low-grade covert intravascular coagulation.[5,141] The mechanisms by which FDPs interfere with hemostasis were discussed in chapters 7 and 8. Circulating anticoagulants may assume major importance in the paraprotein disorders.

Primary Fibrino(geno)lysis

Primary fibrino(geno)lysis has been repeatedly noted in patients with metastatic malignancy.[5,19,33,42,116] In this disorder, hemorrhage, as was discussed in detail in chapters 7 and 8, is caused by plasmin-induced biodegradation of many clotting factors, including fibrinogen, factor V, factor VIII:C, and the impairment of hemostasis by circulating FDPs, which interfere with fibrin monomer polymerization, thrombin generation, and platelet function.[141,142] Although primary fibrinolysis happens in malignancy, DIC is a more common cause of hemorrhage in patients with cancer. Many malignant tissues are capable of spontaneous fibrinolytic

Table 12-13. Malignancies Associated With Primary Fibrino(geno)lysis

Sarcomas
Breast
Colon
Gastric
Thyroid

activity and activation of the fibrinolytic system, and this has been noted in patients with carcinoma of the breast, thyroid, colon, and stomach, but the greatest activity is seen in patients with disseminated sarcoma.[3-5,33] If patients with carcinoma of the breast, thyroid, colon, or stomach develop a systemic hemorrhagic syndrome, the cause is most probably DIC and only rarely is it primary activation of the fibrinolytic system and a primary fibrino(geno)lytic syndrome.[5] The opposite is true, however, in patients with disseminated sarcoma.[5] If these patients develop a systemic hemorrhagic syndrome, the most common cause is primary fibrino(geno)lysis, and only rarely is it from DIC.[3,4,33] Kwaan et al noted a decrease in tumor fibrinolytic activity in patients with liver metastases and ascribed this phenomena to increased levels of fibrinolytic inhibitors that appear with liver involvement.[143] Primary fibrino(geno)lytic hemorrhage is treated with agents that inhibit the fibrinolytic system. My approach is to give epsilon aminocaproic acid as an initial 5- to 10-g slow intravenous push followed by 1 to 2 g/hour for 24 hours or until bleeding stops.[5,144] After 24 hours the patient may be given oral therapy if necessary. Those using this agent should be aware of the hypotension, hypokalemia, and ventricular arrhythmias that may develop. The use of epsilon aminocaproic acid is contraindicated in the patient with DIC.[105] A newer and more potent antifibrinolytic now available and possibly associated with fewer undesirable effects is tranexamic acid, and the usual dose is 500 mg orally or intravenously every eight to 12 hours. Tumors associated with primary fibrinolysis are summarized in Table 12-13.

Platelets and Bleeding

Thrombocytopenia

Thrombocytopenia is clearly the most common cause of hemorrhage in patients with both solid tumors and hematologic malignancies.[5,17] Thrombocytopenia is commonly the result of bone marrow suppression by radiation therapy or chemotherapy, with alkylating agents clearly being the worst offenders.[145-147] Drugs inducing thrombocytopenia may be classified as mild, moderate, and severe, and these are summarized in Table 12-14. Thrombocytopenia also commonly results from bone marrow invasion by tumor and generally correlates well with marrow invasion.[5,7,12,17] Marrow metastases should be suspected when unexplained thrombocy-

Table 12-14. Intensity of Thrombocytopenia With Antineoplastic Drugs

Mild thrombocytopenia
  L-asparaginase
  Bleomycin
  Cis-platinum
  Diethylstilbesterol
  Prednisone
  Tamoxifen
  Vincristine

Moderate thrombocytopenia
  Actinomycin-D
  Cyclophosphamide
  5-fluorouracil
  6-mercaptopurine
  Methotrexate
  Procarbazine

Severe thrombocytopenia
  Busulfan
  Chlorambucil
  Cytosine arabinoside
  Melphalan
  Nitrogen mustard
  Nitrosourea compounds
  Vinblastine

topenia develops in patients with malignancy and carefully searched for by examination of the bone marrow aspirate or biopsy, although biopsy is more reliable than aspirate alone in detecting and evaluating bone marrow involvement by carcinoma.[5,148-152]

Aside from bone marrow suppressive therapy and marrow metastases, patients with cancer may develop other types of thrombocytopenia. When splenomegaly develops as a part of the malignant process, hypersplenism and later thrombocytopenia may follow.[5,147,153] Development of splenic metastases is more common than generally recognized, especially in carcinoma of the lung, breast, prostate, colon, and stomach,[5,154,155] which may lead to reactive hypersplenism and thrombocytopenia.[5,17,147] If clinically feasible, splenectomy may be of benefit in these situations. If splenectomy is considered, in an attempt to control thrombocytopenia secondary to hypersplenism, a preoperative infusion of epinephrine may help in predicting the response to this procedure.[3-5,106] When thrombocytopenia from decreased bone marrow production or increased splenic sequestration becomes significant, platelet concentrates provide the mainstay of management.[147] Platelet counts below 10×10^9/L (10,000/mm^3) are commonly associated with spontaneous and serious hemorrhage, whereas platelet counts greater than 30×10^9/L (30,000/mm^3) are usually not associated with this complication unless the patient undergoes trauma or surgical stress.[147,156] My general approach is to infuse platelet concentrates in most situations in which a platelet count is less than 10×10^9/L (10,000/mm^3) unless the patient develops signs of bleeding

above this level or when surgery or other invasive procedures are planned.[5,147] Platelet concentrates are now readily available and provide the most efficient modality of platelet replacement therapy. An ideal platelet concentrate contains about 1.2×10^{11} platelets, and generally one unit of platelet concentrate will elevate the platelet count by approximately 5 to 7×10^9/L (5,000 to 7,000/mm^3) in an adult and by approximately 10 to 12×10^9/L (10,000 to 12,000/mm^3) in an infant.[157] In practice, 8 to 10 units of platelet packs are usually administered to the severely thrombocytopenic adult every time the platelet count decreases to below 10×10^9/L (10,000/mm^3). Appropriately reduced numbers are used for children and infants.[157] If long-term platelet transfusions are foreseen and proper facilities are available, HLA-compatible platelets should be used if possible, especially in patients with leukemia who may be candidates for bone marrow transplantation.[3-5] Directed single-donor platelets are preferred over random-donor platelets.

Autoimmune thrombocytopenia purpura (ITP) occasionally happens in patients with solid tumors but is more commonly noted in patients with lymphoid malignancies.[147,158] When ITP happens in association with malignancy, the approach to management should be the use of steroids and possibly splenectomy if indicated and as was outlined in chapter 5. In cases of ITP refractory to the usual forms of therapy, the use of intravenous vincristine or intravenous gamma globulin may be potentially useful.[159,160] Another type of increased platelet destruction that may sometimes be associated with malignancy is thrombotic thrombocytopenic purpura (TTP).[5,147,161,162] This rare syndrome is commonly fatal when it develops in the patient with cancer but may respond to vigorous plasmapheresis, plasma exchange, or the use of intravenous prostacyclins,[161] as was discussed in chapter 5.

Platelet Function Defects

Abnormalities of platelet function are commonly found in association with both solid and hematologic malignancies. Because of frequent episodes of intravascular coagulation and resulting elevated FDPs noted in patients with cancer, the coating of platelet surfaces by these fragments probably is the most common cause of platelet dysfunction in patients with malignancy.[3,4,141] However, other platelet function abnormalities are also noted in these patients. Platelet factor 3 is commonly decreased in patients with cancer.[163] Other platelet function defects have also been consistently noted and include defective platelet aggregation to ADP and other presumptive evidence of platelet dysfunction as manifest by a prolonged thromboplastin generation test, prolonged template bleeding times, positive results of tourniquet tests, and poor clot retraction.[7,163-165] It is unclear whether these defects develop secondary to the malignancy itself, whether they happen from partial release of platelet contents after contact with malignant tissue, or whether they develop in response to circulating activated clotting factors. The malignant paraprotein disorders are frequently associated with platelet

Table 12-15. Hemorrhagic Syndromes Seen With Metastatic Malignancy (Descending Order of Probability)

Thrombocytopenia
Disseminated intravascular coagulation
Decreased clotting factors
Primary fibrino(geno)lysis
Platelet dysfunction
Vascular defects
Circulating anticoagulants

function abnormalities that develop from coating of platelet surfaces by circulating immunoglobulins.[5,166,167] Consistent platelet aggregation abnormalities are found in the myeloproliferative syndromes[3,5,45] and in preleukemia.[5,163] The exact significance of these many platelet function defects in contributing to hemorrhage in patients with solid tumors is unclear. These platelet function defects, however, may correlate better with the development of hemorrhage in patients with cancer than does the actual platelet count.[3,5,163,164] At the very least, these defects must be presumed to be active in aggravating bleeding in patients with cancer who have an already severely compromised hemostasis system or attendant thrombocytopenia.[3,5]

Clinical clues to platelet dysfunction include the noting of easy or spontaneous bruising, gingival bleeding, petechiae and purpura, and other minor forms of mucosal membrane bleeding in association with a normal platelet count. A prolonged template bleeding time is a reasonable screening test for the possibility of platelet dysfunction in patients with malignancy. When noting a prolonged template bleeding time in patients with malignancy, platelet aggregation or lumi-aggregation should be done to document the presence or absence of this defect and to delineate the type and severity of defect present.[168] Unless secondary to intravascular coagulation, bleeding resulting from or aggravated by platelet dysfunction calls for platelet concentrate replacement therapy, which should be approached in essentially the same manner as that outlined for thrombocytopenia (see chapter 5). The patient with malignancy and a documented associated platelet function defect should be strongly cautioned regarding the use of common drugs known to interfere with platelet function (see chapter 4). Mechanisms of hemorrhage in metastatic malignancy are summarized in Table 12-15.

Malignant Paraprotein Disorders

Defects in hemostasis associated with malignant paraprotein disorders are well known, because these commonly lead to significant clinical hemorrhage and subsequent serious treatment difficulties in patients with these disorders. Alterations of hemostasis in malignant paraprotein disorders are expressed as either hemorrhage, thrombosis, or a combination of the two; however, hemorrhage is more common than thrombosis.[3,166]

The actual incidence of hemorrhage in malignant paraprotein disorders varies somewhat depending on the particular paraprotein present. About 15% of patients with IgG myeloma experience hemorrhage, whereas those with IgA myeloma have a 40% chance of hemorrhage.[3,166] Patients with Waldenström's macroglobulinemia or IgM myeloma have a greater than 60% chance of significant hemorrhage.[6,166,169]

Hemorrhage occurs for many reasons in patients with malignant paraprotein disorders, and some of these are not caused by alterations of the hemostasis system. The most common reasons for hemorrhage are abnormalities in hemostasis, which are manifestations of circulating paraprotein. Uremia and attendant abnormal platelet function account for significant hemorrhage in many of these patients. Liver failure or hypersplenism may also be associated with defects in hemostasis in patients with malignant paraprotein disorders.[3,48,166] Hypersplenism is a frequent accompaniment of malignant paraprotein disorders, and significant thrombocytopenia resulting from splenic sequestration of platelets may reach alarming proportions. Many patients with malignant paraprotein disorders develop liver disease with resultant decreased synthesis of the vitamin K–dependent factors, abnormal fibrinogen (dysfibrinogenemia), abnormal fibrinolytic activity, and other coagulation protein defects associated with diffuse myelomatous involvement of the liver. Disseminated intravascular coagulation has been reported in myeloma and may account for significant hemorrhage in some patients. Thrombocytopenia resulting from chemotherapy or radiation therapy may also lead to hemorrhage in patients with malignant paraprotein disorders. Significant thrombocytopenia obviously may result from bone marrow replacement in multiple myeloma, light chain disease, or Waldenström's macroglobulinemia.

Thrombocytopenia

Thrombocytopenia is commonly seen in malignant paraprotein disorders but is often not pronounced enough to account for clinically significant bleeding. Thrombocytopenia can happen via several mechanisms in myeloma, primarily by the development of hypersplenism and increased platelet sequestration, liver disease, radiation therapy, chemotherapy, or bone marrow replacement.

Platelet Dysfunction

Platelet function defects are more common causes of hemorrhage in malignant paraprotein disorders than is thrombocytopenia.[5,166] Many patients with multiple myeloma show a prolonged template bleeding time that correlates well with clinical bleeding, but many patients will have normal or shortened bleeding times even with marked defects in platelet function. Results of platelet aggregation or lumi-aggregation studies are usually markedly abnormal in most patients with circulating paraprotein, and these studies correlate better with predisposition to clinical hemorrhage.[3,5,166] Platelet aggregation abnormalities in a patient with multiple myeloma both before and after plasmapheresis are shown in

Figure 12-1. Platelet Dysfunction in Myeloma (Preplasmapheresis)

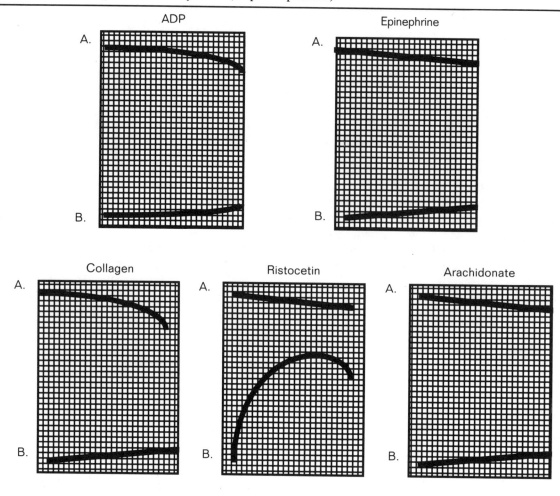

A. = Release Reaction
B. = Aggregation

Figures 12-1 and 12-2. Abnormalities of platelet function in multiple myeloma have not been clearly defined but usually result from coating of platelet membrane surfaces by paraprotein.[3,5,166] Platelet aggregation abnormalities are seen in about 80% of patients with myeloma. These defects do not correlate well with the type of paraprotein[3,166] but do appear to correlate with the quantity of paraprotein circulating. Platelet factor 3 release has been normal more often than abnormal in my patient population with myeloma and associated abnormal platelet lumi-aggregation.[48] It is thought that platelet membrane coating by paraprotein is not an antigen-antibody reaction but simply a chemical paraprotein-protein interaction with platelet membrane receptor sites. Poor correlation exists between platelet aggregation abnormalities and template bleeding times in multiple myeloma or other malignant paraprotein disorders. Up to 80% of patients with malignant paraprotein disorders have markedly abnormal aggregation and release. Epinephrine-induced aggregation is abnormal in about 90% of patients, ADP-induced aggregation and release is abnormal in about 60% of

patients, and collagen-induced aggregation is abnormal in about 60% of patients with malignant paraprotein disorders.[170] The most sensitive indicator of abnormal platelet aggregation in multiple myeloma is epinephrine-induced platelet aggregation.[3,5,166] Some individuals show markedly abnormal platelet lumi-aggregation but will have normal template bleeding times and the absence of clinical bleeding.

Other causes of abnormal platelet function in multiple myeloma include uremia, the development of liver disease, and circulating FDPs. Malignant paraproteins may coat the vasculature, interfere with normal endothelial function, or precipitate in the vasa vasorum causing interference with vascular function. Paraprotein may also interfere with in vivo collagen-induced platelet aggregation. All these occurrences may account for not only prolonged template bleeding times but also interference with the normal platelet-endothelial cell interaction.

Coagulation Proteins

Malignant paraprotein may interfere with coagulation proteins. Probably the most publicized change of the coagu-

Figure 12-2. Platelet Dysfunction in Myeloma (Postplasmapheresis)

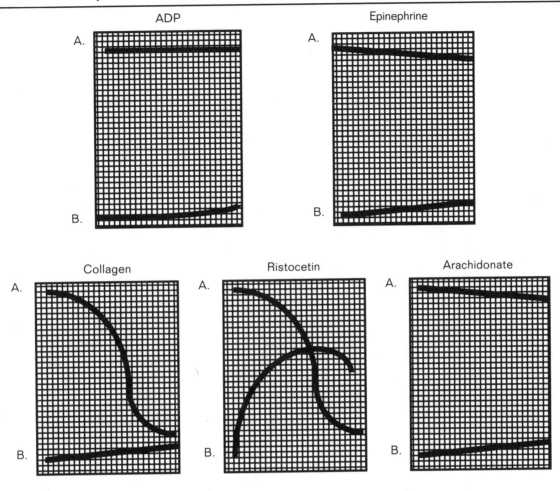

A. = Release Reaction
B. = Aggregation

lation system in malignant paraprotein disorders is inhibition of a single specific clotting factor, such as factor VIII:C. In reality, however, this phenomenon is rare and the least common cause of hemorrhage by paraprotein–coagulation protein interactions. When specific inhibition of blood coagulation factors by paraprotein does happen, it is usually somewhat selective. For example, IgG paraprotein is commonly directed against factors II, VII, X, or thrombin; alternatively IgA and IgM paraprotein are more commonly directed against the larger coagulation proteins, usually factors V and VIII:C activity. The most common coagulation protein interaction is inhibition of fibrin monomer polymerization. Paraprotein selectively attacks fibrin monomer and impedes polymerization into a stable fibrin clot. It is unclear if paraprotein coats the intact fibrinogen molecule and impedes the generation of fibrin monomer after exposure to thrombin or, alternatively, if paraprotein attacks fibrin monomer only after its generation from fibrinogen.[166,167] It has been proposed, but not proven, that the Fab segment is the primary site of attachment to fibrin monomer by para-

protein. An abnormal thrombin time or reptilase time is a good indication of inhibition of fibrin monomer polymerization in paraprotein disorders and correlates well with clinical hemorrhage resulting from this phenomenon.[3,5,166] An abnormal thrombin time or reptilase time is often noted in more than 50% of patients with malignant paraprotein disorders.[3,166] An abnormal thrombin time or reptilase time is correlated with clinical bleeding but not with the quantity or type of paraprotein present. Acquired von Willebrand's syndrome may be noted in association with malignant paraprotein diseases, whereas in myeloma, this association has been noted to be because of an inhibition by paraprotein of von Willebrand factor.[171-173]

Other Defects

Low-grade DIC is present in some patients with malignant paraprotein disorders, although this is uncommon.[3,5,166] Enhanced fibrinolytic activity is present in many patients with malignant paraprotein disorders, which is manifest by circulating elevated FDPs, circulating plasmin, and the absence of soluble fibrin monomer complexes. The mechanism for this activity, however, is unclear. To further complicate these defects, rare patients develop circulating heparinoids that have, on occasion, been responsible for severe fatal hemorrhage.[136-138]

Management

Therapy for hemorrhage in patients with malignant or benign paraprotein disorders presents difficult management problems. The exact alterations of hemostasis associated with hypersplenism, uremia, liver infiltration, and bone marrow infiltration are usually best controlled by proper management of the paraprotein disorder itself. This also applies to paraprotein inhibition of platelet function, coagulation protein defects, or interference by paraprotein of fibrin monomer polymerization. Often, these defects will correct partly, and sometimes completely, with decreases in the myeloma cell population induced by chemotherapy or radiation therapy. When bleeding becomes severe and rapid control of hemorrhage is called for, vigorous plasmapheresis is usually effective for rapidly lowering the paraprotein concentration and restoring normal or near normal hemostasis.[174] As mentioned earlier, the use of DDAVP has been useful in aborting bleeding associated with acquired von Willebrand's syndrome in myeloma.

Chemotherapy

Chemotherapeutic agents may alter hemostasis by a variety of mechanisms.[3,5] The most common and significant of these include the thrombocytopenia commonly associated with bone marrow suppressive cytotoxic drugs or the initiation or enhancement of DIC by cytotoxic drugs or hormones in conditions involving both solid tumors and acute promyelocytic or myelomonocytic leukemia. Antineoplastic agents that may significantly interfere with hemostasis and their mechanisms are listed in Table 12-16.

L-Asparaginase therapy is often accompanied by substantial hypofibrinogenemia, which is a common complication of this drug. Although earlier investigators attributed this phenomena to decreased fibrinogen synthesis,[175] others have shown this to result from the synthesis of functionally abnormal fibrinogen. This probably arises from reactions between L-asparaginase and asparagine residues of the fibrinogen molecule.[176] L-Asparaginase may also induce a DIC-type syndrome. Mithramycin therapy may be associated with hemorrhage in more than 50% of patients receiving this drug. Although mithramycin causes thrombocytopenia, hemorrhage more often results from impaired platelet function, hyperfibrino(geno)lysis, and decreased levels of factors II, V, VIII:C, and X.[3,177] In view of these findings, the triggering of DIC by mithramycin seems probable. Actinomycin D is also associated with hemorrhage. Actinomycin D is a potent vitamin K antagonist and causes defective (PIVKA) synthesis of factors II, VII, IX, and X.[178] Mitomycin is asso-

Table 12-16. Antineoplastic Drugs Altering Hemostasis

Drug	Mechanism
Actinomycin-D	Vitamin K antagonist
L-asparaginase	Dysfibrinogenemia, hypofibrinogenemia
Melphalan	Platelet dysfunction, hypofibrinogenemia
Mithramycin	Thrombocytopenia, DIC syndrome
Adriamycin	Primary fibrinolysis
Daunomycin	Primary fibrinolysis
Methotrexate	Platelet dysfunction

ciated with the development of a microangiopathic hemolytic anemia.[179-182] Adriamycin[183] and Daunomycin[184] cause primary activation of the fibrinolytic system and sometimes clinical hemorrhage. Melphalan, cytosine arabinoside, rubidomycin, vincristine, and vinblastine induce platelet dysfunction that may contribute to bleeding in patients receiving these antineoplastics.[3,185] Thrombosis due to single or multiple agent chemotherapy or hormonal therapy has been repeatedly reported.[5,186-190]

Bone Marrow Transplantation

The most common defect in hemostasis associated with bone marrow transplantation is hepatic veno-occlusive disease. This syndrome occurs three to four weeks' posttransplantation, is probably due to aggressive preconditioning radiochemotherapy, and is characterized by sudden weight gain, hepatomegaly, ascites, hyperbilirubinemia, and hepatic encephalopathy. This syndrome is preceded by three to four days of thrombocytopenia, usually refractory to platelet transfusions. It was initially thought that hepatic veno-occlusive disease posttransplantation may be related to graft vs host disease; however, there is probably no such relationship. The initial symptomatology of hepatic veno-occlusive disease can be confused with graft vs host disease. The incidence in major transplantation centers is about 40% with the highest incidence being noted in aggressively preconditioned patients with acute leukemia or in patients who have pretransplantation transaminasemia. The mortality may be from 30% to 45%.[191,192] Shulman and associates found an overall incidence of 21% among transplant patients, with a mortality of 33%.[193] This study evaluated the molecular and cellular events associated with veno-occlusive disease by use of immunofluorescent staining with anti–factor VIII, antifibrinogen, and antibody to platelet glycoprotein Ib. In the 11 patients studied, eight had widespread hepatic changes and three had patchy lesions. The lesions were associated with marked widening of the subendothelial zone of terminal hepatic venules and sublobular veins by fragmented red blood cells within an edematous background. The central lobar area had severe congestion with hemorrhagic necrosis of hepatocytes. Of eight patients with late veno-occlusive disease, five had diffuse fibrous obliteration of most central venules associated with atrophy of central lobar hepatocytes, sinusoidal widening, and fibrosis. The remaining three patients with late veno-occlusive disease had only focal fibrotic obliterative changes of the central venules. Immunohistochemical stains revealed that nine of the 11 patients with early veno-occlusive disease demonstrated intense immunostaining of the adventitial portion of the central vein walls (intima) with anti–factor VIII and some patients had additional immunostaining for anti–factor VIII in the subendothelial zone. A significant number of patients with early veno-occlusive disease had anti-fibrinogen staining on both the central venules and in the central lobar areas. However, none of the patients showed immunostaining for antibody to platelet glycoprotein Ib. This study indicates that in the early stages of veno-occlusive disease the coagulation system is activated around and within the walls of the central venules. Veno-occlusive disease and its sequelae, the deposition of interstitial collagens, can be considered a form of localized wound healing confined to the central lobar area of the liver acinus. The liver immunohistochemical studies suggest that coagulation proteins are first deposited within the adventitial zone of affected terminal hepatic venules before involving the subendothelial zone. Shulman and associates were unable to explain the lack of antiplatelet glycoprotein Ib but suggested this may have resulted from either postmortem autolysis or lysis of platelet thrombi following aggregation.

An additional complication that has, on occasion, been associated with bone marrow transplantation is nonbacterial thrombotic endocarditis. Jerman and Fick described two patients treated with bone marrow transplantation who subsequently developed fatal nonbacterial thrombotic endocarditis.[194] These particular patients developed typical findings of DIC, soft systolic cardiac murmurs, hematuria, and signs of cerebral embolic events. The overall incidence of nonbacterial thrombotic endocarditis in bone marrow transplant recipients may approximate 10%.[195]

Summary

Patients with malignancy may experience many alterations of hemostasis, which are multifaceted and must be taken into account when trying to control hemorrhage or thrombosis in patients with cancer. Hemorrhage or thrombosis is often the final fatal event in many patients with metastatic solid tumor or hematologic malignancies. Patients with malignancy present a major clinical challenge in this new era of oncologic awareness, and more aggressive care has led to prolonged survival for patients and a longer timeframe during which these complications may develop. These alterations of hemostasis must be approached in a sequential and logical manner with respect to diagnosis; only in this way can responsible, effica-cious, and rational therapy be delivered to patients. By far the most common alteration of hemostasis in malignancy is that of hemorrhage associated with thrombocytopenia, induced by drugs, radiation, or bone marrow invasion. Hemorrhage resulting from DIC is also common and may present as hemorrhage, thrombosis, thromboembolus, or any combination of these. Many antineoplastic drugs and radiation therapy may lead to or significantly enhance hemorrhage in patients with malignancy. Thrombosis, also commonly seen in patients with malignancy, is often a manifestation of low-grade DIC, conspicuous as an intravascular thrombotic or thromboembolic event instead of an intravascular proteolytic (hemorrhagic) event. When suspecting this, confirmatory laboratory evidence must be sought, and the patient treated appropriately. When approaching the patient with malignancy and either hemorrhage or thrombosis, all the potential defects in hemostasis must be taken into account, defined from the laboratory standpoint, and treated in as precise and logical a manner as possible.

References

1. Trousseau A: Phlegmasia alba dolens. Clinique Medicale de L'Hotel Dieu de Paris 3, ed 2. Paris, Balliere, 1865.

2. Morrison M: An analysis of the blood picture in 100 cases of malignancy. J Lab Clin Med 17:1071, 1932.

3. Bick RL: Alterations of hemostasis associated with malignancy: etiology, pathophysiology, diagnosis and management. Semin Thromb Hemost 5:1, 1978.

4. Bick RL: Alterations of hemostasis associated with malignancy, ch 11. In: G Murano, RL Bick (Eds): Basic Concepts of Hemostasis and Thrombosis. CRC Press, Boca Raton, FL, 1980, p 213.

5. Bick RL: Alerations of hemostasis in malignancy, ch 10. In: Disorders of Hemostasis and Thrombosis: Principles of Clinical Practice. Thieme, Inc., New York, 1985, p 262.

6. Amundsen MA, JA Spitell, JH Thompson: Hypercoagulability associated with malignant disease and with the postoperative state. Ann Intern Med 58:608, 1963.

7. Davis RB, A Theologides, BJ Kennedy: Comparative studies of blood coagulation and platelet aggregation in patients with cancer and non-malignant disease. Ann Intern Med 71:67, 1969.

8. Edwards EA: Migrating thrombophlebitis associated with carcinoma. N Engl J Med 240:1031, 1949.

9. Fisch C, AW Jones, WD Gambill: Acute thrombophlebitis associated with carcinoma of the stomach. Gastroenterology 18:290, 1951.

10. Innerfield I, A Anrist, JW Benjamin: Plasma antithrombin patterns in disturbances of the pancreas. Gastroenterology 19:843, 1951.

11. Goldsmith GH: Hemostatic disorders associated with malignancy, ch 11. In: OD Ratnoff, CD Forbes (Eds): Disorders of Hemostasis. WB Saunders, Philadelphia, 1991, p 352.

12. Miller SP, J Sanchez-Avalos, T Stefanski: Coagulation disorders in cancer, I: clinical and laboratory studies. Cancer 20:1452, 1967.

13. Perlow S, JL Daniels: Venous thrombosis and obscure abdominal malignancy. Arch Intern Med 97:184, 1956.

14. Sproul EF: Carcinoma and venous thrombosis: the frequency of association of carcinoma in the body or tail of the pancreas with multiple venous thrombosis. Am J Cancer 34:566, 1938.

15. Fumarola D, G del Bono: The blood coagulation patterns in malignancy. Prog Med Napoli 14:327, 1958.

16. Pineo GF, MC Brain, AS Gallus: Tumors, mucus production, and hypercoagulability. Ann N Y Acad Sci 230:262, 1974.

17. Slickter SJ, LA Harker: Hemostasis in malignancy. Ann N Y Acad Sci 230:252, 1974.

18. Astedt B, L Svanberg, IM Nilsson: Cancer, FDP, and radiotherapy. Br Med J 2:47, 1972.

19. Phillips LL, V Skrodelis, CA Furey: The fibrinolytic enzyme system in prostatic cancer. Cancer 12:721, 1959.

20. Yip ML, S Lee, HJ Sacks: Nonspecificity of the protamine sulfate test for intravascular coagulation. Am J Clin Pathol 57:487, 1972.

21. Boughton BJ, A Simpson: Plasma fibronectin in acute leukemia. Br J Haematol 51:487, 1982.

22. Rickles FR, RL Edwards, C Barb: Abnormalities of blood coagulation in patients with cancer. Fibrinopeptide A generation and tumor growth. Cancer 51:301, 1983.

23. Douglas JT, GDO Lowe, CD Forbes: Beta-thromboglobulin and platelet counts: effect of malignancy, infection, age, and obesity. Thromb Res 25:459, 1982.

24. Yodo Y, T Abe: Fibrinopeptide A (FPA) level and fibrinogen kinetics in patients with malignant disease. Thromb Haemost 46:706, 1981.

25. Choate JJ, DF Mosher: Fibronectin concentration in plasma of patients with breast cancer, colon cancer, and acute leukemia. Cancer 51:1142, 1983.

26. Walenga JM, J Fareed, G Mariani: Diagnostic efficacy of a simple radioimmunoassay test for fibrinogen/fibrin fragments containing the B-beta 15-42 sequence. Semin Thromb Hemost 10:252, 1984.

27. Fareed J, JM Walenga, RL Bick: Impact of automation on the quantitation of low molecular weight markers of hemostatic defects. Semin Thromb Hemost 9:355, 1983.

28. Bick RL: Disseminated intravascular coagulation and related syndromes, ch 6. In: Disorders of Hemostasis and Thrombosis: Principles of Clinical Practice. Thieme, Inc., New York, 1985, p 157.

29. Bick RL: Disseminated intravascular coagulation: a clinical review. Semin Thromb Hemost 14:299, 1988.

30. Bick RL, T Adams: Fibrinolytic activity in myeloproliferative disorders. Clin Res 21:264, 1973.

31. Bick RL: Clinical relevance of antithrombin III. Semin Thromb Hemost 8:276, 1982.

32. Baker WF: Clinical aspects of disseminated intravascular coagulation: a clinician's point of view. Semin Thromb Hemost 15:1, 1989.

33. Cliffton EE, CE Grossi: Fibrinolytic activity of human tumors as measured by the fibrinplate method. Cancer 8:1146, 1955.

34. Enck RE, CN Rios: Tamoxifen treatment of metastatic breast cancer and antithrombin III levels. Cancer 53:2607, 1984.

35. Boggust WA, DJ O'Brien, RA O'Meara: The coagulative factors of normal human and human cancer tissue. Irish J Med Sci 6:131, 1963.

36. O'Meara RAQ: Coagulation properties of cancers. Irish J Med Sci 394:474, 1958.

37. Pineo GF, F Regorczi, MWC Hatton: The activation of coagulation by extracts of mucin: a possible pathway of intravascular coagulation accompanying adenocarcinomas. J Lab Clin Med 82:255, 1973.

38. Gore I: Thrombosis and pancreatic cancer. Am J Pathol 29:1093, 1953.

39. Owen CA, HC Oels, EJW Bowie: Chronic intravascular coagulation syndrome. Thromb Diath Haemorrh 36:197, 1969.

40. Rapaport SI, CG Chapman: Coexistent hypercoagulability and acute hypofibrinogenemia in a patient with prostatic carcinoma. Am J Med 27:144, 1959.

41. Brown RC, DC Campbell, JH Thompson: Increased fibrinolysis with malignant disease. Arch Intern Med 109:129, 1962.

42. Omar JB, HS Saxena, HS Mitel: Fibrinolytic activity in malignant diseases. J Assoc Physicians India 19:293, 1971.

43. Moolten SE, L Vroman, GMS Broman: Role of blood platelets in thromboembolism. Arch Intern Med 84:667, 1949.

44. Levin J, CL Conley: Thrombocytosis associated with malignant disease. Arch Intern Med 114:487, 1964.

45. Adams T, L Shultz, L Goldberg: Platelet function abnormalities in the myeloproliferative disorders. Scand J Haematol 13:215, 1974.

46. Bick RL: Hypercoagulability and thrombosis, ch 12. In: Disorders of Thrombosis and Hemostasis. Thieme, Inc., New York, 1985, p 294.

47. Patterson WP, QS Ringenberg: The pathophysiology of thrombosis in cancer. Semin Oncol 17:140, 1990.

48. Bick RL: Treatment of bleeding and thrombosis in the patient with cancer, ch 5. In: T Nealon (Ed): Management of the Patient With Cancer. WB Saunders, Philadelphia, 1976, p 48.

49. Kumar S, B Monorama: Pre-leukemic acute myelogenous leukemia. Acta Haematol 3:21, 1970.

50. Lisiewicz J: Mechanisms of hemorrhage in leukemias. Semin Thromb Hemost 4:241, 1978.

51. Coleman RW, RN Rubin: Disseminated intravascular coagulation due to malignancy. Semin Oncol 17:172, 1990.

52. Lisiewicz J: Disseminated intravascular coagulation in acute leukemia. Semin Thromb Hemost 14:339, 1988.

53. Boggs DR, MM Wintrobe, CE Cartwright: Acute leukemias: analysis of 322 cases and review of the literature. Medicine 41:163, 1962.

54. Evans HE, IJ Wolman: Problems in the diagnosis and management of acute leukemia in childhood. Clin Pediatr 10:571, 1971.

55. Moszczynski P, J Lisiewicz: The liver function in leukemic patients in the light of enzymatic studies. Pol Tyg Lek 29:1925, 1974.

56. Holt JM, EG Gordon-Smith: Retinal abnormalities in diseases of the blood. Br J Ophthalmol 53:145, 1969.

57. Hersh EM, GP Bodey, BA Nies: Causes of death in acute leukemia: a ten-year study of 414 patients from 1954–1963. JAMA 193:105, 1965.

58. Han T, L Stutzman, E Cohen: Effect of platelet transfusion on hemorrhage in patients with acute leukemia. Cancer 19:1937, 1966.

59. Moszczynski P, J Lisiewicz: Early symptoms of acute and chronic leukemias in 300 patients. Med Wiejska 8:249, 1973.

60. Kuznik BI, EL Kuzmiehco, GP Alnikov: On the role of leukocytes in the process of blood coagulation in chronic lymphocytic leukemia. Probl Gematol Pereliv Krovi 14:3, 1969.

61. Seifter EJ, WR Bell: Platelet disorders, ch 2. In: Coagulation Disorders in the Cancer Patient. Futura Publishing Co, Mt Kisco, New York, 1984, p 15.

62. Lisiewicz J: Chronic granulocytic leukemia, ch 3. In: Hemorrhage in Leukemias. Polish Medical Publishers, Warsaw, 1976, p 82.

63. Brakman P, J Synder, ES Henderson: Blood coagulation and fibrinolysis in acute leukemia. Br J Haematol 18:135, 1970.

64. Ventura GJ, JP Hester, DO Dixon: Analysis of risk factors for fatal hemorrhage during induction therapy of patients with acute promyelocytic leukemia. Hematol Pathol 3:23, 1989.

65. Foon KA, RE Champlin, RP Gale: Acute myelogenous leukemia and the myelodysplastic syndromes, ch 56. In: CM Haskell (Ed): Cancer Treatment. WB Saunders, Philadelphia, 1990, p 589.

66. Rosove MH, GE Schwartz: Hematologic complications of cancer and its treatment, ch 77. In: CM Haskell (Ed): Cancer Treatment. WB Saunders, Philadelphia, 1990, p 850.

67. Caen J, Z Sinakoz, V Sultan: Les troubles du functionnement des plaquettes dans les leukemies myeloides chroniques. Nouv Rev Fr Hematol 6:719, 1966.

68. Cardamone JM, J Edson, JK McArthur: Abnormalities of platelet function in the myeloproliferative disorders. JAMA 221:270, 1972.

69. Sultan Y, J Delobel, J Caen: Anomalies de l'hemostase primaire au cours des leucemies myeloides chroniques et des autres syndromes myeloproliferatifs. Actual Hematol (Paris) 3:95, 1969.

70. Miyagawa K, Kawakita Y: Ultrastructure of blood platelets in various hematologic disorders. Acta Haematol (Japan) 32:64, 1969.

71. Bick RL, WL Wilson: Essential (hemorrhagic) thrombocythemia: a clinical and laboratory study of 14 patients. Am J Clin Pathol 81:799, 1984.

72. Bick RL: Essential (primary) thrombocythemia. Hematology Check Sample #H-86-4, vol 3, no 4. American Society of Clinical Pathologists, Chicago, 1989.

73. Wehmeier A, RE Scharf, S Fricke: Bleeding and thrombosis in chronic myeloproliferative disorders: relation of platelet disorders to clinical aspects of the disease. Haemostasis 19:251, 1989.

74. Rosner F, JV Dobbs, DN Ritz: Disturbances of hemostasis in acute myeloblastic leukemia. Acta Haematol 43:65, 1970.

75. Cowan DM, MJ Haut: Platelet function in acute leukemia. J Lab Clin Med 79:893, 1972.

76. Lisiewicz J, P Moszcynski: Disturbances of hemostasis in patients with various leukemia types in the light of results of basic tests of blood coagulation and fibrinolysis. Przegl Lek 29:389, 1972.

77. Diebold J, TP Camilieri, J Delarue: Les lesions hepatiques au cours des leucoses. Etude histopathologique. Ann Anat Pathol (Paris) 14:41, 1969.

78. Lisiewicz J: Chronic lymphocytic leukemia, ch 4. In: Hemorrhage in Leukemias. Polish Medical Publishers, Warsaw, 1976, p 104.

79. Lazarachick J, AA Pappas, J Kizer: Acquired von Willebrand's syndrome due to an inhibitor specific for von Willebrand factor antigens. Am J Hematol 21:305, 1986.

80. Mohri H: Acquired von Willebrand's disease and storage pool disease in chronic myelocytic leukemia. Am J Hematol 22:391, 1986.

81. Budde U, JA Dent, SD Berkowitz: Subunit composition of plasma von Willebrand factor in patients with the myeloproliferative syndrome. Blood 68:1213, 1986.

82. Fabris F, A Casonato, MG Del Ben: Abnormalities of von Willebrand factor in myeloproliferative disease: a relationship with bleeding diathesis. Br J Haematol 63:75, 1986.

83. Goudemand J, B Samor, C Caron: Acquired Type II von Willebrand's disease: demonstration of a complexed inhibitor of the von Willebrand factor–platelet interaction and response to treatment. Br J Haematol 68:227, 1988.

84. Meschengieser S, A Blanco, N Maugeri: Platelet and intraplatelet von Willebrand factor antigen and fibrinogen in myelodysplastic syndromes. Thromb Res 46:601, 1987.

85. Mohri H, T Noguchi, F Kodama: Acquired von Willebrand disease due to inhibitor of human myeloma protein specific for von Willebrand factor. Am J Clin Pathol 87:663, 1987.

86. Tatewaki W, H Takahashi, K Wada: Plasma von Willebrand factor proteolysis in patients with chronic myeloproliferative disorders: no possibility of ex vivo degradation by calcium-dependent proteolysis. Thromb Res 56:191, 1989.

87. Takahashi H, R Nagayama, Y Tanabe: DDAVP in acquired von Willebrand syndrome associated with multiple myeloma. Am J Hematol 22:421, 1986.

88. Lisiewicz J, P Moszcynski: Leukocytosis and fibrinolytic activity of the blood in the leukemic patients. Rev Med Intern 1:37, 1975.

89. Tatarsky J, Z Sinakos, MJ Larrieu: Leukocytes et fibrinolyse. II. Etudes des leukocytes pathologiques. Nouv Rev Fr Hematol 7:95, 1967.

90. Kirchmayer S, I Stalowa, B Biernacka: Measurements of proteolytic activity of leukoblasts: a new diagnostic method. Pol Arch Med Wewn 44:365, 1970.

91. Wado H, T Nagano, M Tomeoku: Coagulant and fibrinolytic activities in the leukemic cell lysates. Thromb Res 30:315, 1982.

92. Gralnick HR, HK Tan: Acute promyelocytic leukemia: a model for understanding the role of the malignant cells in hemostasis. Hum Pathol 5:661, 1974.

93. Eiseman G, M Stefanini: Thromboplastic activity of leukemic white cells. Proc Soc Exp Biol Med 86:763, 1954.

94. Girolami A, EE Cliffton: Fibrinolytic and proteolytic activity in acute and chronic leukemia. Am J Med Sci 51:638, 1966.

95. Polliack A: Acute promyelocytic leukemia with disseminated intravascular coagulation. Am J Clin Pathol 56:155, 1971.

96. Galloway MJ, MJ Mackie, BA McVerry: Combinations of increased thrombin, plasmin, and non-specific protease activity in patients with acute leukemia. Haemostasis 13:322, 1983.

97. Matsuoka M, Y Onishi: Pathologic cells as procoagulant substances of disseminated intravascular coagulation syndrome in acute promyelocytic leukemia. Thromb Res 8:263, 1976.

98. Sultan C, M Gounault, B Varet: Relationship between the cell morphology of acute myeloblastic leukemia and occurrence of a syndrome of disseminated intravascular coagulation. XIV International Congress of Hematology, São Paulo, 1972, abstract 603.

99. Huth K, H Loffler, U Lechlemayer: Verbrauchskoagulopathie bei unreifzelligen keukosen. Verh Dtsch Ges Inn Med 74:147, 1968.

100. van Creveld J, JA Mochtar: Fibrinolysis in acute leukemia. Pediatr Ann 194:65, 1960.

101. Fisher S, B Ramot, B Kreisler: Fibrinolysis in acute leukemia. Israel Med J 19:195, 1960.

102. Cooperberg AA, GMA Neiman: Fibrinogenopenia and fibrinolysis in acute myelogenous leukemia. Ann Intern Med 42:706, 1955.

103. Pisciotta AV, EJ Schulz: Fibrinolytic purpura in acute leukemia. Am J Med 19:824, 1955.

104. Sznajd J, J Naskalski, J Lisiewicz: Antiheparin activity of myeloperoxidase and ribonuclease of chronic granulocytic leukemia leukocytes. Pol Arch Med Wewn 42:207, 1969.

105. Bick RL: Disseminated intravascular coagulation, ch 2. In: Disseminated Intravascular Coagulation and Related Syndromes. CRC Press, Boca Raton, FL, 1983, p 31.

106. Bick RL: Disseminated intravascular coagulation and related syndromes, ch 8. In: G Murano, RL Bick (Eds): Basic Concepts of Hemostasis and Thrombosis. CRC Press, Boca Raton, FL, 1980, p 163.

107. Bick RL: Disseminated intravascular coagulation and related syndromes. A review. Am J Hematol 5:265, 1978.

108. Gralnick HR, J Bagley, E Abrell: Heparin treatment for the hemorrhagic diathesis of acute promyelocytic leukemia. Am J Med 52:167, 1974.

109. Bennett RM: Acute leukemia. In: Rappaport H (Ed): Proc Tutorial in Hematopathology. University of Chicago Press, Chicago, 1980.

110. Shustrova NM: On the permeability of vascular walls in some disorders of the blood system. Doctoral dissertation, Alma-Ata, U.S.S.R., 1965.

111. Trunova LE: The pathogenesis of the hemorrhagic system in acute leukemia. Vrach Delo 11:41, 1965.

112. Valkov J: Histologic studies of extramedullary hematopoiesis in leukemias and its relationship to the blood vessels. Med Fizkult 42:35, 1963.

113. Luzzatto G, AI Schaffer: The prethrombotic state in cancer. Semin Oncol 17:147, 1990.

114. Didisheim P, EJW Bowie, CA Owen: Intravascular coagulation fibrinolysis (ICF) syndrome and malignancy: historical review and report of two cases with metastatic carcinoid and with acute myelomonocytic leukemia. Thromb Diath Haemorrh 36:215, 1969.

115. Goodnight SH: Bleeding and intravascular clotting in malignancy: a review. Ann N Y Acad Sci 230:271, 1974.

116. Soong BCF, SP Miller: Coagulation disorders in cancer: fibrinolysis and inhibitors. Cancer 25:867, 1970.

117. Frick PG: Acute hemorrhagic syndrome with hypofibrinogenemia in metastatic cancer. Acta Haematol (Basel) 16:11, 1956.

118. Leavy RA, SB Kahn, I Brodsky: Disseminated intravascular coagulation: a complication of chemotherapy in acute promyelocytic leukemia. Cancer 26:142, 1970.

119. Henderson ES: Acute myelogenous leukemia. In: WJ Williams, E Beutler, AJ Erslev, RW Rundles (Eds): Hematology. McGraw Hill, New York, 1977, p 830.

120. Brassinne C, A Coone, M Jijs: Characterization of two direct fibrinogenolytic activities and one proteolytic inhibitor activity in the human prostate. Thromb Res 8:803, 1976.

121. Mertins BF, LF Green, EJW Bowie: Fibrinolytic split products and ethanol gelation test in preoperative evaluation of patients with prostatic disease. Mayo Clin Proc 49:642, 1974.

122. Bick RL: Basic mechanisms of hemostasis pertaining to DIC, ch 1. In: Disseminated Intravascular Coagulation and Related Syndromes. CRC Press, Boca Raton, FL, 1983, p 1.

123. Bull B, M Rubenberg, J Dacie: Microangiopathic hemolytic anemia: mechanisms of red cell fragmentation. Br J Haematol 14:643, 1968.

124. Folkman J: Tumor angiogenesis: therapeutic implications. N Engl J Med 285:1182, 1971.

125. Cheung DK, JH Raaf: Selection of patients with malignant ascites for a peritoneovenous shunt. Cancer 50:1204, 1982.

126. Bick RL: Alterations of hemostasis associated with surgery, cardiopulmonary bypass surgery, and prosthetic devices, ch 13. In: OD Ratnoff, CD Forbes (Eds): Disorders of Hemostasis. WB Saunders, Philadelphia, 1991, p 382.

127. Lerner RG, JC Nelson, P Corines, LRM del Guercio: Disseminated intravascular coagulation: complication of LeVeen peritoneovenous shunts. JAMA 240:2064, 1984.

128. Harmon DC, Z Demirjian, L Ellman: Disseminated intravascular coagulation with the peritoneovenous shunt. Ann Intern Med 90:714, 1979.

129. Stein SF, JT Fulenwider, JD Ansley: Accelerated fibrinogen and platelet destruction after peritoneovenous shunting. Arch Intern Med 141:1149, 1981.

130. Qazi R, ED Savlov: Peritoneovenous shunt for palliation of malignant ascites. Cancer 49:600, 1982.

131. Bick RL: Disseminated intravascular coagulation: a clinical/laboratory study of 48 patients. In: DA Walz, LE McCoy (Eds): Contributions to Hemostasis. Ann N Y Acad Sci 370:843, 1981.

132. Feinstein DI: Treatment of disseminated intravascular coagulation. Semin Thromb Hemost 14:351, 1988.

133. Bick RL, WR Schmalhorst, E Shanbrom: Prothrombin complex concentrates: use in controlling the hemorrhagic diathesis of chronic liver disease. Am J Dig Dis 20:741, 1975.

134. Margolius A, DP Jackson, OD Ratnoff: Circulating anticoagulants: a study of 40 cases and review of the literature. Medicine (Baltimore) 40:145, 1961.

135. Ikkala E: Transfusion therapy in congenital deficiencies of plasma factor XIII. Ann N Y Acad Sci 202:200, 1972.

136. Bick RL: Circulating heparin activity in multiple myeloma. Blood 64:924, 1984.

137. Palmer RN, ME Rick, PD Rick: Circulating heparan sulfate anticoagulant in a patient with a fatal bleeding disorder. N Engl J Med 310:1696, 1984.

138. Khoory MS, ME Nesheim, EJW Bowie: Circulating heparan sulfate proteoglycan anticoagulant from a patient with a plasma cell disorder. J Clin Invest 65:666, 1980.

139. Bussel JB, PG Steinherz, DR Miller: A heparin-like anticoagulant in an 8-month-old boy with acute monoblastic leukemia. Am J Hematol 16:83, 1984.

140. Nenci GG, M Berrettini, P Parise: Persistent spontaneous heparinemia in systemic mastocytosis. Folia Haematol 109:453, 1982.

141. Bick RL: The clinical significance of fibrinogen degradation products. Semin Thromb Hemost 8:302, 1982.

142. Bick RL: Congenital and acquired coagulation protein defects associated with hemorrhage or thrombosis, ch 24. In: J Powers (Ed): Diagnostic Hematology: Clinical and Technical Aspects. CV Mosby, St. Louis, 1989, p 375.

143. Kwaan HC, R Lo, AJS McFadzean: Antifibrinolytic activity in primary carcinoma of the liver. Clin Sci 18:251, 1959.

144. Bick RL: Syndromes associated with hyperfibrino(geno)lysis, ch 3. In: Disseminated Intravascular Coagulation and Related Syndromes. CRC Press, Boca Raton, FL, 1983, p 105.

145. Livingston RB, SK Carter: Single agents in cancer chemotherapy. Plenum Press, New York, 1970.

146. Rubin P, GW Casareh: Clinical radiation pathology. WB Saunders, Philadelphia, 1968, p 778.

147. Bick RL: Platelet defects, ch 4. In: Disorders of Hemostasis and Thrombosis: Principles of Clinical Practice. Thieme, Inc., New York, 1985, p 65.

148. Berkheiser SW: The incidence of malignant cells in routine bone marrow examination. Cancer 8:958, 1955.

149. Hansen HH, FM Muggia, OS Selawry: Bone marrow examination in 100 consecutive patients with bronchogenic carcinoma. Lancet 1:443, 1971.

150. Jamshidi K, WR Swaim: Bone marrow biopsy with unaltered architecture: a new biopsy device. J Lab Clin Med 77:335, 1971.

151. Jonsson U, RW Rundles: Tumor metastases in bone marrow. Blood 6:16, 1951.

152. Lanier PF: Sternal marrow in patients with metastatic cancer. Arch Intern Med 84:891, 1949.

153. Harker LA, CA Finch: Thrombokinetics in man. J Clin Invest 48:963, 1969.

154. Marymount JH, S Gross: Patterns of metastatic cancer in the spleen. Am J Clin Pathol 40:58, 1963.

155. Miale JB: Laboratory medicine hematology. CV Mosby, St. Louis, 1972, p 53.

156. Gardner GF: Platelet transfusion. In: MG Baldini, S Elbe (Eds): Platelets: Production, Function and Storage. Grune and Stratton, New York, 1974, p 393.

157. Heustis DW, JR Bove, S Busch: Practical blood transfusion. Little, Brown and Company, Boston, 1969.

158. Ey FS, SH Goodnight: Bleeding disorders in cancer. Semin Oncol 17:87, 1990.

159. Ahn YS, WJ Harrington, RC Seelman: Vincristine therapy of idiopathic and secondary thrombocytopenias. N Engl J Med 291:376, 1974.

160. Marmont AM, EE Damasio, E Gori: Vinblastine sulfate in idiopathic thrombocytopenic purpura. Lancet 2:94, 1971.

161. Nalbandian RM, RL Henry, RL Bick: Thrombotic thrombocytopenic purpura. Semin Thromb Hemost 5:216, 1979.

162. Brook J, BE Konwaler: Thrombotic thrombocytopenic purpura: association with metastatic gastric carcinoma and a possible autoimmune disorder. Calif Med 102:222, 1965.

163. Friedman IA, SO Schwartz, SL Leifhold: Platelet function defects with bleeding. Arch Intern Med 113:177, 1964.

164. Perry S: Coagulation defects in leukemia. J Lab Clin Med 50:229, 1957.

165. Sanchez-Avalos J, BCF Soong, SP Miller: Coagulation disorders in cancer. II. Multiple myeloma. Cancer 23:1388, 1969.

166. Bick RL: Acquired circulating anticoagulants and defective hemostasis in malignant paraprotein disorders, ch 10. In: G Murano, RL Bick (Eds): Basic Concepts of Hemostasis and Thrombosis. CRC Press, Boca Raton, FL, 1980, p 205.

167. Lachner H: Hemostatic abnormalities associated with dysproteinemias. Semin Hematol 10:125, 1973.

168. Bick RL, T Adams, WR Schmalhorst: Bleeding times, platelet adhesion, and aspirin. Am J Clin Pathol 65:69, 1976.

169. Patterson WP, CW Caldwell, DC Doll: Hyperviscosity syndromes and coagulopathies. Semin Oncol 17:210, 1990.

170. Bick RL, CA Klein, LF Fekete: Alterations of hemostasis associated with malignant paraprotein disorders. Transactions of the American Society of Hematology, 1976, p 163.

171. Silberstein LE, J Abrahm, SJ Shattil: The efficacy of intensive plasma exchange in acquired von Willebrand's disease. Transfusion 27:234, 1987.

172. Bovill EG, WB Ershler, EA Golden: A human myeloma-produced monoclonal protein directed against the active subpopulation of von Willebrand factor. Am J Clin Pathol 85:115, 1986.

173. Horellou MH, E Baumelou, N Sitbon: Four cases of acquired Willebrand factor deficiency associated with monoclonal dysglobulinemia. Ann Med Interne (Paris) 134:707, 1983.

174. Schwab PJ, JL Fahey: Treatment of Waldenström's macroglobulinemia by plasmapheresis. N Engl J Med 263:574, 1960.

175. Bettigole RF, ES Himelstein, HF Oettgen: Hypofibrinogenemia due to L-asparaginase: studies of fibrinogen survival using autologous ^{131}I-fibrinogen. Blood 35:195, 1970.

176. Brodsky I, JF Conroy: The effects of chemotherapy on hemostasis. Cancer Chemother 2:85, 1972.

177. Monto RW, RW Talley, MJ Caldwell: Observation on the mechanisms of hemorrhagic toxicity in mithramycin therapy. Cancer Res 29:697, 1969.

178. Olson RE: Vitamin K–induced prothrombin formation antagonism by actinomycin-D. Science 145:926, 1964.

179. Hayano K, H Fukui, Y Otsuka: Three cases of renal failure associated with microangiopathic hemolytic anemia after mitomycin C therapy. Nippon Jinzo Gakkai Shi 30:835, 1988.

180. Jain S, AE Seymour: Mitomycin C associated hemolytic uremic syndrome. Pathology 19:58, 1987.

181. Sheldon R, D Slaughter: A syndrome of microangiopathic hemolytic anemia, renal impairment, and pulmonary edema in chemotherapy-treated patients with adenocarcinoma. Cancer 58:1428, 1986.

182. McCarthy JT, BA Staats: Pulmonary hypertension, hemolytic anemia, and renal failure. A mitomycin-associated syndrome. Chest 89:608, 1986.

183. Bick RL, LF Fekete, WL Wilson: Adriamycin and fibrinolysis. Thromb Res 8:467, 1976.

184. Bick RL, L Fekete, G Murano: Daunomycin and fibrinolysis. Thromb Res 9:201, 1976.

185. Klener P, P Kubisz, J Suranova: Influence of cytotoxic drugs on platelet functions and coagulation. Thromb Hemost 37:53, 1977.

186. Feffer SE, LS Carmosino, RL Fox: Acquired Protein C deficiency in patients with breast cancer receiving cyclophosphamide, methotrexate, and 5-fluorouracil. Cancer 63:1303, 1989.

187. Milne A, S Talbot, D Bevan: Thrombosis during cytotoxic chemotherapy. Br Med J 297:624, 1988.

188. Levin MN, M Gent, J Hirsh: The thrombogenic effect of anticancer drug therapy in women with Stage II breast cancer. N Engl J Med 318:404, 1988.

189. Goodnough CT, H Saito, A Manni: Increased incidence of thromboembolism in Stage IV breast cancer patients treated with a five drug chemotherapy regimen. Cancer 54:1264, 1984.

190. Weiss RB, DC Tormey, JF Holland: Venous thrombosis during multimodal treatment of primary breast carcinoma. Cancer Treat Rep 65:677, 1981.

191. Farbstein MJ, KG Blume: Acute leukemia, ch 10. In: KG Blume, LD Petz (Eds): Clinical Bone Marrow Transplantation. Churchill Livingstone, New York, 1983, p 271.

192. Sullivan KM: Graft-versus-host disease, ch 5. In: KG Blume, LD Petz (Eds): Clinical Bone Marrow Transplantation. Churchill Livingstone, New York, 1983, p 91.

193. Shulman HM, AM Gown, DJ Nugent: Hepatic veno-occlusive disease after bone marrow transplantation. Am J Pathol 127:549, 1987.

194. Jerman MR, RB Fick: Nonbacterial thrombotic endocarditis associated with bone marrow transplantation. Chest 90:919, 1986.

195. Kuramoto K, S Matsushita, H Yamanouchi: Nonbacterial thrombotic endocarditis as a cause of cerebral and myocardial infarction. Jpn Circ J 48:1000, 1984.

C H A P T E R
13

Hypercoagulability and Thrombosis

ypercoagulability and thrombosis are poorly understood phenomena. In about 50% of patients undergoing thrombotic or thromboembolic events, a definitive cause is not identifiable. Despite sophistication in blood coagulation laboratories and in clinical hemostasis practice, the etiology of hypercoagulability and thrombosis often is a mystery. The advent of new molecular marker profiling, however, may change this trend and allow for predicting which patients are at increased risk for thrombosis. The discovery of new inhibitor systems and new congenital deficiencies may now allow for defining the etiology in many patients experiencing arterial or venous thrombotic events, as these newer assays become more generally available.[1-3] Formerly, methods of laboratory hemostasis testing did not allow for clear conclusions regarding the origin of thrombotic events. Many changes in the hemostasis system reported to occur in association with hypercoagulability and thrombosis may not be of etiologic significance but may simply be the result of an already occurring thrombotic event, although when measuring hemostasis parameters, the event may be subclinical. Therapy for hypercoagulability and thrombosis also has been largely empiric, which is expected since clinicians are just beginning to understand etiologic aspects and to develop accurate diagnostic tools for the assessment of hypercoagulable and thrombotic disorders. Generally, as was described more than 100 years ago, three primary factors contribute to thrombus formation: changes in the blood flow, changes in the circulating blood, and changes in the vessel wall.[4]

Blood Flow Changes

With respect to changes in the blood flow, very little is known about venous thrombosis and the initiation of thrombus formation. Several theories exist about altered blood flow and thrombus formation. The most popular of these is that of Hume and coworkers, who proposed that during periods of stasis, especially in venous valve pockets, activation of factors XII, XI, and IX occurs.[5] Because of activation of these early contact activation factors, factor Xa is generated, which in turn generates thrombin activity, which then propagates thrombus formation via two mechanisms: fibrin formation and induction of platelet aggregation with subsequent availability of platelet factor 3 and ADP. This process then cascades into more platelet aggregation and more blood coagulation. Another popular theory is that during stasis a large amount of endothelial sloughing occurs with exposure of subendothelial collagen and the later activation of platelets, factor XII to factor XIIa, and factor XI to factor XIa. Any one of these three events could then lead to thrombin generation and thrombus formation.[6] It is possible, however, that these hypotheses are only several of many potential changes in coagulation and platelet function leading to thrombus formation in association with systemic stasis. These theories are shown in Figures 13-1 and 13-2.

Circulating Blood Changes

Changes in the circulating blood, both before and after thrombosis, are well defined, but the meaning of many of these changes discovered in the hemostasis laboratory is unclear. Some changes are difficult to assess because they have been measured after thrombosis has occurred. Although many of these are thought to be measured before thrombosis, some changes might have been measured when subclinical thrombus formation and fibrin deposition were already happening. Table 13-1 lists the changes in circulating blood that could, theoretically, lead to hypercoagulability and thrombosis.

Increased platelet reactivity as measured by many techniques has been noted in association with various thrombotic and thrombohemorrhagic disorders associated with hypercoagulability.[7,8] Generally, increased platelet reactivity is noted in patients with acute thrombosis.[9] However, this has usually been assessed after the thrombosis has occurred. Platelet hyperactivity is most often normal in patients with aged

Figure 13-1. Stasis in Venous Valve Pockets

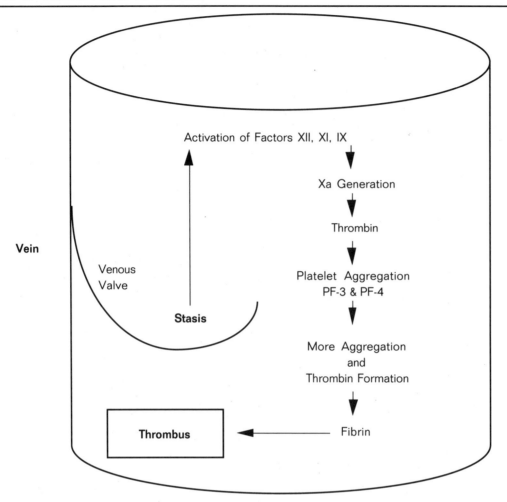

arterial thrombi, which suggests that platelet hyperreactivity plays an unclear role in the etiology of arterial thrombotic and thromboembolic problems. Increased platelet reactivity is seen in many patients with recurrent deep venous thrombosis,[10] but this is usually assessed after thrombosis has been clinically detected. The postoperative state is associated with an increased chance of thrombosis, and in a general surgical postoperative population, increased platelet reactivity can often be measured.[11] In postpartum women, the risk of thrombosis is increased, and in many postpartum patients increased platelet reactivity is shown. Additionally, increased platelet reactivity has been found in many patients with disseminated malignancy, which was discussed in detail in chapter 12. Increased platelet reactivity is seen in patients with diabetes mellitus, a disorder commonly associated with hypercoagulability and propensity to thrombus formation,[12] as well as in many individuals with generalized atherosclerosis. Whether any correlation exists between increased platelet reactivity, as measured by many techniques, and the chance of a clinical thrombotic event is controversial. The only conclusion that can be drawn now is that increased platelet reactivity is probably an important influencing factor in thrombus formation, especially when coupled with other changes in the hemostasis system. However, proof that isolated increased platelet reactivity clearly leads to clinical thrombosis is lacking.[4,13]

Changes in circulating coagulation factors have also been well documented in both thrombosis and situations leading to thrombus formation (hypercoagulability). Increased coagulation factors are often noted postoperatively in general surgical patients, postoperatively in patients with fractures or trauma, in patients with chronic inflammatory disorders such as ulcerative colitis, and in patients with disseminated malignancy, acute thrombosis, and recurrent deep venous thrombosis or pulmonary emboli.[4,14-16] Like the finding of increased platelet reactivity, however, many increases in coagulation factors have been measured after the thrombosis has occurred, and the significance of these findings is unclear with respect to these changes being of etiologic significance or simply being a result of subclinical fibrin deposition. The coagulation factors most commonly increased in these disorders are fibrinogen, factor VIII, factor V, and factor VII.[17] Many investigators have measured increased thromboplastin generation in these same disorders. Poor cor-

Figure 13-2. Stasis and the Endothelium

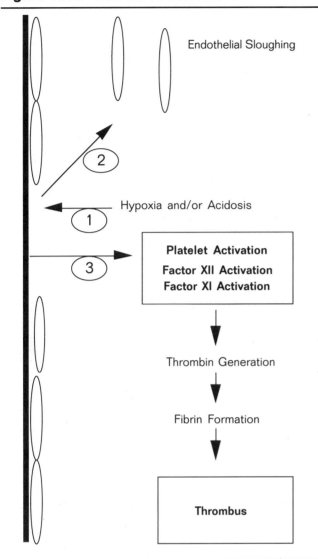

Endothelial Sloughing

Hypoxia and/or Acidosis

Platelet Activation
Factor XII Activation
Factor XI Activation

Thrombin Generation

Fibrin Formation

Thrombus

Table 13-1. Alterations in Circulating Blood Leading to Hypercoagulability and Thrombosis

Increased platelet reactivity
Increased coagulation factors
Decreased coagulation inhibitors
Decreased fibrinolytic activity
Increased fibrinolytic inhibitors
Increased or abnormal lipids

increased fibrino(geno)lysis (hemorrhage) depend on a fragile balance between the procoagulant system and associated inhibitors and the fibrinolytic system and its inhibitors.[21-23] Primary inhibitors of the procoagulant and fibrino(geno)lytic system consist of AT III, protein C, protein S, heparin cofactor II, alpha-2-macroglobulin, alpha-1-antitrypsin, C1 esterase inhibitor, and alpha-2-antiplasmin (Table 13-3).[24] Antithrombins were first described in 1939 by Brinkhous and coworkers.[25] The first large survey of antithrombins was reported by Seegers and associates in 1952.[26]

The most important of the antithrombins is antithrombin III. Antithrombin III has activity not only against thrombin but also against other serine proteases generated during coagulation, including factors Xa, IXa, XIa, and XIIa, plasmin, and kallikrein,[27-29] as well as against protein C and protein S (Table 13-4). This activity is markedly accelerated by heparin, especially for activity against thrombin and factor Xa.[30,31] Differing molecular weights of heparin have differing inhibitory effects on AT III, with higher–molecular weight forms of heparin accelerating inhibitory activity for factor IIa and lower–molecular weight activity fractions and fragments concomitantly decreasing anti–factor IIa inhibitory activity and increasing anti–factor Xa inhibitory activity. The kinetics of these reactions have been described for USP heterogenous heparin.[32,33] When the hemostasis system is driven in the procoagulant direction with attendant generation of serine proteases and later fibrin formation, AT III consumption occurs, since it combines irreversibly with activated clotting factors.[34] Pathologic consumption of AT III happens in conditions associated with the pathologic acceleration of procoagulant activity and the pathologic generation of thrombin and other serine proteases, such as in deep venous thrombosis,

Table 13-2. Conditions Associated With Elevated Clotting Factors, Hypercoagulability, and Thrombosis

Acute arterial thrombosis
Autoimmune diseases
Chronic inflammatory disorders
Deep venous thrombosis
Disseminated malignancy
Fractures
Hemolysis
Postoperative state
Pregnancy
Trauma

relation exists between any individual increased clotting factor and the development of clinical thrombosis.[4] Factor VIII:C and fibrinogen are the coagulation factors most often noted to be increased and are increased in pregnancy, chronic inflammatory disorders, disseminated malignancy, in postoperative patients, and during intravascular hemolytic episodes,[4] all of which are associated with an increased risk of thrombosis. The conditions or situations associated with hypercoagulability, thrombosis, and elevated clotting factors are summarized in Table 13-2.

Coagulation Inhibitors

It is generally accepted that coagulation occurs in a cybernetic manner with fibrin deposition and subsequent lysis happening as a continuous process.[18-20] The manifestations of normal hemostasis vs increased fibrin deposition (thrombosis) or pulmonary embolism, and DIC. To a large extent this same consumption occurs with protein C. Since AT III, a major serine protease inhibitor, is important in protecting against thrombus formation, an increased propensity to thrombus formation and an inadequate response to later heparinization occur in situations associated with significant decreases in AT III. Decreases in protein C and protein S are also associated with increased thrombotic tendencies.

Antithrombin III is an alpha-2-globulin with a molecular weight of about 65,000 d,[35,36] and its specific characteristics have been described in detail.[37,38] Antithrombin III is purified by chromatography with heparin sepharose.[39,40] Without heparin, AT III inactivates thrombin and other serine proteases in a progressive, irreversible manner following second-order kinetics.[41] Antithrombin III inactivates other serine proteases, including factors Xa, IXa, XIa, XIIa, and kallikrein, although with less efficiency than for its inhibition of thrombin.[27-29,42-44] About 70% of the total inhibition of the serine protease procoagulant system may be ascribed to AT III, and approximately 25% to 30% may be attributed to

Table 13-3. Physiologic Inhibitors of the Procoagulant and Fibrinolytic Systems

Antithrombin III
Heparin cofactor II
Protein C
Protein S
Alpha-2-macroglobulin
Alpha-2-antitrypsin
Alpha-2-antiplasmin
C1 esterase inhibitor

other inhibitors.[35,45] However, others have suggested that greater than 90% of the total inhibition of the procoagulant system may be ascribed to AT III.[46,47] The relative general contributions of AT III, protein C, protein S, heparin cofactor II, and alpha-2-macroglobulin in inhibiting the procoagulant system are still unclear and are to be defined. In the presence of heparin, the inactivation of thrombin and factor Xa by AT III is markedly accelerated and almost instanta-

Figure 13-3. Antithrombin III Activity (Model I)

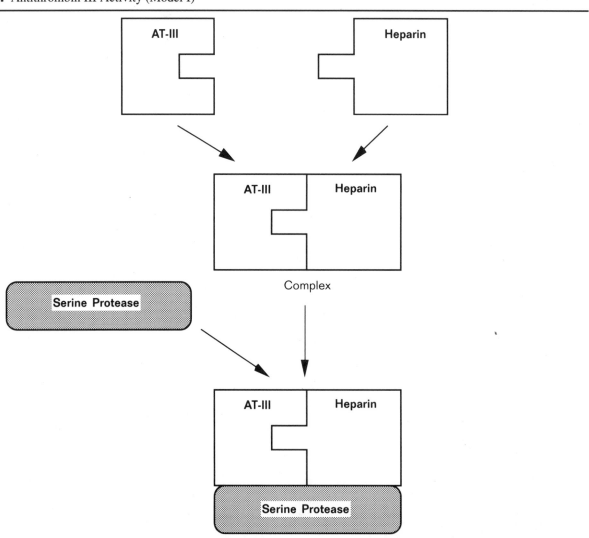

Figure 13-4. Antithrombin III Activity (Model II)

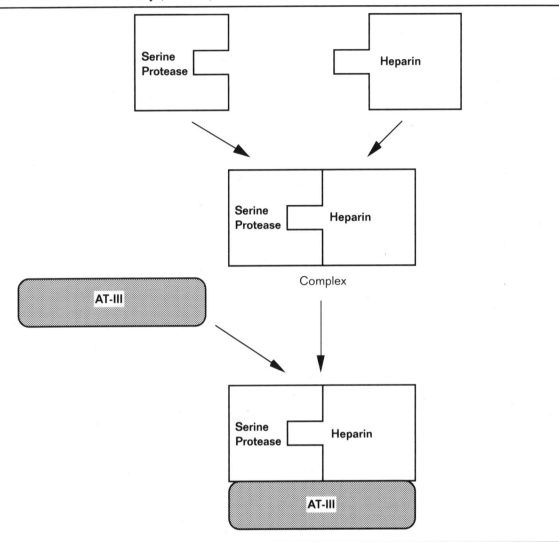

neous. Rosenberg and Damus showed that heparin interacts with AT III by binding to lysine residues of the AT III molecule, markedly enhancing its inhibitory activity.[34] Heparin also combines with thrombin and factor Xa, however, and whether the neutralization of thrombin and factor Xa by AT III is caused by the interaction of heparin with AT III or the particular serine protease involved remains controversial.[48-51] Another proposed mechanism is that a molecule of heparin may bind to AT III and thrombin.[52] In the presence of heparin, the preferential target of AT III is thrombin, followed by factor Xa. Proposed mechanisms of action of AT III are summarized in Figures 13-3 and 13-4. Differing molecular weight subspecies of heparin have different activities with respect to the interaction of AT III and factor Xa or interaction with the vasculature (vascular proteoglycans).[53-56] Anti–factor IIa (thrombin) activity of heparin appears to be greatest with higher–molecular weight forms. As the molecular weight decreases, the anti–factor IIa activity decreases, and the anti–factor Xa activity increases. During these processes, heparin is not consumed.[57] After the for-

mation of AT III and serine protease complex, heparin disassociates from the complex, acting as a catalyst. The kinetics of the heparin and serine protease interaction have been well elucidated, providing evidence that only minute amounts of heparin need to be present to accelerate the inhibitory activity of AT III.[32,41,58] Endogenous heparin is rarely, if ever, detected in the blood in significant amounts except in selected pathologic conditions, such as particular malignancies.

Table 13-4. Proteins Inhibited by Antithrombin III

Factor IIa (thrombin)
Factor Xa
Factor IXa
Factor XIa
Factor XIIa
Kallikrein
Protein C
Protein S
Plasmin

Table 13-5. Mechanisms of Antithrombin III Deficiency

Decreased synthesis
    Congenital
    Acquired

Dysfunctional synthesis
    Congenital
    Acquired

Increased consumption
    Disseminated intravascular coagulation
    Deep venous thrombosis
    Pulmonary embolus
    Diffuse vaso-occlusive diseases

Proteinuria and nonselective loss of antithrombin III

Increased nonselective protein catabolism

When exogenous heparin is delivered to the blood compartment, it is rapidly absorbed by the surface of endothelial cells, and endothelial-bound heparin may be far more important physiologically than circulating heparin for preventing thrombus formation in humans.[59-62] Some vascular proteoglycans, other than heparin, are also able to absorb AT III and enhance the rate of inhibition of thrombin, factor Xa, and possibly other serine proteases by AT III.[56,63] The obvious major physiologic significance of this activity is implied but not yet conclusively proven.

The physiologic range of AT III in normal human blood is narrow.[24,64,65] Only moderate decreases of AT III are associated with thrombus formation or thromboembolus.[24,66] Infants have about 50% of normal adult AT III levels; however, adult levels are attained at an early age.[67] The mechanisms by which a potential deficiency of AT III may occur are as follows: (1) a defect in synthesis that may occur in the congenital form and in several acquired forms, such as liver disease; (2) increased consumption of AT III resulting from the generation of pathologic levels of serine proteases, such as in DIC, extensive deep venous thrombosis, massive pulmonary embolization, and diffuse small and large venous and arterial thrombo-occlusive events; (3) loss of AT III from the intravascular compartment, such as in selected renal diseases; and (4) increased protein catabolism.[24,66] These mechanisms are listed in Table 13-5.

Antithrombin III Defects

Hereditary Deficiency

Hereditary thrombophilia was initially the term used to describe congenital AT III deficiency but is now generically used for all the hypercoagulable or prethrombotic disorders caused by a congenital deficiency. Hereditary thrombophilia also includes congenital heparin cofactor II, protein C, protein S, plasminogen, and other deficiencies. Congenital defi-

ciency of AT III is usually inherited as an autosomal dominant trait, although variant inheritance has also been described.[68] In most patients with classic hereditary deficiency of AT III, the synthesis of a biologically normal AT III molecule is reduced,[68] although this deficiency may also be caused by a dysfunctional AT III molecule.[68,69] Thus, the absence form (CRM−) and dysfunctional form (CRM+) exist. One variant has been described that is not associated with a thrombotic tendency.[70] The prevalence of hereditary deficiency of AT III is not known for certain because screening and widespread use of quantitative AT III assays have happened only recently. At the present time, however, the incidence appears to be between 1 in 2,000 to 1 in 5,000.[71,72] However, this incidence may change with more widespread availability and use of easy automated synthetic substrate AT III assays in patients with hypercoagulability and thrombosis. Maybe of more clinical relevance, however, is the question of how many individuals with deep venous thrombosis or pulmonary embolus seen in a general population experience these events because of hereditary AT III deficiency. The answer to this question will have to await large population studies. Currently it appears that the prevalence of hereditary antithrombin deficiency in a general patient population with thrombotic or thromboembolic events is about 3% to 4%.[24,73,74]

Patients with hereditary deficiency of AT III have a markedly increased risk of venous thrombotic events and pulmonary embolism.[24,66,75-79] These events typically appear in the mid- to late-teenage years. The most common sites of thrombosis are the deep veins of the lower extremities and the mesenteric veins.[80] The usual presentation is that of recurrent deep venous thrombosis with or without pulmonary embolization.[24,66,79] From the family studies reported, it appears that the deficiency of AT III need not be especially severe for thrombotic events to happen. Some individuals have deep venous thrombosis and pulmonary emboli at between 50% and 70% biologic activity, whereas others with low AT III levels may not have thrombosis.[24,75-79] Heterozygotes are also at risk for severe venous thrombotic and thromboembolic events. Many patients with hereditary thrombophilia treated with oral anticoagulants have an increase in AT III levels after the initiation of therapy.[24,81-83] Other patients are unresponsive to oral anticoagulant therapy and show no significant increases in AT III levels.[24,84-86] A typical family with congenital deficiency of AT III is presented in Table 13-6. One individual in this family was treated with oral anticoagulants, and two were treated with combination platelet suppressive therapy (aspirin and dipyridamole). The increases in AT III levels were identical among the three patients. These AT III increases presumably occur because of blunting low levels of intravascular procoagulant drive (and presumed fibrin deposition), decreasing intravascular concentrations of serine protease, and, thus, increasing AT III biologic activity. Patients with hereditary thrombophilia who do not show the desired AT III response to oral anticoagulant therapy may be given a trial of combi-

Table 13-6. A Typical Family With Congenital Antithrombin III Deficiency

Mother

    52-year-old white woman with a lifelong history of recurrent deep venous thrombosis and two episodes of pulmonary embolus.

    Antithrombin III level at presentation was 79% by biologic and immunologic assay. (Patient was taking warfarin therapy at time of these determinations.)

Son

    18-year-old white man with a five-year history of deep venous thrombosis.

    He had experienced three episodes of pulmonary emboli; the first being at age 13 years.

    Antithrombin III level at presentation was 59% by biologic and immunologic assay.

Daughter

    16-year-old white girl with seven episodes of deep venous thrombosis, the first being at age 12 years, but no pulmonary emboli.

    Antithrombin III level at presentation was 52% by biologic and immunologic assay.

Father

    Not available for study.

Table 13-7. Characteristics of Congenital Antithrombin III Deficiency

Clinical features

    Autosomal dominant trait

    Absence form and dysfunctional form exist

    Venous thrombosis begins in mid- to late-teenage years

    Pulmonary emboli are common

    Mesenteric vessels particularly susceptible

    Thrombosis occurs commonly in heterozygotes

    Thrombosis may occur at antithrombin III levels below 75%

Laboratory features

    Low AT III levels by biologic assay

    Low immunologic AT III levels in absence form

    Normal immunologic levels in dysfunctional form

    Global tests of coagulation are normal

    Tests of fibrinolysis are normal

    Template bleeding time is normal

    Platelet aggregation is normal

    APTT may not prolong adequately or at all during intravenous heparin therapy

Therapy

    Oral anticoagulants

    Antiplatelet agents (aspirin plus dipyridamole)

    AT III concentrates

    Heparin often ineffective

nation platelet suppressive therapy to see if this will enhance AT III levels. The AT III biochemical characteristics of this family and two similar families have been reported.[87] Antithrombin III concentrates are now available for treating hereditary AT III deficiency. Table 13-7 summarizes the characteristics of congenital AT III deficiency.

Deep Venous Thrombosis and Pulmonary Embolism

Many risk factors are associated with the development of deep venous thrombosis and pulmonary embolism, including age, blood group, obesity, the use of oral contraceptives, estrogens, and many specific clinical events such as malignancy, the postoperative or postpartum state, cardiovascular disease, and a history of deep venous thrombosis and varicose veins.[88] Cigarette smoking and venous thrombotic disease are inversely correlated, although a positive correlation between arterial thrombosis and smoking exists. About 70% of individuals with deep venous thrombosis or pulmonary embolus had decreased levels of AT III before the initiation of anticoagulant therapy. However, most of these individuals have decreased AT III levels because of consumption when the thrombus developed, and only a few individuals, 3% to 4%, had the thrombotic event as a result of a deficiency of AT III. A general correlation exists between the severity of the intravascular thrombotic event (such as deep venous thrombosis and pulmonary emboli) and the degree of decrease in AT III levels in most acquired cases. Generally, the intensity of decrease correlates with DIC, iliofemoral thrombosis, pulmonary embolization, bilateral calf thrombo-

sis, and single calf thrombosis in descending order of decrease of AT III.[63,89] Table 13-8 lists the AT III levels before and after therapy in 40 individuals with deep venous thrombosis with and without pulmonary embolism.[3,24,90] Table 13-9 shows correlations noted in our laboratories between the extent of decrease in AT III and the site and severity of thrombotic events. Most instances of a deep venous thrombotic event and decreased levels of AT III are caused by consumption instead of a hereditary deficiency.

My usual routine is to obtain a pretreatment AT III level in any individual in whom a deep venous thrombosis or pulmonary embolism is present or strongly suspected.[3,24] The purpose of this determination is to gain information regarding the potential efficacy of heparin therapy and to detect those individuals who may have hereditary deficiency of AT III.[3,24] Some AT III assay systems may give erroneously

Table 13-8. Deep Venous Thrombosis and Antithrombin III Consumption

	AT III level (% NHP)	Percentage of patients abnormal (%)
Pretreatment	77	67
Posttreatment*	105.3	25
Normal range	89 to 125	

* Subcutaneous calcium heparin, 80 to 100 units/kg three times a day

Table 13-9. Severity of Thrombotic Event and Antithrombin III Levels

Severity	Event	AT III level (% NHP)	SD
I	Single calf thrombus	109	18.3
II	Bilateral calf thrombi	104.8	25.3
III	Isolated pulmonary embolus	83.2	20.2
IV	Iliofemoral thrombus	81.5	6.4
V	Deep venous thrombosis plus pulmonary embolus	66.5	9.9
VI	Acute DIC	62.6	18.5
Normal values	89% to 125%		

high results, leading to a missed diagnosis of AT III deficiency.[89,91,92] If the AT III level is significantly decreased, it is again measured one to two months later in the steady state when no detectable intravascular thrombosis is present to find out whether the early decrease was because of acquired consumption or hereditary deficiency.[24] Decreases in AT III have sometimes been noted following heparin therapy. Specifically, in several studies a 10% to 15% decrease in AT III levels was associated with the use of intravascular heparin, but this was without any apparent risk of thrombosis. Usually, however, individuals with low AT III levels before heparin therapy tend to have normal levels within 24 hours after therapy. I aim for a plasma heparin level of between .01 and .1 units/mL when instituting subcutaneous heparin therapy in my hematology practice.[4,24,74,93] However, in the individuals depicted in Table 13-8, 25% still have abnormally decreased AT III levels following the initiation of heparin therapy. Only two individuals out of 40, however, had a later decrease of pretreatment AT III levels following the initiation of heparin therapy.[24]

Oral Contraceptives

Many reports have discussed AT III levels in patients taking oral contraceptives.[94-99] Many conflicting data are found and are summarized in a review article giving rational perspective to the issue of oral contraceptives, thromboembolism, and the hemostasis system.[100] Many investigators have found decreased levels of AT III, and others have found unchanged levels of AT III in women ingesting oral contraceptives.[100] These marked descrepancies are probably caused by differences in testing techniques.[24] Antithrombin III measurements in serum instead of plasma have yielded more consistent decreases in oral contraceptive users; however, serum systems are not adequate to quantitate the ability of the patient to inactivate thrombin and other serine proteases, since they measure AT III remaining after clotting.[101,102] Other discrepancies are found in studies measuring AT III levels in oral contraceptive users by both immunologic and biologic techniques. In one such study, the biologic activity was decreased in 55% of women, whereas the immunologic

level was abnormal in only 12%.[103] Estrogens may reduce AT III levels by about 15%, and the greater reductions are correlated with higher doses of estrogens.[104,105] Studies have shown specific binding between estrogens as well as other steroids and AT III.[106] One might deduce a potential relationship between decreases in AT III levels and thrombotic tendencies in women taking oral contraceptives. However, the data are too conflicting for any firm conclusions regarding the clinical relevance of decreased AT III levels in women taking oral contraceptive agents.

Attentive studies using reliable plasma AT III determinations, preferably by synthetic substrate assays, will become more commonly used and this issue more carefully understood. The use of serum AT III levels is to be condemned, because these determinations are without clinical relevance.[24,100-102]

Coronary Artery Disease

The relationships between thrombosis, coronary artery ischemia, and coronary artery disease are controversial.[107,108] The role of AT III with respect to atherogenesis and myocardial infarction is even less clear. Antithrombin III levels are decreased in many individuals with coronary artery disease and in individuals at high risk for coronary artery disease. Yue and coworkers examined a large population of patients and found excellent correlation between AT III levels and individuals at low risk for ischemia, those at high risk for ischemia, those with chronic ischemic heart disease taking heparin, those with chronic ischemic disease not taking heparin, and those with acute myocardial infarction.[109] Antithrombin III levels decreased concomitantly in each of these groups of patients. O'Brien and colleagues reported a significant decrease in AT III levels in patients after myocardial infarction and in patients with generalized atherosclerotic vaso-occlusive peripheral vascular disease.[110] Banerjee and coworkers reported decreased AT III levels in women and men with generalized atherosclerosis.[111] Innerfield and coworkers reported decreased AT III levels in patients with coronary artery occlusion.[112] However, Hedner and Nilsson reported normal AT III levels in patients with myocardial infarction.[113] All these studies, except that of Innerfield et al, relied only on clinical diagnosis, and angiographic proof of coronary artery disease has been lacking. Bick and Faulstick studied 102 individuals with angiographically documented coronary artery disease.[114] In these 102 individuals, plasma levels of biologic AT III activity were determined at the time of coronary artery catheterization and when the catheter was removed. In these patients undergoing coronary artery angiography, only 10 (9.8%) had decreased AT III levels. After catheterization, however, 17% of patients had decreased AT III levels, which further supports the suggestion that angiographic dyes generally alter AT III levels.[115] An attempt to correlate AT III levels with the type of intracoronary lesion was attempted, but no significant differences were found when patients were segregated into those with specific coronary artery involvement (lesions of the left anterior descending coronary artery, circumflex artery, or right coronary artery) or when compared to class of coronary artery disease (class 1 through 4).[114] Thus, the role of antithrombins in coronary artery disease is conflicting and unclear, but most patients with documented coronary artery disease, proven by angiographic studies, have normal AT III levels. Determinations of AT III levels in patients with coronary artery disease are without clear-cut clinical relevance.[24,114]

Renal and Liver Disease

Patients with proteinuria lose AT III and other plasma proteins in the urine.[116] Urinary AT III levels can be correlated with urinary proteinuria and urinary albumin.[117] As anticipated, plasma AT III levels correlate inversely with urinary proteinuria.[118] Deep vein thrombosis and pulmonary embolism are well-recognized risks in patients with nephrotic syndrome.[119] However, these patients have many other conditions also constituting high-risk factors for this complication, including high concentrations of various clotting factors, prolonged bed rest, and stasis.[120,121] It is unclear whether a causal relationship exists between decreases of AT III and the increased risk of thrombosis and thromboembolic disease in patients with nephrotic syndrome. Glucocorticoid therapy may enhance AT III levels in patients who have AT III deficiency secondary to urinary proteinuria because of steroid-induced stimulation of AT III synthesis or a direct effect of steroids on renal protein loss.[122]

Antithrombin III levels are often decreased in patients with chronic liver disease[24,64] and normal in patients with acute hepatitis, unless the patient with acute fulminant hepatitis develops fulminant DIC.[123-125] The significance of this finding is unclear, since patients with chronic liver disease and hepatic failure have no apparent increased risk of thrombosis. The decrease in AT III may be counterbalanced by the severe defects in hemostasis and subsequent hypocoagulability often associated with acute and chronic liver disease.[126-128] If the patient with chronic liver disease has a catastrophic event, such as being provided with a trigger for DIC (eg, sepsis or massive transfusions), then this low-level procoagulant-inhibitor balance may be easily disrupted, and later catastrophic thrombohemorrhagic disease may result.

Disseminated Intravascular Coagulation

Disseminated intravascular coagulation syndromes are intermediary mechanisms of disease commonly recognized throughout all medical disciplines (see chapter 7).[123-125,129] Disseminated intravascular coagulation is usually associated with a triggering disease process and is rarely an isolated event. The recognized triggers for DIC are generally associated with low AT III levels, including severe burns complicated by infection, malignancy, acute promyelocytic leukemia, septicemia, and obstetric accidents.[123-125,129-132] These decreases are expected since AT III has activity against thrombin and other serine proteases generated during blood coagulation. In a situation such as DIC, in which hemostasis is driven in the procoagulant direction with attendant (massive?) generation of serine proteases including thrombin and factor Xa, AT III consumption occurs because of irreversible binding with these activated clotting factors. Indeed, radioactive AT III represents a useful probe for the study of in vivo thrombin formation and subsequent fibrin deposition.[133] Pathologic consumption of AT III is expected in conditions associated with abnormal acceleration of procoagulant activity and the pathologic generation of thrombin and other serine proteases, such as in DIC.[123-125,129,134-137] Several studies have shown significant decreases in AT III levels in patients with DIC.

Antithrombin III determinations are useful for diagnosing disseminated intravascular clotting processes, and monitoring AT III levels after initiation of heparin therapy (usually given subcutaneously) in DIC may represent an effective means of establishing efficacy of therapy in DIC for blunting or stopping the intravascular clotting process. Pretreatment and posttreatment AT III levels in 50 individuals with DIC are depicted in Table 13-10, and Table 13-11 shows the reliability of laboratory tests in patients with DIC,[135,138] which has also been found by others.[137] I rely on AT III levels in conjunction with elevated D-dimer levels, FDPs, circulating soluble fibrin monomer, thrombocytopenia, hypofibrinogenemia, and the elevation of fibrinopeptide A levels for the reliable diagnosis of DIC.[1,3,6,123] The return to normal or near normal posttreatment AT III levels, fibrinopeptide A levels, and platelet markers (either platelet factor 4 or beta-thromboglobulin) provide useful indices in assessing the efficacy of heparin or other therapy in patients with DIC.[1,3,6]

Antithrombin III Concentrates

Antithrombin III concentrates have been used investigationally in patients with DIC and have recently become available for patients with the congenital deficiency state. These concentrates may be of value in therapy for patients with DIC, consumption associated with acute or chronic liver disease, the control of hereditary deficiency of AT III deficiency, and in eradicating thrombogenicity of prothrombin complex concentrates. Most investigational clinical

Table 13-10. Antithrombin III Consumption in Disseminated Intravascular Coagulation

	AT III level % NHP	SD	Percentage of patients abnormal
Pretherapy	63.1	25	92
Posttherapy*	106.7	32	18
P value	< .001		
Normal range	89% to 125%		

* Subcutaneous heparin

Table 13-11. Laboratory Tests in Fulminant Disseminated Intravascular Coagulation (Descending Order of Reliability)

Elevated D-dimer
Elevated FDPs
Decreased AT III
Thrombocytopenia
Elevated fibrinopeptide A
Elevated platelet factor 4
Positive protamine sulfate
Long prothrombin time
Low fibrinogen
Long thrombin time
Long APTT
Long reptilase time

experience with AT III concentrates has been directed toward therapy for DIC and for control of consumption or frank DIC in association with acute liver failure. Vogel and coworkers treated 22 patients who had acute liver disease with AT III concentrates when AT III levels fell to below 80% of normal.[139] They found antithrombin therapy to be successful in stopping intravascular consumption at a dose of 250 units delivered over three hours. They also concluded that AT III concentrates are useful for improving the prognosis in patients with acute liver failure. Egbring and coworkers[140] and Braude and coworkers[141] treated a total of six patients with acute hepatic failure, and both groups concluded that AT III concentrates are effective in prolonging survival in patients with acute liver failure. Kakkar reported on the therapeutic use of AT III concentrates for four postoperative patients with AT III levels less than 50% of normal, and none of these patients had a postoperative thromboembolic event.[142] Kakkar also studied 50 patients who were randomly assigned to AT III concentrate or placebo plus low-dose heparin treatment, which was delivered preoperatively for total hip replacement. The results were promising.[142] Egbring and associates treated 10 patients who had hereditary and acquired AT III deficiency and reported these concentrates to be beneficial in treating thromboembolic disease in all patients.[143] They concluded that patients with AT III levels of less than 75% of normal would not respond adequately to heparin therapy. Bick and coworkers treated five patients with acute DIC with an AT III concentrate. All five patients survived, and the use of AT III was thought to be effective therapy and a potential alternative to heparin or mini-heparin therapy.[6,134] Schipper and coworkers[144] and Thaler and coworkers[145] in two independent studies each treated five patients who had DIC with AT III concentrates. The Schipper study concluded that the concentrate was effective, as determined by decreased fibrinopeptide A levels and increased fibrinogen levels but uncorrectable fibrinogen survival, for a period of 48 hours after the infusion. However, the Thaler study was ended without clear-cut conclusions about efficacy. Dunn and coworkers showed that endotoxin-induced DIC in dogs can be successfully treated with the use of AT III concentrates.[146] They concluded that AT III appeared to be as effec-

tive as heparin in controlling DIC and may have distinct advantages over heparin for general survival and bleeding risk. Potential thrombogenicity of prothrombin complex concentrates may be controlled by the addition of AT III to this therapeutic fraction before its infusion into patients.[147]

Antithrombin III concentrates are probably the specific antiprocoagulant therapy of choice for patients with acute DIC,[6,24,123,148] but prospective randomized clinical trials using AT III concentrates in patients with acute DIC and patients with consumption resulting from acute hepatic failure are needed to determine if efficacy is present and equal to or better than current modalities of therapy. The clinical use of AT III concentrates has recently been reviewed by Vinazzer.[149]

Clinical Indications

With the development and ready availability of simple and reproducible AT III determinations by synthetic substrate assay, this laboratory testing modality is generally available at a minimum expense for most clinical laboratories and should certainly be available at institutions dealing with patients with thrombohemorrhagic disorders.[3,24] Synthetic substrate methods for the determination of AT III are clearly the methods of choice, and clot-based or immunologic methods should no longer be used in the clinical laboratory.[3,38,66,90,150,151]

Antithrombin III levels should be considered in the following situations: (1) Patients who may be at high risk for thrombotic or thromboembolic disease should be identified. Generally, if AT III is less than 75% of normal activity, the individual is assumed to have an increased risk of thrombotic or thromboembolic disease, and proper prophylactic therapy should be considered. (2) The potential responsiveness to heparin therapy should be determined. Patients with lower AT III levels may respond less than ideally, or not at all, to heparin therapy. Patients who have an AT III level of less than 40% of normal biologic activity will usually not respond to heparin therapy at any dose. Alternatively, if the biologic AT III level is greater than 60% of normal activity, patients will usually respond to heparin. If a patient has less than 40% of normal biologic activity of AT III, another form of therapy should be considered when appropriate. (3) When patients and families with hereditary AT III deficiency are identified, all family members should also be studied to find other affected individuals. Prophylactic therapy with oral anticoagulants should be considered. For those individuals not responding to oral anticoagulants, a combination of aspirin and dipyridamole may be effective. Of course, determination of efficacy of therapy in individuals with hereditary AT III deficiency calls for additional subsequent AT III determinations. (4) The efficacy of therapy in DIC should be determined by the AT III level. Posttreatment AT III determinations are a reliable index to note if one has established control of the intravascular clotting process in patients with DIC following delivery of subcutaneous or intravenous heparin. The determination of AT III is a useful diagnostic tool for patients with DIC.

Thus, AT III determinations are an important part of the battery of tests used to establish a diagnosis of DIC. After the institution of appropriate therapy, AT III determinations are used to establish whether the intravascular coagulation process has been blunted or stopped. The role of AT III determinations in rendering information regarding efficacy of therapy in other thrombotic or thromboembolic disorders has not yet been clearly established.

Patient populations considered candidates for AT III are determined by the following[24]: (1) patients with a history of deep venous thrombosis or pulmonary embolus; (2) patients with active deep venous thrombosis or pulmonary embolus; (3) patients developing a recurrent thrombotic event during heparin therapy; (4) preoperative patients with a family history of deep venous thrombosis or pulmonary embolus; (5) patients with DIC or a related syndrome; (6) patients with significant proteinuria; (7) patients with a family history of deep venous thrombosis or pulmonary embolus; (8) patients showing inadequate prolongation of an activated partial thromboplastin time or other global clotting tests while taking intravenous heparin; (9) patients receiving subcutaneous or intrapulmonary heparin; (10) possibly patients who are considering taking oral contraceptives, although indications in this instance are not clearly established. These indications are summarized in Table 13-12.

Heparin Cofactor II

Heparin cofactor II was first discovered by Briginshaw and Shanberge when they noticed that besides the rapid inhibition of thrombin by heparin, which could be reversed by addition of polybrene or protamine, a slow, time-dependent inhibition occurred, which represented an irreversible decrease in thrombin. This second inhibitory effect was called heparin cofactor A.[152,153] Briginshaw and Shanberge also noted that unlike the activity of AT III, heparin cofactor A had no inhibitory effect on factor Xa. Later, Tollefson and

Table 13-12. Clinical Indications for Obtaining Antithrombin III Determinations

Patients with a history of unexplained deep venous thrombosis or pulmonary embolus

Patients with unexplained active deep venous thrombosis or pulmonary embolus

Patients developing a recurrent thrombotic event during heparin therapy

Preoperative patients with a personal or family history of unexplained deep venous thrombosis or pulmonary embolus

Patients with disseminated intravascular coagulation syndromes

Patients with a family history of unexplained thrombosis or pulmonary embolus

Patients demonstrating inadequate prolongation of the APTT or other global clotting tests while taking heparin therapy

Possibly patients considering taking oral contraceptives; indications in this instance are not clearly established

associates further isolated and characterized this thrombin-inhibiting glycoprotein and called it heparin cofactor II (HC II).[154] These investigators showed that not only heparin but also dermatan sulfate accelerated the thrombin-inhibiting activity of HC II, and they noticed that HC II inhibited the amidolytic and proteolytic activities of thrombin by forming a covalent 1:1 molar complex with thrombin.[155,156] Since these original investigations, much has been learned about HC II. Heparin cofactor II is a glycoprotein with a molecular weight of about 64,000 d. The inhibitory activity of HC II is accelerated by heparin, including heparins with low AT III affinity, dermatan sulfate, the semisynthetic heparinoid pentosan polysulfate, dextran sulfate, and other sulfated polysaccharides.[157] The thrombin inhibitory activity of HC II is dependent on the sulfated portion of heparin and other polysaccharides that activate or accelerate HC II activity. Vitronectin (S protein) protects thrombin and factor Xa from heparin-induced inhibition of AT III and has been found to protect thrombin from HC II neutralization when HC II activation is by heparin or pentosan sulfate.[158] S protein does not, however, protect thrombin inactivation if HC II activation is by dermatan sulfate. Thus, S protein appears to be a general inhibitor of the anticoagulant activity of various glycosaminoglycans and their activation of AT III or HC II. The plasma half-life of HC II is about 2.5 days. Unlike AT III, HC II is not capable of significant inhibition of factors Xa, XIa, IXa, or plasmin. In addition to thrombin inhibition, heparin cofactor II inhibits chymotrypsin. The inhibition of thrombin by HC II is not limited to the activity of thrombin on fibrinogen, but thrombin-induced platelet aggregation and release are also inhibited.[159] Similar to AT III, HC II is inactivated by stimulated polymorphonuclear leukocytes, presumably by release of proteolytic elastases and cathepsins.[160] The partial proteolysis of HC II by polymorphonuclear leukocytes is accompanied by peptide by-products having potent chemotactic activity, which suggests HC II may also play a role in the inflammatory process.

Congenital Deficiency

Many assays are available for assessing HC II activity, and concomitant with availability have been the finding of patients with congenital deficiency and the definition of acquired HC II defects.[161,162] Although many different assays are now available, two are particularly easy for the routine clinical hematology laboratory. The first assay, described by Abildgaard,[163] measures the thrombin-inactivating effect of plasma in the presence of dermatan sulfate. Patient plasma is incubated with thrombin in the presence of dermatan sulfate, and residual thrombin activity is measured by a synthetic chromogenic substrate. The other assay, described by Vinazzer and Pangraz,[164] utilizes inactivation of AT III by anti–AT III IgG, and the subsequent inactivation of thrombin by heparin plus HC II incubation is measured.

Following the availability of specific assays, the first case of congenital HC II was reported by Tran and associates in 1985.[165] The patient was a 42-year-old woman with left middle cerebral artery thrombosis and a HC II level of 50% of normal. Of four additional family members, two had had thrombotic events and were also found to have low HC II levels. Since this original report, other patients and families have been found.[165,166] In the families in whom molecular defects in HC II (dysfunctional HC II) have been searched for, none have as yet been found. Thus, all congenital deficiencies are currently quantitative and not qualitative. Some studies have shown low HC II activity in asymptomatic individuals and families, and because of this finding it appears the clinical manifestations of hereditary HC II deficiency can span from arterial or venous thrombosis to asymptomatic states.[167,168]

Acquired Deficiency

Since HC II is a normal physiologic inhibitor of thrombin, it would be expected that in situations associated with activation of the coagulation system and subsequent thrombin generation, HC II would be consumed, much like AT III. Heparin cofactor II is markedly decreased in DIC,[169] and in instances where simultaneous AT III determinations have been determined, the HC II decreases parallel the decrease in AT III levels. Heparin cofactor II activity has only been studied in a small population of patients with deep venous thrombosis,[170] and the HC II levels were neither decreased nor influenced by the later addition of either heparin or warfarin anticoagulation. Heparin cofactor II activity has been studied in patients with nephrotic syndrome and found to generally remain normal, unlike AT III activity, which is commonly decreased in nephrotic syndrome.[171] In patients with chronic renal failure[172] undergoing hemodialysis, however, HC II activity was noted to be significantly decreased before dialysis and increased in some patients after dialysis. Heparin cofactor II is decreased

when a systemic activation of coagulation occurs but appears to not decrease with local activation, as in deep venous thrombosis.

Protein C

Protein C is a newly rediscovered vitamin K–dependent protein that is a major inhibitor of the procoagulant system and may equal or exceed the importance of AT III.[173,174] Protein C was first discovered in 1960 by Mammen, Thomas, and Seegers, who also noted its inhibitory nature.[175] Protein C was rediscovered in 1976 by Stenflo.[176] Seegers and coworkers,[177] in 1976, quickly showed that their early protein C, originally called autoprothrombin II-A, and Stenflo's rediscovered protein C were the same inhibitory protein. Since the rediscovery of protein C, great interest has centered around its modes of inhibitory action and its role in disease states. Protein C is a vitamin K–dependent protein synthesized in the hepatocyte with a molecular weight of about 56,000 d.[174,176] Protein C exerts its primary inhibitory activity by inactivating factors V and VIII:C.[174,178] To perform this inactivation, protein C must first be activated by thrombin.[173,174] The thrombin that activates protein C to protein CA (activated form) must first be bound to endothelial thrombomodulin. Following binding to endothelial thrombomodulin, thrombin derives the ability to activate protein C,[174,177] loses the ability to convert fibrinogen to fibrin, and loses the ability to activate platelets.[177] Protein CA (activated) is a serine protease, and its activity is inhibited by AT III.[177] The inhibitory activity of protein C in degrading factors V and VIII:C is markedly enhanced by protein S, another vitamin K–dependent factor.[179] This factor was discovered in 1977 by DiScipio in Seattle, hence the designation protein S.[180] The exact mechanisms by which protein S accentuates the activity of activated protein C in degrading factors V and VIII:C, which must occur in the presence of phospholipid, is unclear.[71] Mechanisms of action of protein C are summarized in Figure 13-5.

Congenital Deficiency

Congenital deficiency of protein C is inherited as an autosomal dominant trait, and the clinical characteristics are similar to congenital AT III deficiency.[58,79,178,181-185] Recurrent deep venous thrombosis and pulmonary embolus typically begin in the late teenage years.[58,79,178,181-185] Two forms of the disease exist: patients may have an absence of the protein (CRM–) or may have a dysfunctional protein (CRM+). Absence of the protein, thus far, appears to be more common than the presence of a dysfunctional protein.[79,186-188] Similar to AT III deficiency, venous thrombi and thromboemboli, especially pulmonary emboli, commonly occur in heterozygous and homozygous patients.[79,183] Most homozygous patients have succumbed to thrombi and thromboemboli during early infancy.[183,185,189,190] One homozygous infant has survived with the prophylactic use of a protein C–containing prothrombin complex concentrate.[189,190] Many patients with protein C deficiency develop skin necrosis

Figure 13-5. Protein C Activity

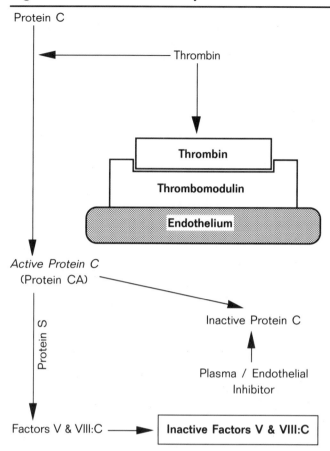

Table 13-13. Features of Congenital Protein C Deficiency

Clinical features
  Autosomal dominant trait
  Absence form and dysfunctional form exist
  Homozygous patients often die of thrombosis in
    early infancy
  Deep venous thrombosis and pulmonary embolus begin in
    mid- to late-teenage years
  Warfarin-induced skin necrosis often seen
  Clotting is common in heterozygotes
  Congenital deficiency may account for 5% to 10% of all
    patients with early clotting problems

Laboratory features
  Low biologic protein C levels
  Low immunologic protein C levels in absence form
  Normal immunologic protein C levels in dysfunctional form

Therapy
  Warfarin
  Prothrombin complex concentrates
  Heparin for acute thrombotic events

venous thrombosis is unclear.[198] Assays for protein C biologic and immunologic activity are readily available and are easily automated by synthetic substrate technique. Hematology laboratories should be encouraged to use this assay in all patients who develop deep venous thrombosis or pulmonary embolus and who present without other obvious causes for these events. Conditions associated with acquired protein C deficiency are listed in Table 13-14.

Protein S

Protein S was discovered by DiScipio and was purified in 1977. The protein is a vitamin K–dependent glycoprotein with a molecular weight of about 70,000 d. The discovery took place in Seattle, hence the designation as protein S.[180] Protein S was first noted to be a cofactor for the protein C inactivation of factor V[199] and was also found to be a cofactor for the protein C–induced inactivation of factor VIII:C.[200,201] Protein S is synthesized by both hepatocytes and megakaryocytes[202] and serves as a cofactor for inactivation of both plasma factor V and platelet (alpha granule) factor V. About 50% of plasma protein S is in the free form, and about 50% is bound to C4b

with warfarin drugs.[183,191,192] Thus, when examining patients with skin necrosis associated with warfarin therapy, the presence of congenital protein C deficiency should be considered strongly and a protein C assay done promptly.

Congenital protein C deficiency may actually be a more common cause of thrombosis or thromboembolus than AT III deficiency.[193] The actual incidence of congenital protein C deficiency will only become known as assays become more widely available. Currently, many protein C assays, some fully automated, are available for the clinical laboratory.[187,194-196] Congenital AT III deficiency probably accounts for about 3% to 5% of all patients presenting with deep venous thrombosis or pulmonary embolus. However, preliminary estimations suggest that congenital protein C deficiency may account for up to 10% of all patients presenting with venous thrombosis or pulmonary embolus. Clinical characteristics of congenital protein C deficiency are summarized in Table 13-13.

Acquired Deficiency

Acquired protein C deficiency is frequently seen in patients with acute DIC, extensive deep venous thrombosis, and severe liver disease.[183,197,198] Protein C levels may also be decreased in postoperative patients, but the role of this decrease in contributing to or causing postoperative deep

Table 13-14. Conditions With Acquired Protein C Deficiency

Disseminated intravascular coagulation
Deep venous thrombosis
Pulmonary embolus
Severe liver disease
Postoperative states

binding protein. About 50% of C4b binding protein appears to be committed to binding protein S. Protein S also serves as a cofactor for protein C enhancement of fibrinolysis.[203,204]

Congenital Deficiency

Congenital protein S deficiency was first reported in 1984 by three independent groups, and as assays became more generally available, more families with protein S deficiency were found.[205,206] It is now known that the deficiency is quite common. The incidence of protein S deficiency in those younger than 45 years of age with unexplained venous thrombosis is 5% to 10%.[207] The inheritance is autosomal dominant, and heterozygous patients have a strong tendency to develop deep venous thrombosis. Homozygotes are severely affected and may develop a form of purpura fulminans shortly after birth.[208] It is also possible that the homozygous state is associated with a high incidence of death in utero. Some heterozygous individuals and families, however, do not appear to demonstrate an increased predisposition to deep venous thrombosis, and thus, an asymptomatic deficiency state also exists.[209]

The clinical course of patients with symptomatic heterozygous protein S deficiency is similar to the clinical course of patients with congenital AT III deficiency or congenital protein C deficiency. Individuals with congenital protein S deficiency may also experience arterial thrombotic and thromboembolic events.[210] Similar to most other congenital coagulation protein abnormalities, the deficiency exists in two different forms: quantitative and qualitative.[211] In the quantitative form, referred to as type II, decreased C4b-bound and free protein S are present. In the qualitative form, decreased free protein S but adequate C4b-bound protein S (type I) are present. Therapy for congenital protein S deficiency is either long-term warfarin therapy or long-term heparin therapy.[212]

Acquired Deficiency

Since protein S is a vitamin K–dependent factor, it, like protein C, is decreased in patients taking warfarin therapy. The level of decrease is similar to that noted for the other vitamin K–dependent factors.[213] This creates the problem of evaluating the etiology of unexplained thrombosis in patients after warfarin has been started for the thrombotic episode. The protein C and S levels drop to about 40% to 60% of normal immediately after warfarin is taken; however, the levels increase to about 70% of normal after warfarin therapy has been in effect for more than two weeks. Thus, if protein C or S is going to be measured for etiologic significance after the patient has taken warfarin, the assays should be done after the patient has been taking the therapy for at least several weeks. In this instance, the levels of both protein S and C should be above 60%, and if they are lower, congenital deficiency should be strongly suspected. Protein S, like protein C, would be expected to decrease in situations where activation of the procoagulant system had occurred, as is the case in DIC. One study showed cleaved protein S

levels to be increased in DIC, suggesting that protein S is not only consumed during the intravascular clotting process but may also undergo proteolysis by the fibrinolytic system.[214] Protein S is decreased in type I diabetes mellitus and increased in type II diabetes mellitus. In the patients with type II diabetes, the increase in free protein S correlated with the increase in cholesterol.[215,216] Protein S levels have been studied in patients with the nephrotic syndrome, a clinical condition known to be associated with thrombosis and thromboembolism.[217-219] However, discrepant results have been reported and several studies have noted increased protein S levels in the nephrotic syndrome. Another study reported increased total protein S antigen in females and decreased free protein S antigen in males with the nephrotic syndrome, and yet another study reported increased levels of total protein S antigen but decreased levels of functional protein S in patients with the nephrotic syndrome. Thus, the behavior of protein S in patients with nephrotic syndrome appears complicated and unclearly understood at present. Free protein S levels are decreased with estrogen therapy. The decrease is most pronounced with high-dose hormonal replacement therapy but also happens with low-dose estrogens in oral contraceptive agents.[220,221] As measured immunologically in the newborn, total protein S is very low but free protein S, although lower than in adults, comprises the majority of the protein S present, because of very low levels of C4b binding protein.[222] Both total and free protein S decrease steadily throughout normal pregnancy, reaching the lowest levels at term, which may account for the increased frequency of postpartum thrombosis.[223] Protein S levels have been studied in a small group of patients with primary (essential) thrombocythemia (ET). Total and free protein S levels were decreased in patients with ET who had experienced vaso-occlusive problems and normal in those who did not have thrombosis or thromboembolus.[224] Protein S levels returned to normal in one patient after initiation of hydroxyurea therapy. Free protein S levels have been reported to occur in patients with untreated acute lymphocytic leukemia and in those receiving L-asparaginase therapy. The L-asparaginase was thought to cause or exaggerate decreased free protein S levels, but a relationship to clinical thrombosis was unclear.[225]

Altered Fibrinolytic Activity

Decreased fibrinolytic and fibrinolytic activator activity should predispose to thrombus formation. Plasminogen, a precursor of plasmin, is synthesized in the liver or eosinophil; however, most physiologically important plasminogen activator activity is from vascular endothelium or via indirect activation by activated Hageman factor.[226] Activation pathways were discussed in detail in chapter 1. Hypoactivity of the fibrinolytic system and predisposition to thrombus formation can arise from either decreased plasminogen levels, decreased plasminogen activator activity, or increased fibrinolytic inhibitor activi-

Table 13-15. Mechanisms of Impaired Fibrinolysis

Decreased plasminogen levels

Decreased plasminogen activators
  Plasma activators
  Endothelial activators
  Abnormal factor XII activation pathway

Increased fibrinolytic system inhibitors
  Alpha-2-antiplasmin
  Alpha-2-macroglobulin

Inhibition of plasminogen activators

Table 13-16. Conditions Associated With Impaired Fibrinolytic Activity

Acute myocardial infarction
Atherosclerosis
Congenital plasminogen defects
Deep venous thrombosis
Diabetes mellitus
Disseminated intravascular coagulation
Liver disease
Malignancy
Oral contraceptive use
Postoperative states
Pregnancy
Pulmonary fibrosis
Scleroderma
Septicemia
Thrombotic thrombocytopenic purpura

ty. Mechanisms of hypoactivity of fibrinolysis are summarized in Table 13-15. Unfortunately, most studies of fibrinolytic activity changes in disease states have been generic, measuring complete fibrinolytic activity. Thus, it is often not known if the decrease in fibrinolytic activity is the result of decreased plasminogen, decreased activation ability, or increased inhibitors, because assays to distinguish between these defects have not formerly been available. Decreased fibrinolytic activity has been noted in acute myocardial infarction and in patients with generalized atherosclerosis.[227,228] Decreased activity is present in diabetes and in patients with scleroderma and thrombotic thrombocytopenic purpura.[229,230] In patients with generalized atherosclerosis, the decrease in fibrinolytic activity may be caused by vascular intimal damage and the loss of fibrinolytic plasminogen activator activity.[56,231-233]

Decreased fibrinolytic activity is present in diabetes and in acute pulmonary embolism. Whether this is of etiologic significance in acute pulmonary embolism or simply because of consumption is unclear.[229] Generally, decreased fibrinolytic activity is also noted in patients with recurrent deep venous thrombosis, patients taking oral contraceptives, and in most postoperative patients.[234,235] The observations of decreased plasminogen levels in patients with deep venous thrombosis, recurrent thrombotic disease, and pulmonary emboli assume major importance if the patient is considered a candidate for thrombolytic therapy.[236] If plasminogen levels are decreased significantly, thrombolytic therapy with streptokinase, TPA, or urokinase may not be efficacious.[236] Conditions associated with decreased fibrinolytic activity are summarized in Table 13-16.

Increased inhibitors of the fibrinolytic system are noted in many disorders. The primary inhibitors of the fibrinolytic system are alpha-2-antiplasmin and alpha-2-macroglobulin. Their mechanisms of inhibitory activity were discussed in chapter 1. These two inhibitors are increased in pulmonary fibrosis, malignancy, infections, acute myocardial infarction, and in thromboembolic disease.[237] Alpha-2-macroglobulin and alpha-1-antitrypsin (other inhibitors of the fibrinolytic system) are increased in the postoperative state, pregnancy, diabetes, and in users of oral contraceptives.[4] Conditions associated with increased fibrinolytic system inhibitors are depicted in Table 13-17.

Inhibitors of the fibrinolytic system are normal in most individuals with recurrent deep venous thrombosis. As with other changes in the circulating blood, the finding of increased inhibitors of fibrinolytic activity (alpha-1-antitrypsin and alpha-2-antiplasmin) have usually been noted after the thrombosis has occurred, and whether these increases are of etiologic significance or because of an acute-phase reaction secondary to an already present thrombotic event remains speculative.[238]

Fibrinolytic activator activity is inhibited in the postoperative state, infections, general inflammatory disorders, scleroderma, and thrombotic thrombocytopenic purpura.[230,239] However, no detectable inhibition against fibrinolytic activator activity is noted in patients with acute thrombosis or thromboembolus. It can only be concluded that, in general, reactive processes are associated with thrombosis and hypofibrinolysis. These processes are caused by several potential mechanisms: (1) decreased plasminogen; (2) decreased plasminogen activator activity; (3) increased fibrinolytic inhibitors; and (4) increased plasminogen activator inhibition. The significance of these findings remains unclear since it is not known whether many of these changes were present before subclinical thrombus formation and,

Table 13-17. Conditions Associated With Elevated Fibrinolytic System Inhibitors

Acute myocardial infarction
Deep venous thrombosis
Diabetes mellitus
Infections
Malignancy
Oral contraceptive use
Postoperative state
Pregnancy
Pulmonary embolus
Pulmonary fibrosis

Table 13-18. Conditions Associated With Inhibition of Plasminogen Activator Activity

General inflammatory conditions
Scleroderma
Thrombotic thrombocytopenic purpura

thus, potentially of etiologic significance or whether they simply developed as a consequence of thrombosis. Conditions associated with inhibition of plasminogen activator activity are summarized in Table 13-18. Assays currently available for components of the fibrinolytic system are listed in Table 13-19.

Congenital Plasminogen Deficiency

Congenital plasminogen deficiency is very rare[240] but may be found to be more common than formerly thought with the availability of reliable and simple plasminogen assays by synthetic substrate methods.[2,150,151,241] The disorder is inherited as an autosomal recessive trait.[242] Both the absence form (CRM−) and the dysfunctional form (CRM+) have been described, and the dysfunctional form is the more common type.[240,242,243] Clinically, patients show similarities to congenital AT III deficiency and congenital protein C or S deficiency. Patients with congenital plasminogen deficiency begin to experience thrombotic events in their late teenage years.[240,242-244] The most common thrombotic events are deep venous thrombosis and pulmonary embolization.[240,242-244] Arterial thrombotic and thromboembolic events are not a prominent characteristic. Venous thrombotic and thromboembolic events occur when the plasminogen level is less than 40% of normal biologic activity.[243] Both homozygous and heterozygous patients can be identified by synthetic substrate assays for biologic activity of plasminogen, and a comparison of biologic activity with immunologic levels is used to identify those patients who have dysfunctional plasminogen vs those with quantitative hypoplasminogenemia (heterozygotes) or

Table 13-19. Assays for Assessment of the Fibrinolytic System

Plasminogen assay
Plasmin assay
Endothelial plasminogen activator
Endothelial plasminogen activator inhibitor
Alpha-2-antiplasmin
Alpha-2-macroglobulin
Fibrin(ogen) degradation products
D-dimer
B-beta 15-42–related peptides

(All are automated by synthetic substrate, ELISA, radioimmunoassay, or laser nephelometry.)

Table 13-20. Features of Congenital Plasminogen Deficiency

Clinical features
    Autosomal recessive trait
    Absence form and dysfunction form exist
    Thrombotic events begin in mid- to late-teenage years
    Deep venous thrombosis is common
    Pulmonary embolization is common
    Arterial thrombotic events are rare
    Thrombosis occurs when plasminogen is less than 40%

Laboratory features
    Low biologic plasminogen activity
    Low immunologic plasminogen in absence form
    Normal immunologic plasminogen in dysfunctional form

Therapy
    Warfarin
    Heparin
    Antiplatelet drugs
    Urokinase

aplasminogenemia (homozygotes). Results of all the usual global tests of coagulation, including the platelet count, prothrombin time, partial thromboplastin time, thrombin time, and bleeding time, will be normal, and the diagnosis depends on specific plasminogen assay for biologic activity.[3,240] Successful therapy has included the use of heparin, warfarin-type drugs, antiplatelet agents, and urokinase.[243,244] The clinical characteristics of congenital plasminogen deficiency are summarized in Table 13-20.

Acquired Plasminogen Deficiency

Congenital deficiency of plasminogen activator appears to be an extremely uncommon problem, and only a few suspected cases have been reported. In the few cases reported, thrombosis, including cerebrovascular thrombosis, has been noted. Likewise, congenital increase in plasminogen activator inhibitor has also been reported but is extremely rare.[245,246] As with congenital plasminogen activator deficiency, congenital elevations of plasminogen activator inhibitor have been associated with familial thrombosis.[247]

Acquired deficiency of plasminogen activator is found in many pathologic conditions. Patients with unstable angina, acute myocardial infarction, and post–percutaneous transluminal coronary angioplasty (post-PTCA) have been noted to be deficient in plasminogen activator activity. In patients with post-PTCA this defect is proposed as a mechanism for restenosis.[248] Patients with diabetes mellitus have been extensively studied for defects in plasminogen activator activity. Although the results are conflicting, patients with non–insulin-dependent diabetes mellitus (NIDDM) have low intrinsic plasminogen activator activity, which increases with blood sugar, exercise, and oral hypoglycemic therapy.[249] Patients with insulin-dependent diabetes have both low and normal plasminogen activator activity, but, like patients with NIDDM, the levels increase with exercise, specific therapeutic agents, and the development of retinopathy.[250]

Decreased plasminogen activator has been noted in both ulcerative colitis and Crohn's disease.[251] Increased levels are found in patients with histiocytosis X and cryptogenic fibrosing alveolitis,[251,252] and cigarette smokers are reported to have higher macrophage plasminogen activator activity than nonsmokers.[253] Interestingly, increased plasminogen activator levels have been noted in breast carcinoma, and the degree of increase is thought to correlate with tumor size and axillary nodal status.[254] Plasminogen activator is decreased in pleural lavage fluid of patients with sarcoidosis; this finding and an increase in procoagulant activity have led to suggestions that these defects may contribute to pulmonary pathophysiology in sarcoidosis.[255] Decreased tissue plasminogen activator activity is associated with alcohol ingestion, and the degree of decrease is related to the amount of alcohol consumed.[256] One study showed decreased plasminogen activator activity in a population of women who both smoked heavily and ingested oral contraceptives.[257] In one study, plasminogen activator was found to be decreased in severe rheumatoid arthritis, and stanozolol therapy induced an increase in plasminogen activator levels.[258] Plasminogen activator and plasminogen activator inhibitor levels are increased in many patients with cirrhosis of the liver.[259,260] Patients with septic shock have elevated plasminogen activator inhibitor levels, and elevation is associated with high mortality. One study suggested this finding to be of significance in the end-organ damage of septic shock that accompanies systemic microvascular occlusion.[261] High values for plasminogen activator inhibitor have been noted in patients with type II diabetes mellitus, and the levels were noted to correlate with high blood glucose, insulin levels, triglyceride and cholesterol levels, and the presence of coronary artery disease. Deep venous thrombosis has been associated with increased plasminogen activator inhibitor levels; however, it is unclear if this was because of thrombosis or of possible etiologic importance.[262]

The use of estrogen-containing oral contraceptives has been associated with a decrease in plasminogen activator inhibition, but an increase has been noted during normal pregnancy. Plasminogen activator activity is inhibited by low-density lipoprotein.[263] The relationship between this inhibition and the development of atherosclerosis, however, is unclear.

Congenital Dysfibrinogenemia

Dysfibrinogenemia represents the presence of a functionally abnormal fibrinogen, the first of which was described by Di Imperato and Dettori in 1958.[264] Since that time, more than 100 different dysfibrinogenemias have been reported.[265,266] The first molecular defect characterized to account

Table 13-21. Congenital Dysfibrinogenemias Accompanied by Thrombosis

Name	Year
Fibrinogen Baltimore	1964
Fibrinogen Bergamo II	1986
Fibrinogen Chapel Hill I	1975
Fibrinogen Charlottesville	1977
Fibrinogen Copenhagen	1979
Fibrinogen Dusard	1984
Fibrinogen Marburg	1977
Fibrinogen Naples	1977
Fibrinogen New York	1975
Fibrinogen Nijmegen	1988
Fibrinogen Oslo I	1967
Fibrinogen Paris II	1968
Fibrinogen Weisbaden	1971

for a dysfibrinogenemia was reported by Blomback and coworkers in 1968.[267] Since that time, many dysfibrinogenemias have been characterized with respect to the underlying defect, but in many, the precise defect remains unclear. The dysfibrinogenemias were discussed in detail in chapter 6. Most individuals with dysfibrinogenemia are either asymptomatic or have a mild to moderate hemorrhagic disorder, although about 10% of the dysfibrinogenemias are accompanied by thrombosis.[265] Although venous thrombosis is the most common manifestation of this subgroup of dysfibrinogenemia, some have been associated with arterial thrombotic disease.[266-268] Most of the dysfibrinogenemias characterized by thrombosis have not been classified; however, of those categorized, some are associated with abnormal fibrin monomer polymerization, impaired activation of fibrinolysis, or resistance to fibrinolysis. Fibrinogen Dusard[269] is associated with defective or decreased activation of plasminogen; fibrinogen Nijmegen[270] is associated with defective plasminogen activator–mediated plasminogen activation; and fibrinogen Bergamo II[271] is characterized by slow fibrin monomer polymerization resulting from a polymerization defect, from an amino acid substitution, found on the carboxy-terminal portion of the gamma chains. The dysfibrinogenemias associated with thrombosis are summarized in Table 13-21.

Anticardiolipin Antibodies

Interest in antiphospholipids began with the discovery of the lupus anticoagulant in about 10% of patients with systemic lupus in 1952.[272] Shortly thereafter, it was recognized that the presence of the lupus anticoagulant was associated with thrombosis instead of bleeding.[273] Many patents without autoimmune disorders also had lupus anticoagulants, and these antiphospholipid antibodies have now been reported in many conditions including malignancy, immune thrombocytopenic purpura, leukemias, infections, in individuals ingesting chlorpromazine or procainamide, and in seemingly normal individuals.[274-278] Because of a noted association between lupus, a biologic false-positive test for syphilis, and the presence of the lupus anticoagulant, in 1983, Harris and coworkers devised a new test for antiphospholipids using cardiolipin.[279] This test and subsequent modifications have now become known as the anticardiolipin antibody test. Generally, IgG, IgA, and IgM anticardiolipin idiotypes are now assessed.[280] Shortly after development of the anticardiolipin antibody assay, it became apparent that these antibodies were not limited to the patient with lupus but were found in patients who did not have lupus as well. These anticardiolipin antibodies have now been associated with thrombosis and thromboembolus of both arterial and venous systems,[281-283] recurrent fetal loss,[284,285] and thrombocytopenia.[286,287] Although associations between the lupus anticoagulant and anticardiolipin antibodies and between lupus anticoagulant and these syndromes exist, it is clear that the lupus anticoagulant and anticardiolipin antibodies are two separate entities. Many individuals with anticardiolipin antibodies do not have a lupus anticoagulant, and many with the lupus anticoagulant do not have the anticardiolipin antibody.[288] Initially, it was thought that primarily IgG anticardiolipin antibody was associated with thrombosis; however, IgA and IgM anticardiolipin antibodies are also associated with thrombosis. The presence of any one anticardiolipin antibody, a combination of two, or all three together may be associated with thrombosis and thromboembolus.[289] Although different types of thrombosis occur, no apparent association between the type of thrombotic event and the type of anticardiolipin antibody present exists.[290]

The mechanism of action of anticardiolipin antibodies in leading or contributing to thrombosis is unknown, but several plausible theories have been suggested. Anticardiolipin antibodies have affinity for important phospholipids involved at many points in the hemostasis system. These antibodies are directed primarily against phosphatidylserine and phosphatidylinositol but not phosphatidylcholine, another important phospholipid in hemostasis.[291] The proposed mechanisms of action of anticardiolipin antibodies in interfering with hemostasis to induce thrombosis are interference with endothelial release of prostacyclin,[292] interference with activation, via thrombomodulin, of protein C or interference with protein S activity as a cofactor,[293] interference with AT III activity,[294] interaction with platelet membrane phospholipids,[295] interference of prekallikrein activation to kallikrein,[296] or interference with endothelial release of plasminogen activator.[297] All these components of normal hemostasis are dependent on phospholipid, except possibly AT III activity. Anticardiolipin antibodies are associated with many types of venous thrombotic problems, including deep venous thrombosis of the upper and lower extremities, pulmonary embolus, intracranial veins, inferior vena cava, hepatic vein, portal vein, renal vein, and retinal veins.[298-300] Arterial thromboses associated with anticardiolipin antibodies have included the coronary arteries, cerebral arteries, retinal arteries, brachial arteries, mesenteric arteries, peripheral (extremity) arteries, and aorta.[301-303] In a recent study, it was found that more than 50% of patients undergoing late graft occlusion following coronary artery bypass grafting had preoperative anticardiolipin antibodies, strongly suggesting that late graft occlusion may be caused by the presence of antiphospholipid antibodies.[304] Anticardiolipin antibodies have also been associated with mitral valvular disease, aortic insufficiency, and endocarditis.[305]

Another recent study reported that 21% of young survivors of acute myocardial infarction had anticardiolipin antibodies. In those surviving, 69% of patients with these antibodies had a later cardiovascular event.[306] Anticardiolipin antibodies are associated with livido reticularis and a syndrome of recurrent deep venous thrombosis, necrotizing purpura, and stasis ulcers.[307] The neurologic syndromes associated with anticardiolipin antibodies have been transient cerebral ischemic attacks, arterial and venous retinal occlusive disease, cerebral arterial and venous thrombosis, migraine headaches, Degos' disease, Guillain-Barré syndrome, chorea, and optic neuritis.[308-310] Anticardiolipin antibodies are associated with a high chance of fetal wastage. The characteristics of this syndrome are frequent spontaneous abortion in the first trimester, recurrent fetal wastage in the second and third trimesters, placental vasculitis, and maternal thrombocytopenia. This syndrome has been successfully treated to normal term by institution of prednisone plus aspirin, low-dose heparin, or plasma exchange. Anticardiolipin antibodies are also associated with a peculiar postpartum syndrome of spiking fevers, pleuritic chest pain, dyspnea and pleural effusion, patchy pulmonary infiltrates, cardiomyopathy, and ventricular arrhythmias. This syndrome characteristically occurs two to 10 days' postpartum.[311]

With respect to thrombosis and the antiphospholipid syndrome, patients can be divided into one of four subgroups: type I syndrome comprises patients with deep venous thrombosis; type II syndrome comprises patients with coronary artery or peripheral arterial (including aorta) thrombosis; type III syndrome comprises patients with retinal or cerebrovascular thrombosis; and type IV syndrome comprises patients with admixtures of the first three types. Patients with type IV syndromes are uncommon, and most fit into one of the first three types. Little overlap occurs between these subtypes, and patients usually conveniently fit onto only one of these groups. The types are summarized in Table 13-22.[290]

Although the type or titer of anticardiolipin antibody and type of syndrome (I through IV) do not appear to correlate, the subclassification of patients with thrombosis and anticardiolipin antibody into these groups is important from the therapy

Table 13-22. Syndromes of Thrombosis Associated With Anticardiolipin Antibodies

Type I syndrome
  Deep venous thrombosis with or without pulmonary embolus

Type II syndrome
  Coronary artery thrombosis
  Peripheral artery thrombosis
  Aortic thrombosis

Type III syndrome
  Retinal artery thrombosis
  Retinal vein thrombosis
  Cerebrovascular thrombosis
  Transient cerebral ischemic attacks

Type IV syndrome
  Mixtures of types I, II, and III
  Type IV conditions are rare

Table 13-23. Suggested Anticoagulant Regimens for Syndromes of Thrombosis Associated With Anticardiolipin Antibodies

Type I syndrome
  Intravenous heparin followed by long-term
    self-administration of subcutaneous calcium heparin*

Type II syndrome
  Intravenous heparin followed by long-term
    self-administration of subcutaneous calcium heparin*

Type III syndrome
  Cerebrovascular
    Long-term warfarin* with a prothrombin time ratio of 1.2
      to 1.5 plus low-dose acetylsalicylic acid twice daily
  Retinal
    Same as for cerebrovascular or pentoxiphylline* at
      400 mg four times daily

Type IV syndrome
  Therapy is dependent on type(s) and site(s) of thrombosis,
    as per above recommendations

* Anticoagulant therapy should not be stopped unless the anticardiolipin antibody has been absent for the preceding four months.

standpoint.[290] Type I syndrome is best managed by long-term subcutaneous heparin or long-term warfarin therapy; type II syndrome is best managed by subcutaneous heparin therapy; and type III syndrome is best managed by low-dose warfarin plus low-dose aspirin (carotid or intracranial) or pentoxiphylline (retinal); and therapy of type IV syndrome depends on the type of thrombosis present.[290] Obviously, patients with thrombosis and anticardiolipin antibodies require long-term anticoagulant therapy. Therapy should be stopped only if the anticardiolipin antibody disappears for several months before considering cessation of anticoagulation.[290] Table 13-23 outlines suggested anticoagulant regimens, based on the type of anticardiolipin thrombosis syndrome.

Vessel Wall Changes

Changes in the vessel wall are probably the most common etiologic factors in arterial thrombus formation.[231,312] These changes can come about via many mechanisms. Collagen can be exposed by local injury to the vessel and by inflammatory vascular changes. Stasis, hypoxia, acidosis, and shock may give rise to endothelial sloughing with exposure to subendothelial collagen and activation of coagulation. Exposed collagen may initiate platelet aggregation and release and may activate the blood coagulation system by the activation of factor XII to factor XIIa and activation of factor XI to factor XIa.[4,6,123,313] Endothelial plasminogen activator activity may be decreased and is usually decreased in many vascular disorders, including scleroderma and thrombotic thrombocytopenic purpura. Much less endothelial plasminogen activator activity is noted in the lower extremities as compared to the upper extremities, which may account for, or at least contribute to, the higher incidence of thrombosis in the lower extremities.[314] Decreased fibrinolytic activator activity is found in about 75% of patients with recurrent deep venous thrombosis, and this is often ascribed to primary vascular damage. The significance of this association, however, is unclear. The distribution and amount of various vascular proteoglycans may be correlated with arterial thrombotic and thromboembolic disease.[315] Excellent summaries of this rapidly evolving topic are available.[56,231]

Laboratory Evaluation

Older techniques for assessing platelet hyperreactivity have primarily been measurements of altered platelet aggregability as measured by the standard platelet aggregometer and noting enhanced slopes of aggregation. These data, however, have not generally been clinically useful. Newer molecular markers of platelet reactivity, such as platelet factor 4 and beta-thromboglobulin, and various platelet or endothelial prostaglandin derivatives, including thromboxane B_2 assays, prostacyclin assays, and cyclo-oxygenase assays, are available. These assays are potentially useful in assessing platelet reactivity in hypercoagulable conditions and in subclinical and clinical thrombotic disorders, including patients with deep venous thrombosis, thromboembolus, unstable angina, alterations of hemostasis associated with malignancy, and arterial thrombotic and thromboembolic events, and other general microvascular disorders.[1-3,316,317] These new molecular markers of platelet reactivity are useful tools for both diagnosis and monitoring of antithrombotic and antiplatelet therapy in individuals with these disorders. Many patients with hypercoagulability or thrombotic disorders have elevated platelet factor 4, beta-thromboglobulin, and thromboxane B_2 levels, which usually decrease after starting effective antithrombotic therapy.[1-3,316,317]

Thus, readily available molecular markers of platelet reactivity include the platelet factor 4 level, beta-thromboglobulin level, and various prostaglandin derivatives, including the immediate breakdown products of thromboxane A_2 (thromboxane B_2), and prostacyclin (6-keto-PGF-1-alpha). Several or all of these markers may be of benefit in diagnosing conditions and in monitoring therapy in patients with hypercoagulable disorders and thrombosis. This is especially true of the platelet factor 4 and beta-thromboglobulin measurement. Platelet survival assessed by many techniques is altered in patients with hypercoagulability or clinical thrombosis.[318]

Many coagulation factors are elevated in patients with hypercoagulability and thrombosis. Generally, however, the measurements of these factors, including fibrinogen, factor VIII:C, factor IX, and other related factors, are not useful for either diagnosis or monitoring of therapy. Decreases in coagulation inhibitors, including AT III, heparin cofactor II, protein C, and protein S, are of major importance in assessing patients with both hypercoagulable states or unexplained thrombosis. These assays are of both diagnostic and therapeutic importance in patients with hypercoagulability and in patients with subclinical or clinical thrombotic and thromboembolic events.[3,24,74,79,183] Automated methods for assessing AT III and proteins C and S are available and are important, especially if a congenital deficiency is found.[3,24,79,174,187] Another advance in the diagnosis of hypercoagulability and thrombosis has been the use of fibrinogen chromatography.[18,319] Much useful information comes from this modality. The procedure is now automated to the point where it can be performed in several hours, although the equipment and time needed is still formidable for the routine clinical hemostasis laboratory. Fibrinogen chromatography when used clinically can detect several fibrinogen subspecies: (1) fibrin monomer (molecular weight of about 320,000 d) is fibrinogen minus fibrinopeptides A and B; (2) fibrinogen dimer has a molecular weight of about 650,000 d and represents one intact fibrinogen molecule complexed with one fibrin monomer; (3) fibrinogen polymer (molecular weight of approximately 400,000 to 1,000,000 d) is fibrinogen complexed with various fibrin(ogen) fragments; (4) fibrinogen-first derivative (molecular weight of 267,000 d) represents fibrinogen that has been cleaved at the carboxy-terminal end of the A-alpha chain by plasmin; (5) X, Y, D, and E fibrin(ogen) fragments are also measured. The applicability of fibrinogen chromatography becomes evident when looking at disorders characterized by the presence of fibrinogen dimer and fibrinogen polymer. Generally, thrombosis is characterized by an increase in fibrin(ogen) complexes of molecular weight of 450,000 d or greater. When these fragments are found, one may presume that increased fibrin deposition is occurring. As a thrombus resolves, because of fibrinolysis, the following are noted: (1) a decrease in fibrinogen/fibrin complexes; (2) an increase in FDP; and (3) an increase in fibrinogen-first derivative.[320] Fibrinopeptide A and fibrinopeptide B

Table 13-24. Molecular Markers for Assessment of Hypercoagulability and Thrombosis

Fibrinopeptide A
Fibrinopeptide B
B-beta 15-42–related peptides
Platelet factor 4
Beta-thromboglobulin
Thromboxanes (TxB-2)
Prostacyclins (6-keto-PGFl-alpha)
Soluble fibrin monomer
Fibrinogen degradation products
D-dimer

(All may be fully automated by synthetic substrates, ELISA, radioimmunoassay, or laser nephelometry)

levels will be decreased. Techniques to detect thrombin generation rapidly using fibrinopeptide A titers are readily available. Fibrinopeptide A is elevated in many hypercoagulable and thrombotic disorders and usually falls with institution of successful antithrombotic therapy.[1-3,316]

Another modality that may prove useful in hypercoagulability and subclinical and clinical thrombosis is the simultaneous determination of B-beta 15-42 and related peptides.[321,322] As plasmin begins to circulate, B-beta peptides 1 through 118 and 1 through 42 begin to circulate. If thrombin has removed fibrinopeptide B (the first 14 amino acids on the B-beta chain), B-beta 15-42 levels also increase. Thus, in patients with circulating thrombin, elevated fibrinopeptide A and B levels will be noted. As plasmin begins to circulate, the elevation of B-beta 15-42 and related peptides will also be noted, allowing for the conclusion that thrombus resolution is beginning. Thus, the molecular profiling of patients with hypercoagulability and subclinical and clinical thrombosis is now becoming available (Table 13-24).

Assays for components of the fibrinolytic system are also available and help in a diagnosis of hypercoagulability and thrombosis. The assays available are for plasminogen, plasmin, endothelial plasminogen activator activity, plasminogen activator inhibitor, and alpha-2-antiplasmin.[3,150,151,323]

The traditional older methods for assessing hypercoagulability and thrombosis, such as the APTT, nonactivated partial thromboplastin time (Kingdon assay), the fibrinogen level, and elevated coagulation factors, have contributed little to the understanding of hypercoagulability and thrombosis and have generally not been associated with useful clinical information. However, newer assays are becoming available by automated techniques including the synthetic substrate equivalent of the APTT, the so-called intrinsic pathway–generated thrombin test (IPGT), the synthetic substrate equivalent of the prothrombin time, the so-called extrinsic pathway–generated thrombin test (EPGT), the AT III level by synthetic substrate assay, protein C levels by synthetic substrate assays, and synthetic substrate assays for fibrinolytic system components.[3,150] Radioimmunoassays

Table 13-25. Newer Assays Available for Assessing Propensity to Hypercoagulability and Thrombosis

Extrinsic pathway–generated thrombin (EPGT)
Intrinsic pathway–generated thrombin (IPGT)
Antithrombin III
Heparin cofactor II
Protein C
Protein S
Plasminogen
Plasmin
Plasminogen activator
Plasminogen activator inhibitor
Alpha-2-antiplasmin
Alpha-2-macroglobulin
Fibrinopeptide A
Fibrinopeptide B
Fibrin(ogen) degradation products
D-dimer
B-beta 15-42–related peptides
Protamine sulfate
Platelet factor 4
Beta-thromboglobulin
Prostaglandins
Thromboxanes
Platelet survival

Table 13-27. Congenital Blood Protein Defects Associated With Hypercoagulability and Thrombosis

Antithrombin III deficiency
Heparin cofactor II deficiency
Protein C deficiency
Protein S deficiency
Plasminogen deficiency
Dysfibrinogenemia
Plasminogen activator deficiency
Hageman factor (factor XII) deficiency
Prekallikrein deficiency?
High–molecular weight kininogen deficiency?
Cystathionine beta-synthetase deficiency

phology, reticulocyte count, general biochemical screening surveys, autoimmune evaluations, paraprotein evaluations, evaluations for occult malignancy, angiography, thrombo-scintography, ventilation perfusion scans, pulmonary angiography, peripheral vascular angiography, and vascular biopsies for morphology and special staining techniques. Nonhemostasis techniques often needed for assessing hypercoagulability and thrombosis are summarized in Table 13-26. Measurements that should be considered to explore congenital defects leading to hypercoagulability and thrombosis are summarized in Table 13-27, and laboratory evaluations for acquired blood defects leading to hypercoagulability and thrombosis are summarized in Table 13-28.

The laboratory diagnosis of hypercoagulability and thrombosis is in its infancy despite recent advances in the coagulation laboratory. Molecular markers of platelet reactivity and altered blood protein function (coagulation, fibrinolysis, and inhibitors) may prove useful in diagnosing conditions and in monitoring patients who are hypercoagulable or have subclinical or clinical thrombosis. It is anticipated that with the widespread use of automated molecular weight profiling, physicians will be able to detect and treat hypercoagulable individuals before they have a life-threatening thrombotic event or before a serious thrombohemorrhagic event leads to irreversible and lifelong morbidity.[324,325]

and potentially ELISA procedures for fibrinopeptide A, fibrinopeptide B, platelet-reactive products, including platelet factor 4 and beta-thromboglobulin, thromboxane B_2, and 6-keto-PGF1-alpha are also available for molecular profiling by automated techniques.[1-3,150,151,316] Newer laboratory tests for the evaluation of hypercoagulability and thrombosis are depicted in Table 13-25.

When assessing patients with hypercoagulability and thrombosis, nonhemostasis testing methods usually must be considered. These include such procedures as complete blood cell count, platelet count, evaluation of platelet mor-

Table 13-26. Additional Nonhemostasis Modalities for Evaluating Hypercoagulability and Thrombosis

Complete blood cell count
Platelet count
Sedimentation rate
Biochemical screening survey
Lipid profile
Orotic acid crystals
Angiography
Thromboscintography
Ascending venography
Pooled gated whole blood venogram
Pulmonary V/P isotope scan
Vascular biopsy
Immunofluorescent stains
Hyperviscosity

Table 13-28. Acquired Blood Protein Defects Associated With Hypercoagulability and Thrombosis

Antithrombin III deficiency
Heparin cofactor II deficiency
Protein C deficiency
Protein S deficiency
Plasminogen deficiency
Dysfibrinogenemia
Plasminogen activator deficiency
Elevated plasminogen activator inhibitor
Lupus anticoagulant
Anticardiolipin antibodies

Summary

This chapter has summarized known alterations of hemostasis in patients with hypercoagulability and subclinical and clinical thrombus formation. It remains unclear whether many of these changes are of etiologic significance or are manifestations (consequences) of already present, clinically undetectable thrombosis. At present, many common laboratory modalities do not allow for a differentiation between cause and effect. Practical techniques consisting of fully automated assays and molecular marker techniques should soon be available to detect subclinical changes in the coagulation system and will become more generally available for detecting prethrombotic events, for monitoring patients who have had a thrombotic event, and for detecting patients potentially predisposed to thrombosis, so that the patient can be treated prophylactically before unalterable morbidity or mortality occurs.

References

1. Bick RL: Clinical implications of molecular markers in hemostasis and thrombosis. Semin Thromb Hemost 10:290, 1984.

2. Bick RL, J Fareed, G Squillaci: Molecular markers of hemostatic processes. Implications in diagnostic and therapeutic management of thrombotic and hemorrhagic disorders. Fed Proc 42:4, 1983.

3. Bick RL: Clinical hemostasis practice: the major impact of laboratory automation. Semin Thromb Hemost 9:139, 1983.

4. Bick RL: Hypercoagulability and thrombosis, ch 13. In: G Murano, RL Bick (Eds): Basic Concepts of Hemostasis and Thrombosis. CRC Press, Boca Raton, FL, 1980, p 237.

5. Hume M, S Sevitt, DP Thomas: Venous thrombosis and pulmonary embolism. Harvard University Press, Cambridge, 1970.

6. Bick RL: Disseminated intravascular coagulation and related syndromes: a clinical review. Semin Thromb Hemost 14:299, 1988.

7. Hellem AJ: Platelet adhesiveness. Ser Haematol 1:99, 1968.

8. Hume M, YK Chan: Examination of the blood in the presence of venous thrombosis. JAMA 200:747, 1967.

9. Bobek K, V Kepelak: Laboratory diagnosis of venous thrombosis. Acta Med Scand 160:121, 1958.

10. Isacson S, IM Nilsson: Coagulation and platelet adhesiveness in recurrent "idiopathic" venous thrombosis and thrombophlebitis. Acta Chir Scand 138:263, 1972.

11. Emmons PR, JRA Mitchell: Postoperative changes in platelet clumping activity. Lancet 1:71, 1965.

12. Hellem AJ: Adenosine diphosphate–induced platelet adhesiveness in diabetes mellitus with complications. Acta Med Scand 190:291, 1971.

13. Becker J: The relation of platelet adhesiveness to postoperative venous thrombosis of the legs. Acta Chir Scand 138:781, 1972.

14. Davidson E, S Tomlin: The levels of the plasma coagulation factors after trauma and childbirth. J Clin Pathol 16:112, 1963.

15. Nicolaides AN, D Irving: Clinical factors and the risk of deep venous thrombosis. In: AN Nicolaides (Ed): Thromboembolism: Etiology, Advances in Prevention and Management. University Park Press, Baltimore, 1975, p 193.

16. Nilsson IM: Thrombosis and treatment of thrombosis. In: IM Nilsson (Ed): Hemorrhagic and Thrombotic Disease. John Wiley & Sons, New York, 1974, p 163.

17. Davis RB, A Theologides, BJ Kennedy: Comparative studies of blood coagulation and platelet aggregation in patients with cancer and non-malignant disease. Ann Intern Med 71:67, 1969.

18. Alkjaersig N, L Roy, AP Fletcher: Analysis of gel exclusion chromatography data by chromatographic plate theory analysis: application to plasma fibrinogen chromatography. Thromb Res 3:525, 1973.

19. Seegers WH: Basic principles of blood coagulation. Semin Thromb Hemost 7:180, 1981.

20. Irwin JF, WH Seegers, TJ Andary: Blood coagulation as a cybernetic system: control of autoprothrombin-C (Xa) formation. Thromb Res 6:431, 1975.

21. Harpel PC, RD Rosenberg: Alpha-2-macroglobulin and antithrombin-heparin cofactor: modulators of hemostasis and inflammatory reactions. Prog Hemost Thromb 3:145, 1976.

22. Mammen EF: Physiology and biochemistry of blood coagulation. In: N Bang, FK Beller, E Deutsch, EF Mammen (Eds): Thrombosis and Bleeding Disorders: Theory and Methods. Academic Press, New York, 1971, p 1.

23. Seegers WH: Use and regulation of blood clotting mechanisms. In: WH Seegers (Ed): Blood Clotting Enzymology. Academic Press, New York, 1971, p 1.

24. Bick RL: Clinical relevance of antithrombin III. Semin Thromb Hemost 8:276, 1982.

25. Brinkhous KM, HP Smith, ED Warner: Inhibition of blood clotting and unidentified substances which act in conjunction with heparin to prevent the conversion of prothrombin to thrombin. Am J Physiol 125:683, 1939.

26. Seegers WH, KD Miller, EB Andrews: Fundamental interaction and effect of storage, other adsorbents, and blood clotting in plasma antithrombin activity. Am J Physiol 169:700, 1952.

27. Seegers WH, ER Cole, CR Harmison: Neutralization of autoprothrombin-C activity with antithrombin. Can J Biochem 42:359, 1964.

28. Seegers WH, H Schroer, M Kagami: Interactivation of purified autoprothrombin I with antithrombin. Can J Biochem 42:1425, 1964.

29. Vennerod AM, K Laake, AK Soleberg: Inactivation and binding of human plasma kallikrein by antithrombin III and heparin. Thromb Res 9:457, 1976.

30. Rosenberg RD: The effect of heparin on Factor IXa and plasmin. Thromb Diath Haemorrh 33:51, 1974.

31. Wessler S: Small doses of heparin and a new concept of hypercoagulability. Thromb Diath Haemorrh 33:81, 1975.

32. Kakkar V: Low dose heparin in the prevention of venous thromboembolism: rationale and results. Thromb Diath Haemorrh 33:87, 1974.

33. Yin E: Effect of heparin on the neutralization of Factor Xa and thrombin by the plasma alpha-2-globulin inhibitor. Thromb Diath Haemorrh 33:43, 1974.

34. Rosenberg RD, P Damus: The purification and mechanism of action of human antithrombin-heparin cofactor. J Biol Chem 248:6490, 1973.

35. Abildgaard U: Purification of two progressive antithrombins of human plasma. Scand J Clin Lab Invest 19:190, 1967.

36. Miller-Anderson M, H Borg, LO Anderson: Purification of antithrombin III by affinity chromatography. Thromb Res 5:439,1974.

37. Messmore HL: Natural inhibitors of the coagulation system. Semin Thromb Hemost 8:267, 1982.

38. Fareed J, HL Messmore, JM Walgena: Laboratory evaluation of antithrombin III: a critical overview of currently available methods for antithrombin III measurements. Semin Thromb Hemost 8:288, 1982.

39. Murano G, L Williams, M Miller-Anderson: Some properties of antithrombin-III and its concentration in human plasma. Thromb Res 18:259, 1980.

40. Thaler E, G Schmer: A simple two-step isolation procedure for human and bovine antithrombin II/III (heparin cofactor): a comparison of two methods. Br J Haematol 31:233, 1975.

41. Abildgaard U: Binding of thrombin to antithrombin III. Scand J Clin Lab Invest 24:23, 1969.

42. Kurachi K, G Schmer, M Hermodson: Inhibition of bovine factor IXa and factor Xa by antithrombin III. Biochemistry 15:368, 1976.

43. Lahiri B, RD Rosenberg, RC Talamo: Antithrombin III: an inhibitor of human plasma kallikrein. Fed Proc 33:642, 1974.

44. Stead N, AP Kaplan, RD Rosenberg: Inhibition of activated factor XII by antithrombin-heparin cofactor. J Biol Chem 251:6481, 1976.

45. Sas G, G Blasko, D Banhegyi: Abnormal antithrombin III (antithrombin III "Budapest") as a cause of familial thrombophilia. Thromb Diath Haemorrh 32:105, 1974.

46. Musumeci Y, R Lanolfi, B Bizza: Amidolytic assay of thrombin bound to alpha-2-macroglobulin in plasma. Haemostasis 6:98, 1977.

47. Shapiro S, D Anderson: Thrombin inhibition in normal plasma. In: R Lundblad, J Fenton, K Mann (Eds): Chemistry and Biology of Thrombin. Ann Arbor Science, Ann Arbor, MI, 1977, p 361.

48. Li E, H Orton, R Feinman: The interaction of thrombin and heparin. Proflavine dye binding studies. Biochemistry 13:5012, 1974.

49. Hook M, I Bjork, J Hopwood: Anticoagulant action of heparin: separation of high-activity and low-activity heparin species by affinity chromatography on immobilized antithrombin. FEBS Lett 66:90, 1976.

50. Walker F, C Esmon: The molecular mechanism of heparin action, II: separation of functionally different heparins by affinity chromatography. Thromb Res 14:219, 1979.

51. Yin E, L Eisenkramer, J Butler: Heparin interaction with activated factor X and its inhibitor. Adv Exp Med Biol 52:239, 1974.

52. Pomerantz M, W Owen: A catalytic role for heparin. Evidence of a ternary complex of heparin cofactor, thrombin, and heparin. Biochim Biophys Acta 535:66, 1978.

53. Barrowcliffe T, E Johnson, C Eggleton: Anticoagulant activities of lung and mucous heparins. Thromb Res 12:27, 1978.

54. Nordeman B, K Nordling, I Bjork: A differential effect of low-affinity heparin on the inhibition of thrombin and factor Xa by antithrombin. Thromb Res 17:595, 1980.

55. Thomas D, R Merton, W Lewis: Studies in man and experimental animals of a low molecular weight heparin fraction. Thromb Haemost 45:214, 1981.

56. Wight T: Vessel proteoglycans and thrombogenesis. Prog Hemost Thromb 5:1, 1980.

57. Carlstrom A, K Lieden, I Bjork: Decreased binding of heparin to antithrombins following the interaction between antithrombin and thrombin. Thromb Res 11:785, 1977.

58. Bertina RM, AW Broekmans, IK van der Linden: Protein C deficiency in a Dutch family with thrombotic disease. Thromb Haemost 48:1, 1982.

59. Jaques L, J Mahadoo: Pharmacodynamics and clinical effectiveness of heparin. Semin Thromb Hemost 4:298, 1978.

60. Jaques L: The chemical and anticoagulant nature of heparin. Semin Thromb Hemost 4:277, 1978.

61. Mahadoo J: Evidence for a cellular storage pool for exogenous heparin. In: R Bradshaw, S Wessler (Eds): Heparin: Structure, Cellular Functions, and Clinical Implications. Academic Press, New York, 1979, p 181.

62. Mahadoo J, L Jaques: Cellular control of heparin in blood. Med Hypotheses 5:835, 1979.

63. Hatton M, L Berry, E Regoeczi: Inhibition of thrombin by antithrombin III in the presence of certain glycosaminoglycans found in the mammalian aorta. Thromb Res 13:655, 1978.

64. Bick RL, I Kovac, L Fekete: A new two-stage functional assay for antithrombin III (heparin cofactor): clinical and laboratory evaluation. Thromb Res 8:745, 1976.

65. Odegard O, M Lie, U Abildgaard: Heparin cofactor activity measured with an amidolytic method. Thromb Res 6:287, 1975.

66. Thaler E, K Lechner: Antithrombin III deficiency and thromboembolism. Clin Haematol 10:369, 1981.

67. Teger-Nilsson A: Antithrombin in infancy and childhood. Acta Paediat Scand 64:624, 1975.

68. Sas G, I Peto, D Banhegyi: Heterogeneity of the "classical" antithrombin deficiency. Thromb Haemost 43:133, 1980.

69. Wolf M, C Boyer, J Lavergne: A new variant of antithrombin III. A study of three related cases. Thromb Haemost 42:186, 1979.

70. Penner J, H Hassouna, M Hunter: A clinically silent antithrombin III deficiency in an Ann Arbor family. Thromb Haemost 42:186, 1979.

71. Odegard O, U Abildgaard: Antithrombin-III: critical review of assay methods: significance of variations in health and disease. Haemostasis 7:127, 1978.

72. Rosenberg RD: Action and interaction of antithrombin and heparin. N Engl J Med 292:146, 1975.

73. Lechner K, E Thaler, N Niessner: Antithrombin-III-Mangel und Thromboseneigung. Wien Klin Wochenschr 89:215, 1977.

74. Bick RL: Deep venous thrombosis: clinical evaluation of 118 consecutive patients. Thromb Haemost 50:305, 1983.

75. Conard J, M Samama, M Horellou: Congenital antithrombin III deficiency in 3 families (7 affected members). Thromb Haemost 42:128, 1979.

76. Tullis J, K Watanabe: Platelet antithrombin deficiency: a new clinical entity. Am J Med 65:472, 1978.

77. van der Meer J, E Stoepman-van Dalen, J Jansen: Anti-thrombin III deficiency in a Dutch family. Am J Clin Pathol 26:532, 1973.

78. von Kaulla E, K von Kaulla: Deficiency of antithrombin III activity with hereditary thrombosis tendency. J Med 3:349, 1972.

79. Mammen EF: Inhibitor abnormalities. Semin Thromb Hemost 9:42, 1983.

80. Dayan L, D Donadio, E David: Maladie thrombo-embolique familiale recidivante par deficit congenital en anti-thrombine III. Etude preliminaire de 3 observations. Nouv Presse Med 7:3229, 1978.

81. Egeberg O: Inherited antithrombin III deficiency and thrombo-embolism. Fifth Congress of the International Society of Thrombosis and Haemostasis, 1975, p 170.

82. Marciniak E, C Farley, P DeSimone: Familial thrombosis due to antithrombin III deficiency. Blood 43:219, 1974.

83. Nagagawa M, H Tsuji, T Kawamura: Familial antithrombin III deficiency and its clinical significance. Blood and Vessel (Tokyo) 11:106, 1980.

84. Johansson L, UY Hedner, I Nilsson: Familial antithrombin III deficiency as pathogenesis of deep venous thrombosis. Acta Med Scand 204:491, 1978.

85. Leone G, V Valori, S Storti: Inferior vena cava thrombosis in a child with familial antithrombin III deficiency. Thromb Haemost 43:74, 1980.

86. Nagy I, H Losonczy: The significance of the chronic anticoagulant treatment in recurrent thromboembolism caused by hereditary antithrombin III deficiency. Fifth Congress of the International Society of Thrombosis and Haemostasis, 1975, p 170.

87. Williams L, G Murano: Human antithrombin III heterogeneity. Blood 57:229, 1981.

88. Meade T: Risk associations in the thrombotic disorders. Clin Haematol 10:391, 1981.

89. Bick RL, BJ McClain: A comparison of the Protopath and DuPont ACA antithrombin III assays in 149 patients with DIC, deep venous thrombosis, and hereditary thrombophilia. Am J Clin Pathol 82:371, 1984.

90. Bick RL, B McClain: A clinical comparison of chromogenic, fluorometric and natural (fibrinogen) substrate assays for determination of antithrombin III. Am J Clin Pathol 77:238, 1982.

91. Bick RL: Discrepant AT-III and fibrinogen levels on the DuPont ACA system. Am J Clin Pathol 80:891, 1983.

92. Bick RL, A Wheeler, A Composano: A comparative study of the DuPont antithrombin III and fibrinogen assay systems. Am J Clin Pathol 83:541, 1985.

93. Bick RL: Monitoring heparin therapy. Diag Dialog 1:1, 1979.

94. Bounameaux N, F Duckert, M Walter: The determination of antithrombin III. Comparison of six methods. Effect of oral contraceptive therapy. Thromb Haemost 39:607, 1978.

95. Conard J, M Samama, Y Salomon: Antithrombin III and the oestrogen content of combined oestro-progesterone contraceptives. Lancet 2:1148, 1972.

96. Conard J, B Casenave, M Samama: AT-III content and antithrombin activity in oestrogen-progesterone and progesterone-only treated women. Thromb Res 18:675, 1980.

97. Kakkar S, P Bentley, P Chan: Oral contraceptives, AT-III, and deep vein thrombosis. Thromb Haemost 42:26, 1979.

98. Peterson R, P Krull, P Finley: Changes in antithrombin-III and plasminogen induced by oral contraceptives. Am J Clin Pathol 53:468, 1970.

99. Zuck T, J Bergin, R Perkins: Antithrombin III and oestrogen content of oral contraceptives. Lancet 1:831, 1973.

100. Mammen E: Oral contraceptives and blood coagulation: a critical review. Am J Obstet Gynecol 142:781, 1982.

101. McKay E: Immunochemical analysis of active and inactive antithrombin III. Br J Haematol 46:277, 1980.

102. Sveger T: Antithrombin III in adolescents. Thromb Res 15:885,1979.

103. Peterson C, R Kelley, B Minard: Antithrombin III. Comparison of functional and immunological assays. Am J Clin Pathol 69:500, 1978.

104. Fagerhol M, U Abildgaard: Immunologic studies in human antithrombin III. Influence of age, sex, and use of oral contraceptives on serum concentration. Scand J Haematol 7:10, 1970.

105. Howie P, A Mallinson, C Prentice: Effect of combined oestrogen-progesterone oral contraceptives, oestrogen, and progesterone on antiplasmin and antithrombin activity. Lancet 2:1329, 1970.

106. Nagaswa H, B Kim, M Steiner: Inhibition of thrombin-neutralizing activity of antithrombin III by steroid hormones. Thromb Haemost 47:157, 1982.

107. Knudsen J, J Gormsen, K Skagen: Changes in platelet function, coagulation, and fibrinolysis in uncomplicated cases of acute myocardial infarction. Thromb Haemost 42:1513, 1979.

108. Mustard J, M Packham: The role of blood and platelets in atherosclerosis and the complications of atherosclerosis. Thromb Diath Haemorrh 33:444, 1975.

109. Yue R, M Gertler, T Starr: Alterations of plasma antithrombin III levels in ischemic heart disease. Thromb Haemost 35:598, 1976.

110. O'Brien J, M Etherington, S Jamieson: Blood changes in atherosclerosis and long after myocardial infarction and venous thrombosis. Thromb Diath Haemorrh 34:483, 1975.

111. Banerjee R, A Sahni, V Kumar: Antithrombin III deficiency in maturity onset diabetes mellitus and atherosclerosis. Thromb Diath Haemorrh 31:339, 1974.

112. Innerfield I, J Goldfischer, H Reichter-Reiss: Serum antithrombins in coronary artery disease. Am J Clin Pathol 65:64, 1976.

113. Hedner U, I Nilsson: Antithrombin III in clinical material. Thromb Res 3:631, 1973.

114. Bick RL, D Faulstick: Antithrombins and coronary artery disease. Am J Clin Pathol 81:773, 1984.

115. Krause W, A Lang: Effect of angiography on blood coagulation. Thromb Haemost 38:73, 1977.

116. Thaler E, E Balzar, H Kopsa: Erworbener Antithrombin-III-Mangel bei Proteinurie. Wien Klin Wochenschr 89:65, 1977.

117. Thaler E, E Balzar, N Kopsa: Acquired antithrombin III deficiency in patients with glomerular proteinuria. Haemostasis 7:257, 1978.

118. Kauffmann R, J Veltkamp, N van Tilburg: Acquired antithrombin III deficiency and thrombosis in the nephrotic syndrome. Am J Med 65:607, 1978.

119. Kendall A, R Lohmann, J Dossetor: Nephrotic syndrome. A hypercoagulable state. Arch Intern Med 127:1021, 1971.

120. Kanfer A, D Kleinknecht, M Boyer: Coagulation studies in 45 cases of the nephrotic syndrome without uremia. Thromb Diath Haemorrh 24:562, 1970.

121. Tomson C, C Forbes, C Prentice: Changes in blood coagulation and fibrinolysis in the nephrotic syndrome. Q J Med 43:399, 1974.

122. Kobayashi N, Y Takeda: Studies of the effects of estradiol, progesterone, cortisol, thrombophlebitis, and typhoid vaccine on synthesis and catabolism of antithrombin-III in the dog. Thromb Haemost 37:111, 1977.

123. Bick RL: Disseminated intravascular coagulation and related syndromes, ch 8. In: G Murano, RL Bick (Eds): Basic Concepts of Hemostasis and Thrombosis. CRC Press, Boca Raton, FL, 1980, p 163.

124. Bick RL: Disseminated intravascular coagulation. Pract Cardiol 7:147, 245, 1981.

125. Bick RL: Disseminated intravascular coagulation and related syndromes. In: J Fareed, HL Messmore, JW Fenton, KM Brinkhous (Eds): Perspectives in Hemostasis. Pergamon Press, New York, 1981, p 122.

126. Bick RL, G Murano: Primary hyperfibrino(geno)lytic syndromes. In: G Murano, RL Bick (Eds): Basic Concepts of Hemostasis and Thrombosis. CRC Press, Boca Raton, FL, 1980, p 181.

127. Bick RL: Syndromes associated with hyperfibrino(geno)lysis, ch 3. In: Disseminated Intravascular Coagulation and Related Syndromes. CRC Press, Boca Raton, FL, 1983, p 105.

128. Lechner K, H Niessner, E Thaler: Coagulation abnormalities in liver disease. Semin Thromb Hemost 4:40, 1977.

129. Bick RL: Disseminated intravascular coagulation and related syndromes. A review. Am J Hematol 5:265, 1978.

130. Corrigan J: Changes in the blood coagulation system associated with septicemia. N Engl J Med 279:851, 1968.

131. Gralnick H, H Tan: Acute promyelocytic leukemia: a model for understanding the role of the malignant cell in hemostasis. Hum Pathol 5:661, 1974.

132. Muller-Berghaus G: Pathophysiology of generalized intravascular coagulation. Semin Thromb Hemost 3:209, 1977.

133. Chandra S, N Bang, C Marks: Radiolabeled AT-III as a probe for the detection of activation of blood coagulation in vivo. Thromb Res 9:9, 1976.

134. Bick RL, ML Dukes, WL Wilson: Antithrombin III (AT-III) as a diagnostic aid in disseminated intravascular coagulation. Thromb Res 10:721, 1977.

135. Bick RL, MD Bick, LF Fekete: Antithrombin III patterns in disseminated intravascular coagulation. Am J Clin Pathol 73:577, 1980.

136. Abildgaard U, M Fagerhol, O Egeberg: Comparison of progressive antithrombin activity and the concentration of three thrombin inhibitors in human plasma. Scand J Clin Lab Invest 26:349, 1970.

137. Spero J, J Lewis, Y Hasiba: Disseminated intravascular coagulation: findings in 346 patients. Thromb Haemost 43:28, 1980.

138. Baker WF: Clinical aspects of disseminated intravascular coagulation: a clinician's point of view. Semin Thromb Hemost 15:1, 1989.

139. Vogel G, P Bottermann, M Clarmann: Antithrombin III treatment in acute liver failure. Thromb Haemost 46:373, 1981.

140. Egbring R, H Klingemann, N Heimburger: Antithrombin III substitution in acute hepatic failure due to CC14 intoxication. Thromb Haemost 46:373, 1981.

141. Braude S, J Arias, R Hughes: Antithrombin III infusion during fulminant hepatic failure. Thromb Haemost 46:369, 1981.

142. Kakkar V: The clinical use of anti-thrombin III. Thromb Haemost 42:265, 1979.

143. Egbring R, B Meneche, F Fuchs: Antithrombin III determination of an amidolytic method before and after AT-III substitution. Thromb Haemost 42:225, 1979.

144. Schipper H, R Lamping, L Kahle: Antithrombin III transfusion in patients with liver cirrhosis. Thromb Haemost 42:327, 1979.

145. Thaler E, H Niessner, G Kleinberger: Antithrombin III replacement therapy in patients with congenital and acquired antithrombin III deficiency. Thromb Haemost 42:327, 1979.

146. Dunn E, R Prager, J Penner: The effect of heparin and antithrombin III on endotoxin-induced disseminated intravascular coagulation (DIC). Transactions of the American Society of Hematology, 1976, p 9.

147. Wickerhauser M: A simple method for preparation of non-thrombogenic prothrombin complex. Thromb Haemost 46:137, 1981.

148. Hellgren M, L Javelin, K Hagnevik: Antithrombin III concentrate as adjuvant in DIC treatment. A pilot study in 9 severely ill patients. Thromb Res 35:459, 1984.

149. Vinazzer H: Therapeutic use of antithrombin III in shock and disseminated intravascular coagulation. Semin Thromb Hemost 15:347, 1989.

150. Fareed J, HL Messmore, EW Bermes: New perspectives in coagulation testing. Clin Chem 26:1380, 1980.

151. Fareed J, HL Messmore, J Walenga: Diagnostic efficacy of newer synthetic substrate methods for assessing coagulation variables: a critical overview. Clin Chem 28:2025, 1983.

152. Briginshaw GF, JN Shanberge: Identification of two distinct heparin cofactors in human plasma: separation and partial purification. Arch Biochem Biophys 161:683, 1974.

153. Briginshaw GF, JN Shanberge: Identification of two distinct heparin cofactors in human plasma: II. Inhibition of thrombin and activated factor X. Thromb Res 4:463, 1974.

154. Tollefson DM, MK Blank: Detection of a new heparin-dependent inhibitor of thrombin in human plasma. J Clin Invest 68:589, 1981.

155. Tollefson DM, DW Majerus, MK Blank: Heparin cofactor II: purification and properties of a heparin-dependent inhibitor of thrombin in human plasma. J Biol Chem 257:2162, 1982.

156. Tollefson DM, CA Pestka, WJ Monafo: Activation of heparin cofactor II by dermatan sulfate. J Biol Chem 258:6713, 1983.

157. Scully MF, VV Kakkar: Identification of heparin cofactor II as the principle plasma cofactor for the antithrombin activity of pentosan polysulfate. Thromb Res 36:187, 1984.

158. Preissner KT, P Sie: Modulation of heparin cofactor II function by S Protein (Vitronectin) and formation of a ternary S Protein-thrombin-heparin cofactor II complex. Thromb Haemost 60:399, 1988.

159. Sie P, F Fernandez, C Caranobe: Inhibition of thrombin-induced platelet aggregation and serotonin release by antithrombin III and heparin cofactor II in the presence of standard heparin, dermatan sulfate and pentosan polysulfate. Thromb Res 35:231, 1984.

160. Sie P, D Dupouy, F Dol: Inactivation of heparin cofactor II by polymorphonuclear leukocytes. Thromb Res 47:657, 1987.

161. Ofosu FA, F Fernandez, D Gauther: Heparin Cofactor II and other endogenous factors in the mediation of the antithrombotic and anticoagulant effects of heparin and dermatan sulfate. Semin Thromb Hemost 11:133, 1985.

162. Tollefson DM: Laboratory diagnosis of antithrombin and heparin cofactor II deficiency. Semin Thromb Hemost 16:162, 1990.

163. Abildgaard U, ML Larsen: Assay of dermatan sulfate cofactor (heparin cofactor II) activity in human plasma. Thromb Res 35:257, 1984.

164. Vinazzer H, U Pangraz: Heparin cofactor II: a simple assay method and results of its clinical application. Thromb Res 48:153, 1987.

165. Tran TH, GA Marbet, F Duckart: Association of hereditary heparin cofactor II deficiency with thrombosis. Lancet 2:413, 1985.

166. Sie P, D Dupouy, J Pichon: Constitutional heparin cofactor II deficiency associated with recurrent thrombosis. Lancet 2:414, 1985.

167. Anderson T, M Larsen, U Abildgaard: Low heparin cofactor II associated with abnormal crossed immunoelectrophoresis pattern in two Norwegian families. Thromb Res 47:243, 1987.

168. Bertina RM, IK van der Linden, L Engesser: Hereditary heparin cofactor II deficiency and the risk of development of thrombosis. Thromb Haemost 57:196, 1987.

169. Chaunsumrit A, MJ Manco-Johnson, WE Hathaway: Heparin cofactor II in adults and infants with thrombosis and DIC. Am J Hematol 31:109, 1989.

170. Toulin P, JF Vitoux, L Capron: Heparin cofactor II in patients with deep venous thrombosis under heparin and oral anticoagulant therapy. Thromb Res 49:479, 1988.

171. Grau E, A Oliver, J Felez: Plasma and urinary heparin cofactor II levels in patients with nephrotic syndrome. Thromb Haemost 60:137, 1988.

172. Toulon P, C Jacquot, L Capron: Antithrombin III and heparin cofactor II in patients with chronic renal failure undergoing regular hemodialysis. Thromb Haemost 57:263, 1987.

173. Esmon CT: Protein C: biochemistry, physiology and clinical implications. Blood 62:1155, 1983.

174. Stenflo J: Structure and function of Protein C. Semin Thromb Hemost 10:109, 1984.

175. Mammen EF, WR Thomas, WH Seegers: Activation of purified prothrombin to autoprothrombin II (platelet cofactor II) or autoprothrombin II-A. Thromb Diath Haemorrh 5:218, 1960.

176. Stenflo J: A new vitamin K–dependent protein: purification from bovine plasma and preliminary characterization. J Biol Chem 251:355, 1976.

177. Seegers WH, E Novoa, RL Henry, H Hassouna: Relationship of "new" vitamin K–dependent protein C and "old" autoprothrombin IIA. Thromb Res 11:633, 1976.

178. Stenflo J: Structure and function of Protein C. Semin Thromb Hemost 10:109, 1984.

179. Walker FJ: Protein S and the regulation of activated Protein C. Semin Thromb Hemost 10:131, 1984.

180. DiScipio RG, MA Hermodson, SG Yates: A comparison of human prothrombin, factor IX (Christmas factor), factor X (Stuart factor), and protein S. Biochemistry 16:698, 1977.

181. Broekmans AW, JJ Veltkamp, R Bertina: Congenital protein C deficiency and venous thromboembolism. N Engl J Med 309:340, 1983.

182. Griffin JH, B Evatt, TS Zimmerman: Deficiency of Protein C in congenital thrombotic disease. J Clin Invest 68:1370, 1981.

183. Griffin JH: Clinical studies on Protein C. Semin Thromb Hemost 10:162, 1984.

184. Marlar RA, J Endres-Brooks: Recurrent thromboembolic disease due to heterozygous protein C deficiency. Thromb Haemost 50:351, 1983.

185. Seligsohn U, A Berger, M Abend: Homozygous protein C deficiency manifested by massive venous thrombosis in the newborn. N Engl J Med 310:559, 1984.

186. Miletich JP: Laboratory diagnosis of Protein C deficiency. Semin Thromb Hemost 16:169, 1990.

187. Comp PC, R Nixon, CT Esmon: Determination of functional levels of protein C, an antithrombotic protein, using thrombin/thrombomodulin complex. Blood 63:15, 1984.

188. Griffin JH, A Bezeaud, B Evatt: Functional and immunologic studies of protein C in thromboembolic disease. Blood 62:301a, 1983.

189. Marlar RA, RH Sills, RR Montgomery: Protein C in commercial factor IX (F IX) concentrations (CONC) and its use in the treatment of "homozygous" protein C deficiency. Blood 62:303, 1983.

190. Sills RH, JR Humbert, RR Montgomery: Clinical course and therapy of an infant with severe "homozygous" protein C deficiency. Blood 62:310, 1983.

191. Broekmans AW, MR Bertina, EA Loelinger: Protein C and the development of skin necrosis during anticoagulant therapy. Thromb Haemost 49:255, 1983.

192. McGehee WG, TA Klotz, DJ Epstein: Coumarin-induced necrosis in a patient with familial protein C deficiency. Blood 62:304, 1983.

193. Mannucci P, A Tripodi: Laboratory screening of inherited thrombotic syndromes. Thromb Haemost 57:247, 1987.

194. American Diagnostica: Activated protein C assay. American Diagnostic Newsletter, Greenwich, CT, 1984.

195. Francis RB, MJ Patch: A functional assay for Protein C in human plasma. Thromb Res 32:605, 1983.

196. Sala N, WG Owen, D Collen: A functional assay of protein C in human plasma. Blood 63:671, 1984.

197. Griffin JH, DF Mosher, TS Zimmerman: Protein C, an antithrombotic protein, is reduced in hospitalized patients with intravascular coagulation. Blood 60:261, 1982.

198. Mannucci PM, S Vigano: Deficiencies of protein C, an inhibitor of blood coagulation. Lancet 2:463, 1982.

199. Walker FJ: Regulation of activated protein C by a new protein. A possible function for bovine protein S. J Biol Chem 255:5521, 1980.

200. Walker FJ, SI Chavin, PJ Fay: Inactivation of factor VIII by activated protein C and protein S. Arch Biochem Biophys 252:322, 1987.

201. Gardiner JE, MA McGann, CW Berridge: Protein S as a cofactor for activated protein C in plasma and in the inactivation of purified factor VIII:C. Circulation 70:205, 1984.

202. Schwarz HP, MJ Heeb, J Wencel-Drake: Localization of protein S, an antithrombotic protein, in human platelets and megakaryocytes. Blood 66:353a, 1985.

203. de Fouw NJ, F Haverkate, RM Bertina: The cofactor role of protein S in the acceleration of whole blood clot lysis by activated protein C in vitro. Blood 67:1189, 1986.

204. D'Angelo A, MS Lockhart, SV D'Angelo: Protein S is a cofactor for activated protein C neutralization of an inhibitor of plasminogen activation released from platelets. Blood 69:231, 1987.

205. Schwarz HP, M Fiscger, P Hopmeier: Plasma protein S deficiency in familial thrombotic disease. Blood 64:1297, 1984.

206. Comp PC, RR Nixon, MR Cooper: Familial protein S deficiency is associated with recurrent thrombosis. J Clin Invest 74:2082, 1984.

207. Gladson KH, JH Griffin, V Hach: The incidence of protein C and protein S deficiency in 139 young thrombotic patients. Blood 66:350, 1985.

208. Griffin JH, MJ Heeb, HP Schwarz: Plasma protein S deficiency and thromboembolic disease. Prog Hematol 15:39, 1987.

209. Broekmans MA, L Engesser, E Briet: Clinical manifestations of hereditary protein S deficiency. Thromb Haemost 54:57, 1985.

210. Sie P, B Boneu, R Bierme: Arterial thrombosis and protein S deficiency. Thromb Haemost 62:1040, 1989.

211. Comp PC, D Doray, D Patton: An abnormal plasma distribution of Protein S occurs in functional Protein S deficiency. Blood 67:504, 1986.

212. Comp PC: Laboratory evaluation of Protein S status. Semin Thromb Hemost 16:177, 1990.

213. Takahashi H, K Wada, S Hayashi: Behavior of protein S during long-term oral anticoagulant therapy. Thromb Res 51:241, 1988.

214. Heeb M, D Mosher, JH Griffin: Activation and complexation of Protein C and cleavage and decrease of Protein S in plasma of patients with intravascular coagulation. Blood 73:455, 1989.

215. Saito M, I Kumabashiri, H Jokaji: The levels of Protein C and Protein S in patients with Type II diabetes mellitus. Thromb Res 52:479, 1988.

216. Schwarz HP, G Schernathaner, JH Griffin: Decreased plasma levels of Protein S in well-controlled Type I diabetes mellitus. Thromb Haemost 57:240, 1987.

217. Vigano-D'Angelo S, A D'Angelo, C Kaufman: Protein S deficiency occurs in the nephrotic syndrome. Ann Intern Med 107:42, 1987.

218. Gouault-Heilmann M, T Gadwlha-Parente, M Levent: Total and free Protein S in nephrotic syndrome. Thromb Res 49:37, 1988.

219. Rostoker C, M Gouault-Heilmann, M Levent: High level of protein C and protein S in nephrotic syndrome. Nephron 46:220, 1987.

220. Melissari E, VV Kakkar: The effects of oestrogen administration on the plasma free Protein S and C4b-binding protein. Thromb Res 49:489, 1988.

221. Huisveld IA, JEH Hospers, JCM Meijers: Oral contraceptives reduce total protein S, but not free Protein S. Thromb Res 45:109, 1987.

222. Malm J, R Bennhagen, L Holmberg: Plasma concentrations of C4b-binding protein and vitamin K–dependent protein S in term and preterm infants: low levels of protein S-C4b-binding protein complexes. Br J Haematol 68:445, 1988.

223. Comp PC, GR Thurnau, J Welsh: Functional and immunological protein S levels are decreased during pregnancy. Blood 68:881, 1986.

224. Conlan MG, WD Haire: Low Protein S in essential thrombocythemia with thrombosis. Am J Hematol 32:88, 1989.

225. Berg L, R Edson, J Villablanca: The effects of L-asparaginase on plasma levels of free protein S. Am J Clin Pathol 93:437, 1990.

226. Verstraete M: The place of long-term stimulation of the endogenous fibrinolytic system: present achievements and clinical perspectives. In: JF Davidson, MM Samama, PC Desnoyers (Eds): Progress in Chemical Fibrinolysis and Thrombolysis, vol 1. Raven Press, New York, 1975, p 289.

227. Bick RL, RC Bishop, E Shanbrom: Fibrinolytic activity in acute myocardial infarction. Am J Clin Pathol 57:359, 1972.

228. Collen D, I Juhan-Vague: Fibrinolysis and atherosclerosis. Semin Thromb Hemost 14:180, 1988.

229. Almer LD, M Pandolfi, S Osterlin: The fibrinolytic system in patients with diabetes mellitus with special reference to diabetic retinopathy. Ophthalmologica 170:353, 1975.

230. Nalbandian RM, RL Henry, RL Bick: Thrombotic thrombocytopenic purpura: an extended editorial. Semin Thromb Hemost 5:216, 1979.

231. Stern DM, PP Nawroth: The vessel wall. Semin Thromb Hemost 13:391, 1987.

232. Astrup T: Tissue activators of plasminogen. Fed Proc 25:42, 1966.

233. Marsh N: Fibrinolysis in disease, ch 6. In: Fibrinolysis. John Wiley and Sons, New York, 1981, p 125.

234. Mansfield AO: Alterations in fibrinolysis associated with surgery and venous thrombosis. Br J Surg 59:754, 1972.

235. Bick RL, WB Thompson: Fibrinolytic activity: changes induced with oral contraceptives. Obstet Gynecol 39:213, 1972.

236. Murano G, RL Bick: Thrombolytic therapy, ch 15. In: G Murano, RL Bick (Eds): Basic Concepts of Hemostasis and Thrombosis. CRC Press, Boca Raton, FL, 1980, p 259.

237. Ganrot PO: Studies on serum protease inhibitors with special reference to -2 macroglobulin. Acta Univ Lund Sect 2:2, 1967.

238. Fischer CL, LW Gill: Acute phase proteins. In: SE Ritzmann, JC Daniels (Eds): Serum Protein Abnormalities. Little, Brown and Company, Boston, 1975, p 331.

239. Hedner U, IM Nilsson: Urokinase inhibitors in serum in a clinical series. Acta Med Scand 189:185, 1971.

240. Mammen EF: Plasminogen abnormalities. Semin Thromb Hemost 9:50, 1983.

241. Conard J, M Samama: Theoretic and practical considerations on laboratory monitoring of thrombolytic therapy. Semin Thromb Hemost 13:212, 1987.

242. Aoki N, M Moroi, Y Sakata: Abnormal plasminogen. A hereditary molecular abnormality found in a patient with recurrent thrombosis. J Clin Invest 61:1186, 1978.

243. Hasegawa DK, BJ Tyler, JR Edson: Thrombotic disease in three families with inherited plasminogen deficiency. Blood 60:213, 1982.

244. Kazama M, C Tahara, Z Suzki: Abnormal plasminogen: a case of recurrent thrombosis. Thromb Res 21:517, 1981.

245. Petaja M, V Rasi, G Myllyla: Familial hypofibrinolysis and venous thrombosis. Br J Haematol 71:393, 1989.

246. Nilsson IM, LA Tengborn: A family with thrombosis associated with high level of tissue plasminogen activator inhibitor. Haemostasis 14:24, 1984.

247. Tabernero MD, A Estelles, V Vicente: Incidence of increased plasminogen activator inhibitor in patients with deep venous thrombosis and/or pulmonary embolism. Thromb Res 56:565, 1989.

248. Kirschstein W, S Simianer, CE Dempfle: Impaired fibrinolytic capacity and tissue plasminogen activator release in patients with restenosis after percutaneous transluminal coronary angioplasty (PTCA). Thromb Haemost 62:772, 1989.

249. Juhan-Vague I, C Roul, MC Alessi, JP Ardissone: Increased plasminogen activator inhibitor activity in non-insulin dependent diabetic patients: relationship with plasma insulin. Thromb Haemost 61:370, 1989.

250. Sundkvist G, B Lilja, LO Almer: Absent elevations in growth hormone, factor VIII related antigen, and plasminogen activator activity during exercise in diabetic patients resistant to retinopathy. Diabetes Res 7:25, 1988.

251. de Jong E, RJ Porte, EA Knot: Disturbed fibrinolysis in patients with inflammatory bowel disease. Gut 30:188, 1989.

252. Robinson BW: Production of plasminogen activator by alveolar macrophages in normal subjects and patients with interstitial lung disease. Thorax 43:508, 1988.

253. Reilly JJ, HA Chapman: Association between alveolar macrophage plasminogen activator activity and indices of lung function in young cigarette smokers. Am Rev Resp Dis 138:1422, 1988.

254. Duffy MJ, P O'Grady, D Devaney: Urokinase-plasminogen activator, a marker for aggressive breast carcinomas. Cancer 62:531, 1988.

255. Hasday JD, PR Bachwich, JP Lynch: Procoagulant and plasminogen activator activities of bronchoalveolar fluid in patients with pulmonary sarcoid. Exp Lung Res 14:261, 1988.

256. Pikaar NA, M Wedel, EJ van der Beek: Effects of moderate alcohol consumption on platelet aggregation, fibrinolysis and blood lipids. Metab Clin Exp 36:538, 1987.

257. Kjaeldgaard A, B Larsson: Long-term treatment with combined oral contraceptives and cigarette smoking associated with impaired activity of tissue plasminogen activator. Acta Obstet Gynecol Scand 65:219, 1986.

258. Belch JJ, B McArdle, R Madhok: Decreased plasma fibrinolysis in patients with rheumatoid arthritis. Ann Rheum Dis 43:774, 1984.

259. Bick RL: Liver disease, ch 7. In: Disorders of Hemostasis and Thrombosis: Principles of Clinical Practice. Thieme, Inc., New York, 1985, p 205.

260. Tran-Thang C, J Fasel-Felley, G Pralong: Plasminogen activators and plasminogen activator inhibitors in liver deficiencies caused by chronic alcoholism or infectious hepatitis. Thromb Haemost 62:651, 1989.

261. Pralong G, T Calandra, M Glauser: Plasminogen activator inhibitor 1: a new prognostic marker in septic shock. Thromb Haemost 61:459, 1989.

262. Paramo JA, MJ Alfaro, E Rocha: Postoperative changes in the plasmatic levels of tissue-type plasminogen activator and its fast-acting inhibitor: relationship to deep venous thrombosis and influence of prophylaxis. Thromb Haemost 54:713, 1985.

263. Edelber JM, M Gonzales-Gronow, SV Pizzo: Lipoprotein(a) inhibition of plasminogen activation by tissue type plasminogen activator. Thromb Res 57:155, 1990.

264. Di Imperato C, AG Dettori: Ipofibrinogenemia congenita con fibrinoastenia. Helv Paediatr Acta 13:380, 1958.

265. Mammen EF: Fibrinogen abnormalities. Semin Thromb Hemost 9:1, 1983.

266. Bithell TC: Hereditary dysfibrinogenemia. Clin Chem 31:509, 1985.

267. Blomback M, B Blomback, EF Mammen: Fibrinogen Detroit: a molecular defect in the N-terminal disulfide knot of fibrinogen? Nature 218:134, 1968.

268. Al-Mondhiry H, D Galanakis: Dysfibrinogenemia and lupus anticoagulant in a patient with recurrent thrombosis. J Lab Clin Med 110:726, 1987.

269. Lijnen HR, J Soria, C Soria: Dysfibrinogenemia (Fibrinogen Dusard) associated with impaired fibrin-enhanced plasminogen activation. Thromb Haemost 51:108, 1984.

270. Engesser L, J Koopman, G DeMunk: Fibrinogen Nijmegen: congenital dysfibrinogenemia associated with impaired t-PA mediated plasminogen activation and decreased binding of t-PA. Thromb Haemost 60:113, 1988.

271. Reber P, M Furlan, A Henschen: Three abnormal fibrinogen variants with the same amino acid substitution (gamma-275 Arg-His): fibrinogens Bergamo II, Essen and Perugia. Thromb Haemost 56:401, 1986.

272. Conley CL, RC Hartmann: A hemorrhagic disorder caused by circulating anticoagulant in patients with disseminated lupus erythematosus. J Clin Invest 31:621, 1952.

273. Bowie EJW, JH Thompson, CA Pascuzzi: Thrombosis in systemic lupus erythematosus despite circulating anticoagulant. J Lab Clin Med 62:416, 1963.

274. Bick RL: Circulating anticoagulants, ch 9. In: Disorders of Hemostasis and Thrombosis: Principles of Clinical Practice. Thieme, Inc., New York, 1985, p 254.

275. Shapiro SS, P Thagarajan: Lupus anticoagulants. Prog Hemost Thromb 6:263, 1982.

276. Espinoza LR, RC Hartmann: Significance of the lupus anticoagulant. Am J Hematol 22:331, 1986.

277. Bell WR, GR Boss, JS Wolfson: Circulating anticoagulant in the procainamide-induced lupus syndrome. Arch Intern Med 137:1471, 1977.

278. Zarrabi MH, S Zucker, F Miller: Immunologic and coagulation disorders in chlorpromazine-treated patients. Ann Intern Med 91:914, 1979.

279. Harris EN, AE Gharavi, ML Boey: Anticardiolipin antibodies: detection by radioimmunoassay and association with thrombosis in systemic lupus erythematosus. Lancet 2:1211, 1983.

280. Weidmann CE, D Wallace, J Peter: Studies of IgG, IgM and IgA antiphospholipid antibody isotypes in systemic lupus erythematosus. J Rheumatol 15:74, 1988.

281. Triplett DA: Clinical significance of antiphospholipid antibodies. American Society of Clinical Pathologists, Hemostasis and Thrombosis Check Sample 10:1, 1988.

282. Hughes GVR, EN Harris, AE Gharavi: The anticardiolipin syndrome. J Rheumatol 13:486, 1986.

283. Asherson RA, EN Harris: Anticardiolipin antibodies: clinical associations. Postgrad Med J 62:1081, 1986.

284. Derue G, H Englert, E Harris: Fetal loss in systemic lupus: association with anticardiolipin antibodies. Br J Obstet Gynecol 5:207, 1985.

285. Lubbe WF, SJ Palmer, WS Butler: Fetal survival after prednisolone suppression of maternal lupus anticoagulant. Lancet 1:1361, 1983.

286. Harris EN, RA Asherson, AE Gharavi: Thrombocytopenia in SLE and related autoimmune disorders: association with anticardiolipin antibodies. Br J Haematol 59:227, 1985.

287. Harris EN, AE Gharavi, U Hedge: Anticardiolipin antibodies in autoimmune thrombocytopenia purpura. Br J Haematol 59:231, 1985.

288. Rosove MH, P Brewer, A Runge: Simultaneous lupus anticoagulant and anticardiolipin assays and clinical detection of antiphospholipids. Am J Hematol 32:148, 1989.

289. Harris EN, GRV Hughes, AE Gharavi: Antiphospholipid antibodies: an elderly statesman dons new garments. J Rheumatol 14:208, 1987.

290. Bick RL: The antiphospholipid thrombosis (APL-T) syndrome: characteristics and recommendations for classification and treatment. Thromb Hemost 65:1343, 1991.

291. Gharavi AE, EN Harris, RA Asherson: Anticardiolipin antibodies: isotype distribution and phospholipid specificity. Ann Rheum Dis 46:1, 1987.

292. Carreras L, S Manchin, R Deman: Arterial thrombosis, intrauterine death and lupus anticoagulant: detection of immunoglobulin interfering with prostacyclin formation. Thromb Haemost 57:374, 1987.

293. Cariou R, G Tobelem, S Bellucci: Effect of lupus anticoagulant on antithrombogenic properties of endothelial cells: inhibition of thrombomodulin-dependent protein C activation. Thromb Haemost 60:54, 1988.

294. Cosgriff TM, BA Martin: Low functional and high antigenic antithrombin III level in a patient with the lupus anticoagulant. Arthritis Rheum 24:94, 1981.

295. Khamashta MA, EN Harris, AE Gharavi: Immune-mediated mechanism for thrombosis: antiphospholipid antibody binding to platelet membranes. Ann Rheum Dis 47:849, 1988.

296. Sanfellipo MJ, CJ Drayna: Prekallikrein inhibition associated with the lupus anticoagulant. Am J Clin Pathol 77:275, 1982.

297. Angeles-Cano E, Y Sultan, JP Clauvel: Predisposing factors to thrombosis in systemic lupus erythematosus. Possible relationship to endothelial cell damage. J Lab Clin Med 94:312, 1979.

298. Elias M, A Eldor: Thromboembolism in patients with the "lupus-like" circulating anticoagulant. Arch Intern Med 144:510, 1984.

299. Hall S, H Buettner, HS Luthra: Occlusive retinal vascular disease in systemic lupus erythematosus. J Rheumatol 11:96, 1984.

300. Boey ML, CB Colaco, AE Gharavi: Thrombosis in SLE: striking association with the presence of circulating "lupus anticoagulant." Br Med J 287:1021, 1983.

301. Asherson RA, EN Harris, AE Gharavi: Aortic arch syndrome associated with anticardiolipin antibodies and the lupus anticoagulant. Arthritis Rheum 28:94, 1985.

302. Asherson RA, SH Morgan, EN Harris: Arterial occlusion causing large bowel infarction: a reflection of clotting diathesis in SLE. Clin Rheumatol 5:102, 1986.

303. Asherson RA, IR MacKay, EN Harris: Myocardial infarction in a young male with systemic lupus erythematosus, deep vein thrombosis and antiphospholipid antibodies. Br Heart J 56:910, 1986.

304. Morton KT, S Gavaghan, G Krilis: Coronary artery bypass graft failure: an autoimmune phenomenon? Lancet 1:1353, 1986.

305. Chartash EK, SA Paget, MD Lockshin: Lupus anticoagulant associated with aortic and mitral valve insufficiency. Arthritis Rheum 29:95, 1986.

306. Hamsten A, R Norberg, M Bjorkholm: Antibodies to cardiolipin in young survivors of myocardial infarction: an association with recurrent cardiovascular events. Lancet 1:113, 1986.

307. Weinstein C, M Miller, R Axtens: Livido reticularis associated with increased titers of anticardiolipin antibodies in systemic lupus erythematosus. Arch Dermatol 123:596, 1987.

308. Levine S, K Welch: The spectrum of neurologic disease associated with anticardiolipin antibodies. Arch Neurol 44:876, 1987.

309. Oppenheimer S, B Hoffbrand: Optic neuritis and myelopathy in systemic lupus erythematosus. Can J Neurol Sci 13:129, 1986.

310. Englert H, C Hawkes, M Boey: Degos' disease: association with anticardiolipin antibodies and the lupus anticoagulant. Br Med J 289:576, 1984.

311. Kochenour N, D Branch, N Rote: A new postpartum syndrome associated with antiphospholipid antibodies. Obstet Gynecol 69:460, 1987.

312. Spaet TH, RB Erichson: The vascular wall in the pathogenesis of thrombosis. In: Proceedings of the Second International Conference on Thrombosis, Basel, 1965, p 67.

313. Wilner GD, HL Nossel, EC Le Roy: Activation of Hageman factor by collagen. J Clin Invest 47:2608, 1968.

314. Nilsson IM, M Pandolfi: Fibrinolytic response of the vascular wall. Thromb Diath Haemorrh 40:231, 1970.

315. Marcum J., F Reilly, R Rosenberg: The role of specific forms of heparan sulfate in regulating blood vessel wall function. Prog Hemost Thromb 8:185, 1986.

316. Fareed J, JM Walenga, RL Bick: Impact of automation on the quantitation of low molecular weight markers of hemostatic defects. Semin Thromb Hemost 9:355, 1983.

317. Fareed J, JM Walenga: Current trends in hemostasis testing. Semin Thromb Hemost 9:380, 1983.

318. Harker L: Platelet survival time: its measurement and use. Prog Hemost Thromb 4:321, 1978.

319. Fletcher AP, N Alkjaersig: Blood hypercoagulability, intravascular coagulation, and thrombosis: new diagnostic concepts. Thromb Diath Haemorrh 45:389, 1971.

320. Fletcher AP, N Alkjaersig: Laboratory diagnosis of intravascular coagulation. In: L Poller (Ed): Recent Advances in Thrombosis. Churchill Livingstone, London, 1973, p 87.

321. Fareed J, RL Bick, C Squallaci: Clinical and experimental studies using a modified radioimmunoassay for B-beta 15-42 related peptides. Thromb Haemost 50:300, 1983.

322. Plow EF, TS Edgington: Surface markers of fibrinogen and its physiologic derivatives related by antibody probes. Semin Thromb Hemost 8:36, 1982.

323. Huseby RM, RE Smith: Synthetic oligopeptide substrates: their diagnostic application in blood coagulation, fibrinolysis, and other pathological states. Semin Thromb Hemost 6:173, 1980.

324. Joist HJ: Hypercoagulability: introduction and perspective. Semin Thromb Hemost 16:151, 1990.

325. Comp PC: Overview of the hypercoagulable states. Semin Thromb Hemost 16:158, 1990.

C H A P T E R
14

Antithrombotic Therapy

nticoagulant therapy is becoming revolutionized with new techniques and dosages of many anticoagulant, antiplatelet agents, and new synthetic agents being the subject of multicenter, double-blind, prospective, randomized, clinical trials. Nonetheless, many earlier and more traditional thoughts regarding anticoagulant therapy, often centered around mystique and lack of scientifically sound information, need to be abandoned because of recent clinical trial results and new information. Furthermore, results of clinical trials may be markedly different depending on the particular method used as an end point of the trial and on the particular preparation of the anticoagulant used.[1] Although the agent may be of the same generic category, different preparations may have markedly different in vivo effects. When interpreting results of clinical trials, the end point of the trial, whether it be clinical thrombosis, radioactive fibrinogen scanning, Doppler ultrasonography, impedence plethysmography, venography, or thromboscintography, may markedly change the statistical end point results. The modalities used for a diagnosis of thrombotic disease in clinical trials are listed in Table 14-1, and the advantages and disadvantages of these techniques are listed in Table 14-2.[1]

Anticoagulant or antiplatelet therapy, in any form, is only prophylactic therapy to prevent further thrombus propagation, recurrent thrombosis, or development of thromboembolism. Anticoagulant or antiplatelet therapy does not ameliorate the existing disease, and anticoagulant therapy will be discussed with this important concept in mind. Generally, this chapter will be limited to indications and doses suggested by prospective, randomized, double-blind, clinical trials with a discussion of newer anticoagulant preparations now available for clinical trials.

Antiplatelet Agents

Many antiplatelet agents have been used in both prospective and retrospective clinical trials to assess efficacy of pro-phylaxis for arterial and venous thrombotic and thromboembolic disease, including thromboembolic disease associated with prosthetic devices. Usually, the doses used have been empiric, and ideal doses are undefined, especially for aspirin and dipyridamole. Only the three most common agents (aspirin, dipyridamole, and sulfinpyrazone) will be discussed. Interpreting data from many clinical trials is difficult because in some studies only one agent was used, in other studies antiplatelet agents in combination with warfarin or heparin were used, and in even others various combinations of antiplatelet agents have been used. Doses and scheduling have been largely empiric, laboratory evaluation has not been uniform, and clinical end points have been variable.[1] To further complicate clinical interpretation of results, side effects and complications of therapy are infrequently addressed and frequently have not been evaluated uniformly. Another variable is the wide variety of hypercoagulable states studied and the end points used for the trials. The dose of aspirin, for example, which is effective for prophylaxis of coronary artery reocclusion, may not be proper for prevention of deep venous thrombosis following hip surgery, since the mechanisms and intensity of hypercoagulability may be different. This discussion addresses the results obtained in prospective, randomized trials and my personal experience.

The antiplatelet action of aspirin is attributed to its ability to inhibit the synthesis of prostaglandins, specifically the enzyme cyclo-oxygenase, therefore decreasing the production of intraplatelet thromboxane A_2, a compound that promotes platelet aggregability.[2] The platelet-inhibiting effect of aspirin lasts for the life span of the circulating platelet, because the enzyme cyclo-oxygenase is irreversibly inhibited. Aspirin may inhibit platelets while they are still within or being made by megakaryocytes. The half-life of circulating platelets is about 10 days. After a single dose of aspirin, only 50% of circulating platelets will function normally after five days. Concern about the ability of aspirin to inhibit endothelial production of prostacyclin via inhibition of cyclo-oxygenase has been translated into concern regarding the potential hypercoagulability that could, at least theoreti-

Table 14-1. Methods Used for the Diagnosis of Deep Venous Thrombosis

Clinical examination
I-125-fibrinogen scanning
Doppler ultrasonography
Impedence plethysmography
Color Doppler flow imaging*
Gated whole blood pooled venogram*
Ascending thromboscintography*
Ascending contrast venography*

* Most reliable methods

cally, be induced by aspirin. Several direct and indirect lines of evidence suggest that aspirin does not induce a hypercoagulable state. Platelet cyclo-oxygenase is far more sensitive to aspirin than vascular cyclo-oxygenase,[3] and prostacyclin production is restored more quickly than thromboxane synthesis.[4,5] Several investigations have shown that after aspirin, the inhibition of thromboxane is severalfold more pronounced than the inhibition of prostacyclin. Clinical observations with large populations taking aspirin for nonthrombotic disease (eg, rheumatoid arthritis) have shown no increased propensity to thrombosis,[6,7] and patients with congenital deficiency of cyclo-oxygenase display a hemorrhagic tendency but have no increased incidence of thrombosis.[8] This implies that the homeostatic role of prostacyclin is less than that of thromboxane. Aspirin produces gastrointestinal side effects after long-term use that are clearly dose-related. These side effects are decreased with concomitant use of cimetidine, enteric-coated aspirin, and liquid antacids.[9,10] Currently, no conclusive proof exists that any particular dose of aspirin is any more effective than any other, and clinical trials have used dosages ranging from 85 mg to more than 1 g per day. Dipyridamole inhibits cyclic-AMP phosphodiesterase, increasing cyclic AMP in the platelet, therefore increasing phosphorylated receptor protein, which enhances calcium binding and decreases platelet aggregability and platelet adhesiveness.[11] The usual side effects of dipyridamole therapy are headaches, dizziness, nausea, flushing, and occasional syncope. Mild gastric distress, similar to that seen with aspirin, may be noted. Sulfinpyrazone also inhibits prostaglandin synthesis, via inhibition of the enzyme cyclo-oxygenase, and has an action similar to aspirin.[2] Like aspirin and dipyridamole, the most common side effects of sulfinpyrazone are gastrointestinal, usually manifest as nausea and emesis. Sulfinpyrazone, like aspirin, will aggravate or reactivate peptic ulcer disease, and this agent, like aspirin, should always be taken with a liquid antacid.[12,13] Usually a patient taking antiplatelet therapy, especially when taking a combination of two antiplatelet agents, will show easy and spontaneous bruising and mild mucosal membrane bleeding, often manifest as gingival bleeding with toothbrushing and periodic melena.[1,13] These are accepted side effects of antiplatelet therapy for the prophylaxis of serious thrombotic or thromboembolic disease.[1,14] Most of these agents have a clinical antiplatelet effect for about five days.[15] If a patient is ingesting these agents and is involved in trauma or needs emergency surgery, platelet concentrates may be indicated to control hemostasis.[13] The mechanisms of aspirin and other antiplatelet agents were given in detail in chapter 1.

Sometimes a combination of two of the three antiplatelet agents is needed for effective prophylaxis against thrombotic or thromboembolic disease, including arterial or venous events.[1,14,16-18] The most common dose for aspirin is 600 mg given twice a day, each dose with 30 mL of liquid antacid, and an ideal nontoxic plasma level is between 4 to 10 mg/dL.[15] Patients taking more than 10 mg/dL commonly develop gastric intolerance, manifest as nausea and emesis,[15] and complain of tinnitus. The usual dosage of dipyridamole is 50 to 75 mg, three or four times a day, and the usual dosage for sulfinpyrazone is 200 mg orally three times a day.[13,14] A combination of two antiplatelet agents, of differing modes of action, are often used to obtain the most effective clinical response.

Table 14-2. Advantages and Disadvantages of Methods to Diagnose Deep Venous Thrombosis

Modality	Reliability	Advantage	Disadvantage
I-125-fibrinogen scanning	Reasonable	Current thrombus detected below groin	Hepatitis, high false-positive and false-negative results
Doppler ultrasonography	High, below knee	Excellent study with experience	Affected by collaterals
Impedence plethysmography	Poor	Unreliable, high false-positive and false-negative results	
Ascending contrast venography	Excellent	Definitive	Painful, rethrombosis rate is 10%
Ascending thromboscintography	Excellent study	Definitive study, can determine age of thrombus, can do V/P scan at same time	None
Gated whole blood pooled venogram	Excellent study	Definitive, antecubital vein used	
Color Doppler flow imaging	Excellent study	Definitive	Unreliable in upper thigh

Like other forms of anticoagulant therapy, antiplatelet therapy is in a state of flux, with many double-blind, prospective, randomized, clinical trials being conducted. The results of these trials will dictate more clear-cut indications for antiplatelet therapy. Changes in platelet reactivity have been observed in patients with existing deep venous thrombosis, and many studies have shown that venous thrombi begin with the development of a platelet (white) thrombus. This finding has led to the obvious suggestion that antiplatelet therapy may be indicated in venous thrombotic and thromboembolic disease.[19-21] The antiplatelet agent that has attracted the most attention in this regard is aspirin. The advantages of aspirin are obvious: it is extremely inexpensive and is relatively free from side effects. Many clinical trials have used aspirin alone or in combination for a wide variety of disorders. Dosages of aspirin, however, have not been standardized, and frequently aspirin has been used in combination with not only another antiplatelet agent but also with warfarin or heparin anticoagulation. Aspirin at a low dose has been shown to be effective prophylaxis for prevention of coronary artery graft rethrombosis and of thrombosis in patients with unstable angina.[22,23] Aspirin has activity in preventing reinfarction and death in patients recovering from acute myocardial infarction.[24,25] High-dose aspirin has been effective in prevention of transient cerebral ischemic attacks (TIAs); this effect was noted in both sexes in one study and only in males in another study.[26,27] In addition, retrospective studies in large patient populations have shown a decrease in the incidence of acute myocardial infarction,[28,29] and aspirin has clearly been shown to decrease thromboembolic disease associated with prosthetic heart valves.[30,31] Other studies have shown favorable benefits of aspirin in decreasing myocardial infarction, although the results did not reach statistical significance.[32] Aspirin as a single agent has been subjected to double-blind, prospective, randomized trials for the prophylaxis of deep venous thrombosis and pulmonary embolus.[33-45] Most trials showed a clear-cut benefit, whereas some were questionable or revealed no benefit. Aspirin in combination with dipyridamole has been used for the prevention of deep venous thrombosis and pulmonary embolus in general surgery, in high-risk medical patients, and in orthopedic surgery in at least 20 trials.[18,34,36-38,46-60] The results were positive in most of these trials and without benefit in others. However, most trials showing no benefit were limited to patients undergoing orthopedic procedures.

The experience with sulfinpyrazone has been less than that with aspirin. Steel demonstrated a significant benefit when studying patients with recurrent venous thrombosis.[61] Several trials have used hydroxychloraquine, with most showing a benefit[62-66] and some showing no benefit.[37,67,68] Although some negative trials have resulted, most trials using aspirin alone or aspirin plus dipyridamole have clearly been shown to be of benefit in decreasing the incidence of deep venous thrombosis and pulmonary embolism following elective surgery, orthopedic surgery, and in medical populations at high risk for deep venous thrombosis and pulmonary embolism.

Dipyridamole as a single agent has been noted to decrease the rate of renal allograft rejection in patients with transplants.[69] Aspirin as a single agent has been shown to normalize platelet survival in patients with prosthetic heart valves.[70] In this same study, sulfinpyrazone was shown to be as effective as dipyridamole. Dipyridamole added to warfarin is more effective than warfarin alone for prevention of systemic thromboembolic disease in patients with prosthetic cardiac valves.[71,72] The combination of aspirin with dipyridamole has been shown to be effective in prevention of rethrombosis of coronary artery grafts. Dipyridamole alone or in combination with aspirin is effective in preventing progression of peripheral arterial occlusive disease.[73] The incidence of failure in a large patient population treated with aspirin and dipyridamole demonstrated a recurrence rate comparable to most experience with warfarin-type drugs and more favorable than that reported by some investigators with warfarin-type drugs. A combination of aspirin and dipyridamole for a six-month period appears to be equally effective as warfarin for the prevention of recurrent deep venous thrombosis and pulmonary embolus in high-risk patients.[14]

Sulfinpyrazone as a single agent has clearly been shown to decrease the chance of transient cerebral ischemic attacks in some studies[74] but has been found to be ineffectual in others.[75] Sulfinpyrazone is effective in decreasing the chance of thromboembolism in patients with rheumatic heart disease,[76] recurrent deep venous thrombosis,[77,78] and shunt thrombosis[79] and is also effective in preventing secondary myocardial infarction.[80,81]

These studies account for most double-blinded, prospective, randomized and nonrandomized trials with antiplatelet agents. Future studies, possibly using combination therapy, should allow for more clear-cut indications. It appears that a combination of two antiplatelet agents, each with a differing mechanism of action, is effective in decreasing incidence or recurrence of deep venous thrombosis or pulmonary embolus. No laboratory monitoring of antiplatelet therapy is necessary, but template bleeding time or platelet aggregation studies can be done to document a clinical response.

Oral Anticoagulants

Oral anticoagulants are of two types, the coumarins and the indanedione derivatives. The indanedione derivatives are no longer generally available and are only used in individuals who are sensitive to the coumarin drugs.[1,14] Coumarin drugs are vitamin K antagonists.[82,83] All the vitamin K antagonists interfere with the normal synthesis of factors II, VII, IX, and X, protein C, and protein S. Their mechanism of interference and the role of vitamin K were discussed in chapter 1. The function of vitamin K is to attach calcium-binding prosthetic groups postribosomally onto the amino-terminal regions of the vitamin K–dependent factors. The calcium-binding prosthetic groups are gamma-carboxyglutamic acid.[84] Without vitamin K (ie, in patients undergoing coumarin or indanedione therapy), factors II, VII, IX, and X, protein C, and protein S are synthesized but are incomplete, lacking the specific calcium-binding sites, and are unable to function as procoagulants or anticoagulants, because they cannot enter into enzyme substrate complex formation as was discussed in chapter 1.[14] These factors, however, are present in plasma in normal immunologic concentration, although their biologic activity is markedly decreased as defined by coagulation-derived assays or global tests of coagulation, such as the prothrombin time. Generally, coumarins are totally absorbed from the gastrointestinal tract and are bound to plasma albumin. The onset of action of most coumarin derivatives is between eight and 12 hours with a maximum anticoagulant effect occurring in about 36 hours. Usually the institution of coumarin derivative therapy calls for overlap with heparin therapy.[14] The duration of action of coumarins is about 72 hours.[1,14,85] Factor VII activity decreases most rapidly and best correlates with the prothrombin time determination. Factor IX and factor X depression best correlate with both the anticoagulant effect and with clinical hemorrhage.[1,14,86] The coumarin derivatives cross the placenta and are not used in pregnant women. Loading doses of coumarin derivatives were used formerly but are no longer indicated and may potentiate hemorrhage.[87] In this regard, a loading dose of coumarin simply serves to accelerate the abnormal synthesis of factor VII but not factors II, IX, or X.

Clinical Trials and Indications

Formerly, coumarin derivatives were widely used in patients with acute myocardial infarction and for prophylaxis of recurrent venous thrombosis and pulmonary embolus.[88-90] For myocardial infarction, the rationale for the immediate (short-term) use of coumarin in these individuals included the following: (1) to prevent venous thrombosis and pulmonary thromboembolism while the patient is at rest; (2) to prevent reinfarction; (3) to prevent systemic embolization; and (4) to prevent extension of existing coronary thrombi in hopes of limiting infarction size. Several early studies showed significant differences between mortality, reinfarction rate, thromboembolic disease following myocardial infarction, and recurrent myocardial infarctions in patients treated with vitamin K antagonists vs those not so treated.[91] Other prospective trials, however, did not show any significant differences in mortality, reinfarction rate, or thromboembolic complications in these individuals, which created controversy regarding the benefit vs risk ratio for use of warfarin drugs in patients with acute myocardial infarction.[90,92] Although three early randomized trials[93-95] showed either significant (one trial) or suggested (two trials) benefit of warfarin in preventing reinfarction, all three trials showed a clear benefit for reducing early pulmonary embolus and stroke in patients with acute myocardial infarction. Four randomized trials have addressed the long-term benefit of war-

farin anticoagulation in survivors of myocardial infarction.[96-99] Although one trial, The Netherlands 60-Plus Reinfarction Study,[99] showed a dramatic reduction of reinfarction (55%) during two years, none of the trials revealed a difference in mortality during study periods of two to seven years. These results, in conjunction with the high hemorrhage rate associated with long-term warfarin therapy, cast serious doubt on the efficacy or advisability of long-term warfarin use in patients with current or previous acute myocardial infarction. Despite these findings, it is justified to administer heparin to patients with acute myocardial infarction to prevent immediate postinfarction venous thromboembolic disease or systemic embolization because of atrial fibrillation or transmural infarct. It also appears prudent to offer long-term warfarin, aspirin, or heparin therapy to patients with postmyocardial infarction who are at increased risk of systemic embolization resulting from transmural infarct or atrial fibrillation, patients with a history of previous venous thromboembolic disease, or patients with severe prolonged congestive heart failure.

Several prospective trials using warfarin for prevention of graft reocclusion after coronary artery bypass grafting (CABG) have been done.[100-102] Two of these studies showed no benefit, and one study showed marginal benefit. These findings, in conjunction with results of trials showing significant efficacy of aspirin, dipyridamole, and combinations of these (using aspirin at 1 g per day and dipyridamole at 225 mg per day) started within one day of surgery, demonstrate that these agents are highly effective at preventing graft reocclusion, which suggests no role for warfarin drugs in this setting.[103-106]

Patients with mechanical cardiac valves (Starr-Edwards, St. Jude, Bjork-Shiley, etc) have a high chance of thromboembolism, and the incidence with valves in the mitral position is generally much higher than in the aortic position. The incidence generally is about 40% in untreated patients and about 15% in treated patients. Warfarin alone is moderately effective in offering prophylaxis against thromboembolism in these patients, and the combination of warfarin plus dipyridamole (400 mg per day) or in combination with aspirin (1 g per day) is more effective than warfarin alone.[107-110] Combination therapy with warfarin plus dipyridamole should particularly be considered in high-risk patients, especially those with atrial fibrillation or previous systemic embolization.[111-113] Patients with mechanical heart valves should be treated with higher doses of warfarin than generally used for most other indications. Patients with bioprosthetic cardiac valves (porcine and bovine) have a lesser incidence of long-term thromboembolism (about 5% to 10%) than those with mechanical heart valves and only need treatment with warfarin for three months after surgery.[114-117] However, the chance of thromboembolism markedly increases in the presence of atrial fibrillation and documented left atrial thrombus, and these particular patients should be strongly considered as candidates for long-term warfarin therapy.[118,119]

Patients with rheumatic mitral valve disease have a high incidence of thromboembolism, varying between 10% and 60%.[120-122] The presence of atrial fibrillation further enhances this already ominous risk.[123,124] The risk is greater with stenosis than with regurgitation and increases with advancing age and compromised cardiac indices.[125,126] Patients with mitral valvular disease with documented systemic embolization or with atrial fibrillation should receive long-term warfarin therapy. If failure occurs, dipyridamole, 400 mg per day, should be added to warfarin.[127,128] Patients with aortic valvular disease or mitral valve prolapse have a much lower chance of systemic embolization than those with mitral valvular disease.[129,130] These individuals are not generally candidates for long-term anticoagulation unless concomitant atrial fibrillation, systemic embolization, or evidence of transient cerebral ischemic episodes are noted, without another documented source.[131,132] Transient cerebral ischemia in patients with mitral valve prolapse is probably best managed with aspirin at 1 g per day.[133,134] If patients fail this regimen (recurrent TIA), however, or develop systemic embolization or atrial fibrillation associated with mitral valve prolapse, they should be treated with long-term warfarin therapy.[135] Any patient with chronic atrial fibrillation, despite etiology, is at high risk for systemic embolization[136,137] and could be considered for long-term warfarin therapy, depending on the clinical particulars of the patient. If a patient with atrial fibrillation, despite etiology, experiences systemic embolization, then strong consideration of long-term warfarin should be entertained.[138,139]

Warfarins have often been used for long-term prophylaxis of venous thrombosis and venous thromboembolism in many high-risk populations. Many uncontrolled trials addressing a variety of thrombotic and thromboembolic disorders, including patients considered at high risk for thromboembolic disease, have been performed. Unfortunately, it is impossible to draw firm conclusions from these studies since they have been retrospective, uncontrolled, nonrandomized, and without uniformity of dosage regimens. Many randomized prospective trials, although not double blind, have addressed a variety of disorders including pulmonary embolization, recurrent deep venous thrombosis, and transient cerebral ischemic attacks. Results show a trend toward decreased mortality in many high-risk patients and, to a lesser degree, a trend toward decreased pulmonary embolization, recurrent deep venous thrombosis, and thromboembolic disease, depending on the end point used.[89,140-143] Although subcutaneous heparin has been shown to be highly effective for prophylaxis of deep venous thrombosis and thromboembolism in most clinical situations associated with high risk for these occurrences, the one instance where heparin is of questionable efficacy and warfarin is of proven efficacy is in patients undergoing emergent surgery for hip fracture. In this instance, prophylaxis is best accomplished with moderate-dose warfarin, as the benefit is clearly greater than the operative or postoperative bleeding risk.[144] Patients undergoing elective hip replacement are better treated with prophylactic subcutaneous heparin, not warfarin.[14]

Table 14-3. General Clinical Indications for Warfarin Therapy*

Surgery for hip fracture, nonelective
Deep venous thrombosis prophylaxis after initial heparin
Recurrent deep venous thrombosis
Deficiency of antithrombin, protein C, or protein S
Anticardiolipin antibody and thrombosis syndrome type III (heparin appears superior for types I and II)
Lupus anticoagulant and thrombosis syndrome
Mitral valve disease with system embolization
Mitral valve disease with chronic atrial fibrillation
Mitral valve prolapse with transient ischemic attacks, systemic embolization, or chronic or paroxysmal atrial fibrillation
Mitral annular calcification with embolism or atrial fibrillation
Bacterial endocarditis with infected prosthetic valve
Mechanical heart valve
Bioprosthetic heart valve; long term if systemic embolization, atrial fibrillation, or left atrial thrombus
Acute myocardial infarction with atrial fibrillation, system embolization, venous thromboembolism, or chronic heart failure
Cardiomyopathy with atrial fibrillation
Congestive heart failure with atrial fibrillation
Thyrotoxic heart disease with atrial fibrillation
Cardioversion for atrial fibrillation
Progressing stroke

* Modified from Dalen JE: Arch Intern Med 146:462, 1986.

It is generally accepted that patients who are at high risk or who are being treated for prophylaxis of recurrent thrombotic or thromboembolic disease should continue taking a regimen of coumarin-type derivatives for three months.[1,14,143] The recurrence rate varies between 3% and 38% depending on the series reported, and sometimes efficacy has been far inferior to that reported with long-term, low-dose heparin or antiplatelet agents.[144,145] Patients who initially receive a regimen of intravenous heparin for a thrombotic event or who receive a regimen of prophylactic subcutaneous heparin that is then switched to long-term warfarin should continue receiving warfarin for an indefinite time if they have a continuing risk factor, such as AT III, protein S, protein C, or plasminogen deficiency, the presence of a lupus anticoagulant, anticardiolipin antibody, or any other inherited or acquired long-term hypercoagulable condition.[14]

Although warfarins have frequently been used in patients with TIAs, no significant benefit has been noted.[146-149] Although warfarins have frequently been used in patients with completed thrombotic stokes, no documented efficacy has been noted.[150,151] The use of warfarin in evolving thrombotic stroke may be marginally effective, but the hemorrhagic complications are often unacceptable.[152,153] Generally accepted indications for warfarin therapy are summarized in Table 14-3.

Risks of Coumarin Therapy

The coumarin derivatives are associated with serious side effects, the most frequently encountered being serious hemorrhage, usually from the gastrointestinal tract. Any vital organ is subject to serious hemorrhage, which will happen frequently in the patient treated with coumarin derivatives in the presence of the usual contraindications to anticoagulant therapy, including significant hypertension, the concomitant ingestion of antiplatelet agents, peptic ulcer disease, a defect in hemostasis, malignancy, or recent surgery or trauma.[14,87,154]

The hemorrhagic risks of coumarins appear to be at least partly dependent on the particular underlying medical condition for which they are used. When evaluating results of clinical trials, many do not mention hemorrhagic complications. When these risks are reported and analyzed, the risks are different for various medical conditions. Whether these differences are caused by methodology of the particular study, different dose intensities used in different trials, different medical conditions being evaluated, or various combinations of these variables is generally unclear. The incidence of coumarin-induced bleeding reported in clinical trials, where such information is available, varies from no bleeding to as high as 47%.[155] The highest occurrence of bleeding is reported in hip surgery (47%), cerebrovascular disease (40%),[156] and cardiac disease (37%).[157] Although many studies have reported hemorrhage to happen frequently in those patients with excessively prolonged prothrombin times, little objective evidence correlates bleeding risk with intensity of anticoagulation, because many patients sustain hemorrhage at seemingly proper levels of anticoagulation.[158,159] The overall and serious or fatal hemorrhagic risks of warfarins, as reported in clinical trials where available, is summarized, according to disease condition being treated, in Table 14-4.[160-162] Most bleeding episodes are from the gastrointestinal tract, but occasionally bleeding from the genitourinary tract is seen. Any organ is susceptible to hemorrhage during warfarin therapy. In patients given warfarin for cerebrovascular disease, central nervous system bleeding is the most common site, and the incidence can be high.

A rare and serious idiosyncratic reaction is coumarin-induced skin and soft tissue necrosis, manifest as a small vessel vasculitis that gives rise to serious skin necrosis and a violet-appearing rash.[163,164] Some individuals who have had this rare and serious complication have been noted to have protein C deficiency[165] and 25% of all cases involve women who have breast gangrene and may slough an entire breast.[14] The clinical and pathologic features of this rare complication have been well described.[163-165]

Laboratory Monitoring

Much new information has appeared in the literature supplying guidelines for monitoring oral anticoagulant therapy. However, many laboratories are still not adopting these

Table 14-4. Bleeding Risks With Warfarin Therapy*

Disease state	Bleeding risk
Deep venous thrombosis	4.3%–37.5%
Hip surgery	6.0%–47.4%
Myocardial infarction	1.3%–12.9%
Ischemic heart disease	3.8%–36.6%
Prosthetic valves	1.2%–20.0%
Cerebrovascular disease	1.4%–39.7%

* Modified from Levine MN, J Hirsh: Semin Thromb Hemost 12:39, 1986.

newer techniques, and this practice in itself may contribute to unnecessary hemorrhage associated with warfarin therapy. It has been shown that reporting prothrombin times and percent activity has little or no meaning.[1,14,166-168] This finding can be readily appreciated in view of the described mechanism of action of the coumarin-type drugs and by asking the question, "percent activity of what factor?" It has been shown that comparing "percent activity" has no meaning when comparing two different reagents, two different coagulation instruments, two different technologists, or two different laboratories. However, the reporting of a prothrombin time as a "prothrombin ratio" that is obtained by dividing the control time into the patient's time is reasonably comparable between two different reagents, two different coagulation instruments, two different technologists, and two different laboratories. Most studies have advocated the use of a prothrombin ratio instead of percent activity.[1,14,166-169]

Recent studies, including the results of many prospective randomized trials, have clearly shown that many clinicians, especially in the United States, have been using excessive doses of coumarin drugs. Many trials in the United Kingdom and Europe have appraised intensity of anticoagulation based on prothrombin times by human brain thromboplastin or the Manchester Comparative Reagent or the British Comparative Thromboplastin Reagent. Based on the results of prospective clinical trials with these reagents, it is recommended that the prothrombin time ratio, the patient time divided by the control time, be expressed as an International Normalized Ratio (INR). The thromboplastins used in the United States are of rabbit brain origin and are generally less sensitive to the vitamin K–dependent factors as compared to the human brain thromboplastin used in the Manchester Reagent or the British Comparative Reagent. Simple conversion tables or formulae are available to convert human brain thromboplastin time ratios to rabbit brain ratios, and these are usually in the package inserts of various reagents. The reagent supplier usually includes an International Sensitivity Index (ISI) of the particular thromboplastin, and equivalency can be calculated by the following formula: International Normalized Ratio (INR) = the Observed Ratio (OR) to the power of ISI, or INR = (OR)^{ISI}.[170,171]

In simple terms, with rabbit brain thromboplastin generally available in the United States, an adequate intensity of anticoagulation for almost all conditions is that amount of warfarin giving a prothrombin time ratio of 1.3 to 1.5 times the control. The exceptions to this general rule are patients with rheumatic valvular heart disease with documented systemic embolization or patients with a mechanical heart valve in whom the intensity of warfarin anticoagulation should be increased to give a prothrombin time ratio of 1.5 to 2.0.[172,173]

When changing therapy from heparin to coumarin-type medications, the regimen is simple and well established. Some overlap is needed since a delayed onset of action of coumarin drugs is noted in heparinized patients. Exact adjustment of the prothrombin ratio must be empiric. The usual procedure in patients taking heparin is to start a regimen of coumarin derivatives at 5 to 10 mg per day for five to seven days and to stop heparin therapy when the prothrombin index is greater than 1.3.[1,14] A dose of 0.75 units of heparin per mL will begin to prolong the prothrombin time. Many drugs interact with coumarin derivatives. Many of these drugs potentiate the activity of coumarin drugs, others interfere with the activity of coumarin drugs, and in addition, coumarin drugs may enhance the action of other drugs. The most common drugs interacting with coumarin derivatives are listed in Table 14-5; more complete lists have been published.[174,175]

The efficacy of coumarin derivatives in thromboembolic disease has been highly effective in limited studies but questionable in others. The contraindications, expense in monitoring, and the real risk of serious or life-threatening hemorrhage are now leading many clinicians to rely more heavily on low-dose heparin for immediate prophylaxis and antiplatelet agents or subcutaneous heparin for long-term prophylaxis of patients at high risk for thrombosis or recurrent thrombotic disease.

Heparin and Heparinlike Preparations

Heparin has been in use for almost half a century, is the most common drug for treatment of acute thrombosis and thromboembolus, and remains one of the most widely used agents for prophylaxis.[178,179] Despite this lengthy clinical experience, speculation, confusion, and general misunderstanding remain regarding the mechanism(s) of action of heparin. Ideal doses, ideal preparations, and ideal methods of delivery are controversial, speculative, and sometimes unknown. USP heparin is a heterogeneous molecular weight preparation, with molecular weights ranging from 4,000 to 40,000 d and the average molecular weight being about 15,000 to 20,000 d.[178,180] Only about 30% of USP heparin binds to AT III, and only 30% is available to accelerate the serine protease inhibitory activity of antithrombin. Little or no in vivo anticoagulant activity is found in 60% to 70% of USP heparin.[178,180,181] Although the ideal doses of heparin are unknown, it is suggested that a plasma heparin level of between .01 and .02 units/mL[180,182-185] is surely adequate for

Table 14-5. Drug Interactions With Warfarins

Potentiate warfarin action	
Aspirin	Oxyphenylbutazone
Amiodarone	Pentoxifylline
Anabolic steroids	Phenothiazines
Antibiotics	Phenylbutazone
Cephalosporins (only those	Quinine
with methylthrotetrazole	Quinidine
side chain)	Sulfisoxazole
Cephoperazone	Sulindan
Cefamandole	Tolazemide
Chloryl hydrate	Tolbutamide
Chloramphenicol	Tolmetin
Chlorpropamide	Vitamin E
Cimetidine	
Clobibrate	**Inhibit warfarin action**
Danazole	Antacids
Dextran	Barbiturates
Diazoxide	Carbamazepine
Disulfiram	Corticosteroids
Erythromycin	Cholystyramine
Estrogens	Etchlorvynol
Ethacrynic acid	Glutethamide
Glucagon	Griseofulvin
Indomethacin	Haldoperidol
Ibuprofen	Meprobamate
Fenoprofin	Nafcillin
Mefenamic acid	Oral contraceptives
Methylphenidate	Primidone
Metronidazole	Rifampin
Miconazole	
Moxalactam	**Enhanced by warfarin**
Naldixic acid	Diphenylhydantoin
Naproxen	Chlorpropamide
	Tolbutamide

prevention of thrombus formation, and at this dose heparin is maximally accelerating the inhibitory activity of AT III.[14,18,180,182,185] Other studies, however, recommend higher plasma heparin levels.[186,187] The essential activity of heparin is thought to be its acceleration of the inhibitory activity of AT III against serine proteases.[182,183,185,188] The mechanism of AT III inhibition of thrombin (factor IIa) vs the antithrombin inhibition activity of factor Xa may differ with the particular preparation of heparin used.[184,189]

Coagulation has been generally accepted to occur in a cybernetic manner with fibrin deposition and lysis happening as a continuous process.[183,190-193] The manifestations of normal hemostasis vs increased fibrin deposition (thrombosis) or increased fibrinolysis (hemorrhage) depends on a fragile balance between the procoagulant system and its associated inhibitors and the fibrinolytic system and its associated inhibitors.[183,192,194-197] The primary inhibitor of the procoagulant system is AT III. Antithrombins were first described by Brinkhous et al in 1939,[198] and the first large survey of antithrombins was reported by Seegers et al in 1952.[199] Antithrombin III has activity not only against thrombin but also against other serine proteases generated during coagulation, including factors Xa, IXa, and XIa, plasmin, kallikrein, and factor XIIa.[183,200-203] The inhibition of factor Xa is thought to correlate most closely with clinical inhibition of thrombus formation, and inhibition of factor Xa appears to be more important than the inhibition of factor IIa for efficacy of heparin.[180,184,189,204,205] Usually, especially for AT III activity against thrombin and factor Xa, this activity is markedly accelerated by the addition of heparin. The kinetics of this heparin-antithrombin–serine protease reaction have recently been described by Wessler,[182] Yin,[185] and Abildgaard.[206] When the hemostasis system is driven in the procoagulant direction with the attendant generation of serine proteases and eventual fibrin formation, AT III consumption happens, since AT III combines irreversibly with activated clotting factors, and the complex is removed from the circulation. Without heparin, antithrombin appears to inactivate thrombin in a progressive, irreversible manner following second-order kinetics.[207] Antithrombin inactivates other serine proteases, although with slower reactivity in the absence of heparin than its inhibition of thrombin.[201-203,208-210] In the presence of heparin, the inactivation of thrombin and factor Xa is markedly accelerated and is almost instantaneous. Differences depend on the differing molecular weights and other characteristics of the particular heparin used.[184,189,204,205] Rosenberg and Damus showed that heparin interacts with antithrombin by binding to lysine residues of the antithrombin molecule, which presumably accelerates the inhibitory activity of antithrombin with respect to serine proteases.[211] Heparin also combines directly with thrombin and factor Xa, however, and whether the neutralization of thrombin and factor Xa by antithrombin is the result of the interaction of heparin with antithrombin or the interaction of heparin with the particular serine protease is still a matter of controversy.[212-215] Alternatively, another proposed mechanism is that a molecule of heparin may act to bind antithrombin to thrombin or factor Xa.[216] These mechanisms may be different with differing heparin preparations and appear to be different for the antithrombin inhibition of thrombin vs the antithrombin inhibition of factor Xa.[184,188,189,204,205] Differing molecular weight subspecies of heparin have different activities for the interaction of AT III and thrombin, AT III and factor Xa, or interaction of AT III and serine proteases with the vasculature.[184,188,189,204,205,217,218] During these processes, heparin appears not to be consumed, and after the formation of the heparin-antithrombin–serine protease complex, heparin dissociates from the complex, acting as a catalyst, and then becomes available to interact with more antithrombin or serine protease.[219] The kinetics of the heparin and serine protease interaction have been well elucidated, supplying evidence that only minute amounts of heparin, from .01 to .02 units per mL, need to be present to maximally accelerate the inhibitory activity of antithrombin.[180,182,183-185,188,206] Endogenous heparin is rarely detected in the blood in significant amounts. It has been suggested, however, that very low doses of heparin or semisynthetic heparin analogues may release endogenous glycosaminogly-

cans that then activate antithrombin to inhibit serine proteases.[183,188,220-223] When exogenous heparin is delivered into the blood compartment it is rapidly absorbed by the surface of endothelial cells. This endothelial-bound heparin may be far more important than heparin circulating in the blood stream for thrombus prevention.[178,224] The subspecies of heparin preparation used and differing routes of delivery may preferentially lead to more or less heparin bound to the endothelium. Thus, theoretically those preparations or modes of delivery that render more endothelial-bound heparin and less heparin in the blood stream may be the most effective for clinical use.[176,178,224]

Some vascular proteoglycans, other than heparin, are also able to interact with AT III and enhance the rate of inhibition of thrombin and factor Xa. This activity appears to be limited to dermatan sulfate and heparan sulfate.[222,225,226] The obvious major physiologic significance of this is implied but not yet conclusively proven. Some evidence exists that the use of ultra–low-dose heparin or semisynthetic heparin analogues may accelerate endogenous vascular glycosaminoglycan-induced, antithrombin-mediated inhibition of serine proteases.[220,221,227]

Most studies have shown that the physiologic range of antithrombin in normal human blood is narrow, and decreases of AT III may be of clinical relevance when choosing to use heparin anticoagulation.[183,188,228,229] Most patients respond to heparin if the biologic AT III level is greater than 60%. Many patients, however, will not respond if biologic AT III levels are less than 40% activity.[183] Formerly, increased anticoagulant activity of heparin has been defined by prolonged global tests of coagulation, primarily the APTT, the activated clotting time, the thrombin time, and other similar tests. Prolongation of these tests, however, does not correlate with efficacy or with clinical bleeding.[230-232] Now that the properties of different heparin preparations are becoming more clear, it is easier to explain this lack of correlation of global clotting tests and clinical efficacy of heparin. No assay yet exists to measure ideally the clinical efficacy of heparin. The anti–factor Xa assay as described by Denson and Bonner with the synthetic substrate S-2222 is probably the most reasonable assay to use now.[188,233]

Clinical Aspects

Heparin can be administered by several routes depending on the desired effect, although it is clear that differing routes may render different clinical efficacy and effects.[14,234] Formerly, the most commonly used route has been intravenous infusion, which has the advantage of an immediate onset of action as defined by global clotting tests. However, this method and these tests do not correlate with efficacy and may inversely correlate with efficacy. If heparin is given intravenously, it should always be given by constant infusion, because intermittent pushes are not only of unclear clinical efficacy but are also associated with a higher chance of hemorrhagic complications.[235,236] A more popular route of heparin administration is subcutaneous injection or so-called "mini-dose" or low-dose heparin therapy. Many clinical trials have now established the efficacy of subcutaneous low-dose heparin therapy for the prophylaxis of deep venous thrombosis and pulmonary embolus.[237-255] Several trials have shown that subcutaneous heparin is equally effective to intravenous heparin in treating an active thrombotic event.[207,256-258] Another trial has shown that "ultra–low-dose" heparin therapy at a dose of 1 mg/kg per hour for three to five days is also highly effective.[220] This dosage schedule only gives a plasma heparin level of .007 units per mL, and this ultra–low-dose heparin may be causing an accelerated endogenous glycosaminoglycan interaction with antithrombin, thereby inhibiting endogenous serine protease generation.[220] There are clear-cut differences in plasma levels, vascular interaction, and anti–factor IIa activity vs anti–factor Xa activity with differing preparations of subcutaneously delivered heparin.

Generally, a medical dose of heparin is delivered as 20,000 to 30,000 units per 24 hours by constant infusion, giving a plasma heparin level of about 1 to 2 units per mL.[1,14] When administered subcutaneously, the usual plasma heparin level is between .01 and .1 units per mL or higher.[1,14] Subcutaneous "mini-dose" heparin therapy is generally delivered as 2,500 to 5,000 units every six to 12 hours, depending on the clinical condition being treated. Heparin need not necessarily be given in the anterior abdominal wall. Alternating injection sites in any subcutaneous tissue is desirable and more comfortable for the patient. The anterior thighs are acceptable and create less pain for the patient. Heparin administered intramuscularly is not recommended, since it may lead to serious intramuscular hematomas. A newer route of delivery is by intrapulmonary inhalation, which also provides adequate plasma heparin levels and in limited trials appears to be highly efficacious for prevention of thrombosis or thromboembolic disease.[259,260]

Significant differences have been found between beef lung vs porcine mucosal heparin when examined by anti–factor Xa assays in vivo and in vitro; however, these differences are not as pronounced when observed by global clotting tests such as the APTT.[184,192,234] With both porcine mucosal or beef lung heparin, the anti–factor Xa activity markedly increases with a decrease in the molecular weight. With beef lung heparin, however, the specific activity of anti–factor Xa is much less than that of porcine mucosal heparin at all molecular weights. The peak heparin levels as measured by anti–factor Xa assay are 50% higher with mucosal heparin than with beef lung heparin, but with either of these preparations the PTT may prolong at a plasma heparin level of about 0.02 units per mL.[180,184,234] Generally low anti–factor Xa activity is found in most batches of beef lung heparin, and most authorities now believe that the anti–factor Xa activity of heparin is by far the essential activity for inhibition of thrombus formation in humans.[184,188,236] The inhibition of thrombin by antithrombin/heparin is dependent on the molecular size of the heparin.[176,178,180,184,189,204,205] The inhibition of factor Xa shows a different dependency, there-

fore suggesting that the heparin-potentiated inhibition of factor Xa and thrombin happen by different mechanisms.[184,189] The inhibition of thrombin and factor Xa differ in plasma vs purified systems, which has been noted by several investigators and has led to the discovery that low-density lipoprotein inhibits heparin.[189,261] These inhibitory effects, however, are more pronounced for high–molecular weight heparin than with low–molecular weight heparin.[189,261] The potentiation of anti–factor Xa activity is inversely proportional to the molecular weight of heparin, with significant inhibitory activity increasing with decreasing molecular weight of the heparin.[176,178,180,184,189,204,205] This correlation is depicted in Figure 14-1. The PTT and other global tests of coagulation also correlate with molecular weight of the heparin preparation, with more prolongation occurring with the higher–molecular weight heparins. This finding, however, does not correlate with efficacy or clinical bleeding. This correlation is depicted in Figure 14-2. These differences may be clinically significant and may relate to the type of assay and the differing molecular weight distribution of heparin subspecies in differing heparin fractions when trying to interpret clinical data in patients who have been given seemingly similar heparin preparations that may not be similar. An extremely low–molecular weight heparin having only 10 to 16 sugar units will greatly potentiate the activity of anti–factor Xa by antithrombin but has no effect on the inhibition of thrombin and, therefore, no prolongation of global tests of coagulation dependent on the inhibition of factor IIa.[205] This extremely low–molecular weight fragment has much less activity for enhancing ADP-induced platelet aggregation than is seen with high–molecular weight forms of heparin. Heparin, when used in extremely high doses, can potentiate platelet aggregation even without ADP.[205,262,263] Platelet aggregating activity as a function of heparin molecular weight is depicted in Figure 14-3.

The anticoagulant effect of heparin is proportional to the anti–factor Xa inhibitory activity and not dependent on the high–molecular weight portion having significant anti–factor IIa activity. The anti–factor IIa activity, however, induces prolongation of global tests of coagulation. Therefore, low–molecular weight fractions and fragments have more antithrombotic activity in clinical efficacy than standard heterogeneous USP heparin. A recent study comparing four heparin preparations injected by the subcutaneous route has shown that the highest anti–factor Xa activity is seen after the injection of low–molecular weight sodium heparin with a maximum effect happening about three to four hours after the injection. With a similar preparation of sodium high–molecular weight heparin, the maximum effects were seen at one hour.[204] Lower anti–factor Xa activity was seen at one hour with calcium heparin, which occurred at three to four hours after the injection. However, low–molecular weight calcium heparin appeared equal to low–molecular weight sodium heparin. These observations may account for why a seemingly uniform dose regimen gives such varying degrees of clinical and laboratory differences in different individual

Figure 14-1. Heparin Molecular Weight and Anti-Factor Xa Activity

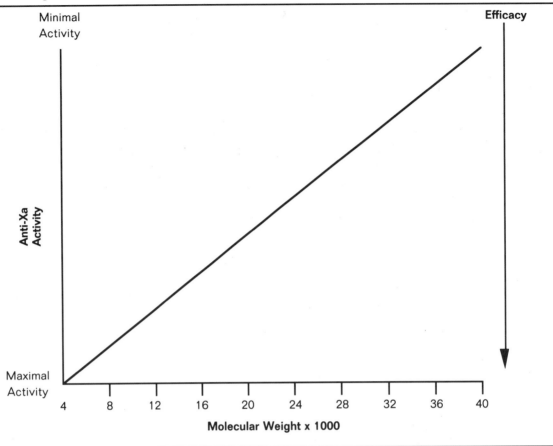

patients. The characteristics of heparin itself may have considerable effects on the plasma heparin levels after subcutaneous injection, with high levels being noted with low–molecular weight heparins as compared to standard high–molecular weight heterogeneous heparins. These preparations may have significant differences in absorption from subcutaneous injection sites with the large–molecular weight species entering the circulation more slowly.

In comparing calcium and sodium heparin salts given subcutaneously, plasma heparin levels were noted to be significantly lower following the administration of a calcium heparin noted in both plasma heparin levels and kaolin-cephalin clotting time assays. No differences were noted between calcium vs sodium salt heparins when delivered intravenously.[264] When using both the Yin assay and the anti–factor Xa assay of Denson and Bonner, calcium heparin levels, although lower than sodium heparin levels, were well above a minimum efficacious range (.01 to .02 units per mL) by both anti–factor IIa and anti–factor Xa assay systems. Sodium heparin may potentiate hemorrhage, whereas an extremely low chance of any hemorrhage, including minor wound hematomas, exists with calcium heparin preparations.[264] This study, comparing calcium and sodium salts of heparin, concluded that calcium heparin is at least equal in efficacy to sodium heparin but is much less likely to produce hemorrhage.

The anti–factor IIa effect vs the anti–factor Xa effect is markedly different depending on the molecular weight subspecies of the heparin. Anti–factor Xa activity increases with decreasing molecular weight of the heparin fragment or fraction, whereas the anti–factor IIa activity increases with increasing molecular weight of the heparin fraction. Those heparins having a higher percentage of low–molecular weight components are thought to be more effective than those having a lesser percentage of low–molecular weight components. Another consideration is that porcine mucosal heparin preparations generally have more anti–factor Xa activity than beef lung preparations, and another difference is that calcium heparins appear to be more effective in anti–factor Xa activity than sodium heparin preparations. Among the standard heparins available today, calcium salt heparin of porcine mucosal origin and a preparation containing the highest percentage of low–molecular weight constituents would comprise the ideal heparin. Preliminary work has been reported on semisynthetic heparin analogues. Thus far, results show semisynthetic heparin analogues to be as effective as low-dose heparin, and these analogues have a strong anti–factor Xa activity and a potent lipoprotein lipase activity.[221,222,227] These semisynthetic analogues may release endogenous glycosaminoglycans and enhance normal physiologic protective mechanisms.[221,222,227] Although having

Figure 14-2. Heparin Molecular Weight and Effect on Global Coagulation Tests

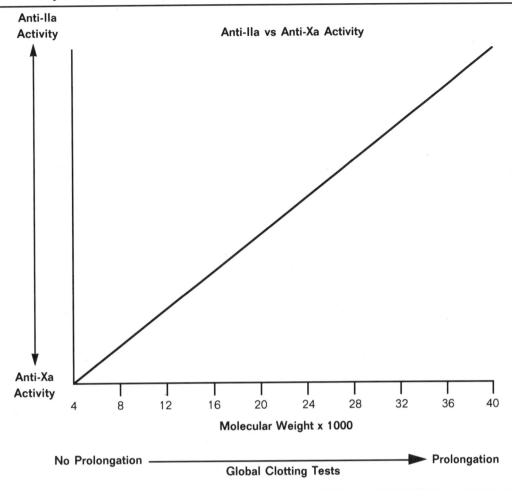

extremely high anti–factor Xa activity, these semisynthetic analogues have minimal to absent in vitro anticoagulant activity as defined by prolongation of global tests of clotting, such as the APTT, thrombin time, activated clotting time, and other tests. Thus, these analogues appear to have minimal to no anti–factor IIa activity. Differences in heparin preparations are summarized in Table 14-6.

No global laboratory test, including the activated partial thromboplastin time, activated clotting time, whole blood recalcification time, or thrombin time, offers any predictability of efficacy or hemorrhage.[1,14] Spontaneous bleeding is rare with heparin therapy at any dose, and generally the hazards of heparin therapy are somewhat dependent on the type of preparation used (low molecular weight vs high molecular weight, subcutaneous vs intravenous, porcine mucosal vs beef lung) and are related to duration of therapy, older age, sex, and surgical trauma.[265] Most bleeding episodes associated with heparin therapy are seen in situations when heparin was given despite a general contraindication to anticoagulant therapy, such as peptic ulcer disease, malignant hypertension, a defect in hemostasis, the simultaneous ingestion of antiplatelet agents, or some type of inva-

sive procedure. Occasionally hematuria is seen in elderly women; however, this side effect need not necessarily be a contraindication for continued therapy.[1,14,266]

Another complication of heparin therapy formerly has been osteoporosis. However, this complication generally only happens when heparin is used for more than six months at a minimum dose of 10,000 units per day, and this dosage regimen is rarely used anymore.[14,267] Heparin, unlike vitamin K antagonists, does not cross the placenta and may be used in pregnant women. About 80% of heparin is degraded by the liver and about 20% by the kidney.[14] In renal or kidney failure, proper adjustments in dose should be made, especially when using high intravenous doses.

Heparin-induced thrombocytopenia is a major complication of heparin therapy, and heparin, in any dose, should always be accompanied by platelet counts at least every three days, and daily for the first week. The incidence of heparin-induced thrombocytopenia varies from less than 1% to greater than 20% depending on the study reported.[14,268-274] Heparin-induced thrombocytopenia is more common with beef lung heparin than with porcine mucosal heparin in a ratio of 4:1.[275] The usual latent period is six to 14 days after

Figure 14-3. Heparin Molecular Weight and Platelet Aggregating Activity

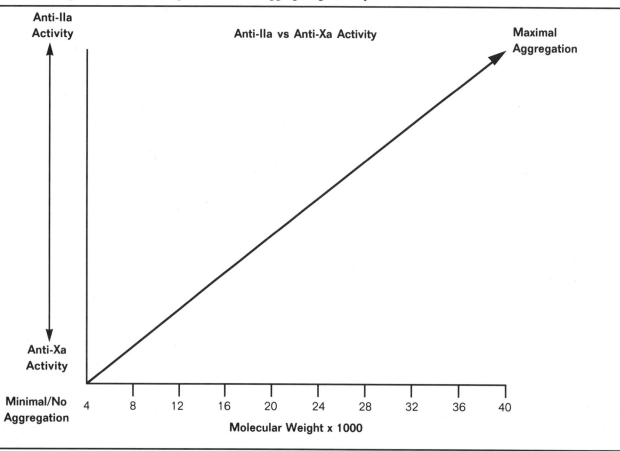

the initiation of heparin, and a typical patient showing heparin-induced thrombocytopenia is depicted in Figure 14-4. Heparin-induced thrombocytopenia happens with intravenous or subcutaneous heparin therapy, and the thrombocytopenia will usually abate 48 hours following the cessation of heparin therapy. Most instances of heparin-induced thrombocytopenia are associated with the easy demonstration of platelet-associated IgG or IgM. It was first hoped that low–molecular weight heparin fragments and fractions would be unassociated with heparin-induced thrombocytopenia, but this may not be the case.[276] Of even greater concern is that serious paradoxic thromboembolism happens in about 50% of patients with severe heparin-induced thrombocytopenia. In about 50% of individuals developing paradoxic thromboembolism, a serious arterial thrombus or thromboembolus occurs. In another 50%, the patient will have an extension of an already existing thrombus, a new deep venous thrombotic event, or a pulmonary embolus. About 10% of individuals developing heparin-induced thrombocytopenia and paradoxic thromboembolism will suffer a major cerebral vascular thrombotic event, myocardial infarction, or mesenteric vascular occlusion.

Many prospective randomized trials have been reported regarding the efficacy of low-dose heparin therapy.[79,234,238-252,254,257] Ultra–low-dose heparin therapy may be

as effective as low-dose heparin therapy, which suggests that perhaps the ideal minimal dose of heparin has not yet been established.[220] Several trials have clearly established that subcutaneous heparin is equally as effective as intravenous heparin therapy in the treatment of active thrombotic events for preventing propagation of existing thrombus, recurrent thrombosis, or thromboembolism.[207,256-258] Low-dose heparin therapy has not only been shown to be highly effective in elective surgery but also in surgery for malignant disease.[238,239,244-246,248] The use of low-dose heparin therapy for prophylaxis in prostatic surgery and in hip surgery remains unclear, with some trials showing good results and others showing no differences in treated vs untreated control patients.[46,237-241,277-283] Large clinical trials evaluating the efficacy of low–molecular weight heparin fragments and fractions are now proceeding, and this preparation appears highly efficacious for prophylaxis of venous thromboembolic disease.[284-288] These preparations are not yet approved for clinical use in the United States. Intrapulmonary heparin is another route of delivery that is currently being explored.[289,290]

Intrapulmonary heparin was first used in 1965 when Bosner subjected nine patients with chronic obstructive pulmonary disease to heparin aerosol at doses of 10,000 to 40,000 units per dose by a bird respirator.[291] No untoward reactions and no bleeding were noted. Of nine patients, four

Table 14-6. Characteristics of Different
Heparin Preparations

Source
Beef lung
Low anti–factor Xa activity
High anti–factor IIa activity
Lower percent low–molecular weight fractions
Higher incidence of hemorrhage?
High incidence of heparin-induced thrombocytopenia
Lower efficacy
Porcine mucosal
High anti–factor Xa activity
Low anti–factor IIa activity
Higher percent low–molecular weight fractions
Low incidence of heparin-induced thrombocytopenia
Higher efficacy

Salt
Calcium
Less hemorrhage
High anti–factor Xa activity
Equal anti–factor IIa activity
Lower plasma levels (SQ)
Sodium
More hemorrhage
Low anti–factor Xa activity
Equal anti–factor IIa activity
Higher plasma levels (SQ)

Molecular weight
High molecular weight
Low anti–factor Xa activity
High anti–factor IIa activity
Prolonged global tests
Lower efficacy
Low molecular weight
High anti–factor Xa activity
Low anti–factor IIa activity
Normal global tests
High efficacy

* Ideal USP (heterogenous molecular weight) heparin = calcium salt,
mucosal origin, and highest percent of low–molecular weight fractions

had relief of bronchospasm and two had slight increases in their whole blood clotting time. Following this, Bardona et al subjected 10 patients with asthma to heparin doses of 20,000 units by intrapulmonary aerosol, and all patients showed subjective improvement, although none showed objective changes in spirometry.[292] More important, none of these patients demonstrated a prolongation of the Lee-White clotting time, and no patient manifested any type of hemorrhage.

In 1969, Young-Chaiyud and associates treated 69 patients with chronic obstructive pulmonary disease with heparin aerosol given by the intrapulmonary route, and the dose in this study was 20,000 units in 1 mL of normal saline.[293] No side effects, including hemorrhage, were noted in any patient.

Of more significance, in 1973, Molino and Bellvardo delivered heparin aerosol by the intrapulmonary route to 86 patients with a variety of cardiovascular and thromboembolic disorders for prophylaxis of recurrent disease, and the dose used was 100 mg (about 10,000 units) delivered at 12-hour intervals for five months.[294] Many of these individuals were followed up for a maximum of five years, and not one recurrent thrombotic or thromboembolic episode or hemorrhage was noted in any of these 86 individuals.

In 1977, Thonnard-Neumann delivered heparin aerosol or intravenous heparin to 60 individuals with migraine or cluster headaches. By the intrapulmonary route 86% of individuals improved, and by the intravenous route 75% of individuals improved. The dose used in this study was 2,500 to 5,000 units weekly by intrapulmonary inhalation, and during this period no change was noted in the prothrombin time or activated partial thromboplastin time, and no hemorrhagic episodes were noted.[295]

In 1979, Kavanagh and Mahadoo subjected human volunteers to massive doses of intrapulmonary heparin, up to 157,500 units per dose, and although in this instance a prolonged clotting time was noted, no bleeding episodes were noted.[296]

Mahadoo and coworkers have delivered intrapulmonary heparin for prophylaxis of deep venous thrombosis and pulmonary emboli following major surgical procedures.[297] In five patients receiving intratrachial installation of heparin, giving a plasma heparin level of .01 to .16 units per mL, two episodes of postoperative wound hematoma were noted in the five treatment episodes. No changes were noted in the whole blood clotting time, activated partial thromboplastin time, platelet count, hematocrit, or fibrinogen level. Following these two wound hematomas, these same investigators then changed the regimen to intrapulmonary heparin (aerosol) and treated eight patients before major surgical procedures with doses of 25,000 units/kg without any wound hematomas or any other type of bleeding being noted. At this dose, no changes in the plasma heparin concentration, whole blood clotting time, AT III level, or platelet count were noted.

In pharmacokinetic animal work done by Jaques and coworkers, doses of intrapulmonary heparin were found to be unassociated with hemorrhage as noted by autopsy studies.[298] Mahadoo and associates using electron microscopy and radioactive-labeled heparin showed that heparin given by the intrapulmonary route appears to undergo immediate uptake by alveolar macrophages and capillaries, which then is distributed throughout the endothelial tree, being attached to the endothelial lining, which may be the ideal place for heparin for inhibition of thrombus formation.[299,300] Jaques and Mahadoo found that the greater the cellular storage pool of heparin, primarily the vascular endothelium, and the greater number of endothelial cells subjected to heparin, the more profound the clinical anticoagulant effect.[224] These same authors have compared the pharmacokinetics of heparin and the efficacy of heparin delivered by the intravenous, intramuscular, subcutaneous, or intrapulmonary route, and these studies have supplied data that now potentially account

Figure 14-4. Typical Course of Platelet Counts in a Patient With Heparin-Induced Thrombocytopenia

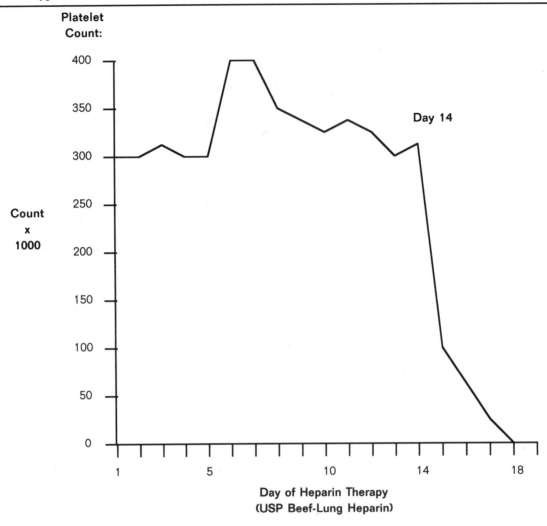

for the variability of clinical efficacy in humans depending on the route of administration.[301,302] Specifically, the heparin cellular storage pool, the vascular endothelium, appears to vary significantly with the route of administration, with evidence suggesting that endothelial-bound heparin is the major fraction involved in prevention of thrombus formation and not the fraction found in plasma, and that the distribution of endothelial-bound heparin appears greatest by the intrapulmonary route and least by the intravenous route.

Laboratory Assessment

The activated partial thromboplastin time, thrombin time, whole blood clotting time, and other global tests of hemostasis that depend on anti–factor IIa activity do not correlate with plasma heparin concentration, clinical efficacy of heparin, or clinical bleeding.[1,14,230,231] This issue was confusing for a long time; however, now that it is clear that the anti–factor IIa activity of heparin has little to do with clinical efficacy and that the anti–factor Xa activity rendered by the low–molecular weight portions is correlated with clinical

efficacy, this paradox becomes understandable. Appreciating the differences between porcine mucosal heparin vs beef lung heparin, and the other differences between calcium and sodium salts of heparin, further clarifies the lack of correlation between global tests of coagulation and plasma heparin levels, bleeding, or efficacy. The APTT was developed as a screening test for hemophilia and was never intended to be used for monitoring heparin therapy.[303] The traditional approach to adjusting a heparin dose, depending on the prolongation of an activated partial thromboplastin time, is of no clinical relevance since it does not correlate with plasma heparin levels, bleeding, or efficacy.[1,14,230,231,303] The same arguments apply to other global tests of coagulation depending on anti–factor IIa activity, including the ACT and thrombin time. If any one test correlates with clinical efficacy of heparin, it is the anti–factor Xa assay described by Denson and Bonner,[233] but this assay system is not yet generally available. When using global tests of coagulation and seeing inadequate prolongation with intravenous doses of heparin or when seeing a patient fail heparin therapy as manifest by a

Table 14-7. Potential Reasons for Heparin Failures

Hereditary or acquired AT III deficiency
Elevated levels of low-density lipoprotein
Elevated levels of lysozyme (muramidase)
Elevated levels of platelet factor 4
Elevated levels of beta-thromboglobulin
Hereditary or acquired heparin cofactor II deficiency
Intravenous nitroglycerin

thrombotic event, the obvious things that should be looked for are AT III deficiency, extremely high levels of lysozyme, platelet factor 4, or extremely high levels of low-density lipoprotein. If any of these factors are found, an alternate mode of therapy should be considered.[180,183,189,261,304] Table 14-7 summarizes common reasons for heparin failures.

Until anti–factor Xa assays become generally available, a simple approach to assessing heparin therapy includes the following criteria. When delivering subcutaneous or intrapulmonary heparin therapy, a plasma heparin level and AT III level are obtained about one hour after the institution of therapy.[14] If the plasma heparin level is greater than .01 units per mL, it is assumed that adequate heparin is present for efficacy, and if the AT III level is greater than 60% it is assumed that adequate AT III is present for anti–factor Xa activity. If these two criteria are met, no further laboratory monitoring is required. This mode of monitoring may change when anti–factor Xa assays using the synthetic substrate S-2222 become more generally available. For those continuing to use global tests of coagulation, prolongation of the test does supply important information, since it can be assumed if prolongation occurs, adequate levels of AT III are available for the heparin–AT III interaction to happen. Clinicians using these global test results, however, should recognize that these results do not correlate with plasma heparin levels, clinical efficacy, or propensity to hemorrhage.

Many new heparin preparations are becoming available, and it is generally recognized that differing preparations have differing modes of activity. Currently, when choosing a USP heterogeneous heparin, the most effective preparations are those with the highest percentage of low–molecular weight material, those with a calcium salt instead of a sodium salt, and those of porcine mucosal instead of beef lung origin. It is expected that within the next several years, low–molecular weight heparin fractions and fragments will become generally available for the treatment and prophylaxis of thrombosis and thromboembolic disease.

Summary

This chapter has summarized current knowledge, apparent indications, and the results of major clinical trials using anticoagulant and antiplatelet therapy. Since many studies have been retrospective in nature, many have been without uniform dosages, and a wide variety of disorders have been studied, efficacy for warfarin therapy, heparin vs mini-dose heparin therapy, and antiplatelet therapy can be expected to undergo significant change in the future. Other changes will be the introduction of new low–molecular weight heparins, semisynthetic heparin analogues, and new antiplatelet agents. The introduction of these newer agents and their use in double-blind prospective randomized trials will eventually provide more clear-cut indications for both long-term prophylactic therapy and the immediate prophylaxis of high-risk patients.

References

1. Bick RL: Anticoagulant and antiplatelet therapy, ch 14. In: G Murano, RL Bick (Eds): Basic Concepts of Hemostasis and Thrombosis. CRC Press, Boca Raton, FL, 1980, p 245.
2. Weiss HJ: The pharmacology of platelet inhibition. Prog Hemost Thromb 1:199, 1972.
3. Burch JW, N Stanford, PW Majerus: Inhibition of platelet prostaglandin synthetase by oral aspirin. J Clin Invest 61:314, 1979.
4. Jaffe EA, BB Weksler: Recovery of endothelial cell prostacyclin production after inhibition by low doses of aspirin. J Clin Invest 63:532, 1979.
5. Buchanan MR, E Dejana, M Gent: Enhanced platelet accumulation onto injured carotid arteries in rabbits following aspirin treatment. J Clin Invest 67:503, 1981.
6. Davis RF, EG Engelman: Incidence of myocardial infarction in patients with rheumatoid arthritis. Arthritis Rheum 17:527, 1974.
7. Linos AJ, JW Worthington, W O'Fallon: Effect of aspirin on prevention of coronary and cerebrovascular disease in patients with rheumatoid arthritis. Mayo Clin Proc 53:581, 1978.
8. Pareti FI, PM Mannucci, A D'Angelo: Congenital deficiency of thromboxane and prostacyclin. Lancet 1:898, 1981.
9. Bowen BK, WG Drause, KJ Ivey: Effect of sodium bicarbonate on aspirin-induced damage and potential difference changes in human gastric mucosa. Br Med J 2:1052, 1977.
10. Kauffman GL, MI Grossman: Prostaglandin and cimetidine inhibit antral ulcers produced by parenteral salicylates. Gastroenterology 74:1049, 1978.
11. Mills DCB, JM Smith: The influence on platelet aggregation of drugs that affect the accumulation of adenosine 3',5'-cyclic monophosphate in platelets. Biochem J 121:185, 1971.
12. Bick RL: Platelet defects, ch 4. In: Disorders of Hemostasis and Thrombosis: Principles of Clinical Practice. Thieme, Inc., New York, 1985, p 65.
13. Hirsh J, E Salzman, L Harker: Aspirin and other platelet active drugs: relationship among dose, effectiveness and side effects. Chest 95:12, 1989.
14. Bick RL: Anticoagulant therapy, ch 13. In: Disorders of Hemostasis and Thrombosis: Principles of Clinical Practice. Thieme, Inc., New York, 1985, p 352.
15. Cohen LS: Clinical pharmacology of acetylsalicylic acid. Semin Thromb Hemost 2:146, 1976.
16. Bick RL: Treatment of bleeding and thrombosis in the patient with cancer. In: T Nealon (Ed): Management of the Patient with Cancer. WB Saunders, Philadelphia, 1976, p 48.

17. Bick RL: Disseminated intravascular coagulation: a clinical review. Semin Thromb Hemost 14:299, 1988.

18. Bick RL, BJ McClain: Deep venous thrombosis: a laboratory evaluation of 118 consecutive patients. Thromb Haemost 50:237, 1983.

19. Hirsh J, JA McBride: Increased platelet adhesiveness in recurrent venous thrombosis and pulmonary embolism. Br Med J 2:797, 1965.

20. Hume M: Platelet adhesiveness and other coagulation factors in thrombophlebitis. Surgery 59:110, 1966.

21. Webster MW, JH Chesebro, V Fuster: Platelet inhibitor therapy: agents and clinical implications. Hematol Oncol Clin North Am 4:265, 1990.

22. Lorenz RL, M Weber, J Kotzur: Improved aortocoronary bypass patency by low-dose aspirin (100 mg daily): effects on platelet aggregation and thromboxane formation. Lancet 1:1261, 1984.

23. Lewis HD, JW Davis, DG Archibald: Protective effects of aspirin against acute myocardial infarction and death in men with unstable angina. N Engl J Med 309:396, 1983.

24. Coronary Drug Project Research Group: Aspirin in coronary heart disease. J Chronic Dis 29:625, 1976.

25. The E.P.S.I.M. Research Group: A controlled comparison of aspirin and oral anticoagulants in prevention of death after myocardial infarction. N Engl J Med 307:701, 1982.

26. Aspirin Myocardial Infarction Study Research Group: A randomized controlled trial of aspirin in persons recovered from myocardial infarction. JAMA 243:661, 1980.

27. Persantin-Aspirin Reinfarction Study Research Group: Persantin and aspirin in coronary heart disease. Circulation 62:449, 1980.

28. Craven LL: Experiences with aspirin in the nonspecific prophylaxis of coronary thrombosis. Miss Val Med J 75:38, 1953.

29. Boston Collaborative Drug Surveillance Group: Regular aspirin intake and acute myocardial infarction. Br Med J 1:436, 1974.

30. Dale J: Prevention of arterial thromboembolism with acetylsalicylic acid in patients with prosthetic heart valves. Thromb Haemost 38:66, 1977.

31. Nunez L, M Gil Aguado, D Celemin: Aspirin or coumarin as the drug of choice for valve replacement with porcine bioprosthesis. Ann Thorac Surg 33:354, 1982.

32. Elwood PC, AL Cochrane, ML Burr: A randomized controlled trial of acetylsalicylic acid in the secondary prevention of mortality from myocardial infarction. Br Med J 1:436, 1974.

33. Medical Research Council: Effect of aspirin on postoperative deep venous thrombosis. Lancet 2:441, 1972.

34. Clagett GP, DF Brier, CB Rosoff: Effect of aspirin on postoperative platelet kinetics and venous thrombosis. Surg Forum 25:473, 1974.

35. Shondorf TH, D Hey: Modified "low-dose" heparin prophylaxis to reduce thrombosis after hip joint operation. Thromb Res 12:153, 1977.

36. Harris WH, EW Salzman, CA Athanasoulis: Aspirin prophylaxis of venous thromboembolism after total hip replacement. N Engl J Med 297:1246, 1977.

37. Hume M, V Bierhaum, TX Kuriakose: Prevention of postoperative thrombosis by aspirin. Am J Surg 133:420, 1977.

38. McKenna R, J Galante, F Bachman: Prevention of venous thromboembolism after total knee replacement by high-dose aspirin or intermittent calf and thigh compression. Br Med J 281:514, 1980.

39. Zerkert F, P Kohn, E Vormittag: Thromboembolic prophylaxe mit acetylsalicylsaure bei operationen wegen huftgelenknaher fracturen. Monatsschr Unfallheilkunde 77:97, 1974.

40. Jennings JJ, WH Harris, A Sarmiento: A clinical evaluation of aspirin prophylaxis of thromboembolic disease after total hip arthroplasty. J Bone Joint Surg 58:926, 1976.

41. Loew P, HK Wellmer, U Baer: Postoperative thromboembolic-prophylaxe mit acetylsalicylsaure. Dtsch Med Wochenschr 99:565, 1974.

42. Soreff J, H Johnsson, L Diener: Acetyl-salicylic acid in a trial to diminish thromboembolic complications after elective hip surgery. Acta Orthop Scand 46:246, 1975.

43. Stamatakis JP, VV Kakkar, D Lawrence: Failure of aspirin to prevent postoperative deep vein thrombosis in patients undergoing total hip replacement. Br Med J 1:1031, 1978.

44. Salzman EW, WH Harris, RW DeSanctis: Reduction in venous thromboembolism by agents affecting platelet function. N Engl J Med 284:1287, 1971.

45. Weber W, U Wolff, G Bromig: Postoperative thromboembolie-prophylaxe mit colfarit. Ther Berichte 43:229, 1971.

46. Harris WH, EW Salzman, C Athanasoulis: Comparison of warfarin, low–molecular weight dextran, aspirin, and subcutaneous heparin prevention of venous thromboembolism following total hip replacement. J Bone Joint Surg 56:1552, 1974.

47. Breddin HK: Current perspectives in the antiplatelet therapy of thrombotic disorders. Semin Thromb Hemost 15:144, 1989.

48. Wood EH, CRM Prentice, DA McGrouther: Trial of aspirin and RA-233 in prevention of postoperative deep vein thrombosis. Thromb Diath Haemorrh 30:18, 1973.

49. McBride JA, AGG Turpie, V Kraus: Failure of aspirin and dipyridamole to influence the incidence of leg scan–detected venous thrombosis after elective hip surgery. Thromb Diath Haemorrh 34:564, 1975.

50. Schondorf TH, D Hey: Combined administration of low-dose heparin and aspirin as prophylaxis of deep vein thrombosis after hip joint surgery. Haemostasis 5:250, 1976.

51. Morris GK, JPA Mitchell: Preventing venous thromboembolism in elderly patients with hip fractures: studies of low-dose heparin, dipyridamole, aspirin, and flurbiprofen. Br Med J 1:535, 1977.

52. Dechavanne M, D Ville, JJ Viala: Controlled trial of platelet anti-aggregating agents and subcutaneous heparin in prevention of postoperative deep vein thrombosis in high risk patients. Haemostasis 4:94, 1975.

53. Silvergleid AJ, R Bernstein, DS Burton: Aspirin-persantin prophylaxis in elective hip replacement. Thromb Haemost 36:166, 1977.

54. Powers PJ, M Gent, RM Jay: A randomized trial of less intense postoperative warfarin or aspirin therapy in the prevention of venous thromboembolism after surgery for fractured hip. Arch Intern Med 149:771, 1989.

55. Parodi JG, A Grandi, E Font: El dipyridamol y el acido acetilsalicilico en la profilaxis de las thrombosis venosas postoperatorias de los membros inferiores. Dia Med 44:92, 1973.

56. Renney JTG, EF O'Sullivan, PF Burke: Prevention of postoperative deep vein thrombosis with dipyridamole and aspirin. Br Med J 2:992, 1976.

57. Plante J, B Boneu, C Vaysse: Dipyridamole-aspirin versus low doses of heparin in the prophylaxis of deep venous thrombosis in abdominal surgery. Thromb Res 14:399, 1979.

58. Weiss V, M Jekiel, J Ritschard: Prevention de la maladie thromboembolique postoperatoire par les anti-agregants en chirurgie gynecologique. Med Hyg 35:943, 1977.

59. Enke A, CH Stock, O Dumke: Doppelblind studie zur postoperativen thrombiose prophylaxe mit dipyridamole-acetyl salicylsaure. Chirurg 47:670, 1976.

60. O'Brien JR, V Tulevski, M Etherington: Two in vivo studies comparing high and low aspirin dosage. Lancet 1:339, 1971.

61. Steele P, J Elles, E Genton: Effects of platelet suppressant, anticoagulant, and fibrinolytic therapy in patients with recurrent venous thrombosis. Am J Med 64:441, 1978.

62. Carter AE, R Eban, RD Perrett: Prevention of postoperative deep venous thrombosis and pulmonary embolism. Br Med J 1:312, 1971.

63. Carter AE, R Eban: Prevention of postoperative deep venous thrombosis in legs by orally administered hydroxychloroquine sulfate. Br Med J 3:94, 1974.

64. Chrisman OD, GA Shook, TC Wilson: Prevention of venous thromboembolism by administration of hydroxychloroquine: a preliminary report. J Bone Joint Surg 58:918, 1976.

65. Hanson EH, P Jessing, H Lindewald: Hydroxychloroquine sulfate in prevention of deep venous thrombosis following fracture of the hip, pelvis, or thoracolumbar spine. J Bone Joint Surg 58:1089, 1976.

66. Wu TK, MJ Tsapogas, FR Jordan: Prophylaxis of deep venous thrombosis by hydroxychloroquine sulfate and heparin. Surg Gynecol Obstet 145:714, 1977.

67. Cooke ED, MHO Dawson, RM Ibbotson: Failure of orally administered hydroxychloroquine sulfate to prevent venous thromboembolism following elective hip operations. J Bone Joint Surg 59:496, 1977.

68. Johansson E, K Forsberg, H Johnsson: Clinical and experimental evaluation of the thromboprophylactic effect of hydroxychloroquine sulfate after total hip replacement. Haemostasis 10:98, 1981.

69. Kincaide-Smith P: Modification of the vascular lesions of rejection in cadaveric renal allografts by dipyridamole and anticoagulants. Lancet 1:920, 1969.

70. Sullivan JM, DE Harken, R Gorlin: Pharmacologic control of thromboembolic complications of cardiac-valve replacement. N Engl J Med 284:1391, 1971.

71. Chesebro JH, V Fuster, LR Elveback: Trial of combined warfarin plus dipyridamole or aspirin therapy in prosthetic heart valve replacement: danger of aspirin compared with dipyridamole. Am J Cardiol 51:1537, 1983.

72. Kawazoe K, T Fujita, H Manabe: Dipyridamole combined with anticoagulant in prevention of early postoperative thromboembolism after cardiac valve replacement. Thromb Res 60:27, 1990.

73. Hess H, A Mietashk, G Deichsel: Drug-induced inhibition of platelet function delays progression of peripheral occlusive arterial disease: a prospective double-blind arteriographically controlled trial. Lancet 1:416, 1985.

74. Evans G: Effects of drugs that suppress platelet surface interaction on incidence of amarrosis fugax and transient cerebral ischemia. Surg Forum 23:239, 1972.

75. The Canadian Cooperative Study Group: A randomized trial of aspirin and sulfinpyrazone in threatened stroke. N Engl J Med 299:53, 1978.

76. Steel P, J Rainwater, E Genton: Controlled trial of sulfinpyrazone in rheumatic heart disease. Thromb Haemost 38:194, 1977.

77. Evans G, M Gent: Effect of platelet suppressive drugs on arterial venous thromboembolism. In: Platelets, Drugs, and Thrombosis Proceedings. S Karger, Basel, 1975, p 258.

78. Steele PP, HS Weily, E Genton: Platelet survival and adhesiveness in recurrent venous thrombosis. N Engl J Med 288:1148, 1973.

79. Kaegi A, FJ Pineo, A Shimizu: Arteriovenous-shunt thrombosis: prevention by sulfinpyrazone. N Engl J Med 290:304, 1974.

80. The Anturane Reinfarction Trial Research Group: Sulfinpyrazone in the prevention of sudden death after myocardial infarction. N Engl J Med 302:250, 1980.

81. The Anturane Reinfarction Italian Study Group: Sulfinpyrazone in post-myocardial infarction. Lancet 1:237, 1982.

82. Raskob GE, CJ Carter, RD Hull: Anticoagulant therapy for venous thromboembolism. Prog Hemost Thromb 9:1, 1989.

83. Mackie MJ, AS Douglas: Drug-induced disorders of coagulation, ch 17. In: OD Ratnoff, CD Forbes (Eds): Disorders of Hemostasis. WB Saunders, Philadelphia, 1991, p 493.

84. Stenflo J: Vitamin K, prothrombin, and gamma-carboxyglutamic acid. N Engl J Med 296:624, 1977.

85. Quick AJ: Hypoprothrombinemia states. In: AJ Quick (Ed): Hemorrhagic Disease and Thrombosis. Lea & Febiger, Philadelphia, 1966, p 60.

86. Loeliger EA, B von der Esch, MJ Mattern: Behaviour of factors II, VII, IX, and X during long-term treatment with coumarin. Thromb Diath Haemorrh 9:74, 1963.

87. Deykin D: Warfarin therapy. N Engl J Med 287:691, 1970.

88. Hyers TM, RD Hull, JG Weg: Antithrombotic therapy for venous thromboembolic disease. Chest 95:37, 1989.

89. Resnekov L, J Chediak, J Hirsh: Antithrombotic agents in coronary artery disease. Chest 95:52, 1989.

90. Prentice CRM: Myocardial infarction. Clin Haematol 10:521, 1981.

91. Ebert RB: Long-term anticoagulant therapy after myocardial infarction: final report of the Veterans Administration cooperative study. JAMA 207:2263, 1969.

92. Ebert RB: Anticoagulants in acute myocardial infarction: results of a cooperative clinical trial. JAMA 225:724, 1973.

93. Drapkin A, C Merskey: Anticoagulant therapy after acute myocardial infarction: relation of therapeutic benefit to patient's age, sex and severity of infarction. JAMA 222:541, 1972.

94. Assessment of short-term anticoagulant administration after cardiac infarction: report of the Working Party on Anticoagulant Therapy to the Medical Research Council. Br Med J 1:335, 1969.

95. Anticoagulants in acute myocardial infarction: results of a cooperative clinical trial. JAMA 225:724, 1973.

96. Second Report of the Working Party on Anticoagulant Therapy in Coronary Thrombosis to the Medical Research Council: An assessment of long-term anticoagulant administration after cardiac infarction. Br Med J 2:837, 1964.

97. United States Veterans Administration: Long-term anticoagulant therapy after myocardial infarction. JAMA 193:157, 1965.

98. Breddin K, D Loew, K Lechner: The German-Austrial Aspirin Trial: a comparison of acetylsalicylic acid, placebo and phenprocoum in secondary prevention of myocardial infarction. Circulation 62:63, 1980.

99. Report of the 60+ Reinfarction Study Research Group: A double-blind trial to assess long-term anticoagulant therapy in elderly patients after myocardial infarction. Lancet 2:989, 1980.

100. McEnany MT, EW Salzman, ED Mundth: The effect of antithrombotic therapy on patency rates of saphenous vein coronary artery bypass grafts. J Thorac Cardiovasc Surg 83:81, 1982.

101. Panteley GA, SH Goodnight, SH Rahimtoola: Failure of antiplatelet and anticoagulant therapy to improve patency of grafts after coronary artery bypass: a controlled, randomized study. N Engl J Med 301:962, 1979.

102. Gohlke H, C Gohlke-Barwolf, P Sturzenhofecker: Improved graft patency with anticoagulant therapy after aortocoronary bypass surgery: a prospective randomized study. Circulation 64:11, 1981.

103. Lorenz RL, M Weber, J Kotzer: Improved aortocoronary bypass patency by low-dose aspirin (100 mg daily). Effects of platelet aggregation and thromboxane production. Lancet 1:1261, 1984.

104. Chesebro JH: Effect of dipyridamole and aspirin on vein graft patency after coronary bypass operations. Thromb Res 60:5, 1990.

105. Rajah SM, MCP Salter, DR Donaldson: Acetylsalicylic acid and dipyridamole improve the early patency of aorta-coronary bypass grafts. J Thorac Cardiovasc Surg 90:373, 1985.

106. Mayer JE, WG Lindsay, W Castaneda: Influence of aspirin and dipyridamole on patency of coronary artery bypass grafts. Ann Thorac Surg 31:204, 1981.

107. Stein PD, A Kantrowitz: Antithrombotic therapy in mechanical and biological prosthetic heart valves and saphenous vein bypass grafts. Chest 95:107, 1989.

108. Chesebro JH, V Fuster, LR Elveback: Trial of combined warfarin plus dipyridamole or aspirin therapy in prosthetic heart valve replacement: danger of aspirin compared with dipyridamole. Am J Cardiol 51:1537, 1983.

109. Rajah SM, N Sreeharan, A Joseph: Prospective trial of dipyridamole and warfarin in heart valve patients. Acta Therapeutica (Brussels) 6:54, 1950.

110. Altman R, F Baullon, J Rouvier: Aspirin and prophylaxis of thromboembolic complications in patients with substitute heart valves. J Thorac Cardiovasc Surg 72:127, 1976.

111. Dale J, E Myhre: Can acetylsalicylic acid alone prevent arterial thromboembolism? A pilot study in patients with aortic ball valve prostheses. Acta Med Scand 645:73, 1981.

112. Sullivan JM, DE Harken, R Gorlin: Effect of dipyridamole on the incidence of arterial emboli after cardiac valve replacement. Circulation (suppl 1):39, 1969.

113. Kasahara T: Clinical effect of dipyridamole ingestion after prosthetic heart valve replacement: especially on the blood coagulation system. J Jpn Assoc Thorac Surg 25:1007, 1977.

114. Williams JB, RB Karp, JW Kirklin: Considerations in selection and management of patients undergoing valve replacement with gluteraldehyde-fixed porcine bioprostheses. Ann Thorac Surg 30:247, 1980.

115. Cohn LH, EN Allred, VJ DiSesa: Early and late risk of aortic valve replacement. A 12-year concomitant comparison of the porcine bioprosthetic and tilting disc prosthetic aortic valves. J Thorac Cardiovasc Surg 88:695, 1984.

116. Jamieson WRE, MT Janusz, RT Miyagishimi: Embolic complications of porcine heterograft cardiac valves. J Thorac Cardiovasc Surg 81:626, 1981.

117. Oyer PE, EB Stinson, RB Griepp: Valve replacement with the Starr-Edwards and Hancock prostheses: comparative analysis of late morbidity and mortality. Ann Surg 186:301, 1977.

118. Ionescu MI, DR Smith, SS Hasan: Clinical durability of the pericardial xenograft valve: ten years experience with mitral replacement. Ann Thorac Surg 34:265, 1982.

119. Gonzales-Lavin L, AP Tandon, S Chi, TC Blair: The risk of thromboembolism and hemorrhage following mitral valve replacement. J Thorac Cardiovasc Surg 87:340, 1984.

120. Wood P: Diseases of the Heart and Circulation. JB Lippincott, Philadelphia, 1956.

121. Ellis LB, DE Harken: Arterial embolization in relation to mitral valvuloplasty. Am Heart J 62:611, 1961.

122. Deverall PB, PM Olley, DR Smith, DA Watson: Incidence of stenosis embolism before and after mitral valvotomy. Thorax 23:530, 1968.

123. Szekely P: Systemic embolism and anticoagulant prophylaxis in rheumatic heart disease. Br Med J 1:209, 1964.

124. Hinton RC, JP Kistler, JJ Falon, AL Freidlich: Influence of etiology of atrial fibrillation on incidence of systemic embolization. Am J Cardiol 40:509, 1977.

125. Dewar HA, D Weightman: A study of embolism in mitral valve disease and atrial fibrillation. Br Heart J 49:33, 1983.

126. Hay WE, SA Levine: Age and atrial fibrillation as independent factors in auricular mural thrombus formation. Am Heart J 24:1, 1942.

127. Levine HJ, SG Pauker, EW Salzman: Antithrombotic therapy in valvular heart disease. Chest 95:98, 1989.

128. Taguchi K, H Matsumara, T Washizu: Effect of antithrombogenic therapy especially high-dose therapy of dipyridamole after prosthetic valve replacement. J Cardiovasc Surg 16:8, 1975.

129. Fuster V, L Badimon, JJ Badimon: Prevention of thromboembolism induced by prosthetic heart valves. Semin Thromb Hemost 14:50, 1988.

130. Myler RK, CA Sanders: Aortic valve disease and atrial fibrillation: report of 122 patients with electrocardiographic, radiographic, and hemodynamic observations. Arch Intern Med 121:530, 1968.

131. Stein P, H Sabbath, J Apitha: Continuing disease process of calcific aortic stenosis. Am J Cardiol 39:159, 1977.

132. Pleet AB, EW Massey, ME Vengrow: Stroke and the bicuspid aortic valve. Neurology 31:1540, 1982.

133. Hanson MR, JR Hodgman, JP Conomy: A study of stroke associated with prolapsed mitral valve. Neurology 23:341, 1978.

134. Barnett HJM, JWD McDonald, DL Sackett: Aspirin: effective in males threatened with stroke. Stroke 9:295, 1978.

135. Greenwood WF, HE Aldriridge, AD McKelvey: Effect of mitral commissurotomy on duration of life, functional capacity, hemoptysis and systemic embolism. Am J Cardiol 11:348, 1963.

136. Rowe JC, EF Bland, HB Sprague: The course of mitral stenosis without surgery: ten and twenty year prospectives. Ann Intern Med 52:741, 1960.

137. Wilson JK, WF Greenwood: The natural history of mitral stenosis. Can Med Assoc J 71:323, 1954.

138. Aberg H: Atrial fibrillation. Acta Med Scand 185:373, 1969.

139. Bjerkelund CJ, OM Orning: The efficacy of anticoagulant therapy in preventing embolism related to DC electroconversion of atrial fibrillation. Am J Cardiol 23:208, 1969.

140. Barker HW, HE Cromer, M Hurn: The use of dicumarol in the prevention of postoperative thrombosis and embolism with special reference to dosage and safe administration. Surgery 17:207, 1945.

141. Pyorala T, V Lampinen: Preoperative anticoagulant treatment in gynecologic surgery. Acta Obstet Gynecol 49:215, 1970.

142. Kakkar VV: Prevention of venous thromboembolism. Clin Haematol 10:543, 1981.

143. Gallus AS: Established venous thrombosis and pulmonary embolism. Clin Haematol 10:583, 1981.

144. Bynum LJ, JE Wilson: Low-dose heparin therapy in the long-term management of venous thromboembolism. Am J Med 67:553, 1979.

145. Engelberg H: Actions of heparin relevant to the prevention of atherosclerosis. In: RL Lundblad, WV Brown, KS Mann, HR Roberts (Eds): Chemistry and Biology of Heparin. Elsevier, New York, 1981, p 555.

146. Baker RN, JA Broward, HC Fang, CM Fisher: Anticoagulant therapy in cerebral infarction: report on cooperative study. Neurology 12:823, 1962.

147. Baker RN, WS Schwartz, AS Rose: Transient ischemic attacks. Neurology 16:841, 1966.

148. Pearce JMS, SS Gubbay, JN Walton: Long-term anticoagulant therapy in transient cerebral ischemic attacks. Lancet 1:6, 1965.

149. Report of the Veterans Administration Cooperative Study of Atherosclerosis, Neurology Section: An evaluation of anticoagulant therapy in the treatment of cerebrovascular disease. Neurology 11:132, 1961.

150. Hill AB, J Marshall, DA Shaw: Cerebrovascular disease: trial of long-term anticoagulant therapy. Br Med J 2:1003, 1962.

151. Enger E, S Boyesen: Long-term anticoagulant therapy in patients with cerebral infarction. A controlled clinical study. Acta Med Scand 178:1, 1965.

152. Carter AB: Anticoagulant therapy in progressive stroke. Br Med J 2:70, 1961.

153. Millikan CH: Anticoagulant therapy in cerebrovascular disease. In: CH Millikan, RG Seikert, JP Whisnant (Eds): Cerebral Vascular Diseases. Grune and Stratton, New York, 1965, p 183.

154. O'Reilly RA: The pharmacodynamics of the oral anticoagulant drugs. Prog Hemost Thromb 2:175, 1974.

155. Hamilton HW, JS Crawford, JH Gardiner: Venous thrombosis in patients with fracture of the upper end of the femur. J Bone Joint Surg (Br) 52:268, 1970.

156. Baker RN: An evaluation of anticoagulant therapy in the treatment of cerebrovascular disease: report of the Veterans Administration cooperative study of atherosclerosis. Neurology 11:132, 1961.

157. Harvald B, T Hilden, E Lund: Long-term anticoagulant therapy after myocardial infarction. Lancet 2:626, 1962.

158. Levine MN, G Raskop, J Hirsh: Hemorrhagic complications of long-term anticoagulant therapy. Chest 89:16, 1986.

159. Forfar JC: A 7-year analysis of hemorrhage in patients on long-term anticoagulant treatment. Br Heart J 42:128, 1979.

160. McDowell F, E McDevitt, IS Wright: Anticoagulant therapy: five years experience with the patient with an established cerebrovascular accident. Arch Neurol 8:209, 1963.

161. Salzman EW, WH Harris, RW DeSanctis: Anticoagulation for prevention of thromboembolism following hip surgery. N Engl J Med 275:122, 1966.

162. Hull R, T Delmore, C Carter: Adjusted subcutaneous heparin versus warfarin sodium in the long-term treatment of venous thrombosis. N Engl J Med 306:189, 1982.

163. Comp PC, JP Elrod, S Karzenski: Warfarin-induced skin necrosis. Semin Thromb Hemost 16:293, 1990.

164. Nalbandian RM, FK Beller, AK Kamp, RL Henry, PL Wolf: Coumarin necrosis of skin treated successfully with heparin. Obstet Gynecol 38:395, 1971.

165. Francis RB: Acquired purpura fulminans. Semin Thromb Hemost 16:310, 1990.

166. Zucker S, E Brosills, GR Cooper: One-stage prothrombin time survey. Am J Clin Pathol 53:340, 1970.

167. Control of anticoagulants. Br Med J 1:126, 1969.

168. Report of the Working Party on Anticoagulant Therapy in Coronary Thrombosis to the Medical Research Council. Br Med J 1:335, 1969.

169. Loeliger EA: International Committee for Standardization in Haematology: Recommendations for reporting prothrombin time in oral anticoagulant therapy. Thromb Haemost 53:155, 1985.

170. World Health Organization: Recommended methodology for using WHA International Reference Preparations for Thromboplastin. WHO, Geneva, 1985.

171. Poller L: A simple nomogram for the derivation of International Normalised Ratios for the standardization of prothrombin times. Thromb Haemost 60:18, 1988.

172. Adams GF, JD Merrett, WM Hutchinson: Cerebral embolism and mitral stenosis: survival with and without anticoagulants. J Neurol Neurosurg Psychiatry 37:378, 1974.

173. Akbarian M, WG Austen, PM Yurchak, JG Scannell: Thromboembolic complications of prosthetic cardiac valves. Circulation 37:826, 1968.

174. Udall JA: Recent advances in anticoagulant therapy. Gen Pract 11:116, 1969.

175. Sigel LT, HC Flessa: Drug interactions with anticoagulants. JAMA 214:2035, 1970.

176. Jaques LB: The premises involved in the clinical use of heparin. Semin Thromb Hemost 4:275, 1978.

177. Choay J: Structure and activity of heparin and its fragments: an overview. Semin Thromb Hemost 15:359, 1989.

178. Casu B: Heparin structure. Haemostasis 20:62, 1990.

179. Hirsh J: Mechanisms of action and monitoring of anticoagulants. Semin Thromb Hemost 12:1, 1986.

180. Thomas DP: Heparin. Clin Haematol 10:443, 1981.

181. Thomas DP: Heparin, low molecular weight heparin, and heparin analogues. Br J Haematol 58:385, 1984.

182. Wessler S: Small doses of heparin and a new concept of hypercoagulability. Thromb Diath Haemorrh 33:81, 1974.

183. Bick RL: Clinical relevance of antithrombin III. Semin Thromb Hemost 8:276, 1982.

184. Barrowcliffe TW, EA Johnson, CA Eggleton: Anticoagulant activities of lung and mucous heparins. Thromb Res 12:27, 1977.

185. Yin ET: Effect of heparin on the neutralization of factor Xa and thrombin by the plasma alpha-2-globulin inhibitor. Thromb Diath Haemorrh 33:43, 1975.

186. Leyvraz PF, J Richard, F Buchmann: Adjusted versus fixed dose subcutaneous heparin in the prevention of deep-vein thrombosis after total hip replacement. N Engl J Med 309:954, 1983.

187. Turpie AGG, JG Robinson, DJ Doyle: Comparison of high-dose with low-dose subcutaneous heparin to prevent left ventricular mural thrombosis in patients with acute transmural anterior myocardial infarction. N Engl J Med 320:352, 1989.

188. Thaler E, K Lechner: Antithrombin III deficiency and thromboembolism. Clin Haematol 10:369, 1981.

189. Losito R, C Losito: Molecular weight of heparin versus biologic activity. Semin Thromb Hemost 11:29, 1985.

190. Alkjaersig N, L Roy, A Fletcher: Analysis of gel exclusion chromatographic data by chromatographic plate theory analysis: application to plasma fibrinogen chromatography. Thromb Res 3:525, 1973.

191. Irwin JF, WH Seegers, TJ Andary: Blood coagulation as a cybernetic system: control of autoprothrombin-C (Xa) formation. Thromb Res 6:431, 1975.

192. Muller-Berghaus G: Pathophysiologic and biochemical events in disseminated intravascular coagulation: dysregulation of procoagulant and anticoagulant pathways. Semin Thromb Hemost 15:88, 1989.

193. Seegers WH, JF Irwin, AB Hivegas: Blood coagulation: a cybernetic system modified in hemophilia. Proceedings of the IX Congress World Federation of Hemophilia, 1974, p 3.

194. Harpel PC, RD Rosenberg: Alpha-2-macroglobulin and antithrombin-heparin cofactor: modulators of hemostasis and inflammatory reactions. Prog Hemost Thromb 3:145, 1976.

195. Mammen EF: Physiology and biochemistry of blood coagulation. In: NU Bang, FK Beller, E Deutsch, EF Mammen (Eds): Thrombosis and Bleeding Disorders: Theory and Methods. Academic Press, New York, 1971, p 1.

196. Murano G: "The Hageman Connection": interrelationships between complement, kinins, and coagulation. Am J Hematol 4:409, 1978.

197. Seegers WH: Use and regulation of blood clotting mechanisms. In: WH Seegers (Ed): Blood Clotting Enzymology. Academic Press, New York, 1971, p 1.

198. Brinkhous KM, HP Smith, ED Warner: Inhibition of blood clotting and unidentified substances which acts in conjunction with heparin to prevent the conversion of prothrombin to thrombin. Am J Physiol 125:683, 1939.

199. Seegers WH, KD Miller, EB Andrews: Fundamental interaction and effect of storage, other adsorbents, and blood clotting in plasma antithrombin activity. Am J Physiol 169:700, 1952.

200. Abildgaard U, K Graven, HC Godal: Assay of progressive antithrombin in plasma. Thromb Diath Haemorrh 34:224, 1970.

201. Seegers WH, ER Cole, CR Harmison: Neutralization of autoprothrombin-C activity with antithrombin. Can J Biochem 42:359, 1964.

202. Seegers WH, H Schroer, M Kagami: Interaction of purified autoprothrombin I with antithrombin. Can J Biochem 42:425, 1964.

203. Vennerod AM, K Laake, AK Soleberg: Inactivation and binding of human plasma kallikrein by antithrombin III and heparin. Thromb Res 9:457, 1976.

204. Johnson EA, TBL Kirkwood, Y Sterling: Four heparin preparations: anti-Xa potentiating effect of heparin after subcutaneous injection. Thromb Haemost 35:586, 1976.

205. Holmer E, U Lindahl, G Backstrom: Anticoagulant activities and effects on platelets of a heparin fragment with high affinity for antithrombin. Thromb Res 18:861, 1980.

206. Abildgaard U: Binding of thrombin to antithrombin III. Scand J Clin Lab Invest 24:23, 1969.

207. Bentley PG, VV Kakkar, MF Scully: An objective study of alternative methods of heparin administration. Thromb Res 18:177, 1980.

208. Kurachi K, G Schmer, M Hermodson: Inhibition of bovine factor IXa by antithrombin III. Biochemistry 15:368, 1976.

209. Lahiri B, RD Rosenberg, RC Talamo: Antithrombin III: An inhibitor of human plasma kallikrein. Fed Proc 33:642, 1974.

210. Stead N, AP Kaplan, RD Rosenberg: Inhibition of activated factor XII by antithrombin-heparin cofactor. J Biol Chem 251:6481, 1976.

211. Rosenberg RD, P Damus: The purification and mechanism of action of human antithrombin-heparin cofactor. J Biol Chem 248:6490, 1973.

212. Hook M, I Bjork, J Hopwood: Anticoagulant action of heparin: separation of high-activity and low-activity heparin species by affinity chromatography on immobilized antithrombin. FEBS Lett 66:90, 1976.

213. Li E, H Orton, R Feinman: The interaction of thrombin and heparin. Proflavine dye binding studies. Biochemistry 13:5012, 1974.

214. Walker F, C Esmon: The molecular mechanism of heparin action: II. Separation of functionally different heparins by affinity chromatography. Thromb Res 14:219, 1979.

215. Yin E, L Eisenkramer, J Butler: Heparin interaction with activated factor X and its inhibitor. Adv Exp Med Biol 52:239, 1974.

216. Pomerantz M, W Owen: A catalytic role for heparin. Evidence of a ternary complex of heparin cofactor, thrombin, and heparin. Biochim Biophys Acta 535:66, 1978.

217. Nordeman B, K Nordling, I Bjork: A differential effect of low-affinity heparin on the inhibition of thrombin and factor Xa by antithrombin. Thromb Res 17:595, 1980.

218. Messmore HL: Clinical potential of low molecular weight heparins. Semin Thromb Hemost 15:405, 1989.

219. Carlstrom A, K Lieden, I Bjork: Decreased binding of heparin to antithrombins following the interaction between antithrombin and thrombin. Thromb Res 11:785, 1977.

220. Negus D, A Friedgood, JJ Cox: Ultra-low dose intravenous heparin in the prevention of postoperative deep-vein thrombosis. Lancet 1:891, 1980.

221. Thomas DP, TW Barrowcliffe, RE Merton: In vivo release of anti-Xa clotting activity by a heparin analogue. Thromb Res 17:831, 1980.

222. Thomas DP, RE Merton, TW Barrowcliffe: Anti-Factor Xa activity of heparan sulfate. Thromb Res 14:501, 1979.

223. Marcum JA, RD Rosenberg: Role of endothelial cell surface heparin-like polysaccharides. Ann N Y Acad Sci 556:81, 1989.

224. Jaques L, J Mahadoo: Pharmacodynamics and clinical effectiveness of heparin. Semin Thromb Hemost 4:298, 1978.

225. Hatton M, L Berry, E Regoeczi: Inhibition of thrombin by antithrombin III in the presence of certain glycosaminoglycans found in the mammalian aorta. Thromb Res 13:655, 1978.

226. Hoppenstaedt D, A Racanelli, J Walenga: Comparative antithrombotic and hemorrhagic effects of dermatan sulfate, heparan sulfate and heparin. Semin Thromb Hemost 15:378, 1989.

227. Kakkar VV, D Lawrence, PG Bentley: A comparative study of low doses of heparin and a heparin analogue in the prevention of postoperative deep vein thrombosis. Thromb Res 13:111, 1978.

228. Bick RL, I Kovacs, L Fekete: A new two-stage functional assay for antithrombin III (heparin cofactor): clinical and laboratory evaluation. Thromb Res 8:745, 1976.

229. Odegard O, M Lie, U Abildgaard: Heparin cofactor activity measured with an amidolytic method. Thromb Res 6:287, 1975.

230. Teiem AN, R Abildgaard: On the value of the activated partial thromboplastin time in monitoring heparin therapy. Thromb Haemost 35:592, 1976.

231. Shapiro GA, SW Huntzinger, JE Wilson: Variation among commercial activated partial thromboplastin time reagents in response to heparin therapy. Am J Clin Pathol 67:477, 1977.

232. Bick RL, BJ McClain: A comparison of five activated partial thromboplastin times and the activated clotting time during heparin therapy. Thromb Haemost 50:236, 1983.

233. Denson KWE, J Bonner: The measurement of heparin. A method based on the potentiation of anti-Factor Xa. Thromb Diath Haemorrh 30:471, 1973.

234. Abbott WM, DF Warnock, WG Austen: The relationship of heparin source to the incidence of delayed hemorrhage. J Surg Res 22:593, 1977.

235. Estes JW, PF Paulin: Pharmacokinetics of heparin: distribution and elimination. Thromb Diath Haemorrh 33:26, 1975.

236. Glazier RL, EB Crowell: Randomized prospective trial of continuous vs intermittent heparin therapy. JAMA 236:1365, 1976.

237. Williams HT: Prevention of postoperative deep vein thrombosis with peri-operative subcutaneous heparin. Lancet 2:950, 1971.

238. Gordon-Smith IC, LP LeQuesne, DJ Grundy: Controlled trial of two regimens of subcutaneous heparin in prevention of postoperative deep-vein thrombosis. Lancet 1:1133, 1972.

239. Kakkar VV, J Spindler, PT Flute: Efficacy of low-doses of heparin in prevention of deep-vein thrombosis after major surgery: a double-blind randomized trial. Lancet 2:101, 1972.

240. Nicolaides AN, PA Dupont, S Desais: Small doses of subcutaneous sodium heparin in preventing deep venous thrombosis after major surgery. Lancet 2:890, 1972.

241. Gallus AS, J Hirsh, RJ Tuttle: Small subcutaneous doses of heparin in prevention of venous thrombosis. N Engl J Med 288:545, 1973.

242. Ballard RM, Bradley-Watson PJ, Johnstone FD: Low doses of subcutaneous heparin in the prevention of deep vein thrombosis after gynecological surgery. J Obstet Gynaecol (Br Commonwealth) 80:469, 1973.

243. Lahnborg G, L Friman, K Bergstrom: Effect of low-dose heparin on incidence of postoperative pulmonary embolism detected by photoscanning. Lancet 1:329, 1974.

244. Scottish Study: A multi-unit controlled study: heparin versus dextran in the prevention of deep vein thrombosis. Lancet 2:118, 1974.

245. Rosenberg IL, M Evans, AV Pollock: Prophylaxis of postoperative leg vein thrombosis by low-dose subcutaneous heparin or perioperative calf muscle stimulation: a controlled clinical trial. Br Med J 1:649, 1975.

246. Gallus AS, J Hirsh, SE O'Brien: Prevention of venous thrombosis with small subcutaneous doses of heparin. JAMA 275:980, 1975.

247. Abernethy EE, JM Hartsuck: Postoperative pulmonary embolism. A prospective study utilizing low-dose heparin. Am J Surg 128:739, 1974.

248. Rem J, F Duckert, R Fridrich: Subkutane klein heparindozen zur thrombose: prophylaxe in der allgemeinen chirurgic und urologie. Schweiz Med Wochenschr 105:827, 1975.

249. International Multicentre Trial: Prevention of fatal postoperative pulmonary embolism by low doses of heparin. Lancet 2:45, 1975.

250. Kakkar VV, ES Field, AN Nicolaides: Low doses of heparin in prevention of deep vein thrombosis. Lancet 2:669, 1971.

251. Corrigan TP, VV Kakkar, DP Fossard: Low-dose subcutaneous heparin: optimal dose regimen. Br J Surg 61:320, 1974.

252. Rosenberg IL, M Evans, AV Pollock: Prevention of postoperative leg vein thrombosis: a comparison of low-dose heparin and electrical calf muscle stimulation. Br Med J 1:153, 1974.

253. Robitaille D, JR Leclerc, G Bravo: Treatment of venous thromboembolism, ch 15. In: Venous Thromboembolic Disorders. Lea & Febiger, Philadelphia, 1991, p 267.

254. Raskob GE, RD Hull: Venous thrombosis, ch 6. In: HC Kwann, MM Samama (Eds): Clinical Thrombosis. CRC Press, Boca Raton, FL, 1989, p 59.

255. Caprini JA, RA Natonson: Postoperative deep venous thrombosis: current clinical considerations. Semin Thromb Hemost 15:244, 1989.

256. Bick RL: Deep venous thrombosis: a clinical evaluation of 118 consecutive patients. Thromb Haemost 50:305, 1983.

257. Andersson G, B Fagrell, K Holmgren: Subcutaneous administration of heparin. A randomized comparison with intravenous administration of heparin to patients with deep vein thrombosis. Thromb Res 34:333, 1984.

258. Parilla H, J Ansell: Anticoagulation by constant subcutaneous heparin infusion. Thromb Haemost 47:1, 1982.

259. Bick RL, E Ross: Clinical use of intrapulmonary heparin. Semin Thromb Hemost 11:213, 1985.

260. Lewandowski K, P Psuja, A Tokarz: Anticoagulant activity in the plasma after a single administration of nebilized heparin or LMW heparin fraction (Fraxiparine) in patients undergoing abdominal surgery. Thromb Res 58:525, 1990.

261. Lane DA, IR MacGregor: Low density lipoprotein: a selective inhibitor of the heparin-accelerated neutralization of factor Xa by antithrombin III. In: RL Lundblad, WV Brown, KG Mann, HR Roberts (Eds): Chemistry and Biology of Heparin. Elsevier, New York, 1981, p 301.

262. Thomas C, CD Forbes, CRM Prentice: The potentiation of platelet aggregation and adhesion by heparin in vitro and in vivo. Clin Sci Mol Med 45:485, 1973.

263. Eika C: On the mechanism of platelet aggregation induced by heparin, protamine, and polybrene. Scand J Haematol 9:248, 1972.

264. Thomas DP, S Sagar, JD Stamatakis: Plasma heparin levels after administration of calcium and sodium salts of heparin. Thromb Res 9:241, 1976.

265. Mant MJ, BD O'Brien, KL Thong: Hemorrhagic complications of heparin therapy. Lancet 1:1133, 1977.

266. Moser RH: Disorders produced by anticoagulants. Clin Pharmacol Ther 9:388, 1968.

267. Griffith GC, G Nichols, JD Asher: Heparin osteoporosis. JAMA 193:91, 1965.

268. Bell WR, PA Tomasulo, BM Alving: Thrombocytopenia occurring during the administration of heparin: a prospective study in 52 patients. Ann Intern Med 85:155, 1976.

269. Warkentin TE, JG Kelton: Heparin-induced thrombocytopenia. Prog Hemost Thromb 10:1, 1991.

270. Ansell J, N Slepchuk, R Kumar: Heparin-induced thrombocytopenia: a prospective study. Thromb Haemost 43:61, 1980.

271. Hackett T, JG Kelton, P Powers: Drug induced platelet destruction. Semin Thromb Hemost 8:138, 1982.

272. King DJ, JG Kelton: Heparin-associated thrombocytopenia. Ann Intern Med 100:535, 1984.

273. Zalcberg JR, K McGrath, R Daver: Heparin-induced thrombocytopenia with associated disseminated intravascular coagulation. Br J Haematol 54:655, 1983.

274. Gollub S, AW Ulin: Heparin-induced thrombocytopenia in man. J Lab Clin Med 59:430, 1962.

275. Stead RB, AI Schafer, RD Rosenberg: Heterogeneity of heparin lots associated with thrombocytopenia and thromboembolism. Am J Med 77:185, 1984.

276. Horellou MH, J Conard, C Lecrubier: Persistent heparin-induced thrombocytopenia despite therapy with low molecular weight heparin. Thromb Haemost 51:134, 1984.

277. Becker J, S Borgstrom, EF Salzman: Incidence of thrombosis associated with EACA administration and with combined EACA and subcutaneous heparin therapy. Acta Chir Scand 136:167, 1970.

278. Morris GK, APJ Henry, BJ Preston: Prevention of deep-vein thrombosis by low-dose heparin in patients undergoing total hip replacement. Lancet 2:797, 1974.

279. Hampson WGJ, FC Harris, HK Lucas: Failure of low-dose heparin to prevent deep-vein thrombosis after hip replacement arthroplasty. Lancet 2:795, 1974.

280. Dechavanne M, F Soudin, JJ Viala: Prevention des thromboses veneuses. Succes de L'heparin a fortes doses lors des coxarthroses. Nouv Presse Med 3:1317, 1974.

281. Hume M, T Kuriakose, ZL Xavier: 125-I fibrinogen and the prevention of venous thrombosis. Arch Surg 107:803, 1973.

282. Venous Thrombosis Study Group: Small doses of subcutaneous sodium heparin in the prevention of deep vein thrombosis after elective hip operations. Br J Surg 62:348, 1975.

283. Evarts M, J Alfidi: Thromboembolism after total hip reconstruction: failure of low doses of heparin in prevention. JAMA 225:515, 1973.

284. Messmore H: Clinical potential of low molecular weight heparins. Semin Thromb Hemost 15:405, 1989.

285. Haas S, G Blumel: An objective evaluation of the clinical potential of low molecular weight heparins in the prevention of thromboembolism. Semin Thromb Hemost 15:424, 1989.

286. Faivre R, E Neuhart, M Mirshahi: Fibrinolytic and thrombolytic parameters in patients with deep vein thrombosis treated by low molecular weight heparin. Semin Thromb Hemost 15:440, 1989.

287. Turpie AGG, J Hirsh, RM Jay: Double-blind randomized trial of Org 10172 low–molecular weight heparinoid in prevention

of deep-vein thrombosis in thrombotic stroke. Lancet 1:523, 1987.

288. Salzman E: Low–molecular weight heparin: is small beautiful? N Engl J Med 315:957, 1986.

289. Bick RL: Intrapulmonary heparin for thrombosis: an eight-year clinical experience. Thromb Haemost 65:1343, 1991.

290. Shulman AG: Heparin for prevention of atherosclerosis. N Engl J Med 319:1154, 1988.

291. Bosner SW: Heparin administration as an aerosol. Vasc Dis 2:131, 1965.

292. Bardona EJ, MJ Edwards, B Pirofsky: Heparin as treatment for bronchospasm of asthma. Ann Allergy 27:103, 1969.

293. Young-Chaiyud P, LJ Kettel, DW Cugell: The effect of heparin aerosols on airway conductance in patients with chronic obstructive pulmonary disease. Am Rev Respir Dis 99:449, 1969.

294. Molino N, C Bellvardo: Consideration on the long-term use of heparin in cardiovasculopathic subjects. A new method of administration: aerosol. Minerva Cardioangiol 22:553, 1973.

295. Thonnard-Neumann E: Migraine therapy with heparin: pathophysiologic basis. Headache 16:284, 1977.

296. Kavanagh LW, J Mahadoo: Heparin by inhalation. In: Heparin: Structure, Cellular Functions, and Clinical Applications. Academic Press, New York, 1979, p 333.

297. Mahadoo J: Personal communication. March 10, 1982.

298. Jaques LB, J Mahadoo, LW Kavanagh: Intrapulmonary heparin: a new procedure for anticoagulant therapy. Lancet 2:1157, 1976.

299. Mahadoo J, LM Hiebert, CJ Wright: Vascular distribution of intratracheally administered heparin. In: D Walz, L McCoy (Eds): Contributions to Hemostasis. Ann N Y Acad Sci 370:650, 1981.

300. Mahadoo J, LM Hiebert, LB Jaques: Endothelial sequestration of heparin administered by the intrapulmonary route. Artery 7:438, 1980.

301. Mahadoo J: Evidence for a cellular storage pool for exogenous heparin. In: Heparin: Structure, Cellular Functions, and Clinical Applications. Academic Press, New York, 1979, p 181.

302. Mahadoo J, LB Jaques: Cellular control of heparin in blood. Med Hypotheses 5:835, 1979.

303. Triplett DA, CS Harms, JA Koepke: The effect of heparin on the activated partial thromboplastin time. Am J Clin Pathol 70:556, 1978.

304. Habbab MA, JI Haft: Heparin resistance induced by nitroglycerine: a word of caution when both drugs are used concomitantly. Arch Intern Med 147:857, 1987.

305. Bick RL, G Murano: Primary hyperfibrino(geno)lytic syndromes. In: G Murano, R Bick (Eds): Basic Concepts of Hemostasis and Thrombosis. CRC Press, Boca Raton, FL, 1980, p 181.

C H A P T E R
15

Thrombolytic Therapy

In contrast to the anticoagulant drugs that are solely prophylactic in that they impede further growth of an existing thrombus and prevent rethrombosis and thromboembolism, thrombolytic agents have the unique ability of inducing the dissolution of intravascular fibrin thrombi and the digestion of fibrinogen and other proteins, resulting in a more immediate recanalization of occluded vessels and immediately improving microcirculatory and macrocirculatory flow.[1]

The most dramatic effects of pharmacologically activated fibrinolysis are usually noted when therapy is started early in the disease, usually in thrombi less than a few days old. However, recent evidence suggests that thrombolytic therapy may be effective in aged arterial and venous thrombi as well. Once thrombi are penetrated by fibroblasts and converted to scar tissue or have been covered by neoendothelialization, the probability of full vessel salvage is generally believed to be poor, but this is not always the case.[1,2] It is, therefore, important to establish a definitive early diagnosis, which is best done by visualizing intravascular thrombi by ascending venography, ascending thromboscintography, angiography, or other indicated techniques.

Thrombolytic therapy originated with the demonstration that certain enzymes will induce the dissolution of preformed fibrin clots in vitro,[3] experimentally induced intravascular thrombi in animals,[4] and superficial venous thrombi in human volunteers.[5] Of the agents tested, five are approved, and the first two enzymes approved were urokinase (UK) and streptokinase (SK). These first agents have received world-wide attention and have undergone many nonrandomized and double-blind, prospective, randomized trials. More recently, three additional newer generation agents, pro-urokinase, tissue plasminogen activator (TPA), and acylated plasminogen streptokinase complex (APSAC), have become available.[6] This chapter summarizes the results of selected clinical trials and outlines the presently accepted therapeutic regimens for the treatment of deep venous thrombosis, massive pulmonary embolism, myocardial infarction, and arterial thrombi.[1,2,6-28] The use of thrombolytic agents in cerebral vascular disease and retinal occlusive disease and the use of plasminogen in hyaline membrane disease have received only limited attention, and these studies have, generally, been associated with less encouraging results.[29,30]

Urokinase and Streptokinase

Urokinase is an enzyme produced by the kidney, found in the urine, and is a potent activator of the fibrinolytic system. Two molecular forms of urokinase are found in current therapeutic preparations: a high–molecular weight protein of 55,000 d and a low–molecular weight protein of 34,000 d. The low–molecular weight species is derived from the high–molecular weight species by proteolysis.[1,2,31] Immunologically, the two forms are indistinguishable. Depending on the method of preparation, either one or the other species, or various proportions of each, are isolated. Kidney tissue cultures and urine are the sources of urokinase and are extremely expensive. Streptokinase is a bacterial enzyme synthesized by group C-beta hemolytic streptococci and has a molecular weight of 47,000 d.[1,2,31] Streptokinase has the advantage of being far less expensive than urokinase, but it is more commonly associated with minor allergic reactions.

Urokinase and streptokinase act on the endogenous fibrinolytic system by converting plasminogen to the potent non-specific proteolytic enzyme plasmin. This activation was discussed in detail in chapter 1. Plasmin, in turn, degrades fibrin clots, fibrinogen, and other plasma proteins, including factors V, VIII, IX, XI, and XII, complement components, growth hormone, ACTH, and insulin.[1,2,32-34] Plasmin is rapidly inactivated by a variety of naturally occurring plasmin inhibitors, the essential one being alpha-2-antiplasmin, which acts rapidly, and alpha-2-macroglobulin, which inhibits more slowly.[34,35] Since plasminogen is present in the thrombus or embolus, lysis happens within the thrombus and on the surface of the thrombus.[1,2,36]

An intravenous infusion of urokinase, streptokinase, or other of the thrombolytic drugs is promptly followed by

Table 15-1. Laboratory Changes With Thrombolytic Therapy

Decreased fibrinogen
Decreased plasminogen
Decreased alpha-2-antiplasmin
Decreased clotting factors (V, VIII:C, IX, XI, XII)
Prolonged activated partial thromboplastin time
Prolonged prothrombin time
Prolonged thrombin time
Elevated plasmin
Elevated fibrin(ogen) degradation products
Elevated B-beta 15-42–related peptides

increased systemic fibrinolytic activity, and the effect may last for up to 12 hours after discontinuation of therapy. This activity is shown by a decrease in plasminogen levels, alpha-2-antiplasmin levels, and fibrinogen levels and a significant increase in circulating fibrin(ogen) degradation products and B-beta 15-42–related peptides.[16,37] Laboratory changes with thrombolytic therapy are summarized in Table 15-1. Urinary and tissue culture urokinase have comparable fibrinolytic activities.[19] The activity of both urokinase and streptokinase is expressed in international units and is a measure of their ability to induce the lysis of a fibrin clot via the plasmin system in vitro. The half-life of both enzymes is short, lasting only 10 to 20 minutes.[1,2,4] Effective blood levels and disappearance rates of streptokinase vary with the availability of the substrate plasminogen. The efficacy of urokinase and streptokinase in the lysis of pulmonary emboli[13-16,18] and the efficacy and lysis of deep venous thrombi[7,8,10,11,17,38] and coronary artery thrombi[23-25] have been established by angiography, perfusion lung scans, pulmonary arteriography, and pulmonary arterial and right heart pressure measurements as well as ascending venography and ascending thromboscintography done before and after therapy.[1,2]

Pro-Urokinase, TPA, and APSAC

These newer thrombolytic agents were developed with the hope that by altering selected biochemical properties of the original agents, streptokinase and urokinase, thrombolytic drugs might be made more fibrin-specific and less attracted to fibrinogen. Theoretically, this effect would decrease the systemic fibrino(geno)lytic activity and lead to fewer hemorrhagic complications.

Pro-urokinase is derived from urine or recombinant technology and is a precursor to urokinase.[39] Since pro-urokinase is a proenzyme, it is only activated when introduced into the blood stream, and the plasma half-life is thought to be much longer than urokinase, so it is available for a longer time to activate plasminogen. Expectations that pro-urokinase would be entirely fibrin-specific have not been realized, but this thrombolytic agent is capable of significant thrombolysis without severe systemic hypofibrinogenemia, hypoplasminogenemia, or depletion of alpha-2-antiplasmin.[39,40]

APSAC is prepared from pasteurized human plasminogen and represents a complex of streptokinase and plasminogen in which the active site of plasminogen has been acylated to make plasminogen inert to activation or inhibition by other plasma proteins.[41] This activation/inhibition site is different from the fibrin binding site of plasminogen. The effect of this manipulation is to provide a longer plasma half-life without hampering fibrin binding. The deacylation half-life for APSAC is about 40 minutes.[42] Although the long half-life of APSAC is clearly an advantage over other older and newer thrombolytic agents, it, like the others, is not fibrin-specific and may be associated with systemic proteolysis.

TPA is the most popular of the new-generation thrombolytic agents, especially as these drugs apply to coronary artery thrombolysis. Currently available TPA is obtained from melanoma cell cultures or recombinant techniques and has a short plasma half-life as compared to APSAC. Fibrin-bound plasminogen is more susceptible to TPA activation than is non–fibrin-bound (systemic) plasminogen, and this agent is possibly more fibrin-specific than other currently available thrombolytic agents.[43]

Indications

The first use of the early available agents, urokinase and streptokinase, centered around deep vein thrombosis, pulmonary embolus, and, later, coronary artery thrombosis. The newer agents were primarily developed for fibrin specificity to abort systemic fibrinolysis with thrombolytic therapy for coronary artery disease. Because of this historical progression, the older agents, streptokinase and urokinase, have been more extensively evaluated in deep vein thrombosis, peripheral arterial thrombotic disease, and pulmonary embolus than the newer agents. There is moderate experience with streptokinase but minimal experience with urokinase in coronary artery disease. Conversely, most experience with the newer agents has centered around coronary artery thrombolysis. Indications for thrombolytic therapy are summarized in Table 15-2.

Pulmonary Embolus

Since streptokinase and urokinase were the first available thrombolytic agents for clinical use, the experience with these two agents is more extensive than with the newer agents. Based on the results obtained in the National Heart and Lung Institute–sponsored Urokinase Pulmonary Embolism Trial (UPET) and the Urokinase-Streptokinase Pulmonary Embolism Trial (USPET), these two thrombolytic agents are clearly indicated in adults for the lysis of acute massive pulmonary emboli or in individuals with pulmonary emboli and unstable hemodynamics, as summarized in Table 15-2.[1,2,13-16,18] Generally, for the best thrombolytic results, treatment should be started immediately, if possible after the

Table 15-2. Indications for Thrombolytic Therapy

Pulmonary embolus

Acute massive pulmonary embolus

Defined as obstruction or significant filling defects involving two or more lobar pulmonary arteries or the equivalent amount of emboli in smaller/other arteries

Other pulmonary embolus

Pulmonary embolus of any size associated with unstable hemodynamics, especially if associated with inability to maintain blood pressure

Deep venous thrombosis

Extensive thrombi of any deep venous system, not indicated in superficial vein thrombosis, may be effective in both fresh (5 days old) or aged (up to 6 months old) venous thrombi

Acute myocardial infarction

Indicated if symptoms are less than 6 hours old and ST segment elevation persists after a trial of sublingual nitroglycerin. The intracoronary route recanalizes about 75% to 80% of occlusions; the intravenous route recanalizes about 50% to 60% of occlusions

Fresh or aged arterial thrombi

May be used intravenously (systemically) or locally

---

onset of pulmonary embolism, and usually no later than five days after pulmonary embolus has happened. Under these circumstances, angiographic and hemodynamic measurements show a more rapid improvement during the first 24 hours of therapy than with heparin.[13,14]

Sharma and coworkers showed that the use of streptokinase and urokinase as compared to heparin significantly enhanced pulmonary capillary volume and diffusion capacity (D-CO) after two weeks and one year.[44] Specifically, these authors studied 40 patients with pulmonary embolism and evaluated the effects of heparin, urokinase, or streptokinase on pulmonary capillary volume and diffusion capacity. The evaluation was done at two weeks and at one year following therapy. The capillary blood volume was found abnormally low in the heparin-treated group at both two weeks and one year.[44] However, pulmonary capillary blood volume and pulmonary diffusion capacity were normal at two weeks and one year in those patients who received fibrinolytic agents. These results clearly show that fibrinolytic agents are useful in the normalization of cardiopulmonary parameters in patients with pulmonary emboli. It is not yet established with certainty, however, that treatment with urokinase or streptokinase will decrease morbidity or mortality when compared to heparin therapy alone.[1,2] In the UPET and USPET trials, urokinase was administered intravenously with a loading dose of 4,400 units/kg per hr over 10 to 20 minutes followed by a continuous infusion of 4,400 units/kg per hr for a period of 12 to 24 hours. Streptokinase was administered intravenously at a loading dose of 250,000 units over 30 minutes followed by a continuous infusion of 100,000 units per hour for 24 hours. At the end of thrombolytic therapy, patients received heparin for seven to 10 days, followed by oral anticoagulants for two to six months. Clinical parameters, including pulmonary angiograms, pulmonary perfusion scans, and cardiorespiratory hemodynamics, were evaluated independently by several panelists, each giving an independent judgment. To establish that the endogenous fibrinolytic system had been activated, the concentrations of fibrinogen, plasminogen, and FDPs were measured in each patient (USPET) at the time of preinfusion, during infusion, and at termination of therapy. As expected, the concentration of fibrinogen and plasminogen decreased, the concentration of FDPs increased, and plasminogen decreased significantly.[1,2,16] Figure 15-1 shows that a more intense thrombolytic state is induced by streptokinase, but any difference in efficacy between streptokinase and urokinase has not been proven, and these differences appear only to be laboratory phenomena.[1,2,16] No dramatic difference was noted in clinical or laboratory parameters between the 12-hour and 24-hour urokinase regimen. Clinically, urokinase and streptokinase are equally effective in pulmonary embolus.

No significant clinical data exist for the use of pro-urokinase or APSAC in pulmonary embolism. Two trials have been completed with TPA in pulmonary embolism.[45-47] In one trial, TPA was compared to urokinase in angiographically documented pulmonary embolus. Thrombolysis by repeat angiography at two hours and assessment of hemodynamics and pulmonary perfusion were monitored for efficacy. The results showed significant thrombolysis and improvement of hemodynamics and pulmonary perfusion in most patients, and results with urokinase and TPA were identical. In another multicenter trial, intravenous vs intrapulmonary TPA, both with concomitant heparin therapy, were compared. Pulmonary emboli were documented by angiography, and efficacy was assessed by repeat angiography and evaluation of hemodynamic status. Most patients showed significant improvement in both reperfusion and hemodynamics, and no significant difference was noted between the two routes of administration. Not only are streptokinase and urokinase effective for thrombolysis of pulmonary emboli, but also the newer agent, TPA, is useful in this clinical setting.

Deep Venous Thrombosis

Many randomized clinical trials have established that streptokinase[7,8,11,17] and urokinase[48-50] are effective and indicated for the lysis of acute extensive thrombi of the deep veins in adults. In one trial, urokinase was infused for one week, and in another trial urokinase was thought to be less effective than streptokinase.[51,52] Generally, however, the two are comparable in efficacy for deep vein thrombosis. The long-term benefits for deep venous thrombosis have been established, and several reports suggest somewhat better salvage of valvular function with streptokinase and heparin than with heparin alone, therefore suggesting that the chance of chronic venous insufficiency and the postphlebitic syndrome are markedly decreased when thrombolytic therapy is used.[1,2,10,38,53]

Figure 15-1. Changes in Fibrinolytic Laboratory Parameters During Thrombolytic Therapy
With Streptokinase and Urokinase

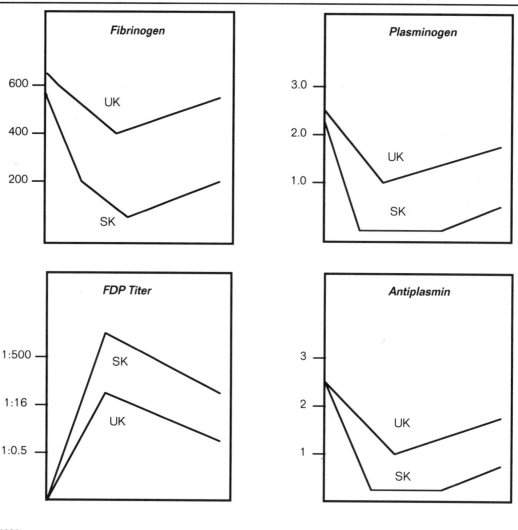

SK = Streptokinase
UK = Urokinase

In studies of deep venous thrombosis, streptokinase was administered intravenously with a loading dose of 250,000 units over 20 to 30 minutes followed by a constant infusion of 100,000 units/hr for 72 hours. At the end of thrombolytic therapy, patients were treated with heparin. Efficacy was documented by serial venography that was evaluated by masked readers. Urokinase dosages have been more variable, ranging from 4,400 units/kg per hour to a fixed dose of 80,000 units per hour for one week. Initially, it was thought that as in pulmonary embolism the best results were obtained when therapy was started within a few days of onset of the thrombotic event.

A recent report by Theiss and coworkers, however, has indicated that old venous thrombi may also be lysed with the use of fibrinolytic therapy when applied to fresh and old thrombi of the iliac and femoral veins.[54] It has been a widely held belief that thrombolytic therapy can clear thrombi from deep veins only when fresh thrombi are present. Because of this belief, which may not be valid, Theiss and coworkers[54] retrospectively analyzed venographic results in 85 patients with thrombosis of the iliac and/or femoral veins with symptoms that had been present between one day and eight weeks before thrombolytic therapy. Streptokinase, urokinase, or both drugs were successfully administered in these patients for a mean of nine days (range, two to 26 days). Total or partial resolutions of the thrombotic occlusions were obtained in 94%, 82%, and 69%, respectively, in those patients who presented with a clot three days old, seven to 14 days old, and 21 to 28 days old, after the first appearance of symptomatology. With a delay from symptomatology of five to eight weeks, the results, however, were uniformly poor with only one partial recanalization seen in the seven patients presenting in this time period. The results of this study suggest that the success rate of thrombolytic therapy of iliofemoral venous thrombosis falls only moderately during the first two weeks after the appearance of symptoms. Patients that begin therapy with a delay of up to two weeks should, therefore, be considered for thrombolytic therapy as though they had presented with a fresh deep venous thrombotic event. With a delay of more than two weeks, but no more than four weeks, the chances of success are clearly reduced, so that thrombolytic therapy should be reserved for particularly young or severely affected patients at this stage of the disease. With a delay of greater than four weeks, a favorable result happens so rarely that thrombolytic therapy, if tried, is only justified in the most desperate cases, such as bilateral iliac thrombosis or thrombosis of the inferior vena cava. The authors also concluded that for aged iliofemoral venous thrombi, fibrinolytic therapy should usually be extended beyond the customary three days and continued until either complete recanalization has been proved with ascending venography or until a significantly prolonged fibrinolytic attempt (10 to 14 days) has guaranteed that all that is possible has been done in a given patient. The investigators also found that the poorest category of patients may often need the successive use of streptokinase and urokinase in those instances where urokinase had not been used first.[54] Another study has also addressed the issue of time-dependent vulnerability of venous thrombi to thrombolytic agents and found, like the Theiss study, thrombi of two weeks of age can be successfully lysed.[55]

Except in the setting of pulmonary embolus, TPA has not been the subject of clinical trials for deep vein thrombosis.[45,46] APSAC has been evaluated in deep vein thrombosis in animal models.[56] Like the other new agents, no significant data as yet exist regarding pro-urokinase for lysis of deep vein thromboses.

Peripheral Arterial Disease

Arterial thrombi have also been successfully treated with thrombolytic therapy. Slanie and coworkers report on local thrombolysis in arterial occlusive disease.[21] These authors studied a series of 38 patients in whom intra-arterial catheters were used to infuse streptokinase or urokinase slightly proximal to an acute thromboembolic occlusion in 20 limbs or to perfuse streptokinase directly into the obstructing thrombus material in 23 extremities with subacute or chronic occlusions by advancing the catheter stepwise until the distal open segment of the artery was reached. The dose of streptokinase used in this study varied between 50,000 and 400,000 units and was administered over one to four hours. Patency was achieved in 16 of 20 acute occlusions and 16 of 23 chronically occluded vessels within this one- to four-hour treatment time. A systemic thrombolytic state of 12 to 24 hours' duration was observed when the total dose of streptokinase exceeded 80,000 units. In nine patients, thrombolysis was immediately followed by angioplasty. This study strongly suggests that the advantage of this technique is rapid, effective, low-cost, highly successful thrombolysis even in chronic femoral/popliteal occlusions

and that local thrombolytic therapy should be applied to patients in whom systemic thrombolysis would be considered contraindicated because of old age or other reasons.[21] Many more trials have now established the efficacy of streptokinase and urokinase for the lysis of acute peripheral arterial thrombi and thromboemboli.[57-66] In the acute setting, the best results are obtained when therapy is started within three days of the event. The results of trials have shown a recanalization rate of about 80%, and streptokinase and urokinase are equally effective in this setting.

Evidence for the efficacy of streptokinase in chronic arterial disease comes from the work of Martin, who reported on 475 arterial occlusions treated with streptokinase given over three days.[22] The occlusions were divided into 257 isolated femoral artery thrombi, 177 iliac artery thrombi, and 41 aortic obstructions. The dose used was a continuous streptokinase regimen at 100,000 units per hour. In subdividing the group of femoral occlusions, 225 were chronic occlusions and 32 were nonchronic occlusions, including reocclusions after transluminal catheter placement, vascular surgery, or thrombotic events following angiography. The success rate was remarkable. In patients undergoing thrombolytic treatment during the first two weeks after femoral occlusion, a clearance rate was established in 75%. Femoral artery occlusions of two to six weeks showed a 57% recanalization rate with streptokinase, and in patients having a six-week-old to three-month-old femoral artery thrombus a 38% recanalization and clearance rate was noted.[22] However, femoral artery occlusions older than six months did not respond to thrombolytic therapy.[22] Recanalization was documented by angiography before and after the administration of streptokinase therapy. Two other studies have addressed the issue of thrombolytic therapy for chronic arterial occlusive disease with favorable results being obtained. Based on these studies, about 30% of aged arterial thrombi may be expected to respond to thrombolytic therapy.

In both acute and chronic peripheral thrombi, local catheterization and thrombolysis are preferable to systemic (intravenous) therapy. Using this approach, more drug-thrombus interaction and usually less of a systemic proteolytic state and potential for distant site hemorrhage are observed. Insufficient clinical data are available for evaluation of the newer thrombolytic drugs, pro-urokinase, APSAC, and TPA, in peripheral artery disease.

Streptokinase and urokinase are useful for treatment of acute and chronic arterial thrombi and thromboemboli. Recanalization is best accomplished with local, instead of systemic, infusion, and the success rate will approach 80% in acute disease and 30% in chronic disease.

Myocardial Infarction and Coronary Artery Thrombolysis

A newer indication for thrombolytic therapy is acute myocardial infarction. This form of treatment has become widely accepted, popular, and appears to be extremely effective. Excellent reviews regarding thrombolytic therapy for acute myocardial infarction have been published.[23-25,67] For many years, it was thought that acute myocardial infarction was secondary to coronary artery spasm and not thrombi. However, DeWood and colleagues finally determined that the prevalence of total coronary artery occlusion during the early hours of myocardial infarction was associated with a high rate of coronary artery thrombus.[68] Specifically, 517 patients (90%) with a documented acute myocardial infarction undergoing angiography and left ventriculography within 24 hours after the onset of symptoms demonstrated intracoronary thrombi. The incidence of intracoronary thrombi, however, fell to 54% if the patients were studied within 12 to 24 hours after the onset of symptoms, which suggests that spontaneous thrombolysis can happen in some patients with acute myocardial infarction. Early attempts to treat coronary artery thrombosis with streptokinase by Fletcher and associates preceded this observation by more than 30 years.[69]

The concept of intracoronary thrombolysis using streptokinase was developed with the major purpose being to salvage myocardium by immediately recanalizing the coronary vasculature and preserving left ventricular function.[1,2,23,24] Generally, patients chosen for intracoronary thrombolysis are those who have a history of onset of chest pain of less than six hours' duration and show typical ST segment elevations that persist after sublingual nitroglycerin.[1,2,23,24] Patients excluded from coronary artery thrombolysis are patients with contraindications to thrombolytic therapy, such as recent surgery, cardiopulmonary resuscitation, or recent cerebral vascular accident.[1,2,23,24] Some physicians also exclude patients with cardiogenic shock, although some studies have suggested that thrombolytic therapy with streptokinase can lead to dramatic reversal of cardiogenic shock.[1,2,23,24] Various dosages are used for intracoronary streptokinase, the most common dose is started with a bolus of 10,000 to 30,000 units followed by a continuous infusion of 2,000 to 4,000 units per minute with the infusion being continued until recanalization of the vessel is documented or until a maximal dose of 500,000 units has been administered.[1,2,23-25] The response to thrombolysis is monitored angiographically every 15 minutes during infusion of streptokinase, although the sudden relief of chest pain, the new onset of arrhythmias, or the rapid resolution of ST segment elevations are clinical markers of potential recanalization.[23,24] Generally, the average time from the onset of intracoronary streptokinase to recanalization is about 30 minutes, and the average dose of streptokinase needed is about 65,000 units.[1,2,23,24] If successful recanalization occurs, a rapid early rise in CK-MB activity is noted with peak levels generally reached eight to 15 hours after the onset of symptoms with successful recanalization of coronary arteries.[1,2,23,24] After streptokinase therapy, heparin is started, since the patient is rendered hypercoagulable and may have a defective fibrinolytic system after thrombolytic activation.[1,2]

Streptokinase

Intravenous

Many trial results have been reported in the literature. Early enthusiasm emanated from the European Cooperative Study Group using streptokinase treatment in acute myocardial infarction. This early study revealed that streptokinase administered to medium-risk patients with myocardial infarction admitted to a coronary care unit within 12 hours after the onset of typical symptomatology had significantly reduced mortality at six months.[67] After this trial, many trials were started and have recently been reviewed by Goa et al.[70] Stampfer and coworkers reported on the effect of intravenous streptokinase in acute myocardial infarction and summarized mortality data obtained in eight randomized trials in which streptokinase was infused intravenously for up to 72 hours after the onset of symptomatology of myocardial infarction.[71] Although the tabulated results of these trials appear favorable, it is important to keep in mind that the summary encompasses selected trials performed within a 10-year period ending in 1979, thus bridging the introduction of the coronary care unit, the use of antiarrhythmic drugs and other ancillary therapy, and the introduction of early ambulatory programs. This renders pooling the data from these eight randomized trials difficult to interpret.[72]

A more recent and impressive trial is the GISSI study in which about 12,000 patients with acute myocardial infarction were randomly assigned between standard coronary care unit support or intravenous streptokinase, delivered as 1,500,000 units over one hour. A net reduction in mortality of 18% was noted in the streptokinase group, and mortality was reduced by 23% in those treated within three hours of symptoms.[73] In a larger study (ISIS-2 Collaborative Trial) of almost 20,000 individuals, patients were randomly assigned to intravenous streptokinase, aspirin, neither drug, or both agents.[74] Results of this trial showed a reduction in mortality with both streptokinase and aspirin groups, and the reduction in mortality in those receiving both drugs was superior to either drug alone. As in other trials, maximal benefit was noted with early therapy, but benefit was also noted in patients receiving therapy at up to 24 hours after onset of symptoms. A slight increase of bleeding was noted in the treated groups, but the benefits clearly outweighed the small (0.5%) risk. Other studies using intravenous streptokinase, the ISAM study and The Netherlands Inter-University study, have shown similar benefits in patients with acute myocardial infarction.[75,76]

Intracoronary

Most trials for assessment of intracoronary streptokinase in acute myocardial infarction are in conjunction with coronary angioplasty (PTCA).[77-81] In these studies, the efficacy of local coronary thrombolysis is well documented. Several early, but small, studies documented efficacy of intracoronary thrombolysis with streptokinase. In one early study, Markis and coworkers studied nine patients with acute myocardial infarction, and about four hours after the onset of chest pain each patient was treated with intracoronary streptokinase.[82] Occluded coronary arteries were opened within 20 minutes, and the effect of thrombolysis on myocardial salvage was assessed by thallium-201 scans. At two weeks and at three months, the patients were restudied, and in most patients the immediate recanalization of thrombosed coronary arteries significantly salvaged jeopardized myocardium.[82]

In other early trials, Khaja and coworkers[83] and Anderson and coworkers[84] studied intracoronary thrombolytic therapy in randomized trials of acute myocardial infarction in 40 and 50 patients, respectively. In the first study, the average time to initiation of therapy was 5.4 hours, and reperfusion was established in 60% of streptokinase-treated patients and only 10% of placebo-treated patients. Antiplatelet therapy was started on the day after intervention. Left ventricular function, angiographic ejection fraction, and regional wall motion measured before and immediately after intervention, as well as radionuclear ejection fraction measurements at the time of treatment, at 12 days, and at five months, showed no significant differences between treatment and placebo groups.[83] In the second group, however, the average time to reinitiation of therapy was four hours.[84] Reperfusion was established in 81% of streptokinase-treated patients, and patients were treated with subcutaneous heparin and antiplatelet agents following this. The ejection fraction and wall motion studies, enzyme changes, and electrocardiogram changes were significantly improved more rapidly in the streptokinase group.[84] In a newer and larger randomized trial, intracoronary streptokinase delivered early demonstrated a clear reduction in mortality at three months, six months, and one year.[85,86] One study did not show clear-cut benefit from intracoronary thrombolysis, but the time to treatment following onset of symptoms was prolonged, and posttherapy heparin was not used.[87]

Timmis and coworkers prospectively examined 116 consecutive patients undergoing thrombolysis for coronary artery thrombus, and hemorrhage, although minor, was documented in about 25% of patients and was related neither to a pre-existing bleeding diathesis nor to the streptokinase dose.[88] As expected, a net reduction in fibrinogen concentration and elevation of FDPs was noted in all patients and did not correlate with bleeding. These authors suggest that sequential fibrinogen profiles may be erroneous because FDP interference with the quantitation of fibrinogen and the bleeding noted is a consequence of the powerful anticoagulant effect of FDPs, specifically the interference with fibrin monomer polymerization and platelet dysfunction, and possibly the concomitant administration of heparin at the conclusion of catheterization.[88] In properly selected patients, however, hemorrhagic complications are generally confined to hematoma formations at arterial puncture sites and localized oozing at venous puncture sites.[1,2] Reperfusion-associated

arrhythmias may happen in as many as 80% of patients treated with intracoronary streptokinase with the most common arrhythmias being accelerated idioventricular rhythm, which occurs in more than 50% of patients who show successful recanalization and frequent premature ventricular contractions.[23,24] Ventricular tachycardia and ventricular fibrillation, however, are extremely rare. Despite long-standing and good experience with intracoronary streptokinase, more and more clinicians are now treating patients with intravenous streptokinase or other thrombolytic agents.[23,24] Intracoronary streptokinase, generally, causes recanalization of coronary arteries in about 75% to 80% of patients when infused directly into the thrombosed coronary artery and when infused within the first six hours of the onset of chest pain and evidence of infarction.[23,24] Conversely, systemic intravenous streptokinase infusion only results in recanalization in about 50% to 60% of patients with acute myocardial infarction.[23,24] Infusion of intravenous streptokinase, however, can be carried out more rapidly than intracoronary streptokinase, since the intravenous route can be started immediately and the intracoronary route requires more team effort, mobilization of equipment, and mobilization of catheterization laboratory personnel and cardiopulmonary bypass standby.[1,2]

Urokinase

The experience with urokinase in acute myocardial infarction is much less extensive than that of streptokinase or the newer agents, especially TPA and APSAC. Some trials have compared streptokinase and urokinase and have generally found them similar in efficacy.[89-91]

In an early European Collaborative trial and several subsequent trials, intravenous urokinase appeared to be equally effective in thrombolysis as streptokinase.[91-95] Since the trials are fewer and smaller, documented reduction in mortality is less clear. In trials comparing intravenous urokinase and streptokinase, results have generally been similar.[89,90] The evaluation of intracoronary urokinase is limited, but one study comparing intracoronary urokinase to streptokinase showed favorable results.[96]

Pro-Urokinase

Most experience with this new agent involve comparison studies also using streptokinase or urokinase, and several have used combinations of pro-urokinase and TPA because of a synergistic action of these two agents.[97,98]

In one study comparing intravenous pro-urokinase to intravenous streptokinase, the results showed better efficacy and less bleeding with pro-urokinase, but no significant differences in mortality or complications of the myocardial infarction were noted between the two drugs.[99] In another comparative trial, intracoronary pro-urokinase was compared to streptokinase by the same route, and results, as in the intravenous trial, showed improved efficacy and less bleeding in the pro-urokinase group.[100] Several trials have used a combination of TPA and pro-urokinase, and the results have been impressive with both efficacy of coronary thrombolysis and lack of serious bleeding.[96,101,102]

APSAC

Acylated streptokinase-plasminogen complex preparations have been extensively evaluated in acute myocardial infarction, and both intracoronary and intravenous routes have been used.[103] The general results of these trials have revealed that intravenous APSAC is equal in efficacy to intracoronary streptokinase and that the intracoronary and intravenous routes of APSAC are generally equivalent for both efficacy and systemic bleeding. Three large trials using intravenous APSAC for acute myocardial infarction have clearly documented efficacy for recanalization (reperfusion), myocardial salvage, and reduced mortality.[104-106] The largest of these trials was the AIMS study, which showed significant reduction in mortality if patients were treated within six hours of symptoms.[104] Based on available data, APSAC appears to be an effective thrombolytic agent for acute myocardial infarction if therapy is started early and is followed by heparin. Earlier aspirations that this agent would be fibrin-specific and unassociated with systemic fibrinolysis have not, however, been realized.

TPA

Like the other newer agents, TPA trials were begun with the hope that this agent would be fibrin-specific and associated with fewer side effects than streptokinase or urokinase. Most trials with TPA have been by the intravenous route and were compared to streptokinase by the same route. The best known of these trials was the TIMI trial.[107] Results of this excellent study revealed intravenous TPA to be significantly more effective at recanalization than intravenous streptokinase, but bleeding complications were similar. Another trial comparing intravenous TPA and streptokinase also revealed superiority of TPA in reperfusion rates but similar bleeding complications.[108] An early placebo-controlled trial showed significant efficacy of TPA in reperfusion. Several larger trials with TPA have addressed the issue of mortality. The largest of these was the ASSET trial[109] and another was reported by van de Werf and Arnold.[110] In these two trials, not only was reperfusion documented but TPA was clearly shown to decrease both early and late (three- and six-month mortality). The GISSI study was another large trial of about 20,000 patients, in which TPA was compared to streptokinase, but no significant differences in mortality were noted.[111] Two other trials comparing TPA and streptokinase also did not show significant differences in efficacy between these drugs.[112,113]

It appears that all of these agents are of generally equal efficacy in coronary thrombolysis, improved hemodynamic parameters, decreased complications, and reduction in mortality. Although the intracoronary route may be slightly more effective in recanalization rates with all thrombolytic agents, the added time element of mobilizing catheterization laboratory personnel and mobilizing cardiac surgery standby counterbalances the clear benefits of the intracoronary route. Although newer agents were generally hoped to be more fibrin-specific and therefore associated with little or no systemic proteolysis, the bleeding risks are generally the same for all agents. For these reasons, most patients with acute myocardial infarction are currently being treated by the more immediate intravenous route with good success. In those centers where trials are being done and where rapid use of the catheterization laboratory is practical, many patients are being treated by the intracoronary route, often in conjunction with PTCA.

Complications of Therapy

Bleeding

Activation of the fibrinolytic system by thrombolytic therapy results in a seriously compromised hemostatic system.[1,2,114,115] This is attributed to a generalized intravascular proteolytic process induced by systemically circulating plasmin. As a consequence, hemorrhage in varying degrees occasionally happens. In initial reports from the USPET and UPET trials, severe spontaneous bleeding, including cerebral, retroperitoneal, and gastrointestinal bleeding, was documented in slightly less than 5% of the patients treated.[1,2] Several fatalities have resulted from cerebral hemorrhage. Less severe spontaneous bleeding, such as superficial hematomas, hematuria, and hemoptysis, have been observed during therapy at about twice the frequency as that happening during heparin therapy alone.[1,2] In several instances, spontaneous bleeding has been traced to concomitant anticoagulant treatment, which is generally contraindicated during thrombolysis.[1,2] Oozing blood from sites of percutaneous trauma is frequent; hence, all invasive procedures, especially arterial punctures and intramuscular injections, must be avoided and intravenous punctures kept to a minimum before and during treatment with streptokinase and urokinase.[1,2] Although the initial UPET and USPET trial reports noted many hemorrhagic complications of therapy, at a National Institutes of Health Consensus Panel Meeting it was noted that the hemorrhagic complications in community hospital settings were much less than those noted during the early trials.[116-118] Although it was first thought that the newer thrombolytic agents, TPA, pro-urokinase, and APSAC, would be more fibrin-specific and generally unassociated with systemic proteolysis, these aspirations have not been realized and hemorrhagic risks with the newer agents are generally similar to those with urokinase and streptokinase.[114,115]

Allergic Reactions

Reactions representing possible anaphylaxis have been observed in about 3% of patients treated with streptokinase

Table 15-3. Contraindications to Thrombolytic Therapy

Active internal bleeding
Hemorrhagic diathesis
Recent (within 2 months) CVA, intracranial, or
    intraspinal surgery
Intracranial neoplasm

Table 15-5. Adverse Reactions to Thrombolytic Therapy

Bleeding
Allergic reactions
Fever
Local phlebitis

for venous thrombosis or pulmonary embolism.[1,2] Allergic reactions to TPA are thus far minimal. The reactions noted with streptokinase ranged in severity from minor breathing difficulty to bronchospasm, periorbital swelling, or angioneurotic edema.[1,2] Other mild or allergic reactions, including urticaria, itching, flushing, nausea, headache, or musculoskeletal pain, have been observed in about 12% of patients, and these mild or allergic reactions are not correlated with the dose of streptokinase.[1,2] Transient elevation or lowering of systolic blood pressure of greater than 25 mm Hg has been observed in less than 2% of patients. Mild allergic reactions including bronchospasm and skin rash have been reported, although rarely, with urokinase.[1,2] With cleaner preparations of streptokinase now available, the allergic reactions should appear much less frequently.[1,2]

Fever

Streptokinase is nonpyrogenic in standard animal tests. However, 30% of patients treated with streptokinase have shown increases in body temperature of 1.5 F or more, and the incidence of a temperature of greater than 104 F has been reported to be about 3.5%.[1,2] Febrile reactions with urokinase happen in about 3% of patients. Like the allergic reactions, the cleaner and newer preparations of streptokinase appear to be associated with far fewer incidences of febrile episodes. TPA has not yet been associated with significant febrile reactions. Table 15-3 lists absolute contraindications for fibrinolytic therapy. Table 15-4 lists warn-

ings for the use of thrombolytic therapy in patients who may be at high risk. Table 15-5 summarizes adverse reactions to streptokinase and urokinase. Table 15-6 summarizes the types of bleeding and proper management for bleeding in patients undergoing thrombolytic therapy. Table 15-7 summarizes the allergic reactions and proper management associated with thrombolytic therapy.

Laboratory Monitoring

Both streptokinase and urokinase are given by fixed-dose regimens, and no laboratory test is noted to correlate with either bleeding or efficacy.[1,2,16] Since the doses of urokinase or streptokinase are fixed doses, the doses are not changed based on laboratory monitoring. The only change required is that associated with clinical bleeding.[1,2,119] Streptokinase is infused intravenously by giving a 250,000-unit loading dose over 30 minutes followed by 100,000 units per hour for 24 to 72 hours. Intracoronary streptokinase, used for acute myocardial infarction, is generally given as a 10,000- to 20,000-unit loading dose followed by 2,000 to 4,000 units per minute for 60 minutes. The intracoronary route is usually not associated with a significant systemic thrombolytic state, such as that noted with intravenous urokinase or streptokinase. The usual intravenous dose of urokinase is 4,400

Table 15-4. Warnings for the Use of Thrombolytic Therapy (Increased Hemorrhagic Risk)

Recent (10 days) surgery, delivery, biopsy, or puncture of
    noncompressible artery
Recent (10 days) gastrointestinal bleed
Recent trauma or cardiopulmonary resuscitation
Severe hypertension
Left heart thrombus (mitral stenosis/atrial fibrillation)
Subacute bacterial endocarditis
Pregnancy
Cerebrovascular disease
Diabetic hemorrhagic retinopathy
Past severe allergy to streptokinase
Septic thrombophlebitis
Occluded A-V cannula with infection
Any other condition in which bleeding constitutes a
    potential hazard

Table 15-6. Bleeding Syndromes With Thrombolytic Therapy

Type of bleeding
    Severe
        Cerebral
        Retroperitoneal
        Gastrointestinal
    Moderate
        Hemoptysis
        Hematuria
    Mild
        Superficial hematoma
        Oozing from intravenous or intra-arterial punctures

Management
    Discontinue therapy immediately
    Volume expanders
    Avoid plasma
    Packed red blood cells
    Aminocaproic acid
    Tranexamic acid

Table 15-7. Allergic Reactions With
Thrombolytic Agents

Reaction
   2.5%
      Minor dyspnea
      Bronchospasm
      Periorbital edema
      Angioneurotic edema
      Urticaria
   12%
      Pruritus
      Flushing
      Nausea
      Headache
      Myalgias
Management
   Mild reactions
      Continue therapy and administer antihistamine and
         corticosteroids
   Severe reactions
      Discontinue therapy and administer intravenous
         corticosteroids, antihistamines, and epinephrine

units/kg per hour for 12 to 24 hours. The newer agents are sometimes associated with less of a systemic proteolytic state, but usual global tests of coagulation are, nevertheless, usually altered and do not constitute a sound reason for changing doses.

Many physicians and laboratory personnel are unclear and confused about appropriate laboratory monitoring procedures that should be done to monitor the use of these agents, especially when used systemically. Again, the dose of these agents is not changed despite changes in laboratory parameters.[1,2,119] No dose adjustment is made based on laboratory tests or changes of laboratory tests; the only dose adjustment ever made is the immediate cessation of the thrombolytic drug should significant clinical bleeding happen.[1,2,119] The recommended monitoring procedures are dictated by previously noting that no laboratory tests or combination of tests in hemostasis correlate with the efficacy of thrombolytic therapy nor has any laboratory test been shown to correlate with predisposition to hemorrhage while receiving these agents.[1,2,16,119] It is possible to keep laboratory testing at a minimum while still supplying useful information for the clinician. The recommended monitoring test for thrombolytic agents is, therefore, the thrombin time.[1,2,119,120]

Before subjecting a patient to systemic thrombolytic therapy, a careful baseline clinical hemostasis history, prothrombin time, activated partial thromboplastin time, hemoglobin, hematocrit, and platelet count must be obtained.[1,119] Most patients deemed candidates have been given heparin before consideration of thrombolytic therapy, and a thrombin time should be drawn before beginning thrombolytic therapy. Thrombolytic therapy should not be started until heparin has been stopped and the thrombin time has returned to less than

two times normal. Once these criteria are met, thrombolytic therapy in the usual doses is started. During thrombolysis the thrombin time will be prolonged; however, no regimented frequency of doing the thrombin time during therapy has yet been devised or recommended, and it is only noted that the thrombin time will usually be prolonged during therapy.[1,2,119] It is reasonable to obtain a thrombin time about four hours after starting therapy to document a systemic thrombolytic effect; however, prolongation of the thrombin time does not correlate with clinical bleeding or efficacy.[1,2,16,119,120] It is important to repeat a thrombin time after cessation of thrombolytic therapy and before reinstituting heparin therapy. Heparin should not be reinstituted until thrombolytic therapy is stopped and the thrombin time has returned to less than two times prolonged. After this is noted, heparin can be safely reinstituted. The reinstitution of some type of anticoagulant therapy is extremely important, since patients are considered to be hypercoagulable following thrombolytic therapy due to a depleted fibrinolytic system.[1,2] Some authors have advocated temporary cessation of thrombolytic therapy if the thrombin time is greater than five times prolonged.[120]

During systemic use of urokinase and streptokinase, the laboratory monitoring test that is recommended and necessary is to obtain a thrombin time after cessation of heparin and before beginning thrombolytic therapy to ascertain that the thrombin time is less than two times prolonged. Thrombolytic therapy is withheld until this criterion is met. There is no advantage to doing multiple thrombin times during thrombolytic therapy because they do not correlate with efficacy or bleeding. A single determination about four hours after starting therapy is reasonable. After cessation of thrombolytic therapy, a repeat thrombin time should be done and heparin not reinstituted until the thrombin time has returned to less than two times prolonged. One exception to this general monitoring procedure is for a patient who has undergone systemic thrombolytic therapy and then becomes a candidate for an invasive procedure, usually transluminal angioplasty or a cardiopulmonary bypass procedure. In this instance, the patient who has previously undergone systemic thrombolytic therapy should also have a fibrinogen level performed, and the fibrinogen level should be documented to be greater than 1 g/L (100 mg/dL) before proceeding with an invasive procedure or angioplasty.[119] In this instance, it is extremely important to choose a fibrinogen determination system that is reliable and not influenced by the presence of FDPs, which may give false elevations of fibrinogen levels in a patient after thrombolytic therapy.[119,121]

Summary

Data reported in several studies show that both the older agents, urokinase and streptokinase, and the newer-generation agents, pro-urokinase, tissue plasminogen activator, and acylated plasminogen-streptokinase complex (APSAC), can induce a systemic thrombolytic state in humans and that their use is definitely superior to heparin alone in accelerating the rate of clot dissolution and vessel recanalization for a wide variety of thrombotic disorders, including acute and chronic venous and arterial thrombosis, acute pulmonary embolus, and coronary artery thrombosis. No well-documented proof suggests that any one agent is clearly superior to any other in efficacy or complication rate. These agents can be safely used, provided therapy is supervised by a physician highly competent in the management of thrombohemorrhagic phenomena.

Although no differences in mortality have been detected between patients with pulmonary embolism taking thrombolytic agents and patients taking heparin, it is apparent that particularly patients with massive pulmonary emboli receive considerable benefit from the rate of return of cardiopulmonary hemodynamics toward normal, including diffusion capacity and capillary blood volume at least up to one year. Thrombolytic therapy has been shown to be highly successful for new and aged venous thrombi, and evidence would suggest that the use of thrombolytic therapy in individuals with deep venous thrombosis will significantly reduce the incidence of postphlebitic syndrome and chronic venous insufficiency. Fresh or aged arterial thrombi can be lysed, including those being present for up to six months. The newer use of intracoronary and intravenous streptokinase, urokinase, TPA, pro-urokinase, and APSAC are highly successful in salvaging myocardium and left ventricular function and reducing short- and long-term mortality in patients with acute myocardial infarction. Generally, patients not responding to conventional anticoagulants are excellent candidates for thrombolytic therapy, which is a much safer alternative than embolectomy.

References

1. Bick RL: Thrombolytic therapy, ch 13. In: Disorders of Hemostasis and Thrombosis: Principles of Clinical Practice. Thieme, Inc., New York, 1985, p 352.

2. Murano G, RL Bick: Thrombolytic therapy, ch 15. In: G Murano, RL Bick (Eds): Basic Concepts of Hemostasis and Thrombosis. CRC Press, Boca Raton, FL, 1980, p 259.

3. Christensen LR: Streptococcal fibrinolysis: a proteolytic reaction due to a serum enzyme activated by streptococcal fibrinolysin. J Gen Physiol 28:363, 1945.

4. Johnson AJ, W Tillett: The lysis in rabbits of intravascular blood clots by the streptococcal fibrinolytic system (streptokinase). J Exp Med 95:449, 1952.

5. Johnson AJ, W McCarty: Some aspects of the mechanism of thrombolysis. Thromb Diath Haemorrh 5:391, 1961.

6. Collen D: Potential approaches for therapeutic intervention on thrombosis by fibrinolytic agents. Semin Thromb Hemost 14:95, 1988.

7. Robertson BR, IM Nilsson, G Nylander: Thrombolytic effect of streptokinase as evaluated by phlebography of deep venous thrombi of the leg. Acta Chir Scand 134:203, 1968.

8. Kakkar VV, C Flanc, CT Howe: Treatment of deep vein thrombosis. A trial of heparin, streptokinase and Arvin. Br Med J 1:806, 1969.

9. Hirsh J: Dosage regimens for streptokinase treatment: evaluation of a standard dosage schedule. Australas Ann Med 19(suppl):12, 1970.

10. Kakkar VV: Results of streptokinase therapy in deep venous thrombosis. Postgrad Med J 49(suppl):60, 1973.

11. Tsapogas JM, RA Peabody, KT Wu: Controlled study of thrombolytic therapy in deep vein thrombosis. Surgery 74:973, 1973.

12. Brogden RN, TM Splight, GS Avery: Streptokinase: a review of its clinical pharmacology, mechanism of action and therapeutic uses. Drugs 5:357, 1973.

13. Sasahara AA, TM Hyers, CM Cole: The urokinase pulmonary embolism trial. Circulation 47(suppl II):1, 1973.

14. Fratantoni JC, P Ness, TL Simon: Thrombolytic therapy: current status. N Engl J Med 293:1073, 1975.

15. Sasahara AA, WR Bell, TL Simon: The phase II urokinase-streptokinase pulmonary embolism trial. Thromb Diath Haemorrh 3:464, 1975.

16. Bell WR: Thrombolytic therapy: a comparison between urokinase and streptokinase. Semin Thromb Hemost 2:1, 1975.

17. Seaman AJ, HH Common, J Rosch: Deep vein thrombosis treated with streptokinase or heparin: a randomized study. Angiology 27:549, 1976.

18. Sherry S: Streptokinase, urokinase: do they really work? Modern Med (Nov 1):72, 1976.

19. Marder VJ, JF Donahoe, WR Bell: Comparison of in vivo biochemical effects of human urokinase prepared from urinary and tissue cultures sources. Thromb Hemost 38:195, 1977.

20. Paoletti R, S Sherry: Thrombosis and Urokinase. Academic Press, New York, 1977.

21. Slanie J, V Ezenhofer, R Karnik: Local thrombolysis in arterial occlusive disease. Angiology 35:231, 1984.

22. Martin M: Systemic streptokinase treatment of arterial occlusions: clinical results, ch 9. In: Streptokinase In Chronic Arterial Disease. CRC Press, Boca Raton, FL, 1982, p 59.

23. Laffel GL, E Braunwald: Thrombolytic therapy: a new strategy for the treatment of acute myocardial infarction: Part I. N Engl J Med 311:710, 1984.

24. Laffel GL, E Braunwald: Thrombolytic therapy: a new strategy for the treatment of acute myocardial infarction: Part II. N Engl J Med 311:770, 1984.

25. Bell WR, AG Meek: Guidelines for the use of thrombolytic agents. N Engl J Med 301:1266, 1979.

26. Cella G, A Palla, AA Sasahara: Controversies of different regimens of thrombolytic therapy in acute pulmonary embolism. Semin Thromb Hemost 13:163, 1987.

27. Samama MM: Deep vein thrombosis of inferior limbs: are thrombolytic agents superior to heparin? Semin Thromb Hemost 13:178, 1987.

28. Acar J, A Vahanian, PL Michel: Thrombolytic treatment in acute myocardial infarction. Semin Thromb Hemost 13:186, 1987.

29. Ambrus CM, TS Choi, DH Weintraub: Studies on the prevention of respiratory distress syndrome of infants due to hyaline membrane disease with plasminogen. Semin Thromb Hemost 2:42, 1975.

30. Terashi A, Y Kobayashi, Y Katayama: Clinical effects and basic studies of thrombolytic therapy on cerebral thrombosis. Semin Thromb Hemost 16:236, 1990.

31. Bang NU: Physiology and biochemistry of fibrinolysis. In:

NU Bang, FK Beller, E Deutsh, EF Mammen (Eds): Thrombosis and Bleeding Disorders. Academic Press, New York, 1971, p 292.

32. McNicol GP: The fibrinolytic system. Postgrad Med J 49(suppl):10, 1973.

33. Bick RL: Syndromes associated with hyperfibrino(geno)lysis, ch 3. In: Disseminated Intravascular Coagulation and Related Syndromes. CRC Press, Boca Raton, FL, 1983, p 105.

34. Bick RL: Physiology of hemostasis and thrombosis, ch 1. In: Disorders of Hemostasis and Thrombosis: Principles of Clinical Practice. Theime, Inc., New York, 1985, p 1.

35. Aoki N, M Moroi, M Matsuda: The behavior of alpha-2-plasmin inhibitor in fibrinolytic states. J Clin Invest 60:361, 1977.

36. Chesterman CN, MJ Allington, A Sharp: Relationship of plasminogen activator to fibrin. Nature 238:15, 1972.

37. Bick RL: Clinical implications of molecular markers in hemostasis and thrombosis. Semin Thromb Hemost 10:290, 1984.

38. Common HH, AJ Seaman, J Rosch: Deep vein thrombosis treated with streptokinase or heparin. Angiology 27:645, 1976.

39. Holmes WE, D Pennica, M Blaher: Cloning and expression of the gene for prourokinase in E. coli. Biotechnology 3:923, 1985.

40. Pannell R, V Gurewich: Prourokinase: a study of its stability in plasma and of a mechanism for its selective fibrinolytic effect. Blood 67:1215, 1986.

41. Fears R: Development of anisoylated plasminogen-streptokinase activator complex from the acyl enzyme complex. Semin Thromb Hemost 15:129, 1989.

42. Smith RA, RJ Dupe, PD English: Acyl-enzymes as thrombolytic agents in a rabbit model of venous thrombosis. Thromb Haemost 47:269, 1982.

43. Bergmann SR, KA Fox, MM Ter-Pogossian: Clot-selective coronary thrombolysis with tissue-type plasminogen activator. Science 220:1181, 1983.

44. Sharma GVRK, VA Burleson, AA Sasahara: Effect of thrombolytic therapy on pulmonary-capillary blood volume in patients with pulmonary embolism. N Engl J Med 303:842, 1980.

45. Verstraete M, GA Miller, H Bounameaux: Intravenous and intrapulmonary recombinant tissue-type plasminogen activator in the treatment of acute massive pulmonary embolism. Circulation 77:353, 1988.

46. Goldhaber SZ, JE Markis, CM Kessler: Perspectives on treatment of acute pulmonary embolism with tissue plasminogen activator. Semin Thromb Hemost 13:171, 1987.

47. Goldhaber SZ, J Heit, G Sharma: Randomized controlled trial of recombinant tissue plasminogen activator versus urokinase in the treatment of acute pulmonary embolism. Lancet 2:293, 1988.

48. Zimmerman R, J Harenberg, H Morley: Thrombolytic therapy of deep vein thrombosis with urokinase. Klin Wochenschr 60:489, 1982.

49. D'Angelo A, PM Mannucci: Outcome of treatment of deep vein thrombosis with urokinase: relationship of dosage, duration of therapy, age of thrombus and laboratory changes. Thromb Haemost 51:236, 1984.

50. Hasler K, D Magdalinski: Urokinase therapy of deep vein thrombosis. Munch Med Wochenschr 126:122, 1984.

51. Trubestein G: Fibrinolytic therapy with streptokinase and urokinase in deep vein thrombosis. Int Angiol 3:377, 1984.

52. Serradimigni A, P Mathiew, J Sainsous: Traitement medical des thromboses veineuses ilio-caves. Arch Mal Coeur 3:347, 1981.

53. Kakkar V, CT Howe, JW Laws: Late results of treatment of deep venous thrombosis. Br Med J 1:810, 1969.

54. Theiss W, A Wirtzfeld, U Fink: The success rate of fibrinolytic therapy in fresh and old thrombosis of the iliac and femoral veins. Angiology 34:61, 1983.

55. Duckert F, G Multer, D Nyman: Treatment of deep venous thrombosis with streptokinase. Br Med J 1:479, 1975.

56. Dupe RJ, PD English, RA Smith: The evaluation of plasmin and streptokinase activator complexes in a new rabbit model of venous thrombosis. Thromb Haemost 46:528, 1981.

57. Katzen BT, A Van Breda: Low dose streptokinase in treatment of arterial occlusions. Am J Roentgenol 136:1171, 1981.

58. Fiessinger JN, M Vayssairat, Y Juillet: Local urokinase in arterial thromboembolism. Angiology 31:715, 1980.

59. Dotter CT, J Rosch, A Seaman: Selective clot lysis with low-dose streptokinase. Radiology 111:31, 1974.

60. Boyles PW, WH Meyer, J Graff: Comparative effectiveness of intravenous and intra-arterial fibrinolysin therapy. Am J Cardiol 6:439, 1960.

61. Kartehner MM, WC Wilcox: Thrombolysis of palmar and digital arterial thrombosis by intraarterial thrombolysin. J Hand Surg 1:67, 1976.

62. Cotton LT, PT Flute, MJ Tsapogas: Popliteal artery thrombosis treated with streptokinase. Lancet 2:1081, 1962.

63. Amery A, W Deloof, J Vermylen: Outcome of recent thromboembolic occlusions of limb arteries treated with streptokinase. Br Med J 4:639, 1970.

64. Cunningham MW, S May, WY Tucker: Response of an abdominal aortic thrombotic occlusion to local low-dose streptokinase therapy. Surgery 93:541, 1983.

65. Flickinger EG, IS Johnsrude, NS Osburg: Local streptokinase infusion for superior mesenteric artery thromboembolism. Am J Roentgenol 140:771, 1983.

66. Jones FE, PJ Black, JS Cameron: Local infusion of urokinase and heparin into renal arteries in impending renal cortical necrosis. Br Med J 4:547, 1975.

67. European Cooperative Study Group for Streptokinase Treatment in Acute Myocardial Infarction. N Engl J Med 301:797, 1979.

68. DeWood MA, J Spores, MD Notske: Prevalence of total coronary occlusion during early hours of transmural myocardial infarction. N Engl J Med 303:897, 1980.

69. Fletcher AP, S Sherry, N Alkjaersig: The maintenance of a sustained thrombolytic state in man: II. Clinical observations on patients with myocardial infarction and other thromboembolic disorders. J Clin Invest 38:1111, 1959.

70. Goa KL, JM Hemwood, JF Stolz: Intravenous streptokinase: a reappraisal of its therapeutic use in acute myocardial infarction. Drugs 39:693, 1990.

71. Stampfer MJ, SZ Goldhaber, S Yosuf: Effect of intravenous streptokinase on acute myocardial infarction. N Engl J Med 307:1180, 1982.

72. Murano G: Editorial comment. Semin Thromb Hemost 9:137, 1983.

73. GISSI: Long-term effects of intravenous thrombolysis in acute myocardial infarction. Final report of the GISSI study. Lancet 2:871, 1987.

74. ISIS-2 Collaborative Group: Randomized trial of intravenous streptokinase, oral aspirin, both or neither among 17,187 cases of suspected acute myocardial infarction: ISIS-2. Lancet 2:349, 1988.

75. The ISAM Study Group Report: Intravenous streptokinase in acute myocardial infarction: preliminary results of a prospective controlled trial (ISAM). Proceedings of the 58th Congress of the American Heart Association, November, 1985.

76. Simoons ML, M van der Brand, C DeZwaan: Improved survival after early thrombolysis in acute myocardial infarction. A randomized trial by the Inter-University Cardiology Institute in the Netherlands. Lancet 2:578, 1985.

77. Rentrop P, F Frit, H Blanke: Effects of intracoronary streptokinase and intracoronary nitroglycerin infusion on coronary angiographic patterns and mortality in patients with acute myocardial infarction. N Engl J Med 311:1458, 1984.

78. Reduto LA, GC Freund, JM Gaeta: Coronary artery reperfusion in acute myocardial infarction: beneficial effects of intracoronary streptokinase on left ventricular salvage and performance. Am Heart J 102:1168, 1981.

79. Merx W, R Dorr, P Rentrop: Evaluation of the effectiveness of intracoronary streptokinase infusion in acute myocardial infarction: postprocedure management and hospital course in 204 patients. Am Heart J 102:1181, 1981.

80. Mathey DG, KH Kuck, V Tilsner: Nonsurgical coronary artery recanalization in acute transmural myocardial infarction. Circulation 63:489, 1981.

81. Rentrop P, H Blanke, R Karsch: Changes in left ventricular function after intracoronary streptokinase infusion in clinically evolving myocardial infarction. Am Heart J 102:1188, 1981.

82. Markis JE, M Malagold, JA Parker: Myocardial salvage after intracoronary thrombolysis with streptokinase in acute myocardial infarction. N Engl J Med 305:777, 1981.

83. Khaja F, JA Walton, JF Brymer: Intracoronary fibrinolytic therapy in acute myocardial infarction. N Engl J Med 308:1305, 1983.

84. Anderson JL, HW Marshall, BE Bray: A randomized trial of intracoronary streptokinase in the treatment of acute myocardial infarction. N Engl J Med 308:1312, 1983.

85. Kennedy JW, JL Ritchie, KB Davis: The Western Washington randomized trial of intracoronary streptokinase in acute myocardial infarction. N Engl J Med 309:1477, 1983.

86. Kennedy JW, JL Ritchie, KB Davis: The Western Washington randomized trial of intracoronary streptokinase in acute myocardial infarction. N Engl J Med 312:1073, 1985.

87. Khaja F, JA Walton, JF Brymer: Intracoronary fibrinolytic therapy in acute myocardial infarction: report of a prospective randomized trial. N Engl J Med 308:1305, 1983.

88. Timmis GC, V Gangadhran, RG Ramos: Hemorrhage and the products of fibrinogen digestion after intracoronary administration of streptokinase. Circulation 69:1146, 1984.

89. Tennant SN, WB Campbell: Intracoronary thrombolysis in acute myocardial infarction: comparison of the efficacy of urokinase to streptokinase. Circulation 69:756, 1984.

90. Doyle DJ, JA Carns, AG Turpie: Intravenous urokinase (UK) and streptokinase (SK) in acute myocardial infarction (AMI). Haemostasis 14:8, 1984.

91. Mathey DG, J Schofer, P Sheehan: Intravenous urokinase in acute myocardial infarction. Am J Cardiol 55:878, 1985.

92. Cernigliaro C, M Sansa, A Campi: Efficacy of intracoronary and intravenous urokinase in acute myocardial infarction. G Ital Cardiol 14:927, 1984.

93. Duckert F, F Burkhart, S Hecker: Controlled trial of urokinase in acute myocardial infarction. A European collaborative study. Lancet 2:624, 1975.

94. Babeau P, P Pras: Urokinase in the treatment of acute myocardial infarction and impending myocardial infarction. Ann Med Interne 128:219, 1977.

95. Witteveen SA, HC Hemker, L Hollaar: Quantitation of infarct size in man by means of plasma enzyme levels. Br Heart J 37:795, 1975.

96. Schwartz F, G Schuler, H Katus: Intracoronary thrombolysis in acute myocardial infarction: duration of ischemia as a major determinant of late results after recanalization. Am J Cardiol 50:933, 1982.

97. Gurewich V: Pro-urokinase: physiochemical properties and promotion of its fibrinolytic activity by urokinase and by tissue plasminogen activator with which it has a complementary mechanism of action. Semin Thromb Hemost 14:110, 1988.

98. Collen D, DC Stump, F Van de Werf: Coronary thrombolysis in patients with acute myocardial infarction by intravenous infusion of synergic thrombolytic agents. Am Heart J 112:1083, 1986.

99. PRIMI Trial Study Group: Randomized double-blind trial of recombinant pro-urokinase against streptokinase in acute myocardial infarction. Lancet 1:863, 1989.

100. Kambara H, C Kawai, N Kajiwara: Randomized double-blinded multicenter study: comparison of intracoronary single-chain urokinase-type plasminogen activator, pro-urokinase (GE-0943), and intracoronary urokinase in patients with acute myocardial infarction. Circulation 78:899, 1988.

101. Bode C, G Schuler, T Nordt: Intravenous thrombolytic therapy with a combination of single-chain urokinase-type plasminogen activator and recombinant tissue-type plasminogen activator in acute myocardial infarction. Circulation 81:907, 1990.

102. Tranchesi B, G Bellotti, D Chamone: Effect of combined administration of saruplase and single-chain alteplase on coronary recanalization in acute myocardial infarction. Am J Cardiol 64:229, 1989.

103. Anderson JL: Summary of U.S. clinical trials program for evaluation of anistreplase. Clin Cardiol 13:33, 1990.

104. AIMS Trial Study Group Report: Effect of intravenous APSAC on mortality after acute myocardial infarction. Preliminary reports of a placebo-controlled clinical trial. Lancet 1:544, 1988.

105. Bassand JP: Multicenter trial of intravenous anisoylated plasminogen streptokinase activator complex (APSAC) in acute myocardial infarction: effect on infarct size and left ventricular function. J Am Coll Cardiol 13:988, 1989.

106. Hogg KJ, JD Germinll, JM Burns: Angiographic patency study of anistreplase versus streptokinase in acute myocardial infarction. Lancet 335:254, 1990.

107. TIMI Study Group: The thrombolysis in myocardial infarction (TIMI) trial. N Engl J Med 312:932, 1985.

108. Verstraete M, M Bory, D Collen: Randomized trial of intravenous recombinant tissue-type plasminogen activator versus intravenous streptokinase in acute myocardial infarction. Lancet 1:842, 1985.

109. Wilcox RG, G Van Der Lippe, CG Olsen: Effects of alteplase in acute myocardial infarction: 6 month results from the ASSET study. Lancet 335:1175, 1990.

110. Van de Werf F, AE Arnold: Intravenous tissue plasminogen activator and size of infarct, left ventricular function, and sur-

vival in acute myocardial infarction. Br Med J 297:1374, 1988.

111. The International Study Group: In-hospital mortality and clinical course of 20,891 patients with suspected acute myocardial infarction randomized between alteplase and streptokinase with or without heparin. Lancet 336:71, 1990.

112. Magnani B: Plasminogen activator Italian multicenter study (PAIMS): comparison of intravenous recombinant single-chain human tissue-type plasminogen activator (rt-PA) with intravenous streptokinase in acute myocardial infarction. J Am Coll Cardiol 13:19, 1989.

113. Rapaport E: Thrombolytic agents in acute myocardial infarction. N Engl J Med 320:861, 1989.

114. Marder V, S Sherry: Thrombolytic therapy: current status. N Engl J Med 318:1512, 1988.

115. Laffel GL, E Braunwald: Thrombolytic therapy: a new strategy for the treatment of acute myocardial infarction. N Engl J Med 311:710, 1984.

116. Medical News: Comments on NIH thrombolytic therapy consensus panel. Greater use of fibrinolytic agents urged. JAMA 243:2275, 1980.

117. Editorial: Thrombolytic therapy in thrombosis. A National Institute of Health Consensus Development Conference. Ann Intern Med 93:141, 1980.

118. Editorial: Are we using fibrinolytic agents often enough? Ann Intern Med 93:136, 1980.

119. Bick RL: Laboratory monitoring of thrombolytic therapy. Summary report of the American Society of Clinical Pathologists. ASCP Press, Chicago, 1984.

120. Conard J, MM Samama: Theoretic and practical considerations on laboratory monitoring of thrombolytic therapy. Semin Thromb Hemost 13:212, 1987.

121. Bick RL, BJ McClain: A comparison of Dade and DuPont fibrinogen assays in patients with DIC, thromboembolic disease, and during thrombolytic therapy. Am J Clin Pathol 82:372, 1984.

Index

Numbers in **boldface** refer to pages on which figures appear; numbers followed by a *t* indicate tabular material.

D

U